Lippincott's Illustrated Reviews: Biochemistry

Sixth Edition

Lippincott's Illustrated Reviews: Biochemistry

Sixth Edition

Denise R. Ferrier, PhD
Professor
Department of Biochemistry and Molecular Biology
Drexel University College of Medicine
Philadelphia, Pennsylvania

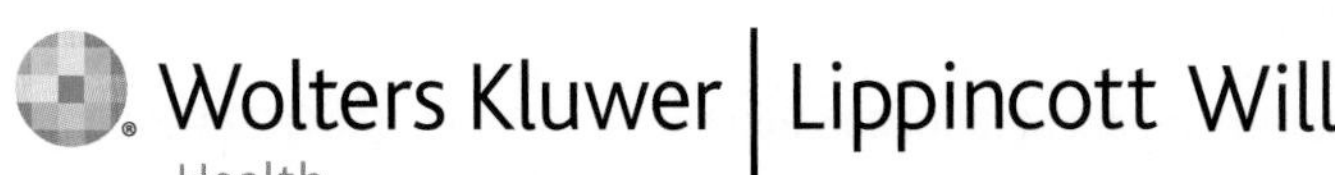

Philadelphia • Baltimore • New York • London
Buenos Aires • Hong Kong • Sydney • Tokyo

Acquisitions Editor: Susan Rhyner
Product Manager: Angela Collins
Development Editor: Kelly Horvath
Marketing Manager: Joy Fisher-Williams
Production Manager: David Saltzberg
Art and Page Design: Debbie McQuade
Cover Design: Holly McLaughlin

Sixth Edition

351 West Camden Street
Baltimore, MD 21201

Two Commerce Square; 2001 Market Street
Philadelphia, PA 19103

Printed in China

9 8 7 6 5 4 3 2 1

Library of Congress Cataloging-in-Publication Data

Ferrier, Denise R.
Biochemistry / Denise R. Ferrier. -- 6th ed.
p. ; cm. -- (Lippincott's illustrated reviews)
Rev. ed. of: Biochemistry / Richard A. Harvey, Denise R. Ferrier. 5th ed. c2011.
Includes bibliographical references and index.
ISBN 978-1-4511-7562-2 (alk. paper)
I. Title. II. Series: Lippincott's illustrated reviews.
[DNLM: 1. Biochemistry--Examination Questions. QU 18.2]

612.3'9--dc23

2012025941

DISCLAIMER
Care has been taken to confirm the accuracy of the information presented and to describe generally accepted practices. However, the authors, editors, and publisher are not responsible for errors or omissions or for any consequences from application of the information in this book and make no warranty, expressed or implied, with respect to the currency, completeness, or accuracy of the contents of the publication. Application of this information in a particular situation remains the professional responsibility of the practitioner; the clinical treatments described and recommended may not be considered absolute and universal recommendations.

The authors, editors, and publisher have exerted every effort to ensure that drug selection and dosage set forth in this text are in accordance with the current recommendations and practice at the time of publication. However, in view of ongoing research, changes in government regulations, and the constant flow of information relating to drug therapy and drug reactions, the reader is urged to check the package insert for each drug for any change in indications and dosage and for added warnings and precautions. This is particularly important when the recommended agent is a new or infrequently employed drug.
Some drugs and medical devices presented in this publication have Food and Drug Administration (FDA) clearance for limited use in restricted research settings. It is the responsibility of the health care provider to ascertain the FDA status of each drug or device planned for use in their clinical practice.

The publishers have made every effort to trace the copyright holders for borrowed material. If they have inadvertently overlooked any, they will be pleased to make the necessary arrangements at the first opportunity.

To purchase additional copies of this book, call our customer service department at **(800) 638-3030** or fax orders to **(301) 223-2320**. International customers should call **(301) 223-2300**.

Visit Lippincott Williams & Wilkins on the Internet: http://www.lww.com. Lippincott Williams & Wilkins customer service representatives are available from 8:30 am to 6:00 pm, EST.

RRS1303

Acknowledgments

I am grateful to my colleagues at Drexel University College of Medicine who generously shared their expertise to help make this book as accurate and as useful to medical students as possible. I am particularly appreciative of the many helpful comments of Dr. Åke Rökaeus of the Karolinska Institute as they have enhanced the accuracy of this work. In addition, the author thanks Dr. Susan K. Fried and Dr. Richard B. Horenstein for their valuable contributions to the Obesity chapter in previous editions of this text. A special thank you to Dr. Alan Katz for his helpful comments on the clinical aspects of the cases in the Appendix. Ms. Barbara Engle was an invaluable sounding board throughout the process.

The editors and production staff of Lippincott Williams & Wilkins were an important source of encouragement. I particularly want to acknowledge the contributions of Susan Ryner, the Acquisitions Editor, and Angela Collins, the Managing Editor. Many thanks are due to Kelly Horvath, Development Editor, for her assistance in the final editing of this book. I also want to thank Deborah McQuade for her work in the assembly of the 6th edition.

This book is dedicated to my
husband John, whose loving
support made the task possible;
to my students, who have taught
me so much over the last 20
years; and to Richard Harvey and
the late Pamela Champe, who
helped me develop as an author.

Contents

Contents

Bonus chapter online! Chapter 34: Blood Clotting [illegible]

UNIT I:
Protein Structure
and Function

Amino Acids

1

I. OVERVIEW

Proteins are the most abundant and functionally diverse molecules in living systems. Virtually every life process depends on this class of macromolecules. For example, enzymes and polypeptide hormones direct and regulate metabolism in the body, whereas contractile proteins in muscle permit movement. In bone, the protein collagen forms a framework for the deposition of calcium phosphate crystals, acting like the steel cables in reinforced concrete. In the bloodstream, proteins, such as hemoglobin and plasma albumin, shuttle molecules essential to life, whereas immunoglobulins fight infectious bacteria and viruses. In short, proteins display an incredible diversity of functions, yet all share the common structural feature of being linear polymers of amino acids. This chapter describes the properties of amino acids. Chapter 2 explores how these simple building blocks are joined to form proteins that have unique three-dimensional structures, making them capable of performing specific biologic functions.

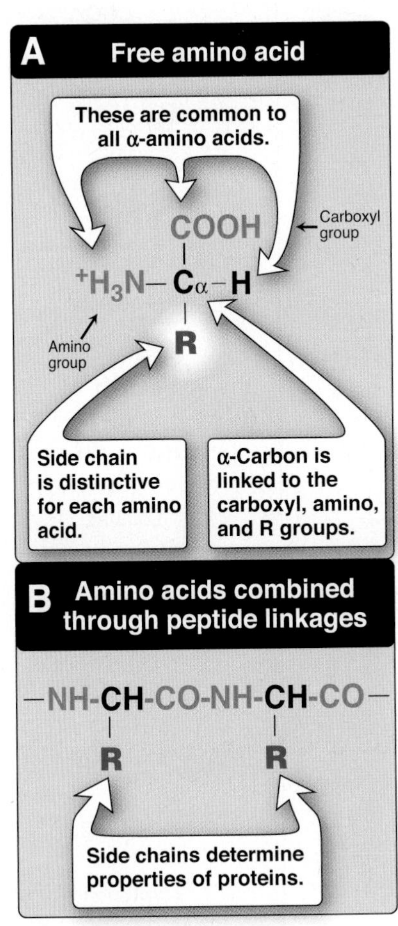

Figure 1.1
Structural features of amino acids (shown in their fully protonated form).

II. STRUCTURE

Although more than 300 different amino acids have been described in nature, only 20 are commonly found as constituents of mammalian proteins. [Note: These are the only amino acids that are coded for by DNA, the genetic material in the cell (see p. 395).] Each amino acid has a carboxyl group, a primary amino group (except for proline, which has a secondary amino group), and a distinctive side chain ("R group") bonded to the α-carbon atom (Figure 1.1A). At physiologic pH (approximately 7.4), the carboxyl group is dissociated, forming the negatively charged carboxylate ion ($-COO^-$), and the amino group is protonated ($-NH_3^+$). In proteins, almost all of these carboxyl and amino groups are combined through peptide linkage and, in general, are not available for chemical reaction except for hydrogen bond formation (Figure 1.1B). Thus, it is the nature of the side chains that ultimately dictates the role an amino acid plays in a protein. It is, therefore, useful to classify the amino acids according to the properties of their side chains, that is, whether they are nonpolar (have an even distribution of electrons) or polar (have an uneven distribution of electrons, such as acids and bases) as shown in Figures 1.2 and 1.3.

A. Amino acids with nonpolar side chains

Each of these amino acids has a nonpolar side chain that does not gain or lose protons or participate in hydrogen or ionic bonds (see Figure 1.2). The side chains of these amino acids can be thought of as "oily" or lipid-like, a property that promotes hydrophobic interactions (see Figure 2.10, p. 19).

1. **Location of nonpolar amino acids in proteins:** In proteins found in aqueous solutions (a polar environment) the side chains of the nonpolar amino acids tend to cluster together in the interior of the protein (Figure 1.4). This phenomenon, known as the hydrophobic

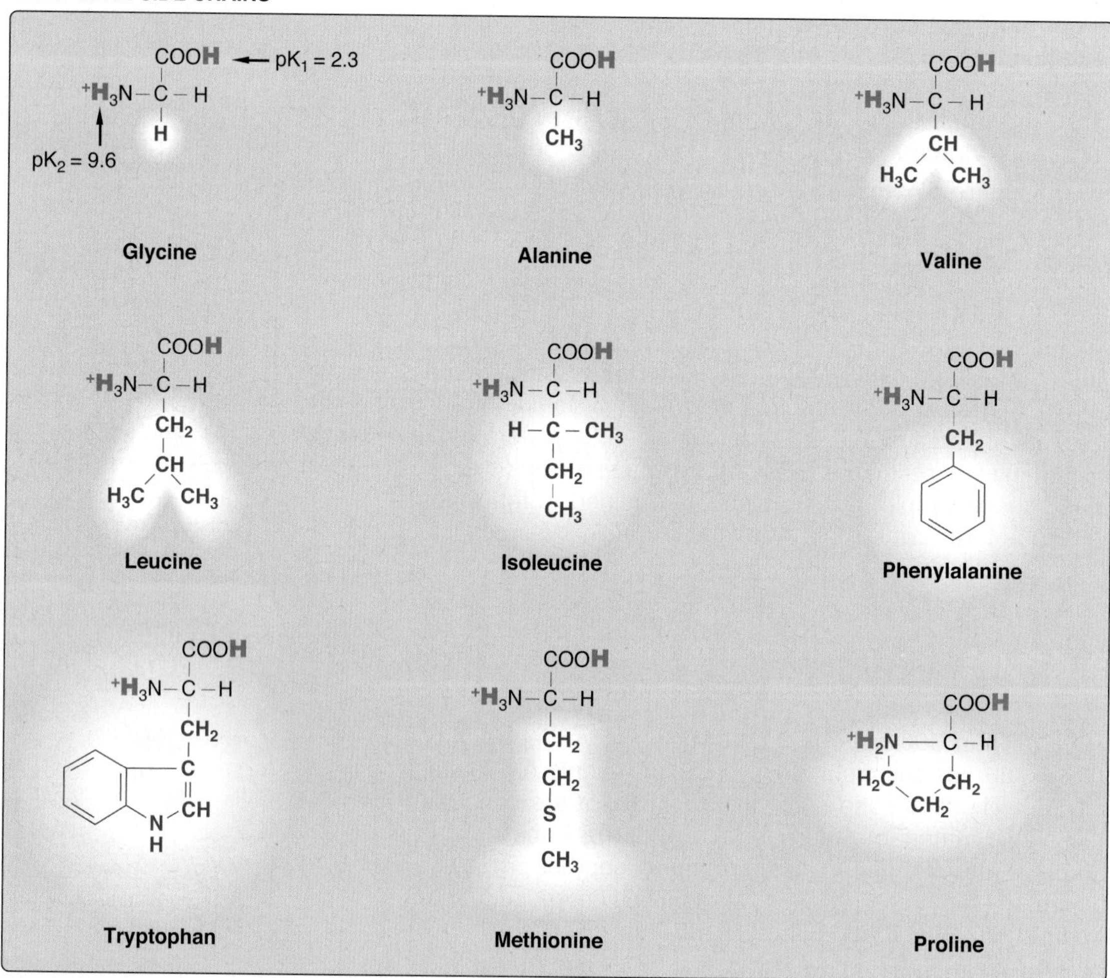

Figure 1.2
Classification of the 20 amino acids commonly found in proteins, according to the charge and polarity of their side chains at acidic pH is shown here and continues in Figure 1.3. Each amino acid is shown in its fully protonated form, with dissociable hydrogen ions represented in red print. The pK values for the α-carboxyl and α-amino groups of the nonpolar amino acids are similar to those shown for glycine.

UNCHARGED POLAR SIDE CHAINS

Serine

Threonine

Tyrosine

$pK_1 = 2.2$

$pK_2 = 9.1$

$pK_3 = 10.1$

Asparagine

Glutamine

Cysteine

$pK_1 = 1.7$

$pK_2 = 8.3$

$pK_3 = 10.8$

ACIDIC SIDE CHAINS

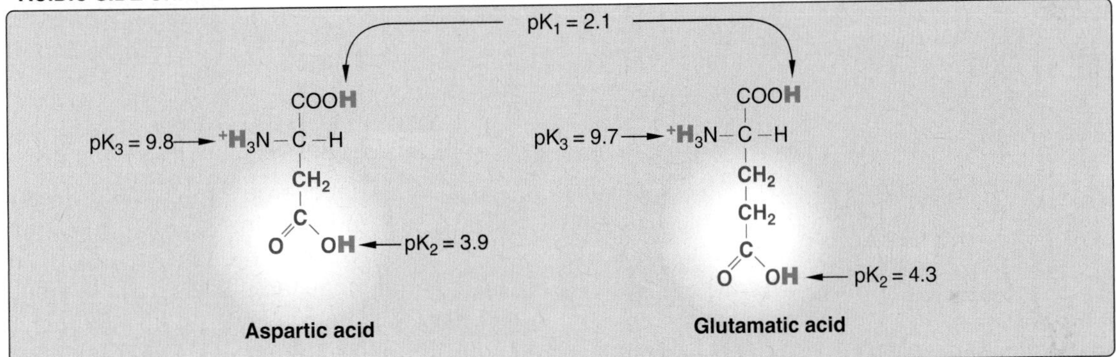

BASIC SIDE CHAINS

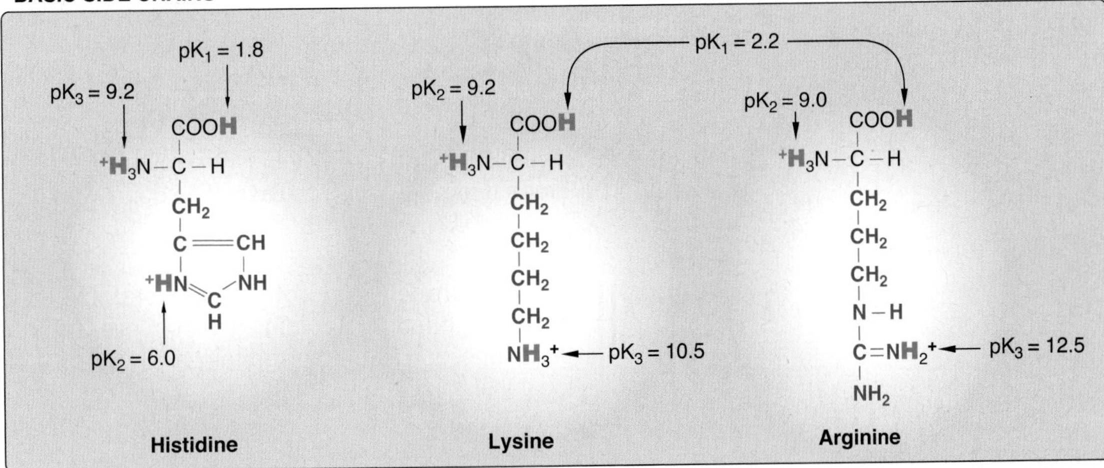

Figure 1.3
Classification of the 20 amino acids commonly found in proteins, according to the charge and polarity of their side chains at acidic pH (continued from Figure 1.2).

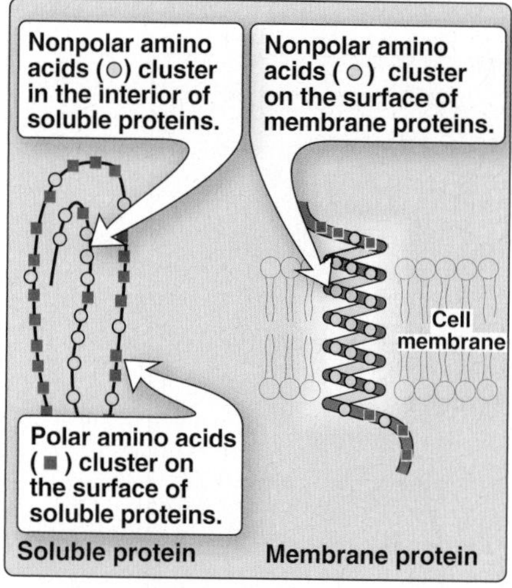

Figure 1.4
Location of nonpolar amino acids in soluble and membrane proteins.

effect, is the result of the hydrophobicity of the nonpolar R groups, which act much like droplets of oil that coalesce in an aqueous environment. The nonpolar R groups, thus, fill up the interior of the folded protein and help give it its three-dimensional shape. However, for proteins that are located in a hydrophobic environment, such as a membrane, the nonpolar R groups are found on the outside surface of the protein, interacting with the lipid environment see Figure 1.4. The importance of these hydrophobic interactions in stabilizing protein structure is discussed on p. 19.

> Sickle cell anemia, a sickling disease of red blood cells, results from the replacement of polar glutamate with nonpolar valine at the sixth position in the β subunit of hemoglobin (see p. 36).

2. **Proline:** Proline differs from other amino acids in that its side chain and α-amino N form a rigid, five-membered ring structure (Figure 1.5). Proline, then, has a secondary (rather than a primary) amino group. It is frequently referred to as an "imino acid." The unique geometry of proline contributes to the formation of the fibrous structure of collagen (see p. 45) and often interrupts the α-helices found in globular proteins (see p. 26).

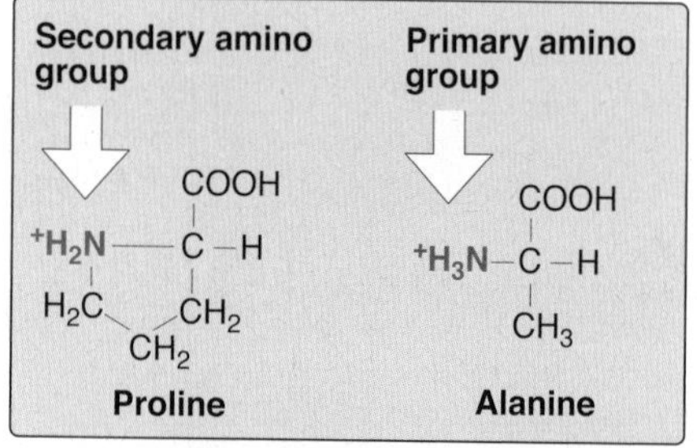

Figure 1.5
Comparison of the secondary amino group found in proline with the primary amino group found in other amino acids such as alanine.

B. Amino acids with uncharged polar side chains

These amino acids have zero net charge at physiologic pH, although the side chains of cysteine and tyrosine can lose a proton at an alkaline pH (see Figure 1.3). Serine, threonine, and tyrosine each contain a polar hydroxyl group that can participate in hydrogen bond formation (Figure 1.6). The side chains of asparagine and glutamine each contain a carbonyl group and an amide group, both of which can also participate in hydrogen bonds.

1. **Disulfide bond:** The side chain of cysteine contains a sulfhydryl (thiol) group (–SH), which is an important component of the active site of many enzymes. In proteins, the –SH groups of two cysteines can be oxidized to form a covalent cross-link called a disulfide bond (–S–S–). Two disulfide-linked cysteines are referred to as "cystine." (See p. 19 for a further discussion of disulfide bond formation.)

> Many extracellular proteins are stabilized by disulfide bonds. Albumin, a blood protein that functions as a transporter for a variety of molecules, is an example.

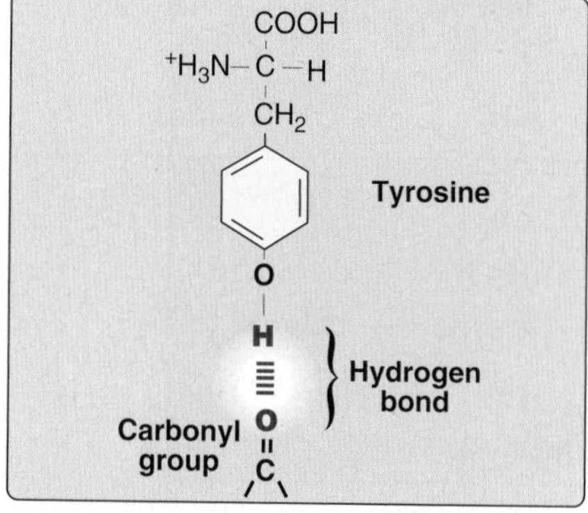

Figure 1.6
Hydrogen bond between the phenolic hydroxyl group of tyrosine and another molecule containing a carbonyl group.

2. **Side chains as sites of attachment for other compounds:** The polar hydroxyl group of serine; threonine; and, rarely, tyrosine, can serve as a site of attachment for structures such as a phosphate group. In addition, the amide group of asparagine, as well as the hydroxyl group of serine or threonine, can serve as a site of attachment for oligosaccharide chains in glycoproteins (see p. 165).

C. Amino acids with acidic side chains

The amino acids aspartic and glutamic acid are proton donors. At physiologic pH, the side chains of these amino acids are fully ionized, containing a negatively charged carboxylate group ($-COO^-$). They are, therefore, called aspartate or glutamate to emphasize that these amino acids are negatively charged at physiologic pH (see Figure 1.3).

D. Amino acids with basic side chains

The side chains of the basic amino acids accept protons (see Figure 1.3). At physiologic pH, the R groups of lysine and arginine are fully ionized and positively charged. In contrast, histidine is weakly basic, and the free amino acid is largely uncharged at physiologic pH. However, when histidine is incorporated into a protein, its R group can be either positively charged (protonated) or neutral, depending on the ionic environment provided by the protein. This is an important property of histidine that contributes to the buffering role it plays in the functioning of proteins such as hemoglobin (see p. 31). [Note: Histidine is the only amino acid with a side chain that can ionize within the physiologic pH range.]

E. Abbreviations and symbols for commonly occurring amino acids

Each amino acid name has an associated three-letter abbreviation and a one-letter symbol (Figure 1.7). The one-letter codes are determined by the following rules.

1. **Unique first letter:** If only one amino acid begins with a given letter, then that letter is used as its symbol. For example, V = valine.

2. **Most commonly occurring amino acids have priority:** If more than one amino acid begins with a particular letter, the most common of these amino acids receives this letter as its symbol. For example, glycine is more common than glutamate, so G = glycine.

3. **Similar sounding names:** Some one-letter symbols sound like the amino acid they represent. For example, F = phenylalanine, or W = tryptophan ("twyptophan" as Elmer Fudd would say).

4. **Letter close to initial letter:** For the remaining amino acids, a one-letter symbol is assigned that is as close in the alphabet as possible to the initial letter of the amino acid, for example, K = lysine. Furthermore, B is assigned to Asx, signifying either aspartic acid or asparagine, Z is assigned to Glx, signifying either glutamic acid or glutamine, and X is assigned to an unidentified amino acid.

1 Unique first letter:

Cysteine	=	Cys	=	C
Histidine	=	His	=	H
Isoleucine	=	Ile	=	I
Methionine	=	Met	=	M
Serine	=	Ser	=	S
Valine	=	Val	=	V

2 Most commonly occurring amino acids have priority:

Alanine	=	Ala	=	A
Glycine	=	Gly	=	G
Leucine	=	Leu	=	L
Proline	=	Pro	=	P
Threonine	=	Thr	=	T

3 Similar sounding names:

Arginine	=	Arg	=	R	("aRginine")
Asparagi**n**e	=	Asn	=	N	(contains N)
Aspartate	=	Asp	=	D	("asparDic")
Glutamate	=	Glu	=	E	("glutEmate")
Glutamine	=	Gln	=	Q	("Q-tamine")
Phenylalanine	=	Phe	=	F	("Fenylalanine")
Tyrosine	=	Tyr	=	Y	("tYrosine")
Tryptophan	=	Trp	=	W	(double ring in the molecule)

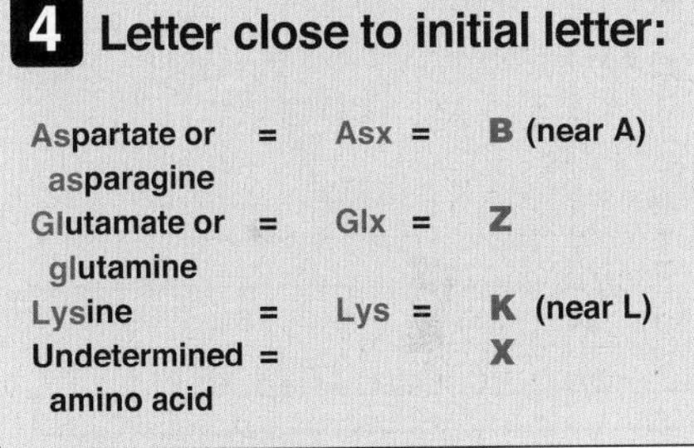

4 Letter close to initial letter:

Aspartate or asparagine	=	Asx	=	B (near A)
Glutamate or glutamine	=	Glx	=	Z
Lysine	=	Lys	=	K (near L)
Undetermined amino acid	=			X

Figure 1.7
Abbreviations and symbols for the commonly occurring amino acids.

F. Optical properties of amino acids

The α-carbon of an amino acid is attached to four different chemical groups (asymmetric) and is, therefore, a chiral, or optically active carbon atom. Glycine is the exception because its α-carbon has two hydrogen substituents. Amino acids with an asymmetric center at the α-carbon can exist in two forms, designated D and L, that are mirror images of each other (Figure 1.8). The two forms in each pair are termed stereoisomers, optical isomers, or enantiomers. All amino acids found in proteins are of the L configuration. However, D-amino acids are found in some antibiotics and in bacterial cell walls. (See p. 252 for a discussion of D-amino acids.)

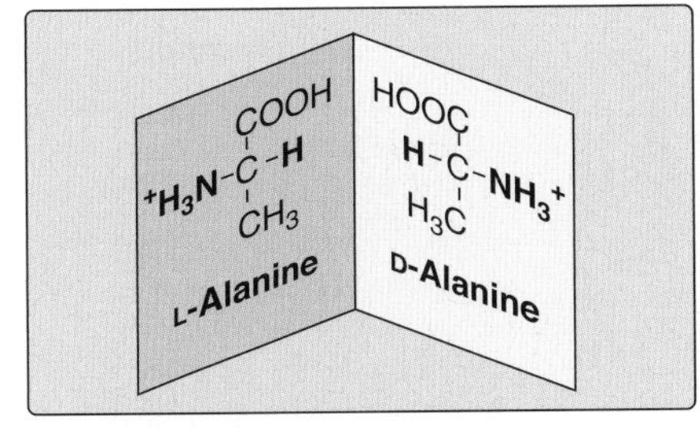

Figure 1.8
D and L forms of alanine are mirror images.

III. ACIDIC AND BASIC PROPERTIES OF AMINO ACIDS

Amino acids in aqueous solution contain weakly acidic α-carboxyl groups and weakly basic α-amino groups. In addition, each of the acidic and basic amino acids contains an ionizable group in its side chain. Thus, both free amino acids and some amino acids combined in peptide linkages can act as buffers. Recall that acids may be defined as proton donors and bases as proton acceptors. Acids (or bases) described as "weak" ionize to only a limited extent. The concentration of protons in aqueous solution is expressed as pH, where pH = log $1/[H^+]$ or $-\log [H^+]$. The quantitative relationship between the pH of the solution and concentration of a weak acid (HA) and its conjugate base (A^-) is described by the Henderson-Hasselbalch equation.

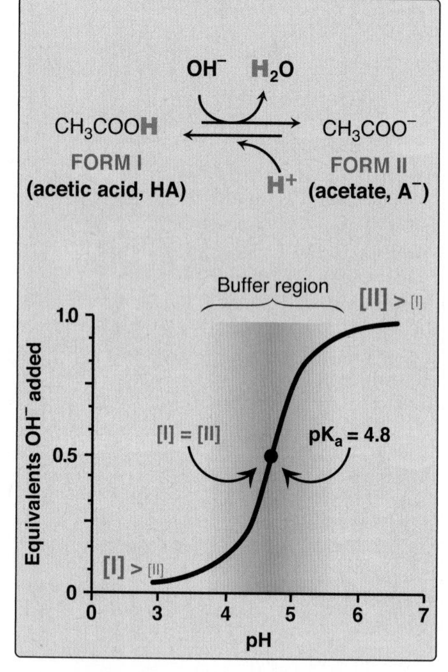

Figure 1.9
Titration curve of acetic acid.

A. Derivation of the equation

Consider the release of a proton by a weak acid represented by HA:

$$\underset{\text{weak acid}}{HA} \leftrightarrows \underset{\text{proton}}{H^+} + \underset{\text{salt form or conjugate base}}{A^-}$$

The "salt" or conjugate base, A^-, is the ionized form of a weak acid. By definition, the dissociation constant of the acid, K_a, is

$$K_a = \frac{[H^+][A^-]}{[HA]}$$

[Note: The larger the K_a, the stronger the acid, because most of the HA has dissociated into H^+ and A^-. Conversely, the smaller the K_a, the less acid has dissociated and, therefore, the weaker the acid.] By solving for the $[H^+]$ in the above equation, taking the logarithm of both sides of the equation, multiplying both sides of the equation by -1, and substituting pH = $-\log [H^+]$ and $pK_a = -\log K_a$, we obtain the Henderson-Hasselbalch equation:

$$pH = pK_a + \log \frac{[A^-]}{[HA]}$$

B. Buffers

A buffer is a solution that resists change in pH following the addition of an acid or base. A buffer can be created by mixing a weak acid (HA) with its conjugate base (A^-). If an acid such as HCl is added to a buffer, A^- can neutralize it, being converted to HA in the process. If a base is added, HA can neutralize it, being converted to A^- in the process. Maximum buffering capacity occurs at a pH equal to the pK_a, but a conjugate acid–base pair can still serve as an effective buffer when the pH of a solution is within approximately ±1 pH unit of the pK_a. If the amounts of HA and A^- are equal, the pH is equal to the pK_a. As shown in Figure

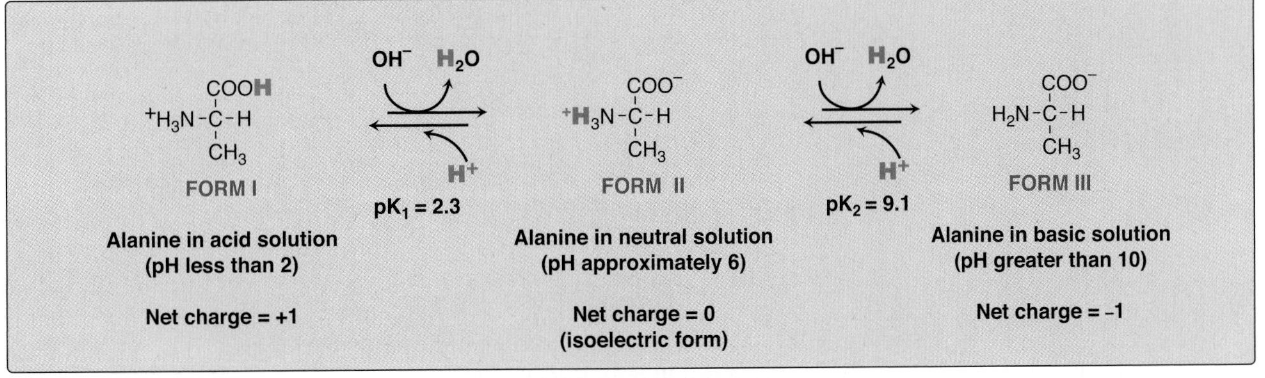

Figure 1.10
Ionic forms of alanine in acidic, neutral, and basic solutions.

1.9, a solution containing acetic acid (HA = CH_3-COOH) and acetate (A^- = CH_3-COO^-) with a pK_a of 4.8 resists a change in pH from pH 3.8 to 5.8, with maximum buffering at pH 4.8. At pH values less than the pK_a, the protonated acid form (CH_3-COOH) is the predominant species in solution. At pH values greater than the pK_a, the deprotonated base form (CH_3-COO^-) is the predominant species.

C. Titration of an amino acid

1. **Dissociation of the carboxyl group:** The titration curve of an amino acid can be analyzed in the same way as described for acetic acid. Consider alanine, for example, which contains an ionizable α-carboxyl and α-amino group. [Note: Its $-CH_3$ R group is nonionizable.] At a low (acidic) pH, both of these groups are protonated (shown in Figure 1.10). As the pH of the solution is raised, the $-COOH$ group of form I can dissociate by donating a proton to the medium. The release of a proton results in the formation of the carboxylate group, $-COO^-$. This structure is shown as form II, which is the dipolar form of the molecule (see Figure 1.10). This form, also called a zwitterion, is the isoelectric form of alanine, that is, it has an overall (net) charge of zero.

2. **Application of the Henderson-Hasselbalch equation:** The dissociation constant of the carboxyl group of an amino acid is called K_1, rather than K_a, because the molecule contains a second titratable group. The Henderson-Hasselbalch equation can be used to analyze the dissociation of the carboxyl group of alanine in the same way as described for acetic acid:

$$K_1 = \frac{[H^+][II]}{[I]}$$

where I is the fully protonated form of alanine, and II is the isoelectric form of alanine (see Figure 1.10). This equation can be rearranged and converted to its logarithmic form to yield:

$$pH = pK_1 + \log \frac{[II]}{[I]}$$

3. **Dissociation of the amino group:** The second titratable group of alanine is the amino ($-NH_3^+$) group shown in Figure 1.10. This is a much weaker acid than the $-COOH$ group and, therefore, has a much smaller dissociation constant, K_2. [Note: Its pK_a is, therefore, larger.] Release of a proton from the protonated amino group of form II results in the fully deprotonated form of alanine, form III (see Figure 1.10).

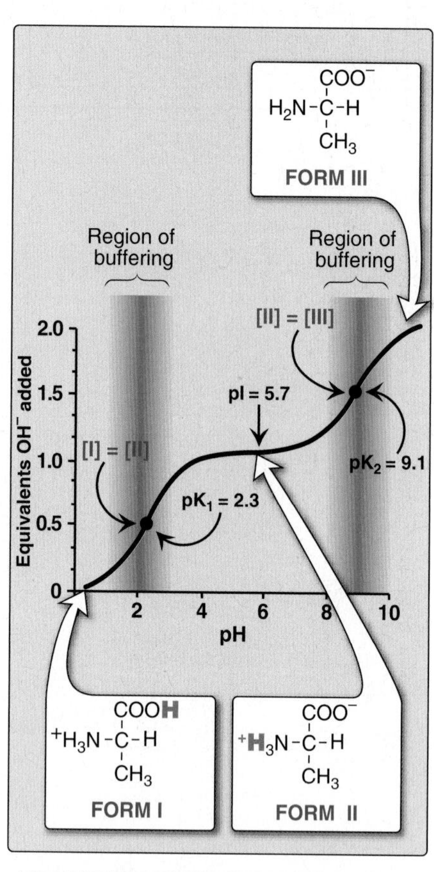

Figure 1.11
The titration curve of alanine.

4. **pKs of alanine:** The sequential dissociation of protons from the carboxyl and amino groups of alanine is summarized in Figure 1.10. Each titratable group has a pK_a that is numerically equal to the pH at which exactly one half of the protons have been removed from that group. The pK_a for the most acidic group ($-COOH$) is pK_1, whereas the pK_a for the next most acidic group ($-NH_3^+$) is pK_2. [Note: The pK_a of the α-carboxyl group of amino acids is approximately 2, whereas that of the α-amino is approximately 9.]

5. **Titration curve of alanine:** By applying the Henderson-Hasselbalch equation to each dissociable acidic group, it is possible to calculate the complete titration curve of a weak acid. Figure 1.11 shows the change in pH that occurs during the addition of base to the fully protonated form of alanine (I) to produce the completely deprotonated form (III). Note the following:

   a. **Buffer pairs:** The $-COOH/-COO^-$ pair can serve as a buffer in the pH region around pK_1, and the $-NH_3^+/-NH_2$ pair can buffer in the region around pK_2.

   b. **When pH = pK:** When the pH is equal to pK_1 (2.3), equal amounts of forms I and II of alanine exist in solution. When the pH is equal to pK_2 (9.1), equal amounts of forms II and III are present in solution.

   c. **Isoelectric point:** At neutral pH, alanine exists predominantly as the dipolar form II in which the amino and carboxyl groups are ionized, but the net charge is zero. The isoelectric point (pI) is the pH at which an amino acid is electrically neutral, that is, in which the sum of the positive charges equals the sum of the negative charges. For an amino acid, such as alanine, that has only two dissociable hydrogens (one from the α-carboxyl and one from the α-amino group), the pI is the average of pK_1 and pK_2 (pI = [2.3 + 9.1]/2 = 5.7) as shown in Figure 1.11. The pI is, thus, midway between pK_1 (2.3) and pK_2 (9.1). pI corresponds to the pH at which the form II (with a net charge of zero) predominates and at which there are also equal amounts of forms I (net charge of +1) and III (net charge of –1).

Separation of plasma proteins by charge typically is done at a pH above the pI of the major proteins. Thus, the charge on the proteins is negative. In an electric field, the proteins will move toward the positive electrode at a rate determined by their net negative charge. Variations in the mobility pattern are suggestive of certain diseases.

6. **Net charge of amino acids at neutral pH:** At physiologic pH, amino acids have a negatively charged group ($-COO^-$) and a positively charged group ($-NH_3^+$), both attached to the α-carbon. [Note: Glutamate, aspartate, histidine, arginine, and lysine have additional potentially charged groups in their side chains.] Substances such as amino acids that can act either as an acid or a base are defined as amphoteric and are referred to as ampholytes (amphoteric electrolytes).

D. Other applications of the Henderson-Hasselbalch equation

The Henderson-Hasselbalch equation can be used to calculate how the pH of a physiologic solution responds to changes in the concentration of a weak acid and/or its corresponding "salt" form. For example, in the bicarbonate buffer system, the Henderson-Hasselbalch equation predicts how shifts in the bicarbonate ion concentration, $[HCO_3^-]$, and CO_2 influence pH (Figure 1.12A). The equation is also useful for calculating the abundance of ionic forms of acidic and basic drugs. For example, most drugs are either weak acids or weak bases (Figure 1.12B). Acidic drugs (HA) release a proton (H^+), causing a charged anion (A^-) to form.

$$HA \rightleftarrows H^+ + A^-$$

Weak bases (BH^+) can also release a H^+. However, the protonated form of basic drugs is usually charged, and the loss of a proton produces the uncharged base (B).

$$BH^+ \rightleftarrows B + H^+$$

A drug passes through membranes more readily if it is uncharged. Thus, for a weak acid, such as aspirin, the uncharged HA can permeate through membranes, but A^- cannot. For a weak base, such as morphine, the uncharged form, B, penetrates through the cell membrane, but BH^+ does not. Therefore, the effective concentration of the permeable form of each drug at its absorption site is determined by the relative concentrations of the charged (impermeant) and uncharged (permeant) forms. The ratio between the two forms is determined by the pH at the site of absorption, and by the strength of the weak acid or base, which is represented by the pK_a of the ionizable group. The Henderson-Hasselbalch equation is useful in determining how much drug is found on either side of a membrane that separates two compartments that differ in pH, for example, the stomach (pH 1.0–1.5) and blood plasma (pH 7.4).

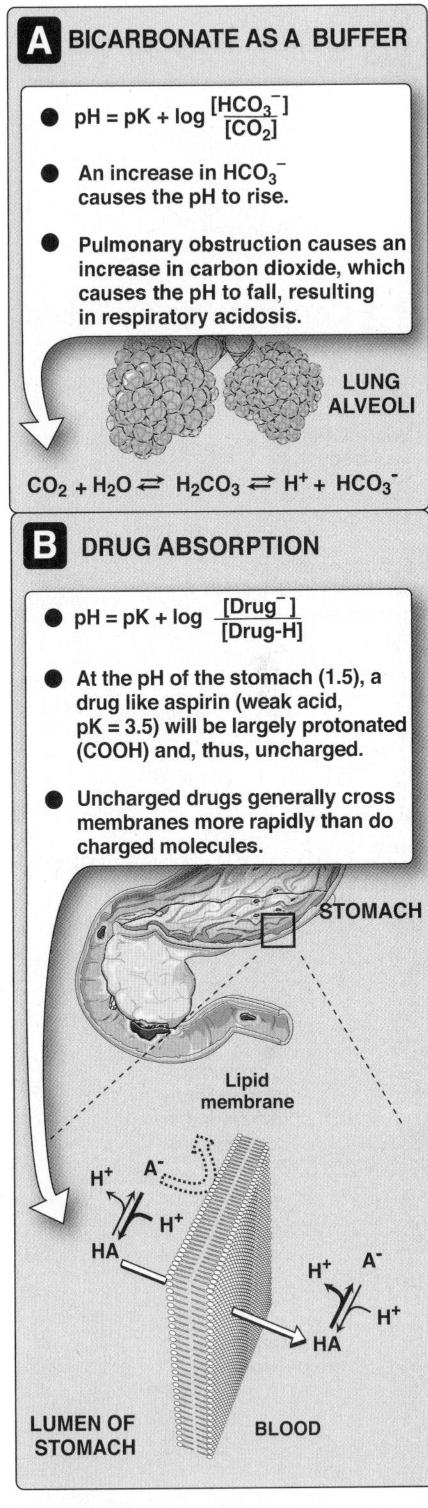

Figure 1.12
The Henderson-Hasselbalch equation is used to predict: A, changes in pH as the concentrations of HCO_3^- or CO_2 are altered, or B, the ionic forms of drugs.

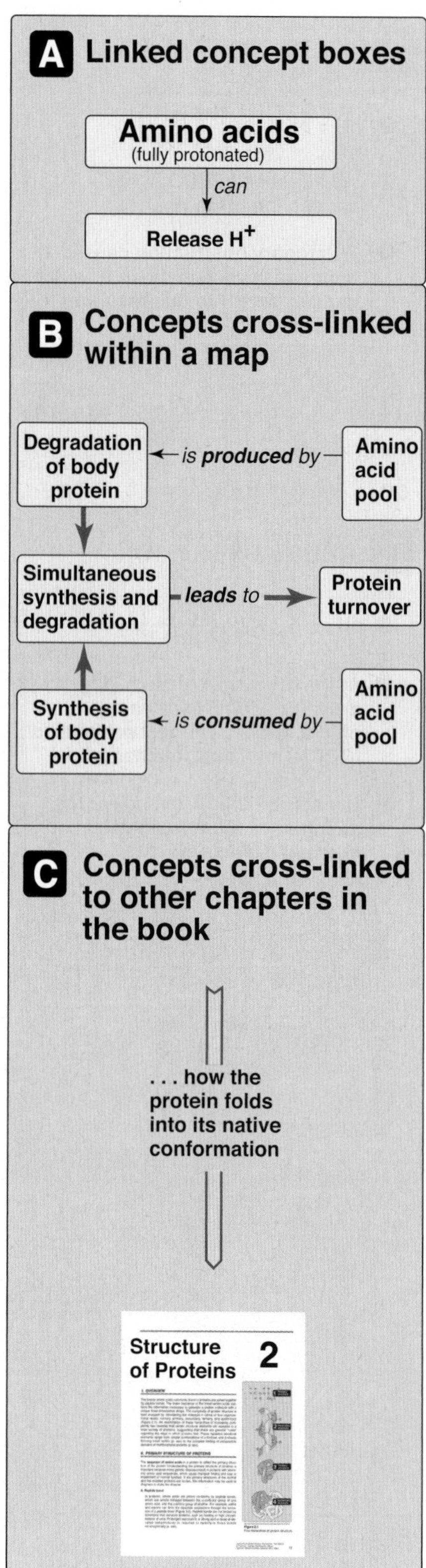

Figure 1.13
Symbols used in concept maps.

IV. CONCEPT MAPS

Students sometimes view biochemistry as a list of facts or equations to be memorized, rather than a body of concepts to be understood. Details provided to enrich understanding of these concepts inadvertently turn into distractions. What seems to be missing is a road map—a guide that provides the student with an understanding of how various topics fit together to make sense. Therefore, a series of biochemical concept maps have been created to graphically illustrate relationships between ideas presented in a chapter and to show how the information can be grouped or organized. A concept map is, thus, a tool for visualizing the connections between concepts. Material is represented in a hierarchic fashion, with the most inclusive, most general concepts at the top of the map and the more specific, less general concepts arranged beneath. The concept maps ideally function as templates or guides for organizing information, so the student can readily find the best ways to integrate new information into knowledge they already possess.

A. How is a concept map constructed?

1. **Concept boxes and links:** Educators define concepts as "perceived regularities in events or objects." In the biochemical maps, concepts include abstractions (for example, free energy), processes (for example, oxidative phosphorylation), and compounds (for example, glucose 6-phosphate). These broadly defined concepts are prioritized with the central idea positioned at the top of the page. The concepts that follow from this central idea are then drawn in boxes (Figure 1.13A). The size of the type indicates the relative importance of each idea. Lines are drawn between concept boxes to show which are related. The label on the line defines the relationship between two concepts, so that it reads as a valid statement, that is, the connection creates meaning. The lines with arrowheads indicate in which direction the connection should be read (Figure 1.14).

2. **Cross-links:** Unlike linear flow charts or outlines, concept maps may contain cross-links that allow the reader to visualize complex relationships between ideas represented in different parts of the map (Figure 1.13B), or between the map and other chapters in this book (Figure 1.13C). Cross-links can, thus, identify concepts that are central to more than one topic in biochemistry, empowering students to be effective in clinical situations and on the United States Medical Licensure Examination (USMLE) or other examinations that require integration of material. Students learn to visually perceive nonlinear relationships between facts, in contrast to cross-referencing within linear text.

V. CHAPTER SUMMARY

Each amino acid has an **α-carboxyl group** and a primary **α-amino group** (except for proline, which has a **secondary amino group**). At physiologic pH, the α-carboxyl group is dissociated, forming the negatively charged carboxylate ion ($-COO^-$), and the α-amino group is protonated ($-NH_3^+$). Each amino acid also contains one of 20 distinctive

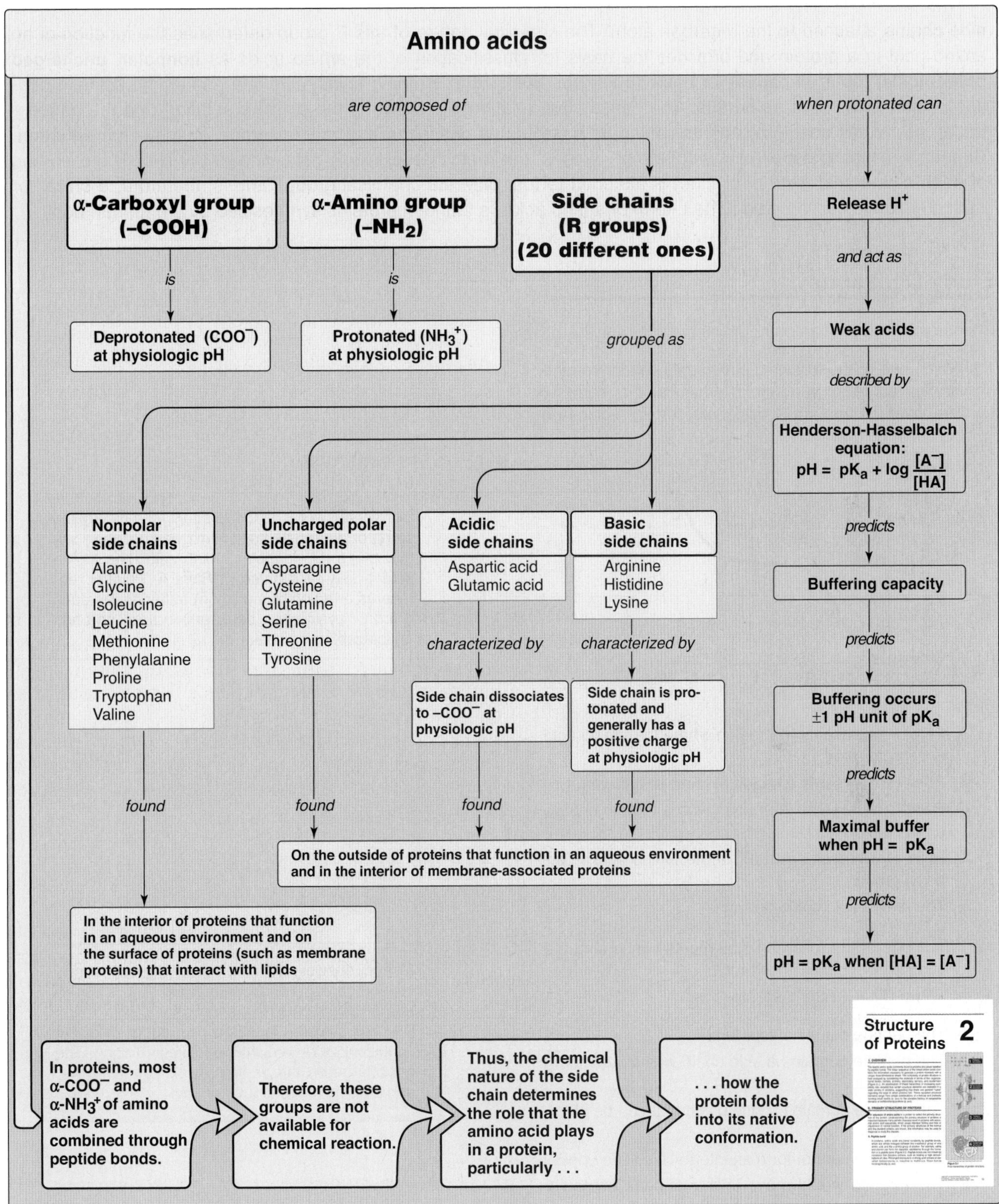

Figure 1.14
Key concept map for amino acids.

side chains attached to the α-carbon atom. The chemical nature of this R group determines the function of an amino acid in a protein and provides the basis for classification of the amino acids as **nonpolar**, **uncharged polar**, **acidic** (**polar negative**), or **basic** (**polar positive**). All free amino acids, plus charged amino acids in peptide chains, can serve as **buffers**. The quantitative relationship between the pH of a solution and the concentration of a weak acid (HA) and its conjugate base (A^-) is described by the **Henderson-Hasselbalch equation**. Buffering occurs within ±1 pH unit of the pK_a and is maximal when pH = pK_a, at which $[A^-]$ = [HA]. The α-carbon of each amino acid (except glycine) is attached to four different chemical groups and is, therefore, a **chiral**, or **optically active** carbon atom. The L-form of amino acids is found in proteins synthesized by the human body.

Study Questions

Choose the ONE best answer.

1.1 Which one of the following statements concerning the titration curve for a nonpolar amino acid is correct? The letters A through D designate certain regions on the curve below.

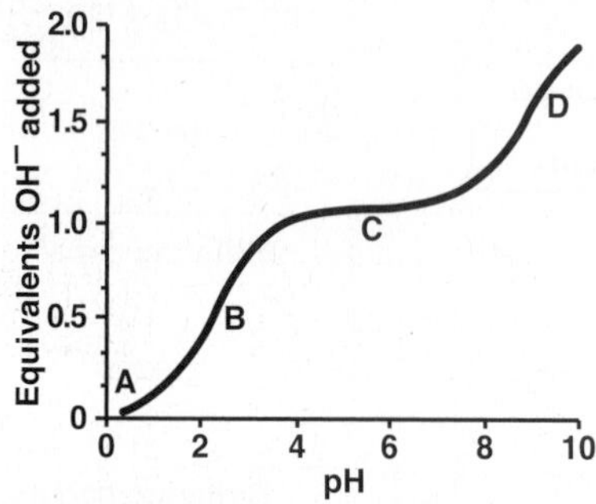

A. Point A represents the region where the amino acid is deprotonated.
B. Point B represents a region of minimal buffering.
C. Point C represents the region where the net charge on the amino acid is zero.
D. Point D represents the pK of the amino acid's carboxyl group.
E. The amino acid could be lysine.

Correct answer = C. C represents the isoelectric point, or pI, and as such is midway between pK_1 and pK_2 for a nonpolar amino acid. The amino acid is fully protonated at Point A. Point B represents a region of maximum buffering, as does Point D. Lysine is a basic amino acid, and has an ionizable side chain.

1.2 Which one of the following statements concerning the peptide shown below is correct?

Val-Cys-Glu-Ser-Asp-Arg-Cys

A. The peptide contains asparagine.
B. The peptide contains a side chain with a secondary amino group.
C. The peptide contains a side chain that can be phosphorylated.
D. The peptide cannot form an internal disulfide bond.
E. The peptide would move to the cathode (negative electrode) during electrophoresis at pH 5.

Correct answer = C. The hydroxyl group of serine can accept a phosphate group. Asp is aspartate. Proline contains a secondary amino group. The two cysteine residues can, under oxidizing conditions, form a disulfide (covalent) bond. The net charge on the peptide at pH 5 is negative, and it would move to the anode.

1.3 A 2-year-old child presents with metabolic acidosis after ingesting an unknown number of flavored aspirin tablets. At presentation, her blood pH was 7.0. Given that the pK_a of aspirin (salicylic acid) is 3, calculate the ratio of its ionized to un-ionized forms at pH 7.0.

Correct answer = 10,000 to 1.

pH = pK_a + log [A–]/[HA]. Therefore, 7 = 3 + x and x = 4. The ratio of A– (ionized) to HA (unionized), then, is 10,000 to 1 because the log of 10,000 is 4.

Structure of Proteins

2

I. OVERVIEW

The 20 amino acids commonly found in proteins are joined together by peptide bonds. The linear sequence of the linked amino acids contains the information necessary to generate a protein molecule with a unique three-dimensional shape. The complexity of protein structure is best analyzed by considering the molecule in terms of four organizational levels: primary, secondary, tertiary, and quaternary (Figure 2.1). An examination of these hierarchies of increasing complexity has revealed that certain structural elements are repeated in a wide variety of proteins, suggesting that there are general "rules" regarding the ways in which proteins achieve their native, functional form. These repeated structural elements range from simple combinations of α-helices and β-sheets forming small motifs, to the complex folding of polypeptide domains of multifunctional proteins (see p. 19).

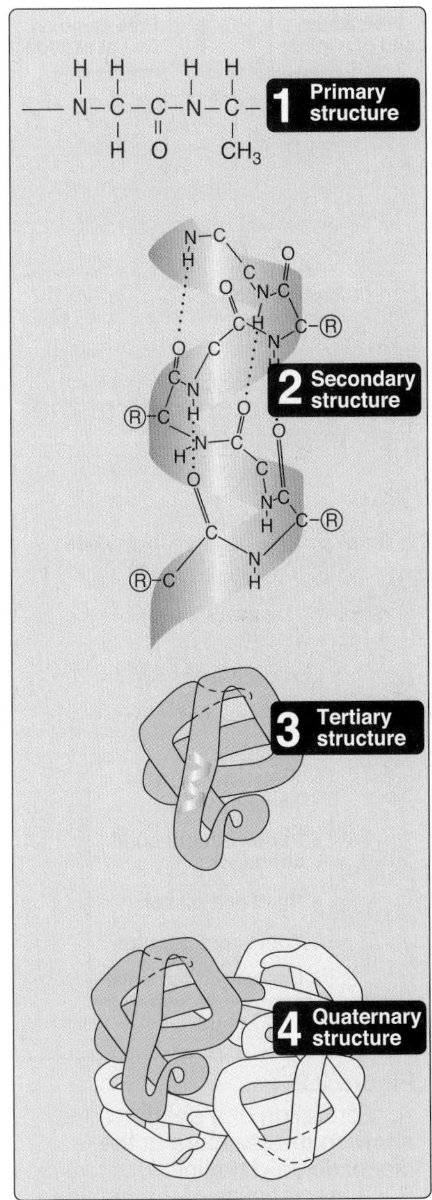

Figure 2.1
Four hierarchies of protein structure.

II. PRIMARY STRUCTURE OF PROTEINS

The sequence of amino acids in a protein is called the primary structure of the protein. Understanding the primary structure of proteins is important because many genetic diseases result in proteins with abnormal amino acid sequences, which cause improper folding and loss or impairment of normal function. If the primary structures of the normal and the mutated proteins are known, this information may be used to diagnose or study the disease.

A. Peptide bond

In proteins, amino acids are joined covalently by peptide bonds, which are amide linkages between the α-carboxyl group of one amino acid and the α-amino group of another. For example, valine and alanine can form the dipeptide valylalanine through the formation of a peptide bond (Figure 2.2). Peptide bonds are resistant to conditions that denature proteins, such as heating and high concentrations of urea (see p. 20). Prolonged exposure to a strong acid or base at elevated temperatures is required to break these bonds nonenzymically.

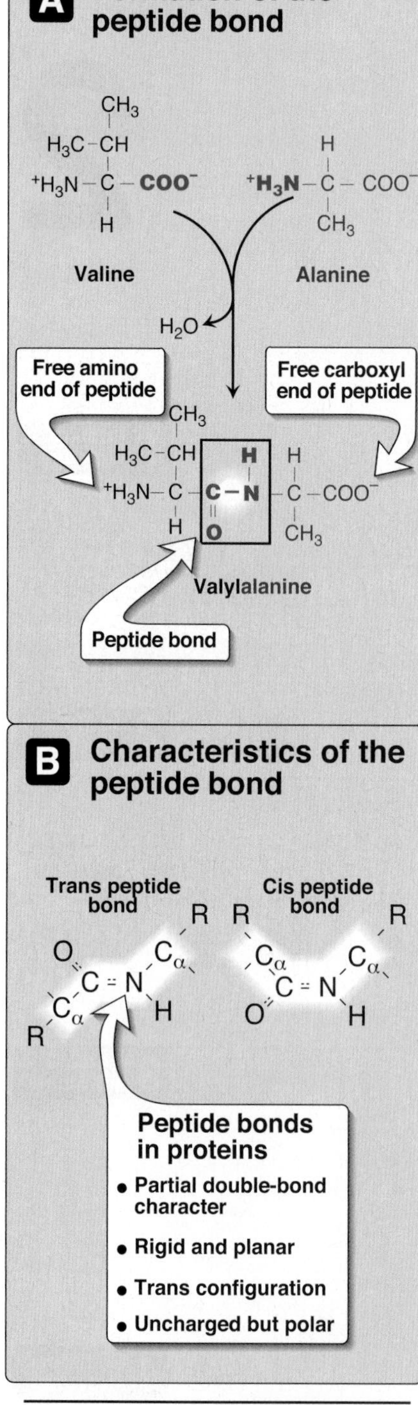

Figure 2.2
A. Formation of a peptide bond, showing the structure of the dipeptide valylalanine.
B. Characteristics of the peptide bond.

1. **Naming the peptide:** By convention, the free amino end (N-terminal) of the peptide chain is written to the left and the free carboxyl end (C-terminal) to the right. Therefore, all amino acid sequences are read from the N- to the C-terminal end of the peptide. For example, in Figure 2.2A, the order of the amino acids is "valine, alanine." Linkage of many amino acids through peptide bonds results in an unbranched chain called a polypeptide. Each component amino acid in a polypeptide is called a "residue" because it is the portion of the amino acid remaining after the atoms of water are lost in the formation of the peptide bond. When a polypeptide is named, all amino acid residues have their suffixes (-ine, -an, -ic, or -ate) changed to -yl, with the exception of the C-terminal amino acid. For example, a tripeptide composed of an N-terminal valine, a glycine, and a C-terminal leucine is called valylglycylleucine.

2. **Characteristics of the peptide bond:** The peptide bond has a partial double-bond character, that is, it is shorter than a single bond and is rigid and planar (Figure 2.2B). This prevents free rotation around the bond between the carbonyl carbon and the nitrogen of the peptide bond. However, the bonds between the α-carbons and the α-amino or α-carboxyl groups can be freely rotated (although they are limited by the size and character of the R groups). This allows the polypeptide chain to assume a variety of possible configurations. The peptide bond is almost always a trans bond (instead of cis, see Figure 2.2B), in large part because of steric interference of the R groups when in the cis position.

3. **Polarity of the peptide bond:** Like all amide linkages, the – C=O and – NH groups of the peptide bond are uncharged and neither accept nor release protons over the pH range of 2–12. Thus, the charged groups present in polypeptides consist solely of the N-terminal (α-amino) group, the C-terminal (α-carboxyl) group, and any ionized groups present in the side chains of the constituent amino acids. The – C=O and – NH groups of the peptide bond are polar, however, and are involved in hydrogen bonds (for example, in α-helices and β-sheets), as described on pp. 16–17.

B. Determination of the amino acid composition of a polypeptide

The first step in determining the primary structure of a polypeptide is to identify and quantitate its constituent amino acids. A purified sample of the polypeptide to be analyzed is first hydrolyzed by strong acid at 110°C for 24 hours. This treatment cleaves the peptide bonds and releases the individual amino acids, which can be separated by cation-exchange chromatography. In this technique, a mixture of amino acids is applied to a column that contains a resin to which a negatively charged group is tightly attached. [Note: If the attached group is positively charged, the column becomes an anion-exchange column.] The amino acids bind to the column with different affinities, depending on their charges, hydrophobicity, and other characteristics. Each amino acid is sequentially released from the chromatography column by eluting with solutions of increasing ionic strength and pH (Figure 2.3). The separated amino acids contained in the eluate from the column are quantitated by heating them with ninhydrin (a reagent that forms a purple compound with most amino acids, ammonia, and amines). The amount of each amino acid is determined spectrophotometrically by measuring the amount of light absorbed by the ninhydrin derivative. The analysis described above is performed using an amino acid analyzer, an automated machine whose components are depicted in Figure 2.3.

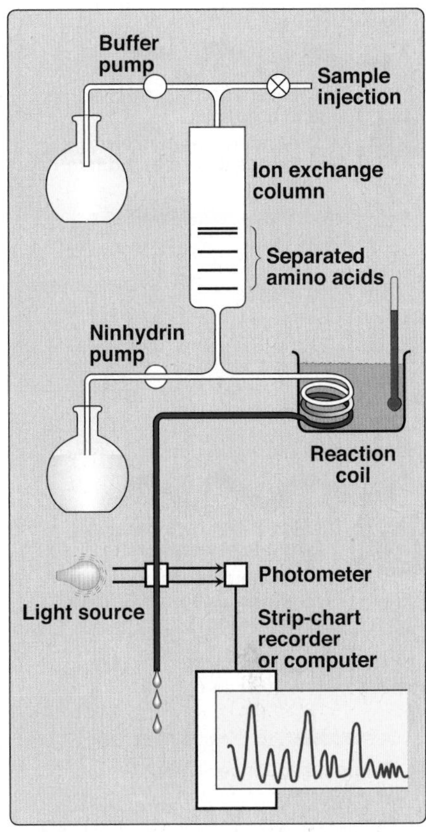

Figure 2.3
Determination of the amino acid composition of a polypeptide using an amino acid analyzer.

C. Sequencing of the peptide from its N-terminal end

Sequencing is a stepwise process of identifying the specific amino acid at each position in the peptide chain, beginning at the N-terminal end. Phenylisothiocyanate, known as Edman reagent, is used to label the amino-terminal residue under mildly alkaline conditions (Figure 2.4). The resulting phenylthiohydantoin (PTH) derivative introduces an instability in the N-terminal peptide bond such that it can be hydrolyzed without cleaving the other peptide bonds. The identity of the amino acid derivative can then be determined. Edman reagent can be applied repeatedly to the shortened peptide obtained in each previous cycle. The process is now automated.

D. Cleavage of the polypeptide into smaller fragments

Many polypeptides have a primary structure composed of more than 100 amino acids. Such molecules cannot be sequenced directly from end to end. However, these large molecules can be cleaved at specific sites and the resulting fragments sequenced. By using more than one cleaving agent (enzymes and/or chemicals) on separate samples of the purified polypeptide, overlapping fragments can be generated that permit the proper ordering of the sequenced fragments, thereby providing a complete amino acid sequence of the large polypeptide (Figure 2.5). Enzymes that hydrolyze peptide bonds are termed *peptidases* (*proteases*). [Note: *Exopeptidases* cut at the ends of proteins and are divided into *aminopeptidases* and *carboxypeptidases*. *Carboxypeptidases* are used in determining the C-terminal amino acid. *Endopeptidases* cleave within a protein.]

E. Determination of a protein's primary structure by DNA sequencing

The sequence of nucleotides in a protein-coding region of the DNA specifies the amino acid sequence of a polypeptide. Therefore, if the nucleotide sequence can be determined, it is possible, from knowledge of the genetic code (see p. 432), to translate the sequence of nucleotides into the corresponding amino acid sequence of that polypeptide. This indirect process, although routinely used to

1 Labeling

2 Release of amino acid derivative by acid hydrolysis

H_2N-CH(CH$_3$)-C(=O)-Lys-His-Leu-Arg-COOH
Peptide
N-terminal alanine

Phenyl-isothiocyanate

HN-CH(CH$_3$)-C(=O)-Lys-His-Leu-Arg-COOH
Labeled peptide

H_2N-Lys-His-Leu-Arg-COOH
Shortened peptide
+
PTH-alanine

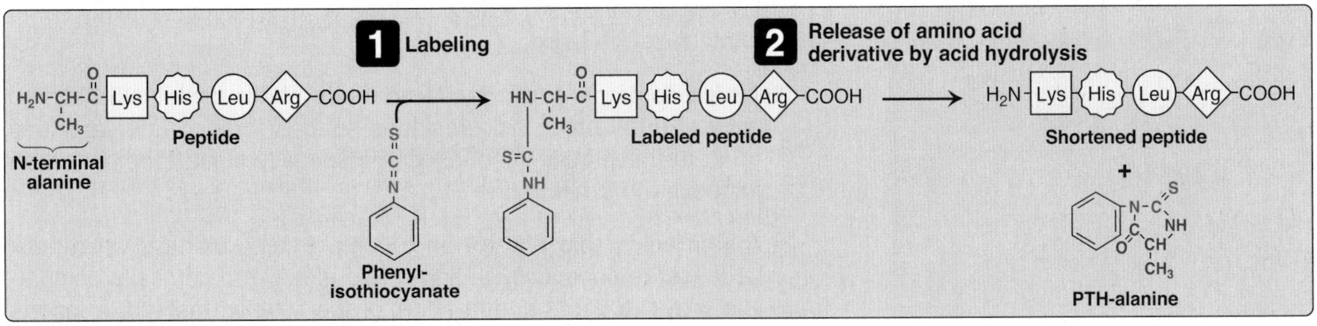

Figure 2.4
Determination of the amino (N)-terminal residue of a polypeptide by Edman degradation. PTH = phenylthiohydantoin.

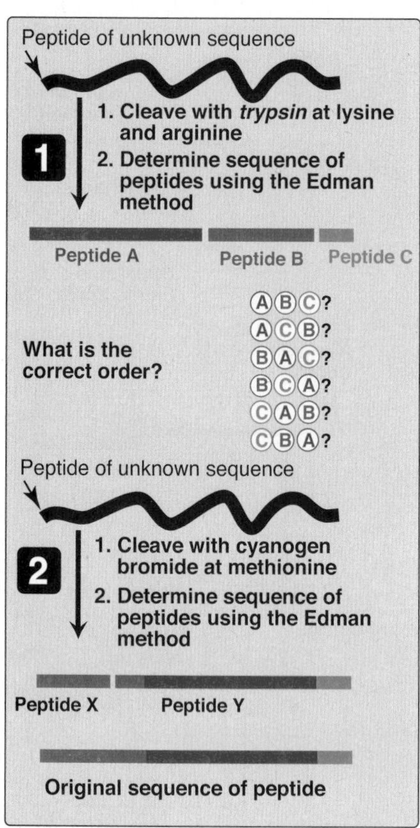

Figure 2.5
Overlapping of peptides produced by the action of *trypsin* and cyanogen bromide.

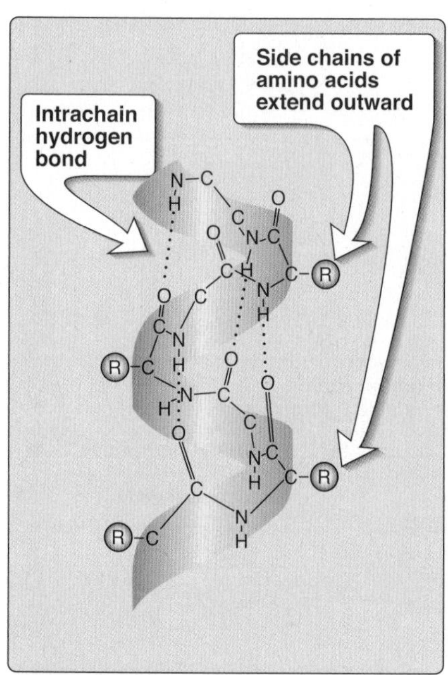

Figure 2.6
α-Helix showing peptide backbone.

obtain the amino acid sequences of proteins, has the limitations of not being able to predict the positions of disulfide bonds in the folded chain and of not identifying any amino acids that are modified after their incorporation into the polypeptide (posttranslational modification, see p. 443). Therefore, direct protein sequencing is an extremely important tool for determining the true character of the primary sequence of many polypeptides.

III. SECONDARY STRUCTURE OF PROTEINS

The polypeptide backbone does not assume a random three-dimensional structure but, instead, generally forms regular arrangements of amino acids that are located near each other in the linear sequence. These arrangements are termed the secondary structure of the polypeptide. The α-helix, β-sheet, and β-bend (β-turn) are examples of secondary structures commonly encountered in proteins. [Note: The collagen α-chain helix, another example of secondary structure, is discussed on p. 45.]

A. α-Helix

Several different polypeptide helices are found in nature, but the α-helix is the most common. It is a spiral structure, consisting of a tightly packed, coiled polypeptide backbone core, with the side chains of the component amino acids extending outward from the central axis to avoid interfering sterically with each other (Figure 2.6). A very diverse group of proteins contains α-helices. For example, the keratins are a family of closely related, fibrous proteins whose structure is nearly entirely α-helical. They are a major component of tissues such as hair and skin, and their rigidity is determined by the number of disulfide bonds between the constituent polypeptide chains. In contrast to keratin, myoglobin, whose structure is also highly α-helical, is a globular, flexible molecule (see p. 26).

1. **Hydrogen bonds:** An α-helix is stabilized by extensive hydrogen bonding between the peptide-bond carbonyl oxygens and amide hydrogens that are part of the polypeptide backbone (see Figure 2.6). The hydrogen bonds extend up and are parallel to the spiral from the carbonyl oxygen of one peptide bond to the – NH – group of a peptide linkage four residues ahead in the polypeptide. This insures that all but the first and last peptide bond components are linked to each other through intrachain hydrogen bonds. Hydrogen bonds are individually weak, but they collectively serve to stabilize the helix.

2. **Amino acids per turn:** Each turn of an α-helix contains 3.6 amino acids. Thus, amino acid residues spaced three or four residues apart in the primary sequence are spatially close together when folded in the α-helix.

3. **Amino acids that disrupt an α-helix:** Proline disrupts an α-helix because its secondary amino group is not geometrically compatible with the right-handed spiral of the α-helix. Instead, it inserts a kink in the chain, which interferes with the smooth, helical structure. Large numbers of charged amino acids (for example,

glutamate, aspartate, histidine, lysine, and arginine) also disrupt the helix by forming ionic bonds or by electrostatically repelling each other. Finally, amino acids with bulky side chains, such as tryptophan, or amino acids, such as valine or isoleucine, that branch at the β-carbon (the first carbon in the R group, next to the α-carbon) can interfere with formation of the α-helix if they are present in large numbers.

B. β-Sheet

The β-sheet is another form of secondary structure in which all of the peptide bond components are involved in hydrogen bonding (Figure 2.7A). The surfaces of β-sheets appear "pleated," and these structures are, therefore, often called β-pleated sheets. When illustrations are made of protein structure, β-strands are often visualized as broad arrows (Figure 2.7B).

1. **Comparison of a β-sheet and an α-helix:** Unlike the α-helix, β-sheets are composed of two or more peptide chains (β-strands), or segments of polypeptide chains, which are almost fully extended. Note also that the hydrogen bonds are perpendicular to the polypeptide backbone in β-sheets (see Figure 2.7A).

2. **Parallel and antiparallel sheets:** A β-sheet can be formed from two or more separate polypeptide chains or segments of polypeptide chains that are arranged either antiparallel to each other (with the N-terminal and C-terminal ends of the β-strands alternating as shown in Figure 2.7B) or parallel to each other (with all the N-termini of the β-strands together as shown in Figure 2.7C). When the hydrogen bonds are formed between the polypeptide backbones of separate polypeptide chains, they are termed interchain bonds. A β-sheet can also be formed by a single polypeptide chain folding back on itself (see Figure 2.7C). In this case, the hydrogen bonds are intrachain bonds. In globular proteins, β-sheets always have a right-handed curl, or twist, when viewed along the polypeptide backbone. [Note: Twisted β-sheets often form the core of globular proteins.]

> The α-helix and β-sheet structures provide maximal hydrogen bonding for peptide bond components within the interior of polypeptides.

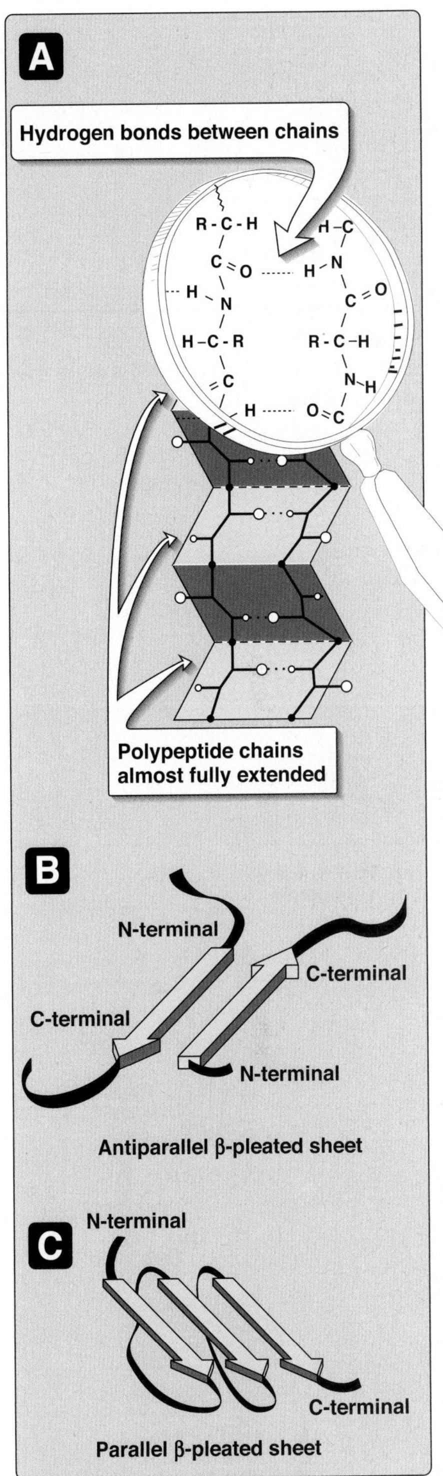

Figure 2.7
A. Structure of a β-sheet. B. An antiparallel β-sheet with the β-strands represented as broad arrows. C. A parallel β-sheet formed from a single polypeptide chain folding back on itself.

C. β-Bends (reverse turns, β-turns)

β-Bends reverse the direction of a polypeptide chain, helping it form a compact, globular shape. They are usually found on the surface of protein molecules and often include charged residues. [Note: β-Bends were given this name because they often connect successive strands of antiparallel β-sheets.] β-Bends are generally composed of four amino acids, one of which may be proline, the amino acid that causes a kink in the polypeptide chain. Glycine, the amino acid with the smallest R group, is also frequently found in β-bends. β-Bends are stabilized by the formation of hydrogen and ionic bonds.

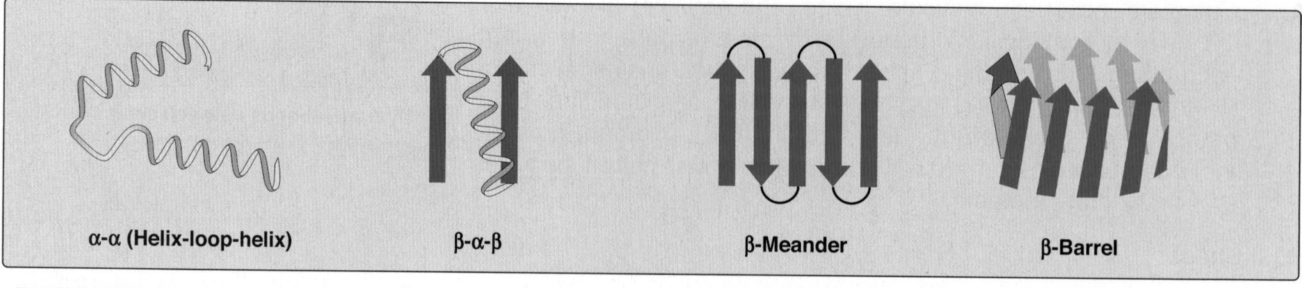

Figure 2.8
Some common structural motifs involving α-helices and β-sheets. The names describe their schematic appearance.

D. Nonrepetitive secondary structure

Approximately one half of an average globular protein is organized into repetitive structures, such as the α-helix and β-sheet. The remainder of the polypeptide chain is described as having a loop or coil conformation. These nonrepetitive secondary structures are not random, but rather simply have a less regular structure than those described above. [Note: The term "random coil" refers to the disordered structure obtained when proteins are denatured (see p. 20).]

E. Supersecondary structures (motifs)

Globular proteins are constructed by combining secondary structural elements (that is, α-helices, β-sheets, and coils), producing specific geometric patterns or motifs. These form primarily the core (interior) region of the molecule. They are connected by loop regions (for example, β-bends) at the surface of the protein. Supersecondary structures are usually produced by the close packing of side chains from adjacent secondary structural elements. Thus, for example, α-helices and β-sheets that are adjacent in the amino acid sequence are also usually (but not always) adjacent in the final, folded protein. Some of the more common motifs are illustrated in Figure 2.8.

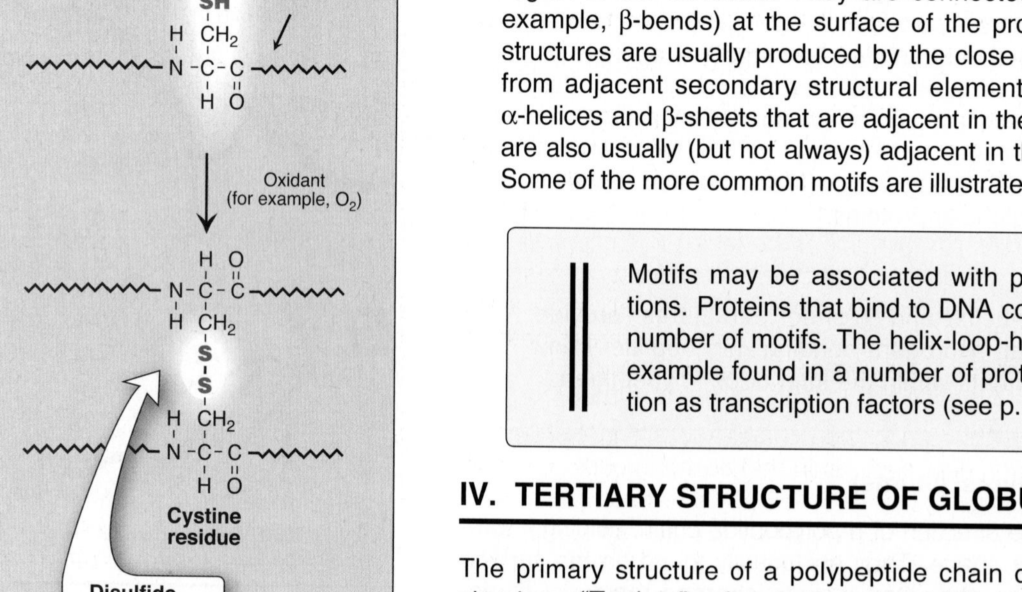

Figure 2.9
Formation of a disulfide bond by the oxidation of two cysteine residues, producing one cystine residue.

> Motifs may be associated with particular functions. Proteins that bind to DNA contain a limited number of motifs. The helix-loop-helix motif is an example found in a number of proteins that function as transcription factors (see p. 450).

IV. TERTIARY STRUCTURE OF GLOBULAR PROTEINS

The primary structure of a polypeptide chain determines its tertiary structure. "Tertiary" refers both to the folding of domains (the basic units of structure and function, see discussion below), and to the final arrangement of domains in the polypeptide. The structure of globular proteins in aqueous solution is compact, with a high density (close packing) of the atoms in the core of the molecule. Hydrophobic side chains are buried in the interior, whereas hydrophilic groups are generally found on the surface of the molecule.

A. Domains

Domains are the fundamental functional and three-dimensional structural units of polypeptides. Polypeptide chains that are greater than 200 amino acids in length generally consist of two or more domains. The core of a domain is built from combinations of super-secondary structural elements (motifs). Folding of the peptide chain within a domain usually occurs independently of folding in other domains. Therefore, each domain has the characteristics of a small, compact globular protein that is structurally independent of the other domains in the polypeptide chain.

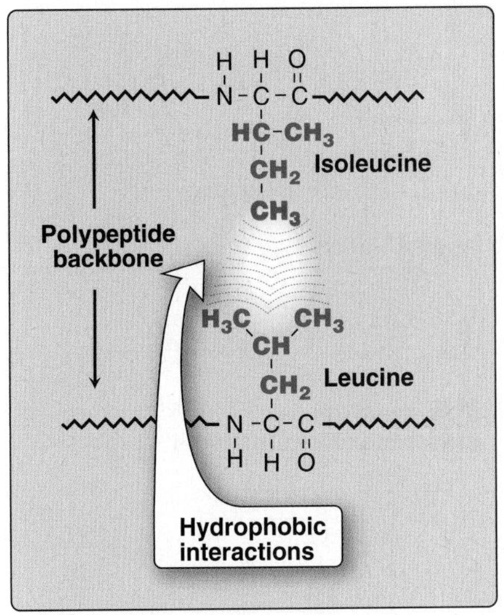

Figure 2.10
Hydrophobic interactions between amino acids with nonpolar side chains.

B. Interactions stabilizing tertiary structure

The unique three-dimensional structure of each polypeptide is determined by its amino acid sequence. Interactions between the amino acid side chains guide the folding of the polypeptide to form a compact structure. The following four types of interactions cooperate in stabilizing the tertiary structures of globular proteins.

1. **Disulfide bonds:** A disulfide bond is a covalent linkage formed from the sulfhydryl group (–SH) of each of two cysteine residues to produce a cystine residue (Figure 2.9). The two cysteines may be separated from each other by many amino acids in the primary sequence of a polypeptide or may even be located on two different polypeptide chains. The folding of the polypeptide chain(s) brings the cysteine residues into proximity and permits covalent bonding of their side chains. A disulfide bond contributes to the stability of the three-dimensional shape of the protein molecule and prevents it from becoming denatured in the extracellular environment. For example, many disulfide bonds are found in proteins such as immunoglobulins that are secreted by cells.

2. **Hydrophobic interactions:** Amino acids with nonpolar side chains tend to be located in the interior of the polypeptide molecule, where they associate with other hydrophobic amino acids (Figure 2.10). In contrast, amino acids with polar or charged side chains tend to be located on the surface of the molecule in contact with the polar solvent. [Note: Recall that proteins located in nonpolar (lipid) environments, such as a membrane, exhibit the reverse arrangement (see Figure 1.4, p. 4).] In each case, a segregation of R groups occurs that is energetically most favorable.

3. **Hydrogen bonds:** Amino acid side chains containing oxygen- or nitrogen-bound hydrogen, such as in the alcohol groups of serine and threonine, can form hydrogen bonds with electron-rich atoms, such as the oxygen of a carboxyl group or carbonyl group of a peptide bond (Figure 2.11; see also Figure 1.6, p. 4). Formation of hydrogen bonds between polar groups on the surface of proteins and the aqueous solvent enhances the solubility of the protein.

4. **Ionic interactions:** Negatively charged groups, such as the carboxylate group ($-COO^-$) in the side chain of aspartate or glutamate, can interact with positively charged groups such as the amino group ($-NH_3^+$) in the side chain of lysine (see Figure 2.11).

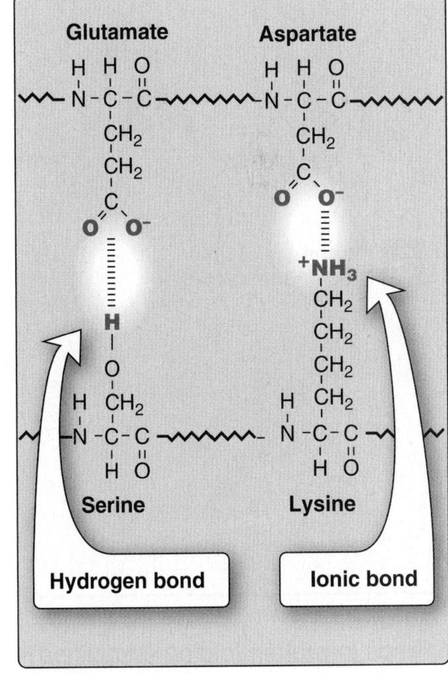

Figure 2.11
Interactions of side chains of amino acids through hydrogen bonds and ionic bonds (salt bridges).

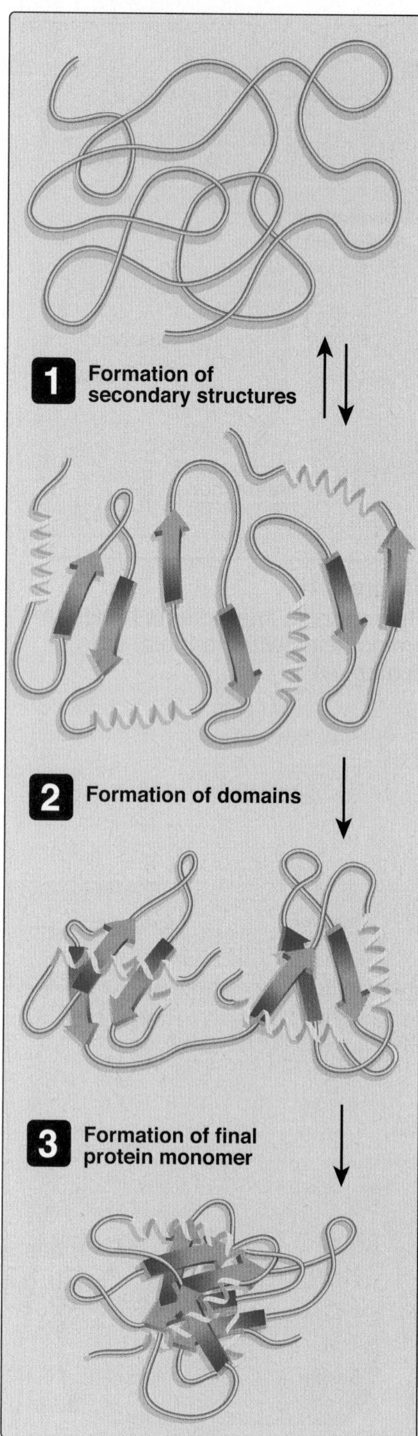

Figure 2.12
Steps in protein folding (simplified).

C. Protein folding

Interactions between the side chains of amino acids determine how a long polypeptide chain folds into the intricate three-dimensional shape of the functional protein. Protein folding, which occurs within the cell in seconds to minutes, involves nonrandom, ordered pathways. As a peptide folds, secondary structures form driven by the hydrophobic effect (that is, hydrophobic groups come together as water is released). These small structures combine to form larger structures. Additional events stabilize secondary structure and initiate formation of tertiary structure. In the last stage, the peptide achieves its fully folded, native (functional) form characterized by a low-energy state (Figure 2.12). [Note: Some biologically active proteins or segments thereof lack a stable tertiary structure. They are referred to as "intrinsically disordered" proteins.]

D. Denaturation of proteins

Protein denaturation results in the unfolding and disorganization of a protein's secondary and tertiary structures without the hydrolysis of peptide bonds. Denaturing agents include heat, organic solvents, strong acids or bases, detergents, and ions of heavy metals such as lead. Denaturation may, under ideal conditions, be reversible, such that the protein refolds into its original native structure when the denaturing agent is removed. However, most proteins, once denatured, remain permanently disordered. Denatured proteins are often insoluble and precipitate from solution.

E. Role of chaperones in protein folding

The information needed for correct protein folding is contained in the primary structure of the polypeptide. However, most proteins when denatured do not resume their native conformations even under favorable environmental conditions. This is because, for many proteins, folding is a facilitated process that requires a specialized group of proteins, referred to as "molecular chaperones," and adenosine triphosphate hydrolysis. The chaperones, also known as "heat shock proteins" (Hsp), interact with a polypeptide at various stages during the folding process. Some chaperones bind hydrophobic regions of an extended polypeptide and are important in keeping the protein unfolded until its synthesis is completed (for example, Hsp70). Others form cage-like macromolecular structures composed of two stacked rings. The partially folded protein enters the cage, binds the central cavity through hydrophobic interactions, folds, and is released (for example, mitochondrial Hsp60). [Note: Cage-like chaperones are sometimes referred to as "chaperonins."] Chaperones, then, facilitate correct protein folding by binding to and stabilizing exposed, aggregation-prone hydrophobic regions in nascent (and denatured) polypeptides, preventing premature folding.

V. QUATERNARY STRUCTURE OF PROTEINS

Many proteins consist of a single polypeptide chain and are defined as monomeric proteins. However, others may consist of two or more polypeptide chains that may be structurally identical or totally unrelated. The arrangement of these polypeptide subunits is called the quaternary structure of the protein. Subunits are held together primarily by noncovalent interactions (for example, hydrogen bonds, ionic bonds, and hydrophobic interactions). Subunits may either function independently of each other or may work cooperatively, as in hemoglobin, in which the binding of oxygen to one subunit of the tetramer increases the affinity of the other subunits for oxygen (see p. 29).

> Isoforms are proteins that perform the same function but have different primary structures. They can arise from different genes or from tissue-specific processing of the product of a single gene. If the proteins function as enzymes, they are referred to as isozymes (see p. 65).

VI. PROTEIN MISFOLDING

Protein folding is a complex process that can sometimes result in improperly folded molecules. These misfolded proteins are usually tagged and degraded within the cell (see p. 444). However, this quality control system is not perfect, and intracellular or extracellular aggregates of misfolded proteins can accumulate, particularly as individuals age. Deposits of misfolded proteins are associated with a number of diseases.

A. Amyloid diseases

Misfolding of proteins may occur spontaneously or be caused by a mutation in a particular gene, which then produces an altered protein. In addition, some apparently normal proteins can, after abnormal proteolytic cleavage, take on a unique conformational state that leads to the formation of long, fibrillar protein assemblies consisting of β-pleated sheets. Accumulation of these insoluble, spontaneously aggregating proteins, called amyloids, has been implicated in degenerative diseases such as Parkinson and Huntington and particularly in the age-related neurodegenerative disorder, Alzheimer disease. The dominant component of the amyloid plaque that accumulates in Alzheimer disease is amyloid β (Aβ), an extracellular peptide containing 40–42 amino acid residues. X-ray crystallography and infrared spectroscopy demonstrate a characteristic β-pleated sheet conformation in nonbranching fibrils. This peptide, when aggregated in a β-pleated sheet configuration, is neurotoxic and is the central pathogenic event leading to the cognitive impairment characteristic of the disease. The Aβ that is deposited in the brain in Alzheimer disease is derived by enzymic cleavages (by *secretases*) from the larger amyloid precursor protein, a single transmembrane protein expressed on the cell surface in the brain and other tissues (Figure 2.13). The Aβ peptides aggregate, generating the amyloid that is found in the brain parenchyma and around blood vessels. Most cases of Alzheimer disease are not genetically based, although at least 5% of cases are familial. A second biologic factor involved in the development of Alzheimer disease is the accumulation of neurofibrillary tangles inside neurons. A key component of these tangled fibers is an abnormal form (hyperphosphorylated and insoluble) of the tau (τ) protein, which, in its healthy version, helps in the assembly of the microtubular structure. The defective τ appears to block the actions of its normal counterpart.

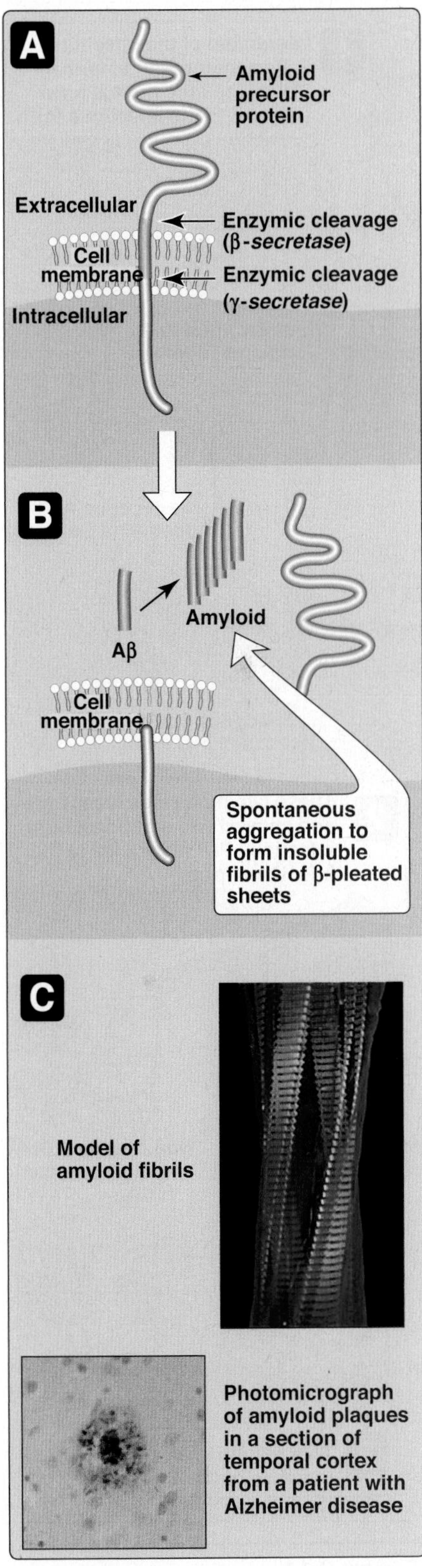

Figure 2.13
Formation of amyloid plaques found in Alzheimer disease (AD). [Note: Mutations to *presenilin*, the catalytic subunit of *γ-secretase*, are the most common cause of familial AD.]

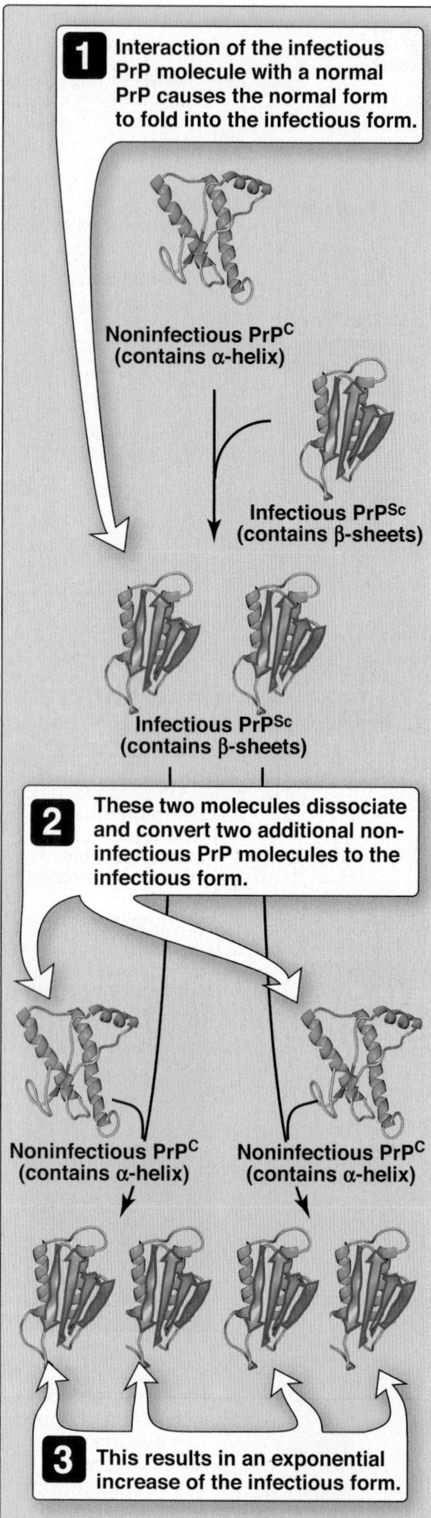

Figure 2.14
One proposed mechanism for multiplication of infectious prion agents. PrP = prion protein; PrP^c = prion protein cellular; PrP^{Sc} = prion protein scrapie.

B. Prion diseases

The prion protein (PrP) has been strongly implicated as the causative agent of transmissible spongiform encephalopathies (TSEs), including Creutzfeldt-Jakob disease in humans, scrapie in sheep, and bovine spongiform encephalopathy in cattle (popularly called "mad cow" disease). After an extensive series of purification procedures, scientists were surprised to find that the infectivity of the agent causing scrapie in sheep was associated with a single protein species that was not complexed with detectable nucleic acid. This infectious protein is designated PrP^{Sc} (Sc = scrapie). It is highly resistant to proteolytic degradation and tends to form insoluble aggregates of fibrils, similar to the amyloid found in some other diseases of the brain. A noninfectious form of PrP^C (C = cellular), encoded by the same gene as the infectious agent, is present in normal mammalian brains on the surface of neurons and glial cells. Thus, PrP^C is a host protein. No primary structure differences or alternate posttranslational modifications have been found between the normal and the infectious forms of the protein. The key to becoming infectious apparently lies in changes in the three-dimensional conformation of PrP^C. It has been observed that a number of α-helices present in noninfectious PrP^C are replaced by β-sheets in the infectious form (Figure 2.14). It is presumably this conformational difference that confers relative resistance to proteolytic degradation of infectious prions and permits them to be distinguished from the normal PrP^C in infected tissue. The infective agent is, thus, an altered version of a normal protein, which acts as a "template" for converting the normal protein to the pathogenic conformation. The TSEs are invariably fatal, and no treatment is currently available that can alter this outcome.

VII. CHAPTER SUMMARY

Central to understanding protein structure is the concept of the **native conformation** (Figure 2.15), which is the functional, fully folded protein structure (for example, an active enzyme or structural protein). The unique three-dimensional structure of the native conformation is determined by its **primary structure**, that is, its amino acid sequence. Interactions between the amino acid side chains guide the folding of the polypeptide chain to form **secondary**, **tertiary**, and (sometimes) **quaternary** structures, which cooperate in stabilizing the native conformation of the protein. In addition, a specialized group of proteins named **chaperones** is required for the proper folding of many species of proteins. **Protein denaturation** results in the unfolding and disorganization of the protein's structure, which are not accompanied by hydrolysis of peptide bonds. Denaturation may be reversible or, more commonly, irreversible. Disease can occur when an apparently normal protein assumes a conformation that is cytotoxic, as in the case of Alzheimer disease and the **transmissible spongiform encephalopathies (TSEs)**, including **Creutzfeldt-Jakob disease**. In **Alzheimer disease,** normal proteins, after abnormal chemical processing, take on a unique conformational state that leads to the formation of neurotoxic **amyloid β peptide (Aβ)** assemblies consisting of β-pleated sheets. In TSEs, the infective agent is an altered version of a normal **prion protein** that acts as a "template" for converting normal protein to the pathogenic conformation.

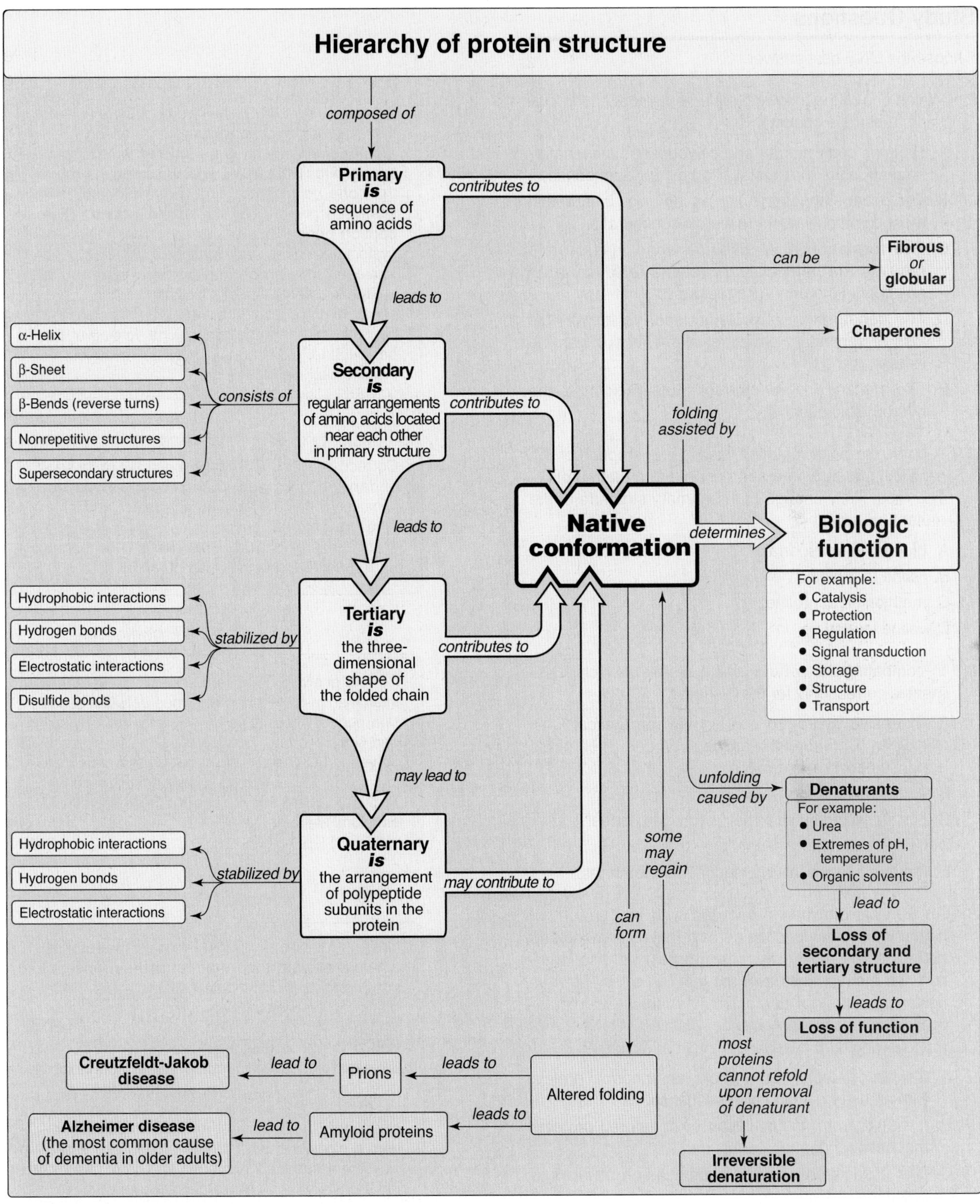

Figure 2.15
Key concept map for protein structure.

Study Questions

Choose the ONE best answer.

2.1 Which one of the following statements concerning protein structure is correct?

A. Proteins consisting of one polypeptide have quaternary structure that is stabilized by covalent bonds.
B. The peptide bonds that link amino acids in a protein most commonly occur in the cis configuration.
C. The formation of a disulfide bond in a protein requires the participating cysteine residues to be adjacent in the primary structure.
D. The denaturation of proteins leads to irreversible loss of secondary structural elements such as the α-helix.
E. The primary driving force for protein folding is the hydrophobic effect.

Correct answer = E. The hydrophobic effect, or the tendency of nonpolar entities to associate in a polar environment, is the driving force of protein folding. Quaternary structure requires more than one polypeptide, and, when present, it is stabilized primarily by noncovalent bonds. The peptide bond is almost always trans. The two cysteine residues participating in disulfide bond formation may be a great distance apart in the amino acid sequence of a polypeptide (or on two separate polypeptides) but are brought into close proximity by the three-dimensional folding of the polypeptide. Denaturation may be reversible or irreversible.

2.2 A particular point mutation results in disruption of the α-helical structure in a segment of the mutant protein. The most likely change in the primary structure of the mutant protein is:

A. glutamate to aspartate.
B. lysine to arginine.
C. methionine to proline.
D. valine to alanine.

Correct answer = C. Proline, because of its secondary amino group, is incompatible with an α-helix. Glutamate, aspartate, lysine, and arginine are charged amino acids, and valine is a branched amino acid. Charged and branched (bulky) amino acids may disrupt an α-helix.

2.3 In comparing the α-helix to the β-sheet, which statement is correct only for the β-sheet?

A. Extensive hydrogen bonds between the carbonyl oxygen (C=O) and the amide hydrogen (N-H) of the peptide bond are formed.
B. It may be found in typical globular proteins.
C. It is stabilized by interchain hydrogen bonds.
D. it is an example of secondary structure.
E. It may be found in supersecondary structures.

Correct answer = C. The β-sheet is stabilized by interchain hydrogen bonds formed between separate polypeptide chains and by intrachain hydrogen bonds formed between regions of a single polypeptide. The α-helix, however, is stabilized only by intrachain hydrogen bonds. Statements A, B, D, and E are true for both of these secondary structural elements.

2.4 An 80-year-old man presented with impairment of higher intellectual function and alterations in mood and behavior. His family reported progressive disorientation and memory loss over the last 6 months. There is no family history of dementia. The patient was tentatively diagnosed with Alzheimer disease. Which one of the following best describes Alzheimer disease?

A. It is associated with β-amyloid, an abnormal protein with an altered amino acid sequence.
B. It results from accumulation of denatured proteins that have random conformations.
C. It is associated with the accumulation of amyloid precursor protein.
D. It is associated with the deposition of neurotoxic amyloid β peptide aggregates.
E. It is an environmentally produced disease not influenced by the genetics of the individual.
F. It is caused by the infectious β-sheet form of a host-cell protein.

Correct answer = D. Alzheimer disease is associated with long, fibrillar protein assemblies consisting of β-pleated sheets found in the brain and elsewhere. The disease is associated with abnormal processing of a normal protein. The accumulated altered protein occurs in a β-pleated sheet configuration that is neurotoxic. The amyloid β that is deposited in the brain in Alzheimer disease is derived by proteolytic cleavages from the larger amyloid precursor protein, a single transmembrane protein expressed on the cell surface in the brain and other tissues. Most cases of Alzheimer disease are sporadic, although at least 5% of cases are familial. Prion diseases, such as Creutzfeldt-Jakob, are caused by the infectious β-sheet form (PrP^{Sc}) of a host-cell protein (PrP^{C}).

Globular Proteins

3

I. OVERVIEW

The previous chapter described the types of secondary and tertiary structures that are the bricks and mortar of protein architecture. By arranging these fundamental structural elements in different combinations, widely diverse proteins can be constructed that are capable of various specialized functions. This chapter examines the relationship between structure and function for the clinically important globular hemeproteins. Fibrous structural proteins are discussed in Chapter 4.

II. GLOBULAR HEMEPROTEINS

Hemeproteins are a group of specialized proteins that contain heme as a tightly bound prosthetic group. (See p. 54 for a discussion of prosthetic groups.) The role of the heme group is dictated by the environment created by the three-dimensional structure of the protein. For example, the heme group of a cytochrome functions as an electron carrier that is alternately oxidized and reduced (see p. 76). In contrast, the heme group of the enzyme *catalase* is part of the active site of the enzyme that catalyzes the breakdown of hydrogen peroxide (see p. 148). In hemoglobin and myoglobin, the two most abundant hemeproteins in humans, the heme group serves to reversibly bind oxygen.

A. Structure of heme

Heme is a complex of protoporphyrin IX and ferrous iron (Fe^{2+}) (Figure 3.1). The iron is held in the center of the heme molecule by bonds to the four nitrogens of the porphyrin ring. The heme Fe^{2+} can form two additional bonds, one on each side of the planar porphyrin ring. In myoglobin and hemoglobin, one of these positions is coordinated to the side chain of a histidine residue of the globin molecule, whereas the other position is available to bind oxygen (Figure 3.2). (See pp. 278 and 282 for a discussion of the synthesis and degradation of heme.)

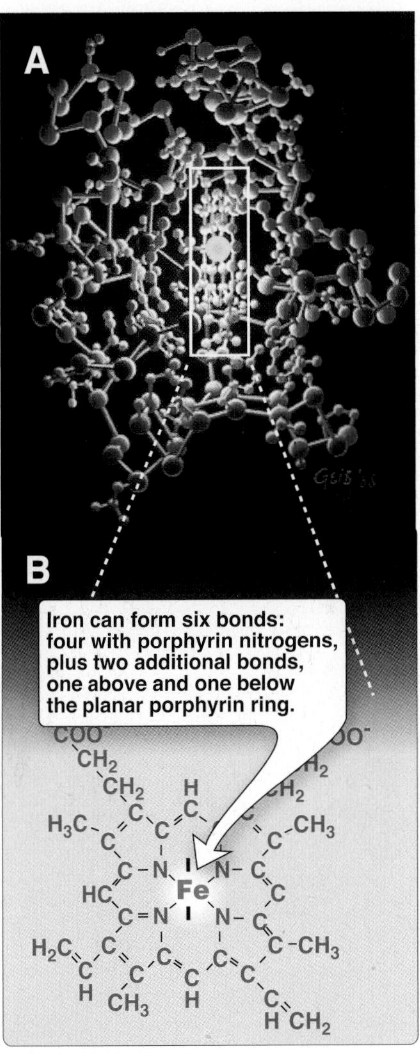

Figure 3.1
A. Hemeprotein (cytochrome c).
B. Structure of heme.

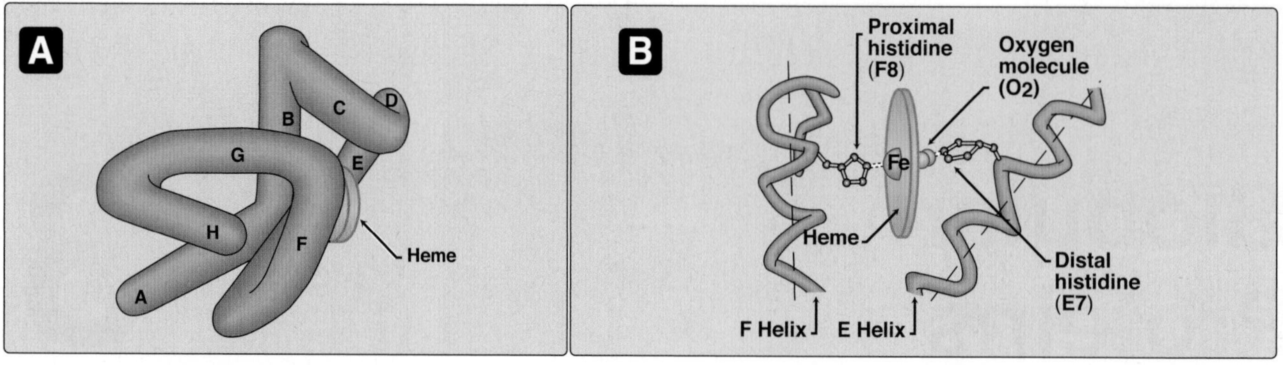

Figure 3.2
A. Model of myoglobin showing helices A to H. B. Schematic diagram of the oxygen-binding site of myoglobin.

B. Structure and function of myoglobin

Myoglobin, a hemeprotein present in heart and skeletal muscle, functions both as a reservoir for oxygen and as an oxygen carrier that increases the rate of transport of oxygen within the muscle cell. [Note: Mouse myoglobin double knockouts (see p. 486) have, surprisingly, an apparently normal phenotype.] Myoglobin consists of a single polypeptide chain that is structurally similar to the individual polypeptide chains of the tetrameric hemoglobin molecule. This homology makes myoglobin a useful model for interpreting some of the more complex properties of hemoglobin.

1. **α-Helical content:** Myoglobin is a compact molecule, with approximately 80% of its polypeptide chain folded into eight stretches of α-helix. These α-helical regions, labeled A to H in Figure 3.2A, are terminated either by the presence of proline, whose five-membered ring cannot be accommodated in an α-helix (see p. 16) or by β-bends and loops stabilized by hydrogen bonds and ionic bonds (see p. 17). [Note: Ionic bonds are also termed electrostatic interactions or salt bridges.]

2. **Location of polar and nonpolar amino acid residues:** The interior of the myoglobin molecule is composed almost entirely of nonpolar amino acids. They are packed closely together, forming a structure stabilized by hydrophobic interactions between these clustered residues (see p. 19). In contrast, polar amino acids are located almost exclusively on the surface, where they can form hydrogen bonds, both with each other and with water.

3. **Binding of the heme group:** The heme group of the myoglobin molecule sits in a crevice, which is lined with nonpolar amino acids. Notable exceptions are two histidine residues (Figure 3.2B). One, the proximal histidine (F8), binds directly to the iron of heme. The second, or distal histidine (E7), does not directly interact with the heme group but helps stabilize the binding of oxygen to the ferrous iron. The protein, or globin, portion of myoglobin thus creates a special microenvironment for the heme that permits the reversible binding of one oxygen molecule (oxygenation). The simultaneous loss of electrons by the ferrous iron (oxidation to the ferric form) occurs only rarely.

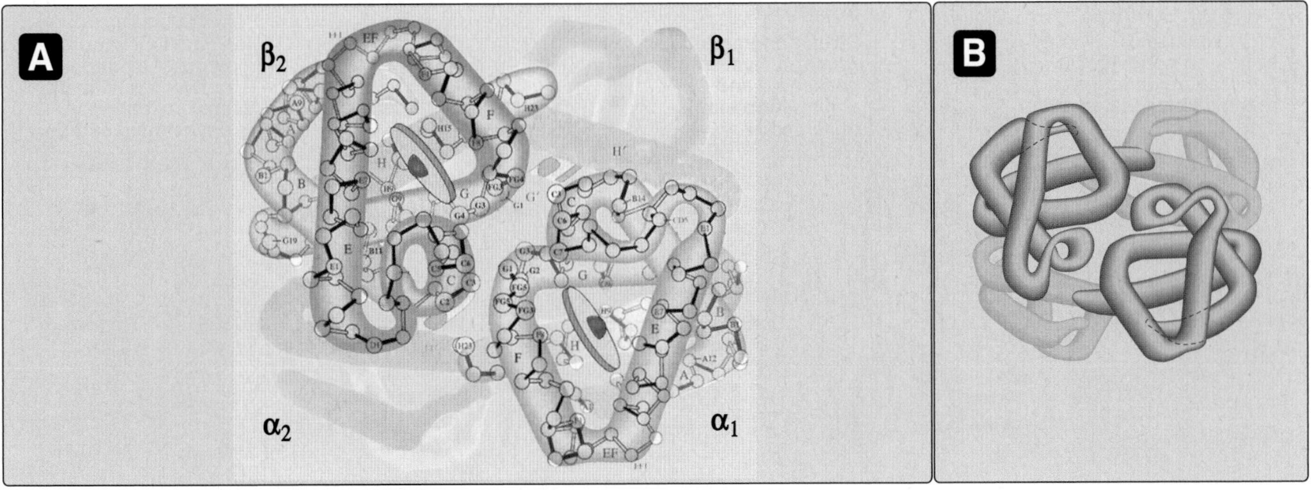

Figure 3.3
A. Structure of hemoglobin showing the polypeptide backbone. B. Simplified drawing showing the helices.

C. Structure and function of hemoglobin

Hemoglobin is found exclusively in red blood cells (RBC), where its main function is to transport oxygen (O_2) from the lungs to the capillaries of the tissues. Hemoglobin A, the major hemoglobin in adults, is composed of four polypeptide chains (two α chains and two β chains) held together by noncovalent interactions (Figure 3.3). Each chain (subunit) has stretches of α-helical structure and a hydrophobic heme-binding pocket similar to that described for myoglobin. However, the tetrameric hemoglobin molecule is structurally and functionally more complex than myoglobin. For example, hemoglobin can transport H^+ and CO_2 from the tissues to the lungs and can carry four molecules of O_2 from the lungs to the cells of the body. Furthermore, the oxygen-binding properties of hemoglobin are regulated by interaction with allosteric effectors (see p. 29).

> Obtaining O_2 from the atmosphere solely by diffusion greatly limits the size of organisms. Circulatory systems overcome this, but transport molecules such as hemoglobin are also required because O_2 is only slightly soluble in aqueous solutions such as blood.

1. **Quaternary structure of hemoglobin:** The hemoglobin tetramer can be envisioned as being composed of two identical dimers, $(\alpha\beta)_1$ and $(\alpha\beta)_2$. The two polypeptide chains within each dimer are held tightly together primarily by hydrophobic interactions (Figure 3.4). [Note: In this instance, hydrophobic amino acid residues are localized not only in the interior of the molecule, but also in a region on the surface of each subunit. Multiple interchain hydrophobic interactions form strong associations between α-subunits and β-subunits in the dimers.] In contrast, the two dimers are

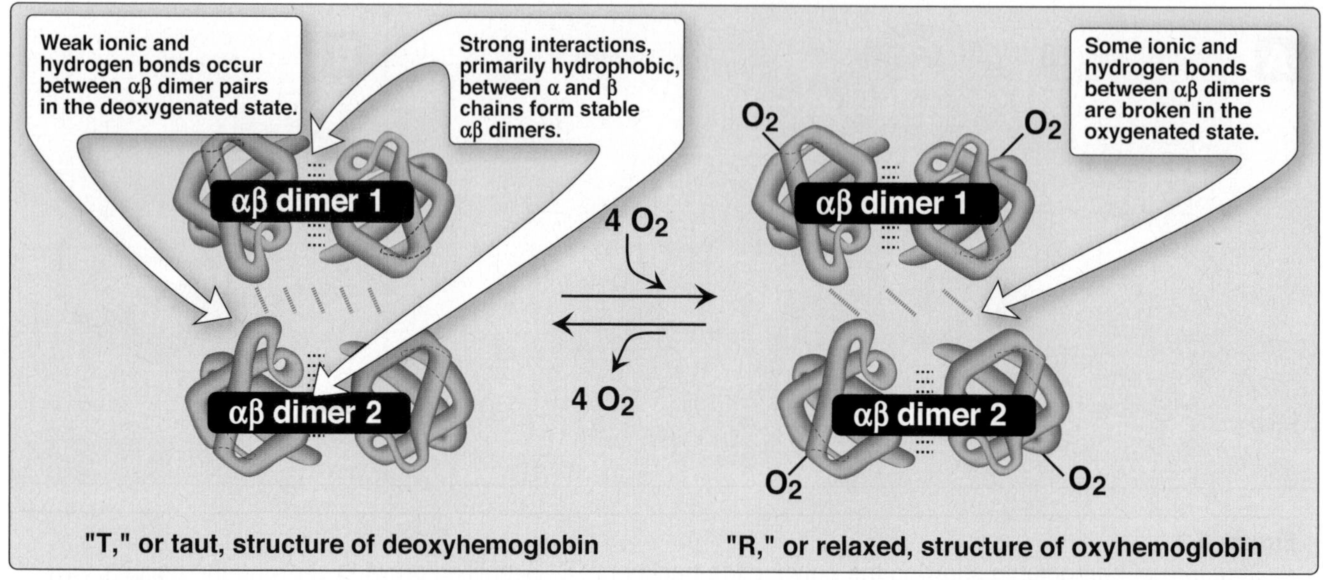

Figure 3.4
Schematic diagram showing structural changes resulting from oxygenation and deoxygenation of hemoglobin.

held together primarily by polar bonds. The weaker interactions between the dimers allows them to move with respect to one other. This movement results in the two dimers occupying different relative positions in deoxyhemoglobin as compared with oxyhemoglobin (see Figure 3.4). [Note: The binding of O_2 to the heme iron pulls the iron into the plane of the heme. Because the iron is also linked to the proximal histidine (F8), there is movement of the globin chains that alters the interface between the αβ dimers.]

a. **T form:** The deoxy form of hemoglobin is called the "T," or taut (tense) form. In the T form, the two αβ dimers interact through a network of ionic bonds and hydrogen bonds that constrain the movement of the polypeptide chains. The T conformation is the low-oxygen-affinity form of hemoglobin.

b. **R form:** The binding of O_2 to hemoglobin causes the rupture of some of the polar bonds between the αβ dimers, allowing movement. This leads to a structure called the "R," or relaxed form (see Figure 3.4). The R conformation is the high-oxygen-affinity form of hemoglobin.

D. Binding of oxygen to myoglobin and hemoglobin

Myoglobin can bind only one molecule of O_2, because it contains only one heme group. In contrast, hemoglobin can bind four O_2 molecules, one at each of its four heme groups. The degree of saturation (Y) of these oxygen-binding sites on all myoglobin or hemoglobin molecules can vary between zero (all sites are empty) and 100% (all sites are full), as shown in Figure 3.5. [Note: Pulse oximetry is a noninvasive, indirect method of measuring the O_2 saturation of arterial blood based on differences in light absorption by oxyhemoglobin and deoxyhemoglobin.]

1. **Oxygen-dissociation curve:** A plot of Y measured at different partial pressures of oxygen (pO_2) is called the oxygen-dissociation curve. [Note: pO_2 may also be represented as PO_2.] The curves for myoglobin and hemoglobin show important differences (see Figure 3.5). This graph illustrates that myoglobin has a higher oxygen affinity at all pO_2 values than does hemoglobin. The partial pressure of oxygen needed to achieve half-saturation of the binding sites (P_{50}) is approximately 1 mm Hg for myoglobin and 26 mm Hg for hemoglobin. The higher the oxygen affinity (that is, the more tightly oxygen binds), the lower the P_{50}.

   a. **Myoglobin:** The oxygen-dissociation curve for myoglobin has a hyperbolic shape (see Figure 3.5). This reflects the fact that myoglobin reversibly binds a single molecule of oxygen. Thus, oxygenated (MbO_2) and deoxygenated (Mb) myoglobin exist in a simple equilibrium:

$$Mb + O_2 \rightleftarrows MbO_2$$

   The equilibrium is shifted to the right or to the left as oxygen is added to or removed from the system. [Note: Myoglobin is designed to bind oxygen released by hemoglobin at the low pO_2 found in muscle. Myoglobin, in turn, releases oxygen within the muscle cell in response to oxygen demand.]

   b. **Hemoglobin:** The oxygen-dissociation curve for hemoglobin is sigmoidal in shape (see Figure 3.5), indicating that the subunits cooperate in binding oxygen. Cooperative binding of oxygen by the four subunits of hemoglobin means that the binding of an oxygen molecule at one heme group increases the oxygen affinity of the remaining heme groups in the same hemoglobin tetramer (Figure 3.6). This effect is referred to as heme–heme interaction (see below). Although it is more difficult for the first oxygen molecule to bind to hemoglobin, the subsequent binding of oxygen occurs with high affinity, as shown by the steep upward curve in the region near 20–30 mm Hg (see Figure 3.5).

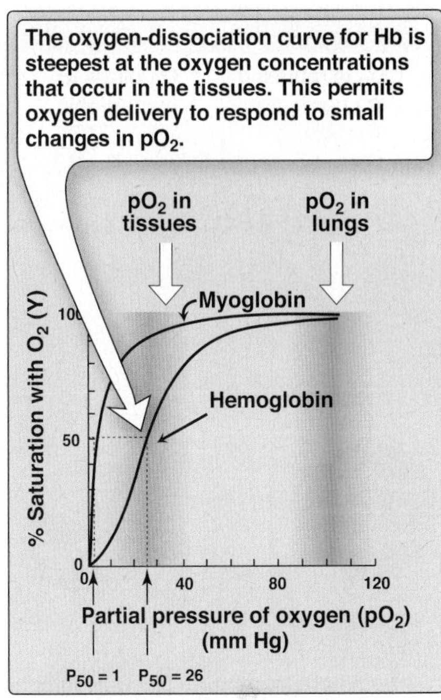

Figure 3.5
Oxygen-dissociation curves for myoglobin and hemoglobin (Hb).

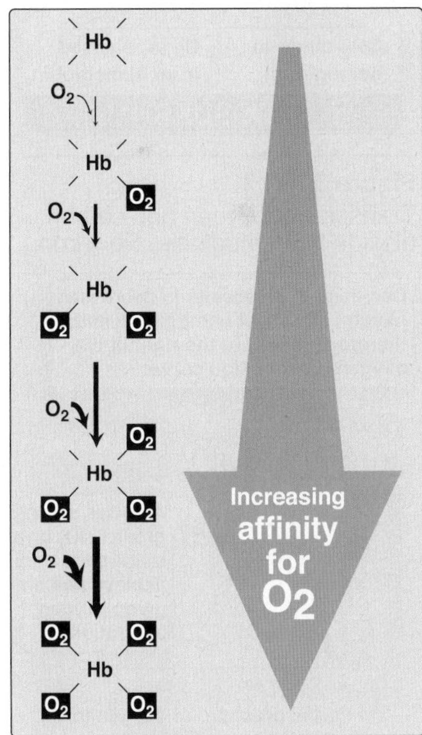

Figure 3.6
Hemoglobin (Hb) binds successive molecules of oxygen with increasing affinity.

E. Allosteric effects

The ability of hemoglobin to reversibly bind oxygen is affected by the pO_2 (through heme–heme interactions as described above), the pH of the environment, the partial pressure of carbon dioxide (pCO_2) and the availability of 2,3-bisphosphoglycerate. These are collectively called allosteric ("other site") effectors, because their interaction at one site on the hemoglobin molecule affects the binding of oxygen to heme groups at other sites on the molecule. [Note: The binding of oxygen to monomeric myoglobin is not influenced by allosteric effectors.]

1. **Heme–heme interactions:** The sigmoidal oxygen-dissociation curve reflects specific structural changes that are initiated at one heme group and transmitted to other heme groups in the hemoglobin tetramer. The net effect is that the affinity of hemoglobin for the last oxygen bound is approximately 300 times greater than its affinity for the first oxygen bound.

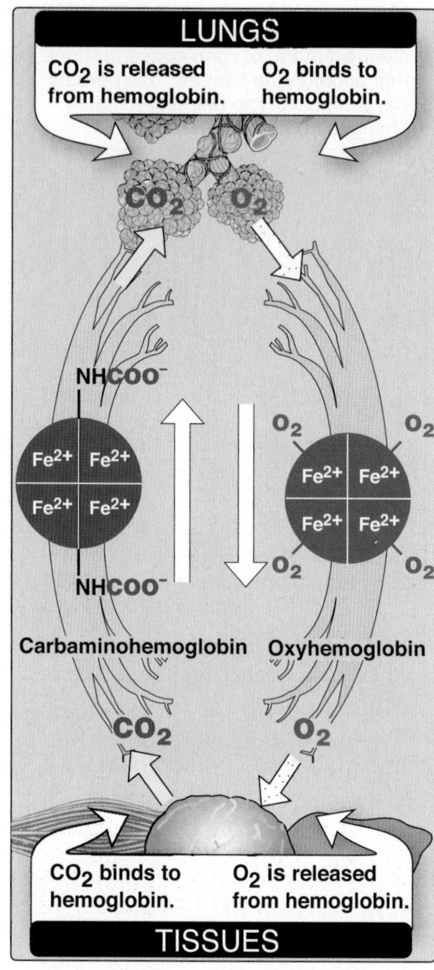

Figure 3.7
Transport of oxygen and carbon dioxide by hemoglobin. Fe = iron.

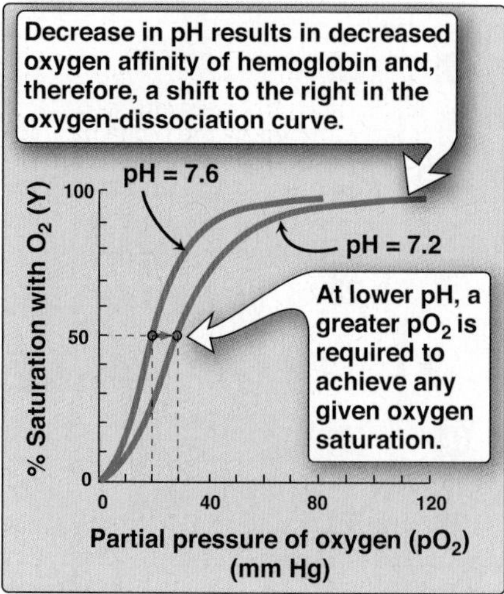

Figure 3.8
Effect of pH on the oxygen affinity of hemoglobin. Protons are allosteric effectors of hemoglobin.

a. **Loading and unloading oxygen:** The cooperative binding of oxygen allows hemoglobin to deliver more oxygen to the tissues in response to relatively small changes in the partial pressure of oxygen. This can be seen in Figure 3.5, which indicates pO_2 in the alveoli of the lung and the capillaries of the tissues. For example, in the lung, the concentration of oxygen is high, and hemoglobin becomes virtually saturated (or "loaded") with oxygen. In contrast, in the peripheral tissues, oxyhemoglobin releases (or "unloads") much of its oxygen for use in the oxidative metabolism of the tissues (Figure 3.7).

b. **Significance of the sigmoidal oxygen-dissociation curve:** The steep slope of the oxygen-dissociation curve over the range of oxygen concentrations that occur between the lungs and the tissues permits hemoglobin to carry and deliver oxygen efficiently from sites of high to sites of low pO_2. A molecule with a hyperbolic oxygen-dissociation curve, such as myoglobin, could not achieve the same degree of oxygen release within this range of partial pressures of oxygen. Instead, it would have maximum affinity for oxygen throughout this oxygen pressure range and, therefore, would deliver no oxygen to the tissues.

2. **Bohr effect:** The release of oxygen from hemoglobin is enhanced when the pH is lowered or when the hemoglobin is in the presence of an increased pCO_2. Both result in a decreased oxygen affinity of hemoglobin and, therefore, a shift to the right in the oxygen-dissociation curve (Figure 3.8), and both, then, stabilize the T (deoxy) form. This change in oxygen binding is called the Bohr effect. Conversely, raising the pH or lowering the concentration of CO_2 results in a greater affinity for oxygen, a shift to the left in the oxygen-dissociation curve, and stabilization of the R (oxy) form.

a. **Source of the protons that lower the pH:** The concentration of both H^+ and CO_2 in the capillaries of metabolically active tissues is higher than that observed in alveolar capillaries of the lungs, where CO_2 is released into the expired air. In the tissues, CO_2 is converted by *carbonic anhydrase* to carbonic acid:

$$CO_2 + H_2O \rightleftarrows H_2CO_3$$

which spontaneously loses a proton, becoming bicarbonate (the major blood buffer):

$$H_2CO_3 \rightleftarrows HCO_3^- + H^+$$

The H^+ produced by this pair of reactions contributes to the lowering of pH. This differential pH gradient (that is, lungs having a higher pH and tissues a lower pH) favors the unloading of oxygen in the peripheral tissues and the loading of oxygen in the lung. Thus, the oxygen affinity of the hemoglobin molecule responds to small shifts in pH between the lungs and oxygen-consuming tissues, making hemoglobin a more efficient transporter of oxygen.

b. **Mechanism of the Bohr effect:** The Bohr effect reflects the fact that the deoxy form of hemoglobin has a greater affinity for protons than does oxyhemoglobin. This effect is caused by ionizable groups such as specific histidine side chains that have a higher pK_a in deoxyhemoglobin than in oxyhemoglobin. Therefore, an increase in the concentration of protons (resulting in a decrease in pH) causes these groups to become protonated (charged) and able to form ionic bonds (salt bridges). These bonds preferentially stabilize the deoxy form of hemoglobin, producing a decrease in oxygen affinity. [Note: Hemoglobin, then, is an important blood buffer.]

The Bohr effect can be represented schematically as:

$$\underset{\text{oxyhemoglobin}}{HbO_2 + H^+} \rightleftarrows \underset{\text{deoxyhemoglobin}}{HbH + O_2}$$

where an increase in protons (or a lower pO_2) shifts the equilibrium to the right (favoring deoxyhemoglobin), whereas an increase in pO_2 (or a decrease in protons) shifts the equilibrium to the left.

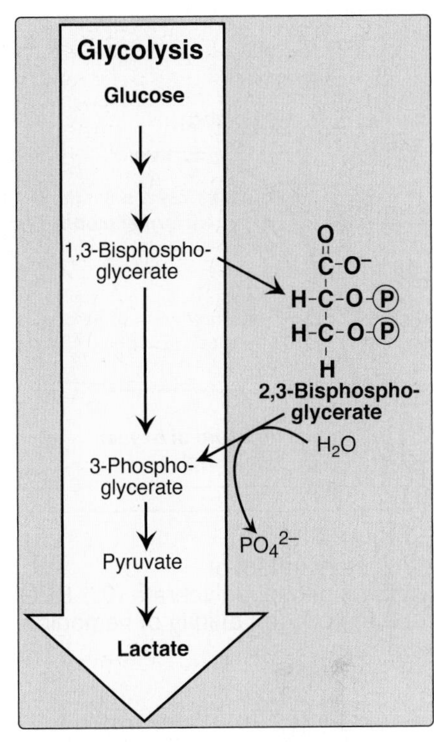

Figure 3.9
Synthesis of 2,3-bisphosphoglycerate. [Note: Ⓟ is a phosphoryl group, PO_3^{2-}.] In older literature, 2,3-bisphosphoglycerate (2,3-BPG) may be referred to as 2,3-diphosphoglycerate (2,3-DPG).

3. **Effect of 2,3-bisphosphoglycerate on oxygen affinity:** 2,3-Bisphosphoglycerate (2,3-BPG) is an important regulator of the binding of oxygen to hemoglobin. It is the most abundant organic phosphate in the RBC, where its concentration is approximately that of hemoglobin. 2,3-BPG is synthesized from an intermediate of the glycolytic pathway (Figure 3.9; see p. 101 for a discussion of 2,3-BPG synthesis in glycolysis).

a. **Binding of 2,3-BPG to deoxyhemoglobin:** 2,3-BPG decreases the O_2 affinity of hemoglobin by binding to deoxyhemoglobin but not to oxyhemoglobin. This preferential binding stabilizes the T conformation of deoxyhemoglobin. The effect of binding 2,3-BPG can be represented schematically as:

$$\underset{\text{oxyhemoglobin}}{HbO_2 + \text{2,3-BPG}} \rightleftarrows \underset{\text{deoxyhemoglobin}}{\text{Hb–2,3-BPG} + O_2}$$

b. **Binding site of 2,3-BPG:** One molecule of 2,3-BPG binds to a pocket, formed by the two β-globin chains, in the center of the deoxyhemoglobin tetramer (Figure 3.10). This pocket contains several positively charged amino acids that form ionic bonds with the negatively charged phosphate groups of 2,3-BPG. [Note: Replacement of one of these amino acids can result in hemoglobin variants with abnormally high oxygen affinity that may be compensated for by increased RBC production (erythrocytosis).] 2,3-BPG is expelled with oxygenation of the hemoglobin.

c. **Shift of the oxygen-dissociation curve:** Hemoglobin from which 2,3-BPG has been removed has a high affinity for oxygen. However, as seen in the RBC, the presence of 2,3-BPG significantly reduces the affinity of hemoglobin for oxygen, shifting the oxygen-dissociation curve to the right (Figure 3.11). This reduced affinity enables hemoglobin to release oxygen efficiently at the partial pressures found in the tissues.

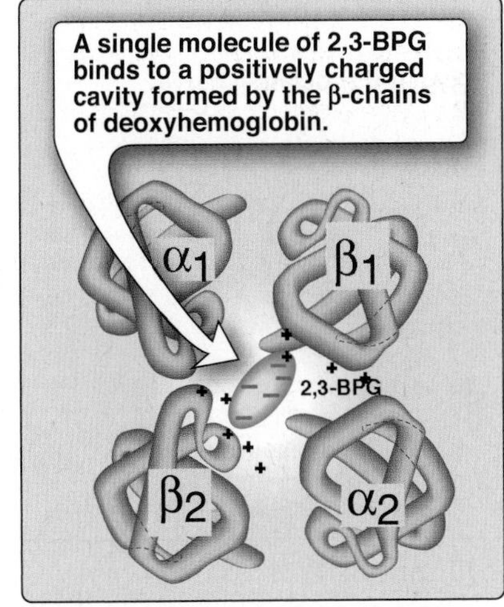

Figure 3.10
Binding of 2,3-bisphosphoglycerate (2,3-BPG) by deoxyhemoglobin.

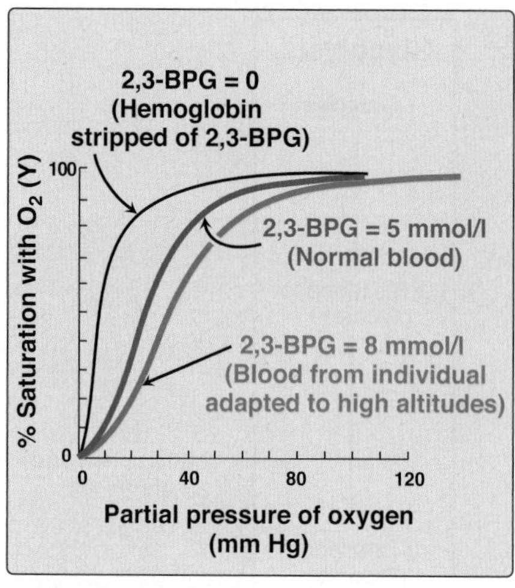

Figure 3.11
Allosteric effect of 2,3-bisphosphoglycerate (2,3-BPG) on the oxygen affinity of hemoglobin.

d. **Response of 2,3-BPG levels to chronic hypoxia or anemia:** The concentration of 2,3-BPG in the RBC increases in response to chronic hypoxia, such as that observed in chronic obstructive pulmonary disease (COPD) like emphysema, or at high altitudes, where circulating hemoglobin may have difficulty receiving sufficient oxygen. Intracellular levels of 2,3-BPG are also elevated in chronic anemia, in which fewer than normal RBCs are available to supply the body's oxygen needs. Elevated 2,3-BPG levels lower the oxygen affinity of hemoglobin, permitting greater unloading of oxygen in the capillaries of the tissues (see Figure 3.11).

e. **Role of 2,3-BPG in transfused blood:** 2,3-BPG is essential for the normal oxygen transport function of hemoglobin. However, storing blood in the currently available media results in a decrease in 2,3-BPG. Stored blood displays an abnormally high oxygen affinity and fails to unload its bound oxygen properly in the tissues. Hemoglobin deficient in 2,3-BPG thus acts as an oxygen "trap" rather than as an oxygen transport system. Transfused RBC are able to restore their depleted supplies of 2,3-BPG in 6–24 hours. However, severely ill patients may be compromised if transfused with large quantities of such 2,3-BPG–"stripped" blood. [Note: The maximum storage time for RBC has been doubled (21 to 42 days, with median time of 15 days) by changes in H^+, phosphate, and hexose sugar concentration and by the addition of adenine (see p. 291). Although the content of 2,3-BPG was not greatly improved in the long-term by these changes, adenosine triphosphate production was increased and improved RBC survival.]

4. **Binding of CO_2:** Most of the CO_2 produced in metabolism is hydrated and transported as bicarbonate ion (see p. 9). However, some CO_2 is carried as carbamate bound to the N-terminal amino groups of hemoglobin (forming carbaminohemoglobin as shown in Figure 3.7), which can be represented schematically as follows:

$$Hb-NH_2 + CO_2 \rightleftarrows Hb-NH-COO^- + H^+$$

The binding of CO_2 stabilizes the T or deoxy form of hemoglobin, resulting in a decrease in its affinity for oxygen (see p. 28) and a right shift in the oxygen-dissociation curve. In the lungs, CO_2 dissociates from the hemoglobin and is released in the breath.

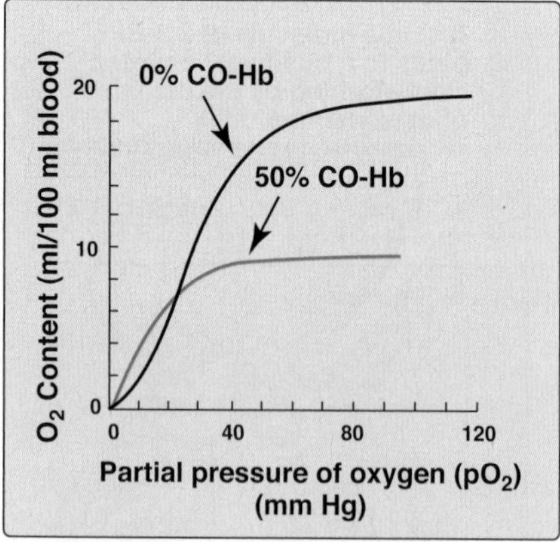

Figure 3.12
Effect of carbon monoxide (CO) on the oxygen affinity of hemoglobin. CO-Hb = carboxyhemoglobin (carbon monoxyhemoglobin).

5. **Binding of CO:** Carbon monoxide (CO) binds tightly (but reversibly) to the hemoglobin iron, forming carboxyhemoglobin. When CO binds to one or more of the four heme sites, hemoglobin shifts to the R conformation, causing the remaining heme sites to bind oxygen with high affinity. This shifts the oxygen-dissociation curve to the left and changes the normal sigmoidal shape toward a hyperbola. As a result, the affected hemoglobin is unable to release oxygen to the tissues (Figure 3.12). [Note: The affinity of hemoglobin for CO is 220 times greater than for oxygen. Consequently, even minute concentrations of CO in the environment can produce toxic concentrations of carboxyhemoglobin in the blood. For example, increased levels of CO are found in the blood of tobacco smokers. CO toxicity appears to result from a

combination of tissue hypoxia and direct CO-mediated damage at the cellular level.] CO poisoning is treated with 100% oxygen at high pressure (hyperbaric oxygen therapy), which facilitates the dissociation of CO from the hemoglobin. [Note: CO inhibits Complex IV of the electron transport chain (see p. 76).] In addition to O_2, CO_2, and CO, nitric oxide gas (NO) also is carried by hemoglobin. NO is a potent vasodilator (see p. 151). It can be taken up (salvaged) or released from RBC, thus modulating NO availability and influencing vessel diameter.

Form	Chain composition	Fraction of total hemoglobin
HbA	$\alpha_2\beta_2$	90%
HbF	$\alpha_2\gamma_2$	<2%
HbA_2	$\alpha_2\delta_2$	2%–5%
HbA_{1c}	$\alpha_2\beta_2$-glucose	3%–9%

Figure 3.13
Normal adult human hemoglobins. [Note: The α-chains in these hemoglobins are identical.] Hb = hemoglobin.

F. Minor hemoglobins

It is important to remember that human hemoglobin A (HbA) is just one member of a functionally and structurally related family of proteins, the hemoglobins (Figure 3.13). Each of these oxygen-carrying proteins is a tetramer, composed of two α-globin (or α-like) polypeptides and two β-globin (or β-like) polypeptides. Certain hemoglobins, such as HbF, are normally synthesized only during fetal development, whereas others, such as HbA_2, are synthesized in the adult, although at low levels compared with HbA. HbA can also become modified by the covalent addition of a hexose (see p. 34).

1. **Fetal hemoglobin:** HbF is a tetramer consisting of two α chains identical to those found in HbA, plus two γ chains ($\alpha_2\gamma_2$; see Figure 3.13). The γ chains are members of the β-globin gene family (see p. 35).

   a. **HbF synthesis during development:** In the first month after conception, embryonic hemoglobins such as Hb Gower 1, composed of two α-like zeta (ζ) chains and two β-like epsilon (ε) chains ($\zeta_2\varepsilon_2$), are synthesized by the embryonic yolk sac. In the fifth week of gestation, the site of globin synthesis shifts, first to the liver and then to the marrow, and the primary product is HbF. HbF is the major hemoglobin found in the fetus and newborn, accounting for about 60% of the total hemoglobin in the RBC during the last months of fetal life (Figure 3.14). HbA synthesis starts in the bone marrow at about the eighth month of pregnancy and gradually replaces HbF. (Figure 3.14 shows the relative production of each type of hemoglobin chain during fetal and postnatal life.) [Note: HbF represents less than 1% of the hemoglobin in most adults and is concentrated in RBC known as F cells.]

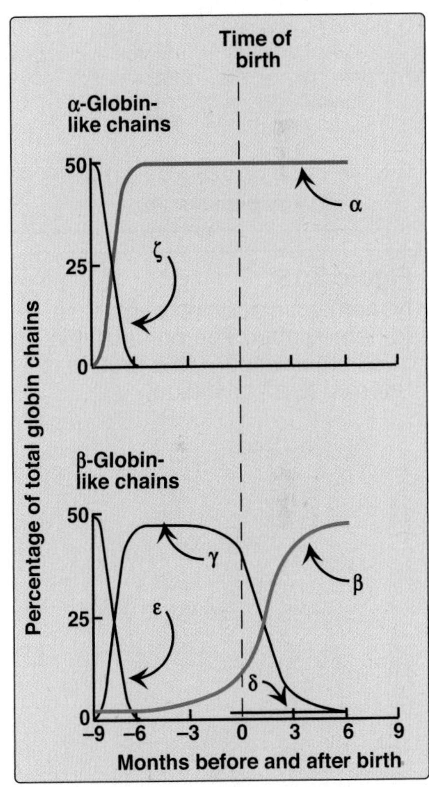

Figure 3.14
Developmental changes in hemoglobin.

   b. **Binding of 2,3-BPG to HbF:** Under physiologic conditions, HbF has a higher affinity for oxygen than does HbA as a result of HbF only weakly binding 2,3-BPG. [Note: The γ-globin chains of HbF lack some of the positively charged amino acids that are responsible for binding 2,3-BPG in the β-globin chains.] Because 2,3-BPG serves to reduce the affinity of hemoglobin for oxygen, the weaker interaction between 2,3-BPG and HbF results in a higher oxygen affinity for HbF relative to HbA. In contrast, if both HbA and HbF are stripped of their 2,3-BPG, they then have a similar affinity for oxygen. The higher oxygen affinity of HbF facilitates the transfer of oxygen from the maternal circulation across the placenta to the RBC of the fetus.

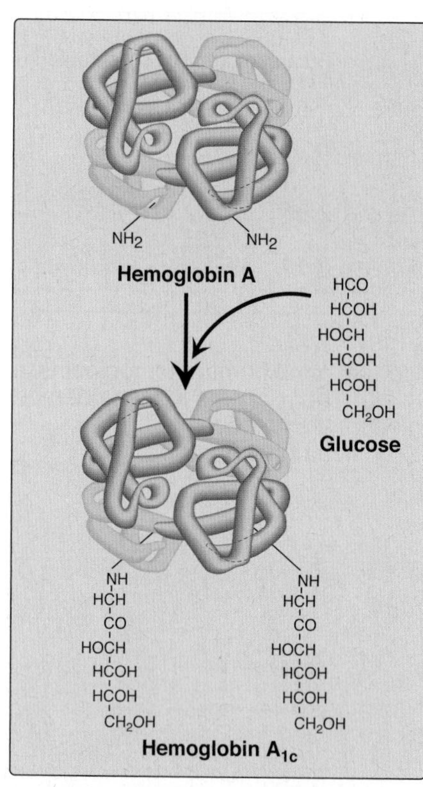

Figure 3.15
Nonenzymic addition of glucose to hemoglobin. The nonenzymic addition of a sugar to a protein is referred to as glycation.

2. **Hemoglobin A_2:** HbA_2 is a minor component of normal adult hemoglobin, first appearing shortly before birth and, ultimately, constituting about 2% of the total hemoglobin. It is composed of two α-globin chains and two δ-globin chains ($\alpha_2\delta_2$; see Figure 3.13).

3. **Hemoglobin A_{1c}:** Under physiologic conditions, HbA is slowly and nonenzymically glycosylated (glycated), the extent of glycosylation being dependent on the plasma concentration of a particular hexose. The most abundant form of glycosylated hemoglobin is HbA_{1c}. It has glucose residues attached predominantly to the NH_2 groups of the N-terminal valines of the β-globin chains (Figure 3.15). Increased amounts of HbA_{1c} are found in RBC of patients with diabetes mellitus, because their HbA has contact with higher glucose concentrations during the 120-day lifetime of these cells. (See p. 340 for a discussion of the use of HbA_{1c} levels in assessing average blood glucose levels in patients with diabetes.)

III. ORGANIZATION OF THE GLOBIN GENES

To understand diseases resulting from genetic alterations in the structure or synthesis of hemoglobins, it is necessary to grasp how the hemoglobin genes, which direct the synthesis of the different globin chains, are structurally organized into gene families and also how they are expressed.

A. α-Gene family

The genes coding for the α-globin and β-globin subunits of the hemoglobin chains occur in two separate gene clusters (or families) located on two different chromosomes (Figure 3.16). The α-gene cluster on chromosome 16 contains two genes for the α-globin chains. It also contains the ζ gene that is expressed early in development as an α-globin-like component of embryonic hemoblobin. [Note: Globin gene famillies also contain globin-like genes that are not expressed, that is, their genetic information is not used to produce globin chains. These are called pseudogenes.]

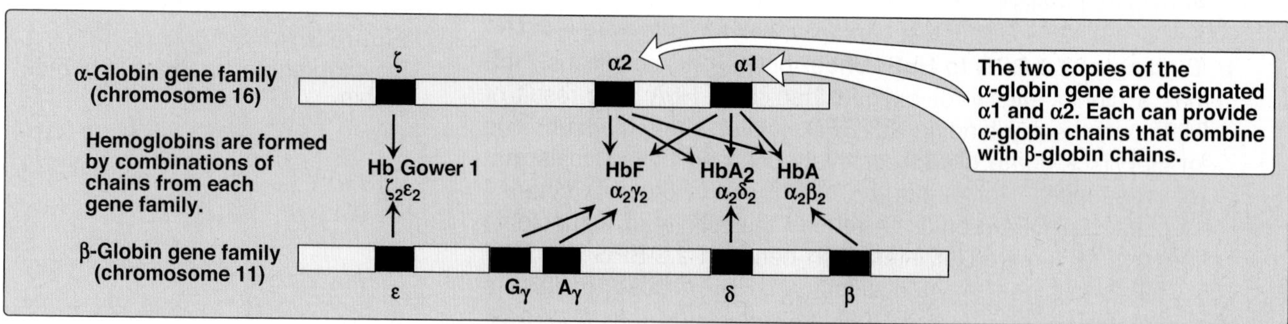

Figure 3.16
Organization of the globin gene families. Hb = hemoglobin.

B. β-Gene family

A single gene for the β-globin chain is located on chromosome 11 (see Figure 3.16). There are an additional four β-globin-like genes: the ε gene (which, like the ζ gene, is expressed early in embryonic development), two γ genes (G_γ and A_γ that are expressed in HbF), and the δ gene that codes for the globin chain found in the minor adult hemoglobin HbA_2.

C. Steps in globin chain synthesis

Expression of a globin gene begins in the nucleus of RBC precursors, where the DNA sequence encoding the gene is transcribed. The RNA produced by transcription is actually a precursor of the messenger RNA (mRNA) that is used as a template for the synthesis of a globin chain. Before it can serve this function, two noncoding stretches of RNA (introns) must be removed from the mRNA precursor sequence and the remaining three fragments (exons) joined in a linear manner. The resulting mature mRNA enters the cytosol, where its genetic information is translated, producing a globin chain. (A summary of this process is shown in Figure 3.17. A more detailed description of gene expresion is presented in Unit VI, p. 395.)

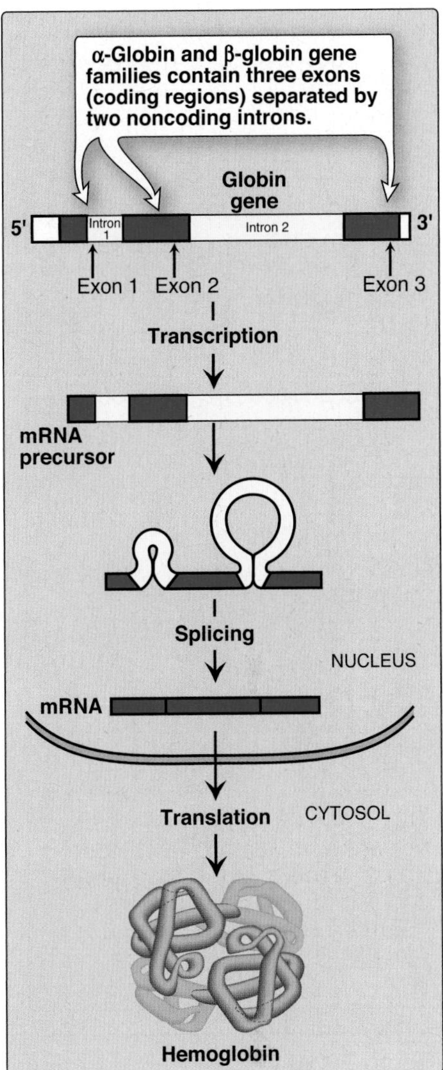

Figure 3.17
Synthesis of globin chains. mRNA = messenger RNA.

IV. HEMOGLOBINOPATHIES

Hemoglobinopathies are defined as a group of genetic disorders caused by production of a structurally abnormal hemoglobin molecule; synthesis of insufficient quantities of normal hemoglobin; or, rarely, both. Sickle cell anemia (HbS), hemoglobin C disease (HbC), hemoglobin SC disease (HbS + HbC = HbSC), and the thalassemias are representative hemoglobinopathies that can have severe clinical consequences. The first three conditions result from production of hemoglobin with an altered amino acid sequence (qualitative hemoglobinopathy), whereas the thalassemias are caused by decreased production of normal hemoglobin (quantitative hemoglobinopathy).

A. Sickle cell anemia (hemoglobin S disease)

Sickle cell anemia, the most common of the RBC sickling diseases, is a genetic disorder of the blood caused by a single nucleotide substitution (a point mutation, see p. 433) in the gene for β-globin. It is the most common inherited blood disorder in the United States, affecting 50,000 Americans. It occurs primarily in the African American population, affecting one of 500 newborn African American infants in the United States. Sickle cell anemia is an autosomal recessive disorder. It occurs in individuals who have inherited two mutant genes (one from each parent) that code for synthesis of the β chains of the globin molecules. [Note: The mutant β-globin chain is designated β^S, and the resulting hemoglobin, $\alpha_2\beta^S{}_2$, is referred to as HbS.] An infant does not begin showing symptoms of the disease until sufficient HbF has been replaced by HbS so that sickling can occur (see below). Sickle cell anemia is characterized by lifelong episodes of pain ("crises"); chronic hemolytic anemia with associated hyperbilirubinemia (see p. 284); and increased susceptibility to infections, usually beginning in infancy. [Note: The lifetime of a RBC in sickle cell anemia is less than 20 days, compared with 120 days

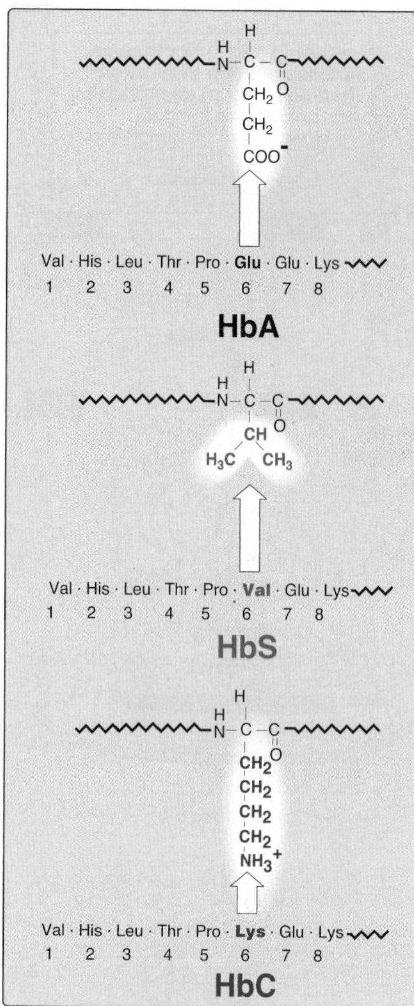

Figure 3.18
Amino acid substitutions in hemoglobin S (HbS) and hemoglobin C (HbC).

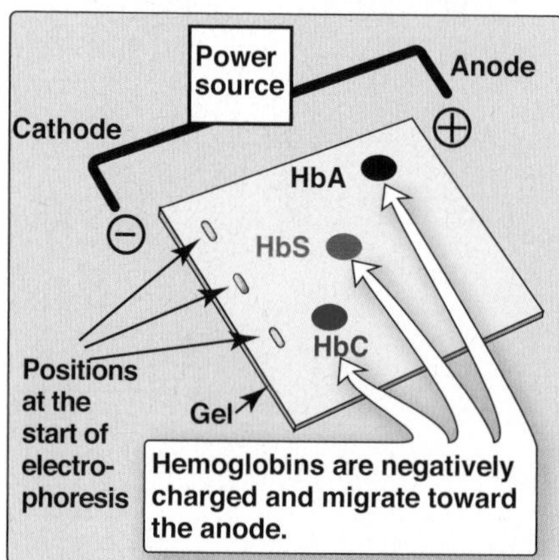

Figure 3.19
Diagram of hemoglobins (HbA), (HbS), and (HbC) after electrophoresis.

for normal RBC, hence, the anemia.] Other symptoms include acute chest syndrome, stroke, splenic and renal dysfunction, and bone changes due to marrow hyperplasia. Heterozygotes, representing 1 in 12 African Americans, have one normal and one sickle cell gene. The blood cells of such heterozygotes contain both HbS and HbA. These individuals have sickle cell trait. They usually do not show clinical symptoms (but may under conditions of extreme physical exertion with dehydration) and can have a normal life span.

1. **Amino acid substitution in HbS β chains:** A molecule of HbS contains two normal α-globin chains and two mutant β-globin chains (β^S), in which glutamate at position six has been replaced with valine (Figure 3.18). Therefore, during electrophoresis at alkaline pH, HbS migrates more slowly toward the anode (positive electrode) than does HbA (Figure 3.19). This altered mobility of HbS is a result of the absence of the negatively charged glutamate residues in the two β chains, thereby rendering HbS less negative than HbA. [Note: Electrophoresis of hemoglobin obtained from lysed RBC is routinely used in the diagnosis of sickle cell trait and sickle cell disease. DNA analysis also is used (see p. 472).]

2. **Sickling and tissue anoxia:** The replacement of the charged glutamate with the nonpolar valine forms a protrusion on the β chain that fits into a complementary site on the β chain of another hemoglobin molecule in the cell (Figure 3.20). At low oxygen tension, deoxyhemoglobin S polymerizes inside the RBC, forming a network of insoluble fibrous polymers that stiffen and distort the cell, producing rigid, misshapen RBC. Such sickled cells frequently block the flow of blood in the narrow capillaries. This interruption in the supply of oxygen leads to localized anoxia (oxygen deprivation) in the tissue, causing pain and eventually death (infarction) of cells in the vicinity of the blockage. The anoxia also leads to an increase in deoxygenated HbS. [Note: The mean diameter of RBC is 7.5 μm, whereas that of the microvasculature is 3–4 μm. Compared to normal RBC, sickled cells have a decreased ability to deform and an increased tendency to adhere to vessel walls and so have difficulty moving through small vessels, thereby causing microvascular occlusion.]

3. **Variables that increase sickling:** The extent of sickling and, therefore, the severity of disease is enhanced by any variable that increases the proportion of HbS in the deoxy state (that is, reduces the affinity of HbS for O_2). These variables include decreased pO_2, increased pCO_2, decreased pH, dehydration, and an increased concentration of 2,3-BPG in RBC.

4. **Treatment:** Therapy involves adequate hydration, analgesics, aggressive antibiotic therapy if infection is present, and transfusions in patients at high risk for fatal occlusion of blood vessels. Intermittent transfusions with packed RBC reduce the risk of stroke, but the benefits must be weighed against the complications of transfusion, which include iron overload (hemosiderosis), bloodborne infections, and immunologic complications. Hydroxyurea (hydroxycarbamide), an antitumor drug, is therapeutically useful because it increases circulating levels of HbF,

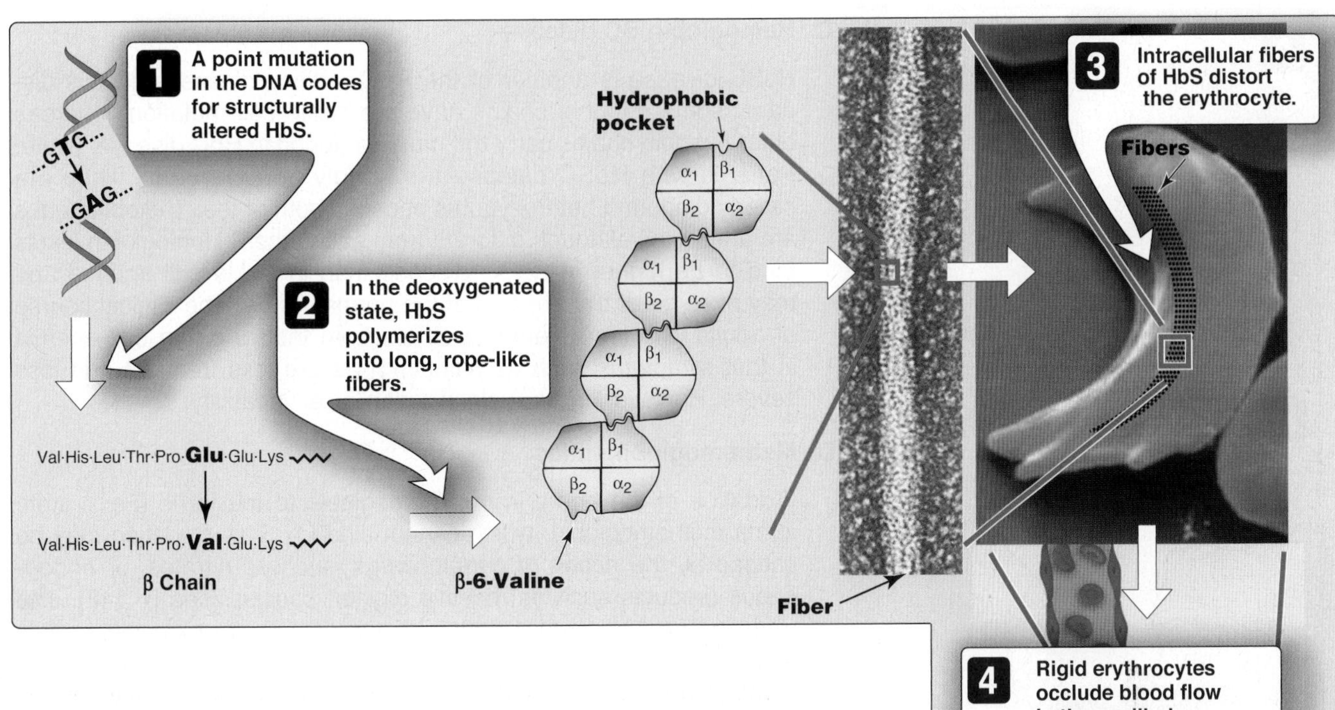

which decreases RBC sickling. This leads to decreased frequency of painful crises and reduces mortality. [Note: The morbidity and mortality associated with sickle cell anemia has led to its inclusion in newborn screening panels to allow prophylactic antibiotic therapy to begin soon after the birth of an affected child.]

5. **Possible selective advantage of the heterozygous state:** The high frequency of the β^S mutation among black Africans, despite its damaging effects in the homozygous state, suggests that a selective advantage exists for heterozygous individuals. For example, heterozygotes for the sickle cell gene are less susceptible to the severe malaria caused by the parasite Plasmodium falciparum. This organism spends an obligatory part of its life cycle in the RBC. One theory is that because these cells in individuals heterozygous for HbS, like those in homozygotes, have a shorter life span than normal, the parasite cannot complete the intracellular stage of its development. This fact may provide a selective advantage to heterozygotes living in regions where malaria is a major cause of death. Figure 3.21 illustrates that in Africa, the geographic distribution of sickle cell anemia is similar to that of malaria.

B. Hemoglobin C disease

Like HbS, HbC is a hemoglobin variant that has a single amino acid substitution in the sixth position of the β-globin chain (see Figure 3.18). In HbC, however, a lysine is substituted for the glutamate (as compared with a valine substitution in HbS). [Note: This substitution causes HbC to move more slowly toward the anode than HbA or HbS does (see Figure 3.19).] Rare patients homozygous for HbC generally have a relatively mild, chronic hemolytic anemia. These patients do not suffer from infarctive crises, and no specific therapy is required.

Figure 3.20
Molecular and cellular events leading to sickle cell crisis. HbS = hemoglobin S.

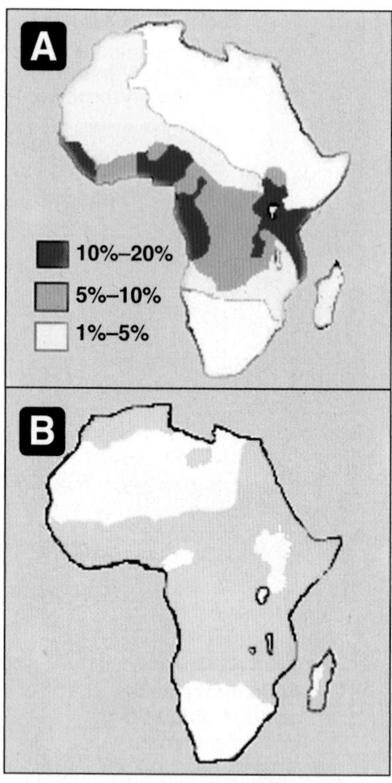

Figure 3.21
A. Distribution of sickle cell in Africa expressed as a percentage of the population with disease.
B. Distribution of malaria in Africa.

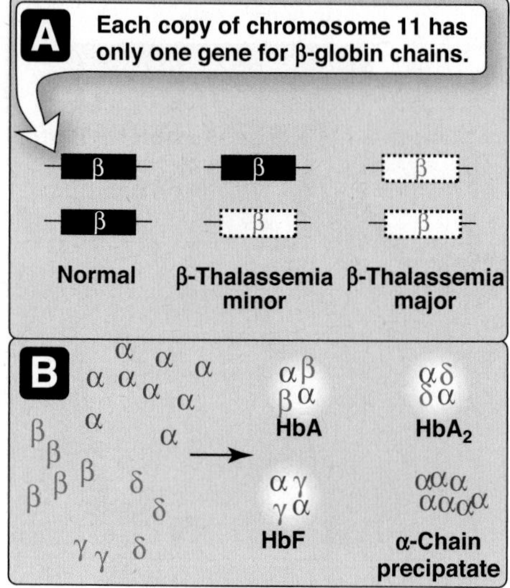

Figure 3.22
A. β-Globin gene mutations in the β-thalassemias. B. Hemoglobin (Hb) tetramers formed in β-thalassemias.

C. Hemoglobin SC disease

HbSC disease is another of the RBC sickling diseases. In this disease, some β-globin chains have the sickle cell mutation, whereas other β-globin chains carry the mutation found in HbC disease. [Note: Patients with HbSC disease are doubly heterozygous. They are called compound heterozygotes because both of their β-globin genes are abnormal, although different from each other.] Hemoglobin levels tend to be higher in HbSC disease than in sickle cell anemia and may even be at the low end of the normal range. The clinical course of adults with HbSC anemia differs from that of sickle cell anemia in that symptoms such as painful crises are less frequent and less severe. However, there is significant clinical variability.

D. Methemoglobinemias

Oxidation of the heme iron in hemoglobin to the ferric (Fe^{3+}) state forms methemoglobin, which cannot bind O_2. This oxidation may be caused by the action of certain drugs, such as nitrates, or endogenous products such as reactive oxygen species (see p. 148). The oxidation may also result from inherited defects, for example, certain mutations in the α- or β-globin chain promote the formation of methemoglobin (HbM). Additionally, a deficiency of *NADH-cytochrome b_5 reductase* (also called *NADH-methemoglobin reductase*), the enzyme responsible for the conversion of methemoglobin (Fe^{3+}) to hemoglobin (Fe^{2+}), leads to the accumulation of HbM. [Note: The RBC of newborns have approximately half the capacity of those of adults to reduce HbM. They are, therefore, particularly susceptible to the effects of HbM-producing compounds.] The methemoglobinemias are characterized by "chocolate cyanosis" (a brownish blue coloration of the skin and mucous membranes and brown-colored blood) as a result of the dark-colored HbM. Symptoms are related to the degree of tissue hypoxia and include anxiety, headache, and dyspnea. In rare cases, coma and death can occur. Treatment is with methylene blue, which is oxidized as Fe^{+3} is reduced.

E. Thalassemias

The thalassemias are hereditary hemolytic diseases in which an imbalance occurs in the synthesis of globin chains. As a group, they are the most common single gene disorders in humans. Normally, synthesis of the α- and β-globin chains is coordinated, so that each α-globin chain has a β-globin chain partner. This leads to the formation of $\alpha_2\beta_2$ (HbA). In the thalassemias, the synthesis of either the α- or the β-globin chain is defective. A thalassemia can be caused by a variety of mutations, including entire gene deletions, or substitutions or deletions of one to many nucleotides in the DNA. [Note: Each thalassemia can be classified as either a disorder in which no globin chains are produced (α^o- or β^o-thalassemia), or one in which some chains are synthesized but at a reduced level (α^+- or β^+-thalassemia).]

1. **β-Thalassemias:** In these disorders, synthesis of β-globin chains is decreased or absent, typically as a result of point mutations that affect the production of functional mRNA. However, α-globin chain synthesis is normal. Excess α-globin chains cannot form stable tetramers and so precipitate, causing the premature death of cells initially destined to become mature RBC. Increase in

$\alpha_2\delta_2$ (HbA$_2$) and $\alpha_2\gamma_2$ (HbF) also occurs. There are only two copies of the β-globin gene in each cell (one on each chromosome 11). Therefore, individuals with β-globin gene defects have either β-thalassemia trait (β-thalassemia minor) if they have only one defective β-globin gene or β-thalassemia major (Cooley anemia) if both genes are defective (Figure 3.22). Because the β-globin gene is not expressed until late in fetal gestation, the physical manifestations of β-thalassemias appear only several months after birth. Those individuals with β-thalassemia minor make some β chains, and usually do not require specific treatment. However, those infants born with β-thalassemia major are seemingly healthy at birth but become severely anemic, usually during the first or second year of life due to ineffective erythropoiesis. Skeletal changes as a result of extramedullary hematopoiesis also are seen.These patients require regular transfusions of blood. [Note: Although this treatment is lifesaving, the cumulative effect of the transfusions is iron overload (a syndrome known as hemosiderosis). Use of iron chelation therapy has improved morbidity and mortality.] The only curative option available is hematopoietic stem cell transplantation.

2. **α-Thalassemias:** In these disorders, synthesis of α-globin chains is decreased or absent, typically as a result of deletional mutations. Because each individual's genome contains four copies of the α-globin gene (two on each chromosome 16), there are several levels of α-globin chain deficiencies (Figure 3.23). If one of the four genes is defective, the individual is termed a silent carrier of α-thalassemia, because no physical manifestations of the disease occur. If two α-globin genes are defective, the individual is designated as having α-thalassemia trait. If three α-globin genes are defective, the individual has hemoglobin H (β_4) disease, a hemolytic anemia of variable severity. If all four α-globin genes are defective, hemoglobin Bart (γ_4) disease with hydrops fetalis and fetal death results, because α-globin chains are required for the synthesis of HbF.

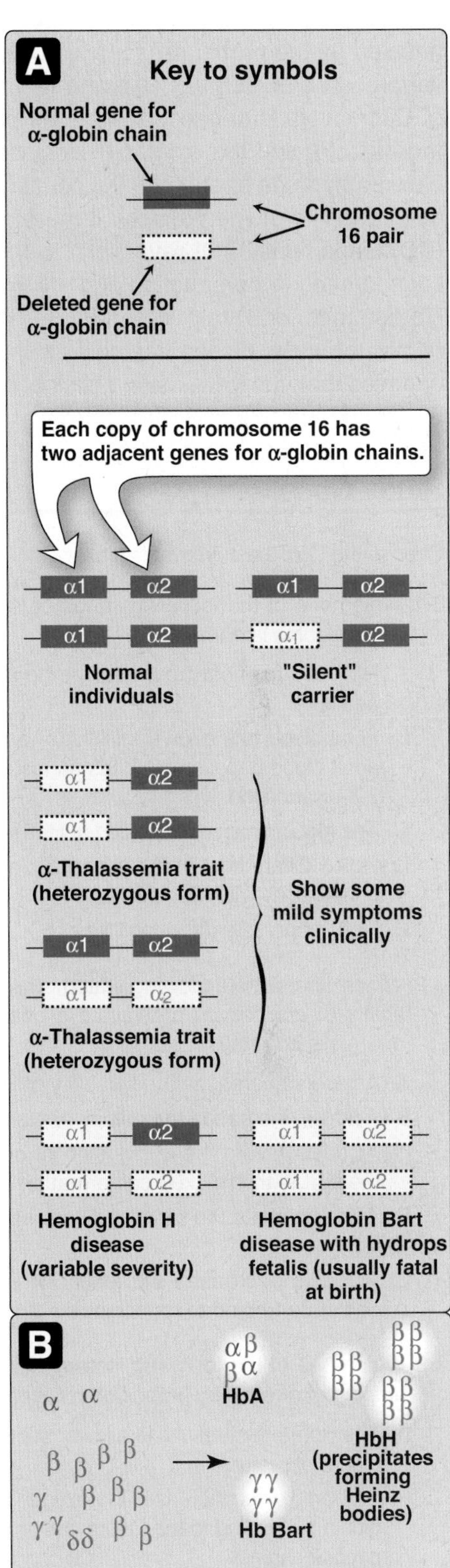

Figure 3.23
A. α-Globin gene deletions in the α-thalassemias. B. Hemoglobin (Hb) tetramers formed in α-thalassemias.

V. CHAPTER SUMMARY

Hemoglobin A (HbA), the major hemoglobin (Hb) in adults, is composed of four polypeptide chains (two α chains and two β chains, $\boldsymbol{\alpha_2\beta_2}$) held together by noncovalent interactions (Figure 3.24). The subunits occupy different relative positions in deoxyhemoglobin compared with oxyhemoglobin. The **deoxy form** of Hb is called the **"T,"** or **taut (tense) conformation**. It has a constrained structure that limits the movement of the polypeptide chains. The T form is the **low-oxygen-affinity form** of Hb. The binding of O_2 to Hb causes rupture of some of the ionic and hydrogen bonds, and movement of the dimers. This leads to a structure called the **"R,"** or **relaxed conformation**. The R form is the **high-oxygen-affinity form** of Hb. The **oxygen-dissociation curve** for Hb is **sigmoidal** in shape (in contrast to that of **myoglobin**, which is **hyperbolic**), indicating that the subunits cooperate in binding O_2. **Cooperative binding** of O_2 by the four subunits of Hb means that the binding of an O_2 molecule at one heme group increases the oxygen affinity of the remaining heme groups in the same Hb molecule. Hb's **ability to bind O_2 reversibly** is affected by the **partial pressure of O_2 (pO_2)** (through heme-heme interactions), the **pH** of the environment, the partial pressure of CO_2 (**pCO_2**), and the availability of **2,3-bisphosphoglycerate (2,3-BPG)**. For example, the release of O_2 from Hb is enhanced when the pH is lowered or the pCO_2 is increased (the **Bohr effect**), such as in **exercising muscle**, and the oxygen-dissociation curve of Hb is shifted to the right. To cope long-term with the effects of **chronic hypoxia** or **anemia**, the concentration of **2,3-BPG** in **red blood cells** increases. **2,3-BPG** binds to the Hb and decreases its oxygen affinity. It therefore also shifts the oxygen-dissociation curve to the right. **Carbon monoxide (CO)** binds tightly (but reversibly) to the Hb iron, forming **carboxyhemoglobin**. **Hemoglobinopathies** are disorders caused either by production of a **structurally abnormal Hb** molecule; synthesis of **insufficient quantities** of normal Hb subunits, or, rarely, both (Figure 3.25). The sickling diseases **sickle cell anemia** (hemoglobin S disease) and **hemoglobin SC disease** as well as **hemoglobin C disease** and the **thalassemias** are representative hemoglobinopathies that can have severe clinical consequences.

Study Questions

Choose the ONE best answer.

3.1 Which one of the following statements concerning the hemoglobins is correct?

A. HbA is the most abundant hemoglobin in normal adults.

B. Fetal blood has a lower affinity for oxygen than does adult blood because HbF has an increased affinity for 2,3-bisphosphoglycerate.

C. The globin chain composition of HbF is $\alpha_2\delta_2$.

D. HbA_{1c} differs from HbA by a single, genetically determined amino acid substitution.

E. HbA_2 appears early in fetal life.

Correct answer = A. HbA accounts for over 90% of the hemoglobin in a normal adult. If HbA_{1c} is included, the percentage rises to approximately 97%. Because 2,3-bisphosphoglycerate (2,3-BPG) reduces the affinity of hemoglobin for oxygen, the weaker interaction between 2,3-BPG and HbF results in a higher oxygen affinity for HbF relative to HbA. HbF consists of $\alpha_2\gamma_2$. HbA_{1c} is a glycosylated form of HbA, formed nonenzymically in red cells. HbA_2 is a minor component of normal adult hemoglobin, first appearing shortly before birth and rising to adult levels (about 2% of the total hemoglobin) by age 6 months.

3.2 Which one of the following statements concerning the ability of acidosis to precipitate a crisis in sickle cell anemia is correct?

A. Acidosis decreases the solubility of HbS.

B. Acidosis increases the affinity of hemoglobin for O_2.

C. Acidosis favors the conversion of hemoglobin from the taut to the relaxed conformation.

D. Acidosis shifts the oxygen-dissociation curve to the left.

E. Acidosis decreases the ability of 2,3-bisphosphoglycerate to bind to hemoglobin.

Correct answer = A. HbS is significantly less soluble in the deoxygenated form, compared with oxyhemoglobin S. A decrease in pH (acidosis) causes the oxygen-dissociation curve to shift to the right, indicating a decreased affinity for oxygen. This favors the formation of the deoxy, or taut, form of hemoglobin, and can precipitate a sickle cell crisis. The binding of 2,3-bisphosphoglycerate is increased, because it binds only to the deoxy form of hemoglobins.

3.3 Which one of the following statements concerning the binding of oxygen by hemoglobin is correct?

A. The Bohr effect results in a lower affinity for oxygen at higher pH values.

B. Carbon dioxide increases the oxygen affinity of hemoglobin by binding to the C-terminal groups of the polypeptide chains.

C. The oxygen affinity of hemoglobin increases as the percentage saturation increases.

D. The hemoglobin tetramer binds four molecules of 2,3-bisphosphoglycerate.

E. Oxyhemoglobin and deoxyhemoglobin have the same affinity for protons.

Correct answer = C. The binding of oxygen at one heme group increases the oxygen affinity of the remaining heme groups in the same molecule. A rise in pH results in increased affinity for oxygen. Carbon dioxide decreases oxygen affinity because it lowers the pH; moreover, binding of carbon dioxide to the N-termini stabilizes the taut, deoxy form. Hemoglobin binds one molecule of 2,3-bisphosphoglycerate. Deoxyhemoglobin has a greater affinity for protons and, therefore, is a weaker acid.

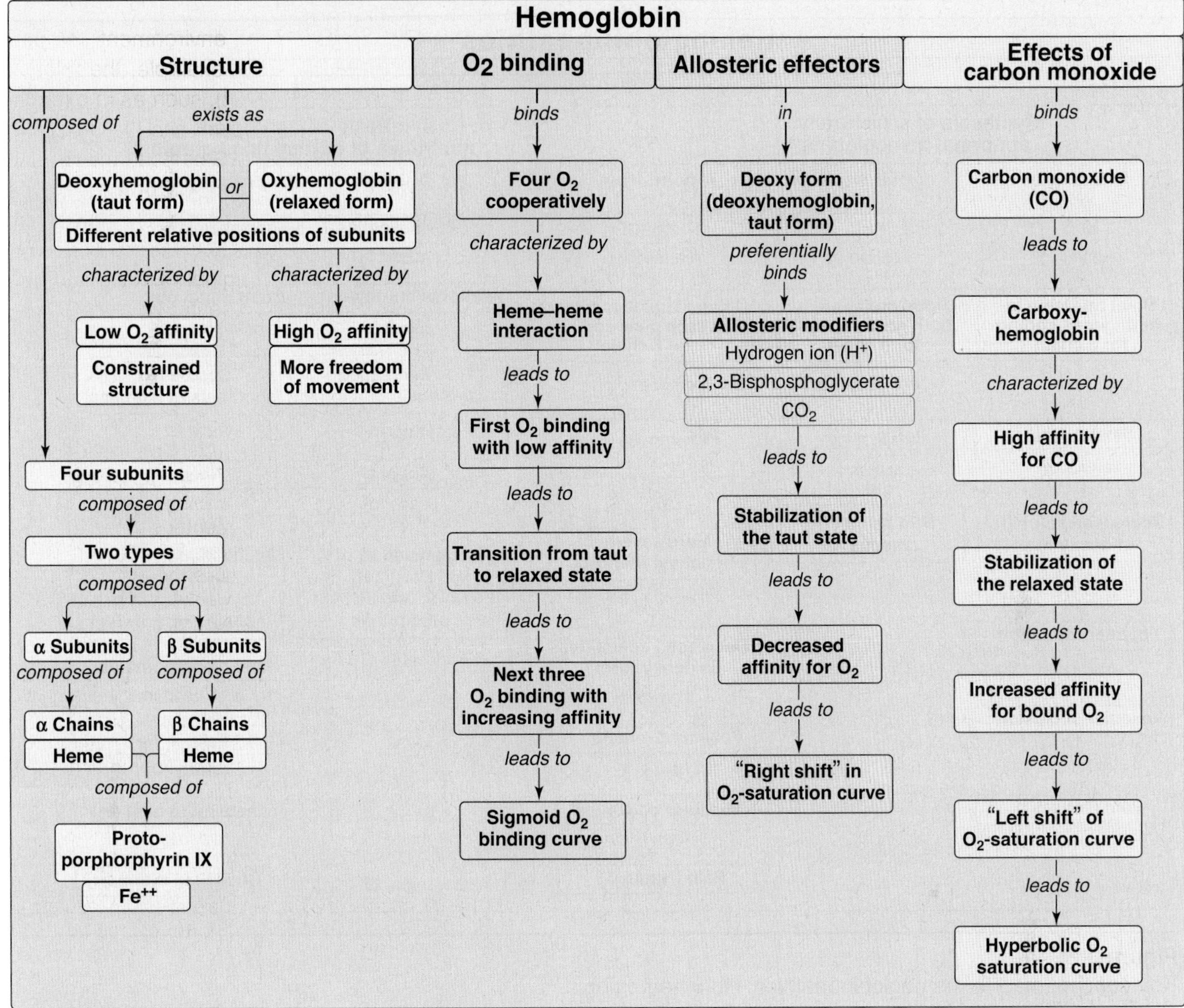

Figure 3.24
Key concept map for hemoglobin structure and function.

Study Questions (continued)

3.4 β-Lysine 82 in HbA is important for the binding of 2,3-bisphosphoglycerate. In Hb Helsinki, this amino acid has been replaced by methionine. Which of the following should be true concerning Hb Helsinki?

A. It should be stabilized in the taut, rather than the relaxed, form.

B. It should have increased O_2 affinity and, consequently, decreased delivery of O_2 to tissues.

C. Its O_2-dissociation curve should be shifted to the right relative to HbA.

D. It results in anemia.

Correct answer = B. Substitution of lysine by methionine decreases the ability of negatively charged phosphate groups in 2,3-bisphosphoglycerate (2,3-BPG) to bind the β subunits of hemoglobin. Because 2,3-BPG decreases the O_2 affinity of hemoglobin, a reduction in 2,3-BPG should result in increased O_2 affinity and decreased delivery of O_2 to tissues. The relaxed form is the high-oxygen-affinity form of hemoglobin. Increased O_2 affinity (decreased delivery) results in a left shift in the O_2-dissociation curve. Decreased O_2 delivery is compensated for by increased RBC production.

3.5 Why is hemoglobin C disease a nonsickling disease?

In HbC, the polar glutamate is replaced by polar lysine rather than by nonpolar valine as in HbS.

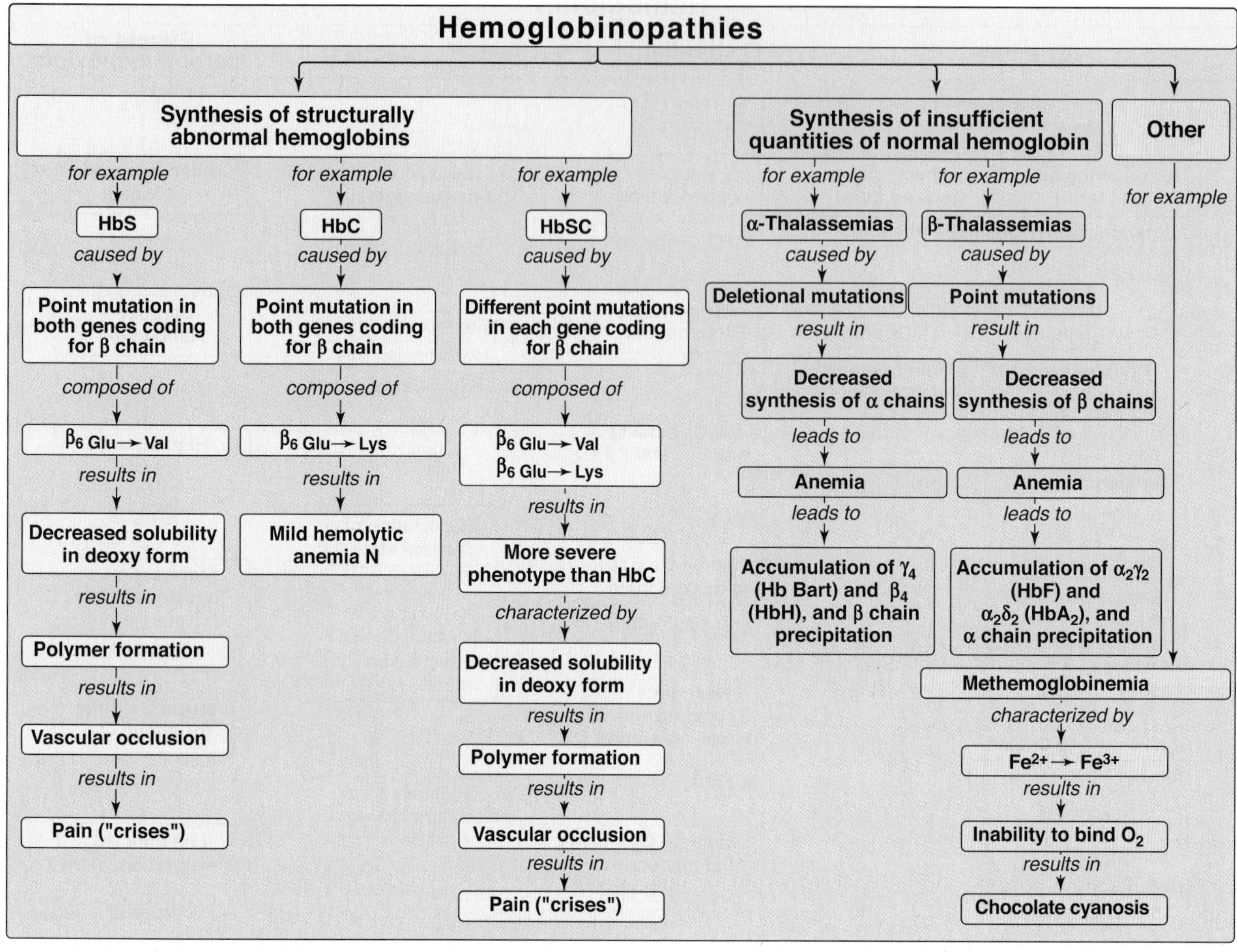

Figure 3.25
Key concept map for hemoglobinopathies. Hb = hemoglobin.

Study Questions (continued)

3.6 A 67-year-old man presented to the emergency department with a 1-week history of angina and shortness of breath. He complained that his face and extremities had a "blue color." His medical history included chronic stable angina treated with isosorbide dinitrate and nitroglycerin. Blood obtained for analysis was brown colored. Which one of the following is the most likely diagnosis?

A. Carboxyhemoglobinemia
B. Hemoglobin SC disease
C. Methemoglobinemia
D. Sickle cell anemia
E. β-Thalassemia

Correct answer = C. Oxidation of the heme component of hemoglobin to the ferric (Fe^{3+}) state forms methemoglobin. This may be caused by the action of certain drugs such as nitrates. The methemoglobinemias are characterized by chocolate cyanosis (a brownish blue coloration of the skin and mucous membranes and chocolate-colored blood) as a result of the dark-colored methemoglobin. Symptoms are related to tissue hypoxia and include anxiety, headache, and dyspnea. In rare cases, coma and death can occur. [Note: Benzocaine, an aromatic amine used as a topical anesthetic, is a cause of acquired methemoglobinemia.]

3.7 What would be true about the extent of red blood cell sickling in individuals with HbS and hereditary persistence of HbF?

Decreased. HbF reduces HbS concentration. It also inhibits polymerization of deoxy HbS.

Fibrous Proteins

4

I. OVERVIEW

Collagen and elastin are examples of common, well-characterized fibrous proteins of the extracellular matrix that serve structural functions in the body. For example, collagen and elastin are found as components of skin, connective tissue, blood vessel walls, and the sclera and cornea of the eye. Each fibrous protein exhibits special mechanical properties, resulting from its unique structure, which are obtained by combining specific amino acids into regular, secondary structural elements. This is in contrast to globular proteins, whose shapes are the result of complex interactions between secondary, tertiary, and, sometimes, quaternary structural elements.

II. COLLAGEN

Collagen is the most abundant protein in the human body. A typical collagen molecule is a long, rigid structure in which three polypeptides (referred to as α chains) are wound around one another in a rope-like triple helix (Figure 4.1). Although these molecules are found throughout the body, their types and organization are dictated by the structural role collagen plays in a particular organ. In some tissues, collagen may be dispersed as a gel that gives support to the structure, as in the extracellular matrix or the vitreous humor of the eye. In other tissues, collagen may be bundled in tight, parallel fibers that provide great strength, as in tendons. In the cornea of the eye, collagen is stacked so as to transmit light with a minimum of scattering. Collagen of bone occurs as fibers arranged at an angle to each other so as to resist mechanical shear from any direction.

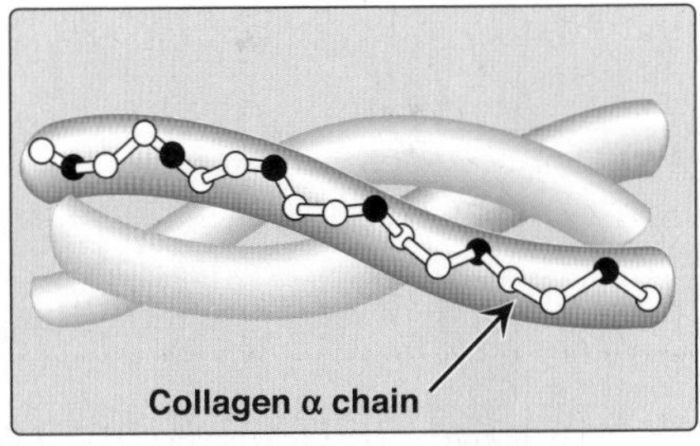

Figure 4.1
Triple-stranded helix of collagen.

A. Types

The collagen superfamily of proteins includes more than 25 collagen types as well as additional proteins that have collagen-like domains. The three polypeptide α chains are held together by interchain hydrogen bonds. Variations in the amino acid sequence of the α chains result in structural components that are about the same size (approximately 1,000 amino acids long) but with slightly different properties. These α chains are combined to form the various types of collagen found in the tissues. For example, the most common collagen, type I, contains two chains called α1 and one chain called α2 ($\alpha1_2\alpha2$), whereas type II collagen contains three α1 chains ($\alpha1_3$). The colla-

TYPE	TISSUE DISTRIBUTION
	Fibril-forming
I	Skin, bone, tendon, blood vessels, cornea
II	Cartilage, intervertebral disk, vitreous body
III	Blood vessels, skin, muscle
	Network-forming
IV	Basement membrane
VIII	Corneal and vascular endothelium
	Fibril-associated*
IX	Cartilage
XII	Tendon, ligaments, some other tissues

Figure 4.2
The most abundant types of collagen. *Known as FACITs: fibril-associated collagens with interrupted triple helices.

gens can be organized into three groups, based on their location and functions in the body (Figure 4.2).

1. **Fibril-forming collagens:** Types I, II, and III are the fibrillar collagens and have the rope-like structure described above for a typical collagen molecule. In the electron microscope, these linear polymers of fibrils have characteristic banding patterns, reflecting the regular staggered packing of the individual collagen molecules in the fibril (Figure 4.3). Type I collagen fibers (composed of collagen fibrils) are found in supporting elements of high tensile strength (for example, tendon and cornea), whereas fibers formed from type II collagen molecules are restricted to cartilaginous structures. The fibers derived from type III collagen are prevalent in more distensible tissues such as blood vessels.

2. **Network-forming collagens:** Types IV and VIII form a three-dimensional mesh, rather than distinct fibrils (Figure 4.4). For example, type IV molecules assemble into a sheet or meshwork that constitutes a major part of basement membranes.

> Basement membranes are thin, sheet-like structures that provide mechanical support for adjacent cells and function as a semipermeable filtration barrier to macromolecules in organs such as the kidney and the lung.

3. **Fibril-associated collagens:** Types IX and XII bind to the surface of collagen fibrils, linking these fibrils to one another and to other components in the extracellular matrix (see Figure 4.2).

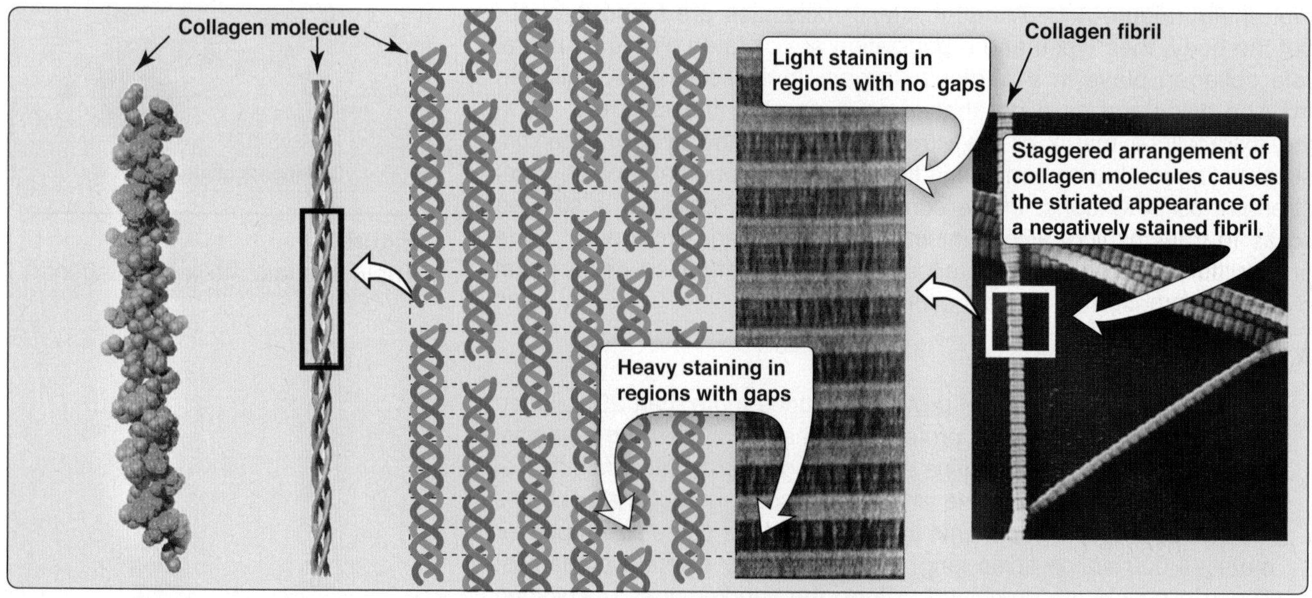

Figure 4.3
Collagen fibrils at right have a characteristic banding pattern, reflecting the regularly staggered packing of the individual collagen molecules in the fibril.

B. Structure

1. **Amino acid sequence:** Collagen is rich in proline and glycine, both of which are important in the formation of the triple-stranded helix. Proline facilitates the formation of the helical conformation of each α chain because its ring structure causes "kinks" in the peptide chain. [Note: The presence of proline dictates that the helical conformation of the α chain cannot be an α helix (see p. 16).] Glycine, the smallest amino acid, is found in every third position of the polypeptide chain. It fits into the restricted spaces where the three chains of the helix come together. The glycine residues are part of a repeating sequence, –Gly–X–Y–, where X is frequently proline, and Y is often hydroxyproline (but can be hydroxylysine, Figure 4.5). Thus, most of the α chain can be regarded as a polytripeptide whose sequence can be represented as $(\text{–Gly–Pro–Hyp–})_{333}$.

2. **Triple-helical structure:** Unlike most globular proteins that are folded into compact structures, collagen, a fibrous protein, has an elongated, triple-helical structure that is stabilized by interchain hydrogen bonds.

3. **Hydroxyproline and hydroxylysine:** Collagen contains hydroxyproline and hydroxylysine, which are not present in most other proteins. These residues result from the hydroxylation of some of the proline and lysine residues after their incorporation into polypeptide chains (Figure 4.6). The hydroxylation is, thus, an example of posttranslational modification (see p. 443). [Note: Generation of hydroxyproline maximizes formation of interchain hydrogen bonds that stabilize the triple-helical structure.]

4. **Glycosylation:** The hydroxyl group of the hydroxylysine residues of collagen may be enzymatically glycosylated. Most commonly, glucose and galactose are sequentially attached to the polypeptide chain prior to triple-helix formation (Figure 4.7).

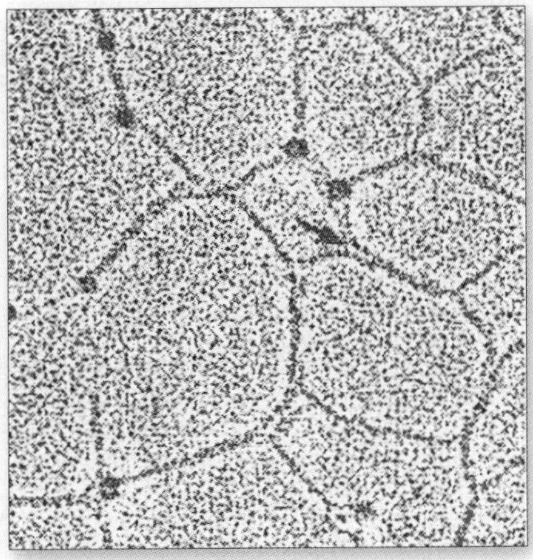

Figure 4.4
Electron micrograph of a polygonal network formed by association of collagen type IV monomers.

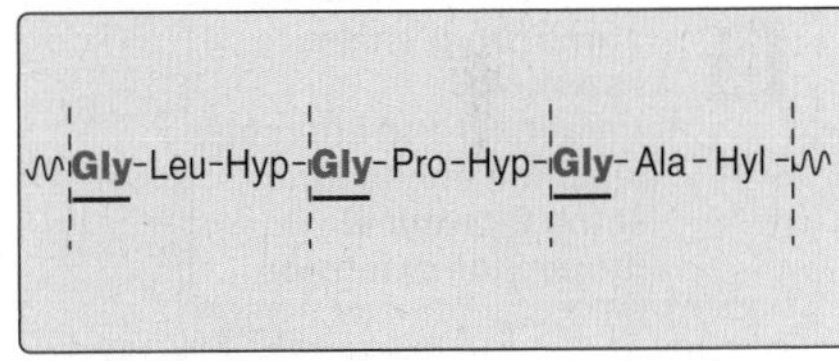

Figure 4.5
Amino acid sequence of a portion of the α1 chain of collagen. [Note: Hyp is hydroxyproline, and Hyl is hydroxylysine.]

C. Biosynthesis

The polypeptide precursors of the collagen molecule are synthesized in fibroblasts (or in the related osteoblasts of bone and chondroblasts of cartilage). They are enzymically modified and form the triple helix, which gets secreted into the extracellular matrix. After additional enzymic modification, the mature extracellular collagen monomers aggregate and become cross-linked to form collagen fibers.

1. **Formation of pro-α chains:** Collagen is one of many proteins that normally function outside of cells. Like most proteins produced for export, the newly synthesized polypeptide precursors of α chains (prepro-α chains) contain a special amino acid sequence at their N-terminal ends. This sequence acts as a signal that, in the absence of additional signals, targets the polypeptide being synthesized for secretion from the cell. The signal sequence facilitates the binding of ribosomes to the rough endoplasmic reticulum (RER), and directs the passage of the prepro-α chain into the lumen of the RER. The signal sequence is rapidly cleaved in the RER to yield a precursor of collagen called a pro-α chain (see Figure 4.7).

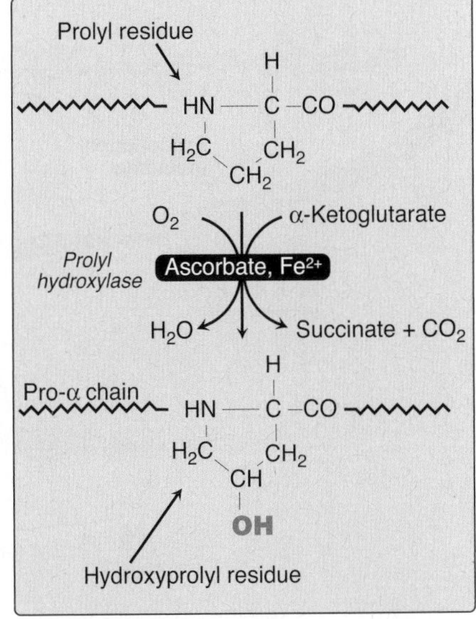

Figure 4.6
Hydroxylation of proline residues of pro-α chains of collagen by *prolyl hydroxylase*.

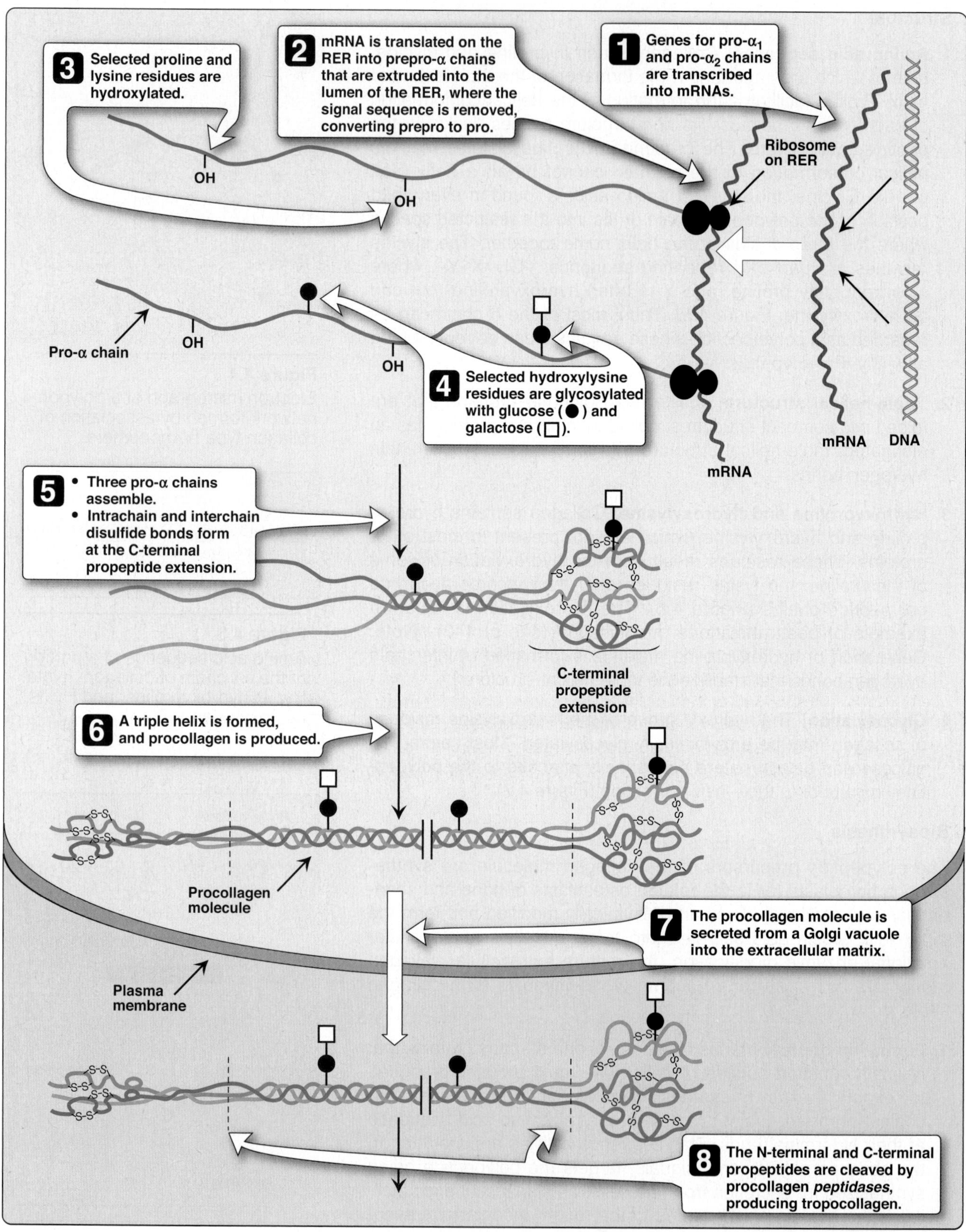

Figure 4.7
Synthesis of collagen. RER = rough endoplasmic reticulum; mRNA = messenger RNA. (continued on the next page)

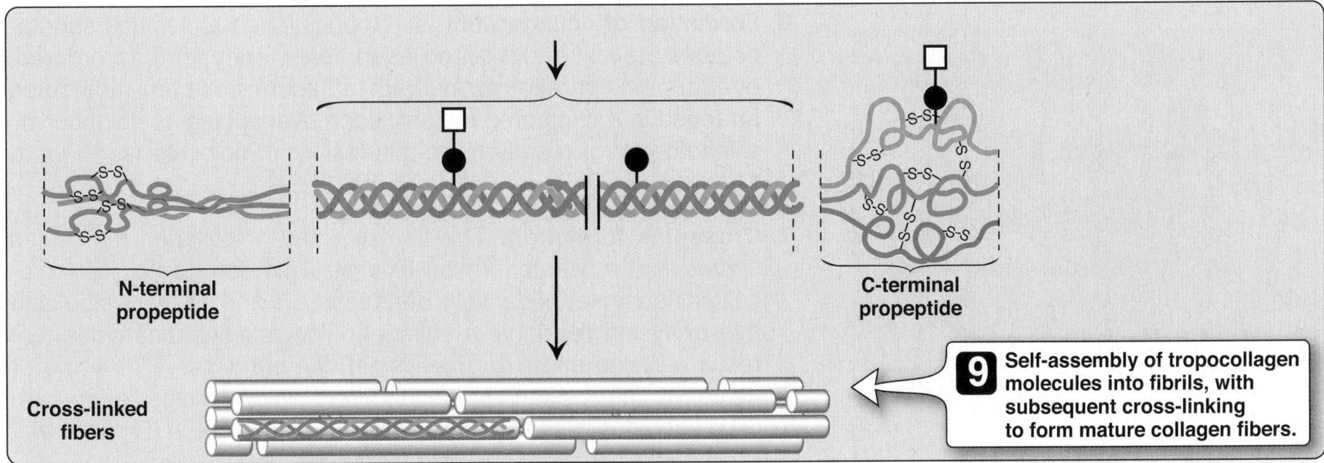

Figure 4.7
Synthesis of collagen. (continued from the previous page)

2. **Hydroxylation:** The pro-α chains are processed by a number of enzymic steps within the lumen of the RER while the polypeptides are still being synthesized (see Figure 4.7). Proline and lysine residues found in the Y-position of the –Gly–X–Y– sequence can be hydroxylated to form hydroxyproline and hydroxylysine residues. These hydroxylation reactions require molecular oxygen, Fe^{2+}, and the reducing agent vitamin C (ascorbic acid, see p. 377), without which the hydroxylating enzymes, *prolyl hydroxylase* and *lysyl hydroxylase*, are unable to function (see Figure 4.6). In the case of ascorbic acid deficiency (and, therefore, a lack of proline and lysine hydroxylation), interchain H-bond formation is impaired, as is formation of a stable triple helix. Additionally, collagen fibrils cannot be cross-linked (see below), greatly decreasing the tensile strength of the assembled fiber. The resulting deficiency disease is known as scurvy. Patients with ascorbic acid deficiency also often show bruises on the limbs as a result of subcutaneous extravasation (leakage) of blood due to capillary fragility (Figure 4.8).

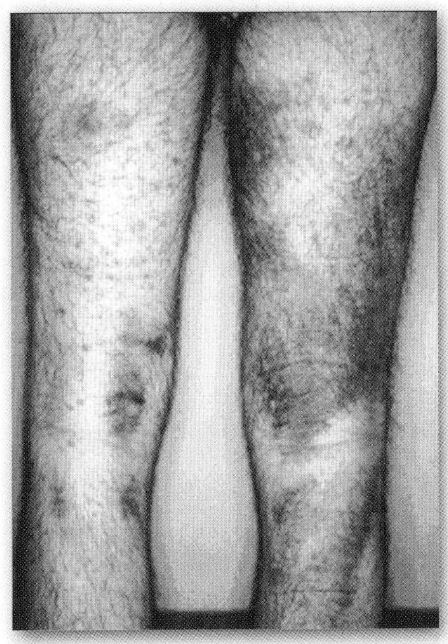

Figure 4.8
The legs of a 46-year-old man with scurvy.

3. **Glycosylation:** Some hydroxylysine residues are modified by glycosylation with glucose or glucosyl-galactose (see Figure 4.7).

4. **Assembly and secretion:** After hydroxylation and glycosylation, three pro-α chains form procollagen, a precursor of collagen that has a central region of triple helix flanked by the nonhelical amino- and carboxyl-terminal extensions called propeptides (see Figure 4.7). The formation of procollagen begins with formation of interchain disulfide bonds between the C-terminal extensions of the pro-α chains. This brings the three α chains into an alignment favorable for helix formation. The procollagen molecules move through the Golgi apparatus, where they are packaged in secretory vesicles. The vesicles fuse with the cell membrane, causing the release of procollagen molecules into the extracellular space.

5. **Extracellular cleavage of procollagen molecules:** After their release, the procollagen molecules are cleaved by *N-* and *C-procollagen peptidases,* which remove the terminal propeptides, releasing triple-helical tropocollagen molecules.

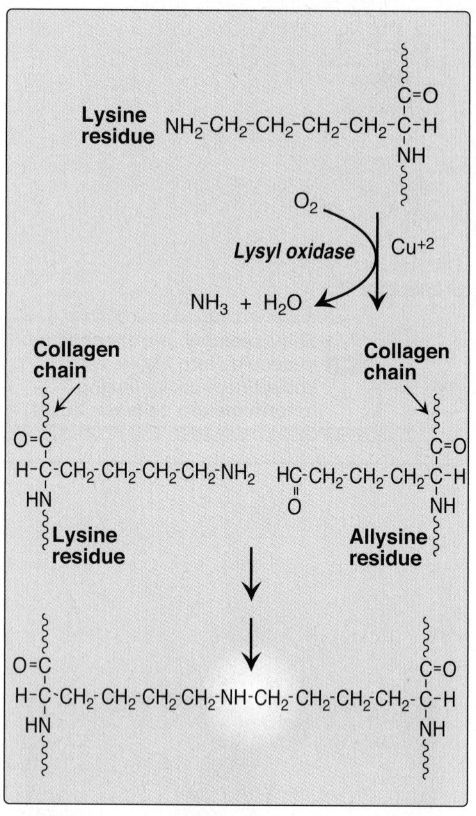

Figure 4.9
Formation of cross-links in collagen. [Note: *Lysyl oxidase* is irreversibly inhibited by a toxin from plants in the genus Lathyrus, leading to a condition known as lathyrism.]

6. **Formation of collagen fibrils:** Tropocollagen molecules spontaneously associate to form collagen fibrils. They form an ordered, overlapping, parallel array, with adjacent collagen molecules arranged in a staggered pattern, each overlapping its neighbor by a length approximately three-quarters of a molecule (see Figure 4.7).

7. **Cross-link formation:** The fibrillar array of collagen molecules serves as a substrate for *lysyl oxidase*. This Cu^{2+}-containing extracellular enzyme oxidatively deaminates some of the lysine and hydroxylysine residues in collagen. The reactive aldehydes that result (allysine and hydroxyallysine) can condense with lysine or hydroxylysine residues in neighboring collagen molecules to form covalent cross-links and, thus, mature collagen fibers (Figure 4.9).

> *Lysyl oxidase* is one of several copper-containing enzymes. Others include *cytochrome oxidase* (see p. 76), *dopamine hydroxylase* (see p. 286), *superoxide dismutase* (see p.148), and *tyrosinase* (see p. 273). Disruption in copper homeostasis causes copper deficiency (X-linked Menkes disease) or overload (Wilson disease).

D. Degradation

Normal collagens are highly stable molecules, having half-lives as long as several years. However, connective tissue is dynamic and is constantly being remodeled, often in response to growth or injury of the tissue. Breakdown of collagen fibers is dependent on the proteolytic action of *collagenases*, which are part of a large family of matrix *metalloproteinases*. For type I collagen, the cleavage site is specific, generating three-quarter and one-quarter length fragments. These fragments are further degraded by other matrix *proteinases*.

E. Collagen diseases: Collagenopathies

Defects in any one of the many steps in collagen fiber synthesis can result in a genetic disease involving an inability of collagen to form fibers properly and, therefore, an inability to provide tissues with the needed tensile strength normally provided by collagen. More than 1,000 mutations have been identified in 23 genes coding for 13 of the collagen types. The following are examples of diseases that are the result of defective collagen synthesis.

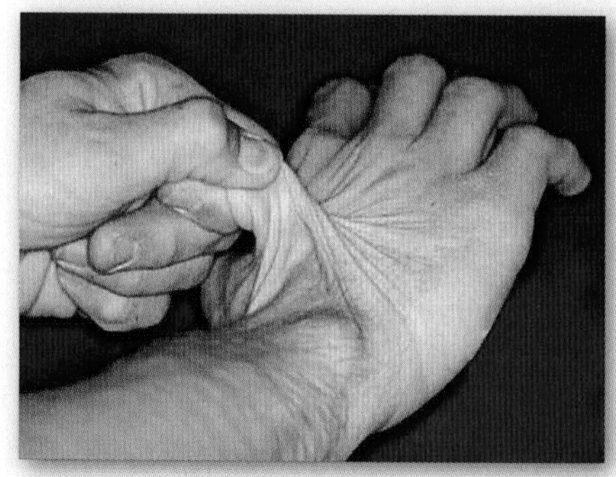

Figure 4.10
Stretchy skin of classic Ehlers-Danlos syndrome.

1. **Ehlers-Danlos syndrome:** Ehlers-Danlos syndrome (EDS) is a heterogeneous group of connective tissue disorders that result from inheritable defects in the metabolism of fibrillar collagen molecules. EDS can be caused by a deficiency of collagen-processing enzymes (for example, *lysyl hydroxylase* or *N-procollagen peptidase*) or from mutations in the amino acid sequences of collagen types I, III, or V. The classic form of EDS, caused by defects in type V collagen, is characterized by skin extensibility and fragility and joint hypermobility (Figure 4.10). The vascular form, due to defects in type III collagen, is the most serious form of EDS because it is associated with potentially lethal arterial rupture. [Note: The classic and vascular forms show autosomal dominant

inheritance.] Collagen containing mutant chains may have altered structure, secretion, or distribution. It frequently is degraded. [Note: Incorporation of just one mutant chain may result in degradation of the triple helix. This is known as a dominant-negative effect.].

2. **Osteogenesis imperfecta:** This syndrome, known as brittle bone disease, is a genetic disorder of bone fragility characterized by bones that fracture easily, with minor or no trauma (Figure 4.11). Over 80% of cases of osteogenesis imperfecta (OI) are caused by dominant mutations to the genes that code for the $\alpha1$ or $\alpha2$ chains in type I collagen. The most common mutations cause the replacement of glycine (in –Gly–X–Y–) by amino acids with bulky side chains. The resultant structurally abnormal α chains prevent the formation of the required triple-helical conformation. Phenotypic severity ranges from mild to lethal. Type I OI, the most common form, is characterized by mild bone fragility, hearing loss, and blue sclerae. Type II, the most severe form, is typically lethal in the perinatal period as a result of pulmonary complications. In utero fractures are seen (see Figure 4.11). Type III is also a severe form. It is characterized by multiple fractures at birth, short stature, spinal curvature leading to a "humped-back" (kyphotic) appearance, and blue sclerae. Dentinogenesis imperfecta, a disorder of tooth development, may be seen in OI.

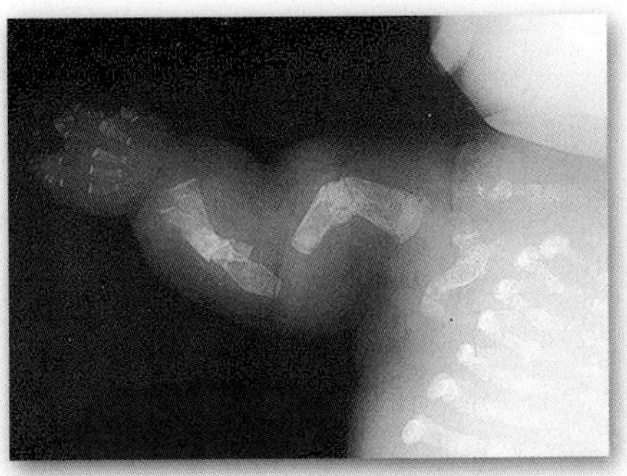

Figure 4.11
Lethal form (type II) of osteogenesis imperfecta in which the fractures appear in utero, as revealed by this radiograph of a stillborn fetus.

III. ELASTIN

In contrast to collagen, which forms fibers that are tough and have high tensile strength, elastin is a connective tissue protein with rubber-like properties. Elastic fibers composed of elastin and glycoprotein microfibrils are found in the lungs, the walls of large arteries, and elastic ligaments. They can be stretched to several times their normal length but recoil to their original shape when the stretching force is relaxed.

A. Structure

Elastin is an insoluble protein polymer synthesized from a precursor, tropoelastin, which is a linear polypeptide composed of about 700 amino acids that are primarily small and nonpolar (for example, glycine, alanine, and valine). Elastin is also rich in proline and lysine but contains scant hydroxyproline and hydroxylysine. Tropoelastin is secreted by the cell into the extracellular space. There, it interacts with specific glycoprotein microfibrils, such as fibrillin, which function as a scaffold onto which tropoelastin is deposited. Some of the lysyl side chains of the tropoelastin polypeptides are oxidatively deaminated by *lysyl oxidase*, forming allysine residues. Three of the allysyl side chains plus one unaltered lysyl side chain from the same or neighboring polypeptides form a desmosine cross-link (Figure 4.12). This produces elastin, an extensively interconnected, rubbery network that can stretch and bend in any direction when stressed, giving connective tissue elasticity (Figure 4.13). Mutations in the fibrillin-1 protein are responsible for Marfan syndrome, a connective tissue disorder characterized by impaired structural integrity in the skeleton, the eye, and the cardiovascular system. With this disease, abnormal fibrillin protein is incorporated into microfibrils along with normal fibrillin, inhibiting the formation of functional microfibrils. [Note: Patients with Marfan syndrome, OI, or EDS may have blue sclerae due to tissue thinning that allows underlying pigment to show through.]

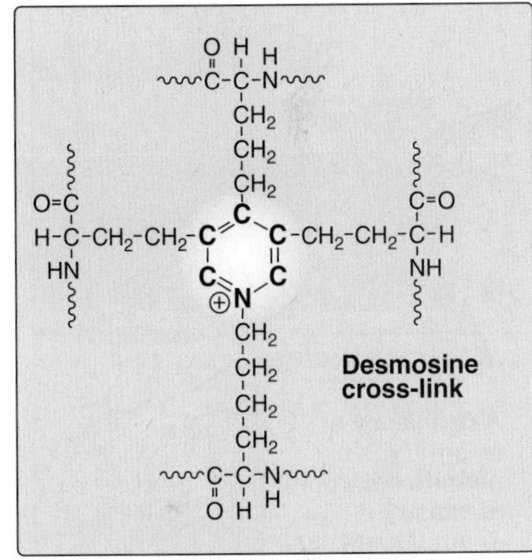

Figure 4.12
Desmosine cross-link in elastin.

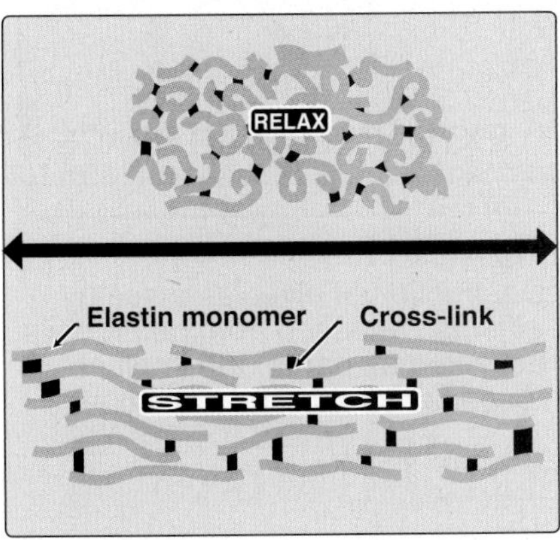

Figure 4.13
Elastin fibers in relaxed and stretched conformations.

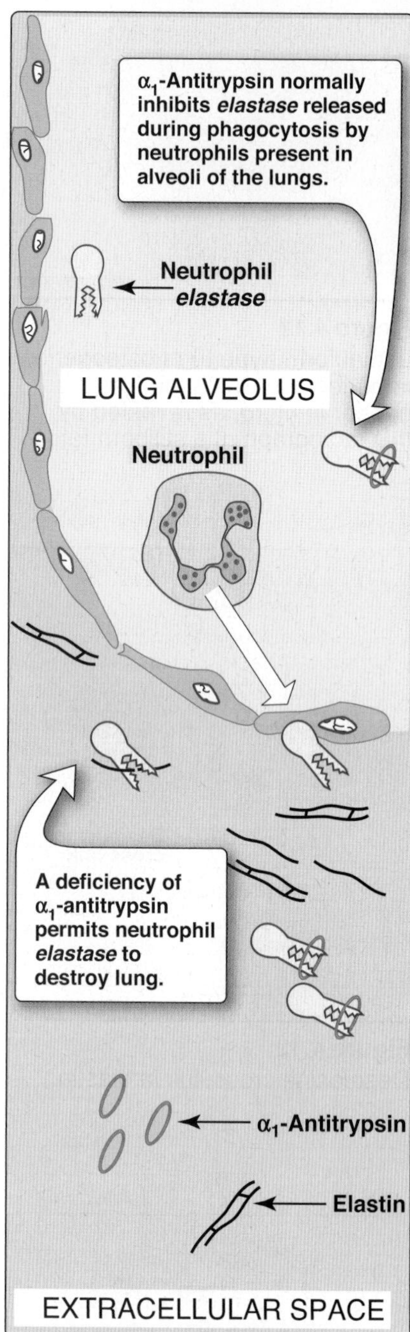

Figure 4.14
Destruction of alveolar tissue by *elastase* released from neutrophils activated as part of the immune response to airborne pathogens.

B. Role of α_1-antitrypsin in elastin degradation

1. **α_1-Antitrypsin:** Blood and other body fluids contain a protein, α_1-antitrypsin (AAT or A1AT), which inhibits a number of proteolytic enzymes (called *proteases* or *proteinases*) that hydrolyze and destroy proteins. [Note: The inhibitor was originally named α1-antitrypsin because it inhibits the activity of *trypsin*, a proteolytic enzyme synthesized as trypsinogen by the pancreas (see p. 248).] AAT has the important physiologic role of inhibiting neutrophil *elastase*, a powerful *protease* that is released into the extracellular space and degrades elastin of alveolar walls as well as other structural proteins in a variety of tissues (Figure 4.14). Most of the AAT found in plasma is synthesized and secreted by the liver. AAT comprises more than 90% of the α_1-globulin fraction of normal plasma. Extrahepatic synthesis occurs in monocytes and alveolar macrophages, and may be important in the prevention of local tissue injury by *elastase*.

2. **Role of α_1-antitrypsin in the lungs:** In the normal lung, the alveoli are chronically exposed to low levels of neutrophil *elastase* released from activated and degenerating neutrophils. The proteolytic activity of *elastase* can destroy the elastin in alveolar walls if unopposed by the action of AAT, the most important inhibitor of neutrophil *elastase* (see Figure 4.14). Because lung tissue cannot regenerate, the destruction of the connective tissue of alveolar walls results in emphysema.

3. **Emphysema resulting from α_1-antitrypsin deficiency:** In the United States, approximately 2%–5% of patients with emphysema are predisposed to the disease by inherited defects in AAT. A number of different mutations in the gene for AAT are known to cause a deficiency of the protein, but one single purine base mutation (GAG to AAG, resulting in the substitution of lysine for glutamic acid at position 342 of the protein) is clinically the most widespread. The mutation causes the normally monomeric AAT to polymerize within the endoplasmic reticulum of hepatocytes, resulting in decreased secretion of AAT by the liver. Consequently, blood levels of AAT are reduced, decreasing the amount that gets to the alveoli. The polymer that accumulates in the liver may result in cirrhosis (scarring of the liver). In the United States, the AAT mutation is most common in Caucasians of Northern European ancestry. An individual must inherit two abnormal AAT alleles to be at risk for the development of emphysema. In a heterozygote, with one normal and one defective gene, the levels of AAT are sufficient to protect the alveoli from damage. [Note: Methionine 358 in AAT is required for the binding of the inhibitor to its target *proteases*. Smoking causes the oxidation and subsequent inactivation of the methionine, thereby rendering the inhibitor powerless to neutralize *elastase*. Smokers with AAT deficiency, therefore, have a considerably elevated rate of lung destruction and a poorer survival rate than nonsmokers with the deficiency.] The deficiency of *elastase* inhibitor can be treated by weekly augmentation therapy, that is, intravenous administration of AAT. The AAT diffuses from the blood into the lung, where it reaches therapeutic levels in the fluid surrounding the lung epithelial cells.

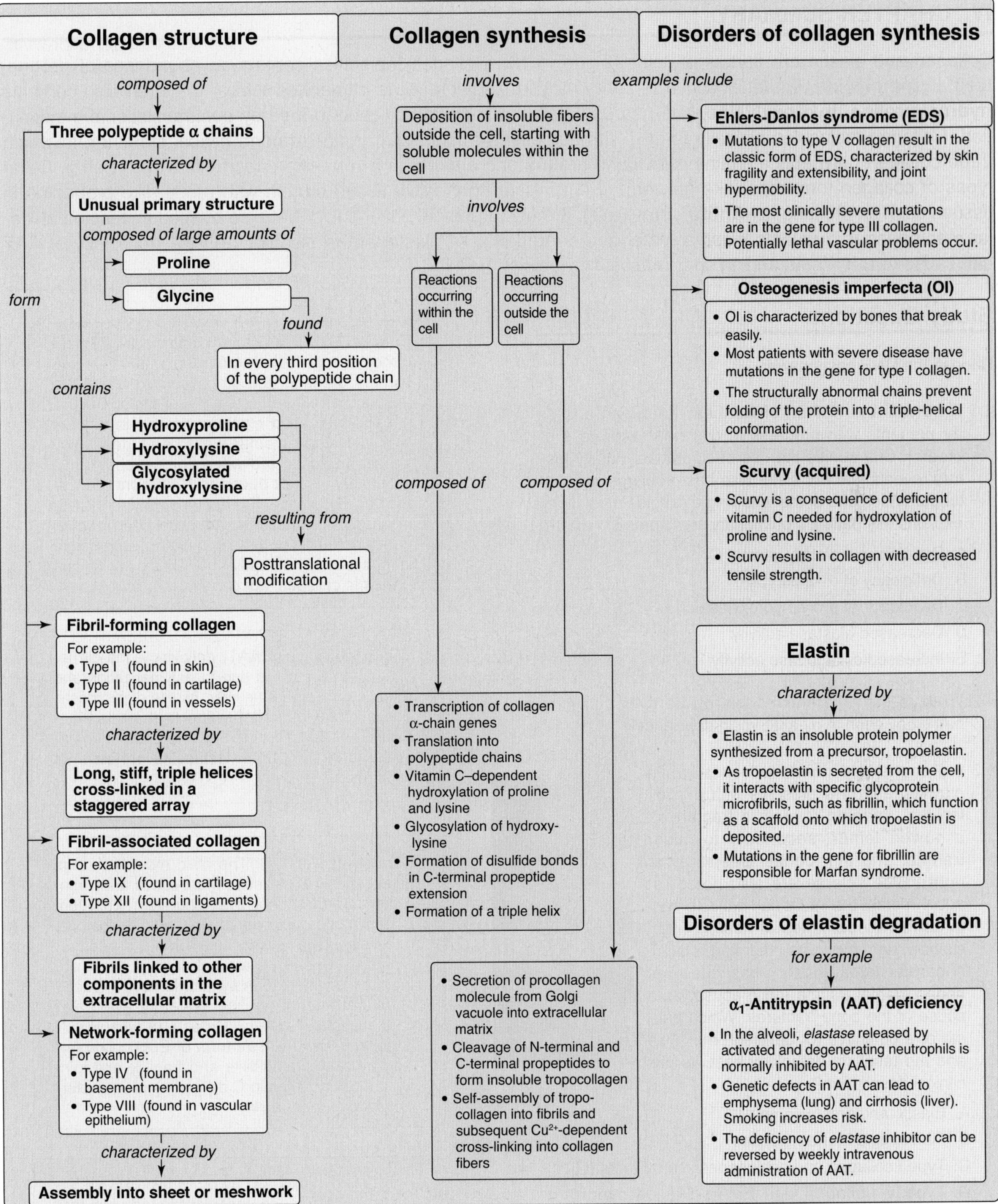

Figure 4.15
Key concept map for the fibrous proteins collagen and elastin.

IV. CHAPTER SUMMARY

Collagen and elastin are fibrous proteins (Figure 4.15). Collagen molecules contain an abundance of **proline**, **lysine**, and **glycine**, the latter occurring at every third position in the primary structure. Collagen also contains **hydroxyproline**, **hydroxylysine**, and **glycosylated hydroxylysine**, each formed by posttranslational modification. Collagen molecules typically form **fibrils** containing a long, stiff, triple-stranded helical structure, in which three collagen polypeptide chains are wound around one another in a rope-like superhelix (**triple helix**). Other types of collagen form mesh-like networks. **Elastin** is a connective tissue protein with rubber-like properties in tissues such as the lung. **α_1-Antitrypsin** (**AAT**), produced primarily by the liver but also by monocytes and alveolar macrophages, prevents *elastase*-catalyzed degradation of elastin in the alveolar walls. A deficiency of AAT can cause **emphysema** and, in some cases, cirrhosis of the liver.

Study Questions

Choose the ONE best answer.

4.1 A 30-year-old woman of Northern European ancestry presents with progressive dyspnea (shortness of breath). She denies the use of cigarettes. Family history reveals that her sister also has problems with her lungs. Which one of the following etiologies most likely explains this patient's pulmonary symptoms?

A. Deficiency in dietary vitamin C
B. Deficiency of α_1-antitrypsin
C. Deficiency of prolyl hydroxylase
D Decreased elastase activity
E. Increased collagenase activity

Correct answer = B. α_1-Antitrypsin (AAT) deficiency is a genetic disorder that can cause pulmonary damage and emphysema even in the absence of cigarette use. A deficiency of AAT permits increased elastase activity to destroy elastin in the alveolar walls. AAT deficiency should be suspected when chronic obstructive pulmonary disease develops in a patient younger than age 45 years who does not have a history of chronic bronchitis or tobacco use or when multiple family members develop obstructive lung disease at an early age. Choices A, C, and E refer to collagen, not elastin.

4.2 What is the differential basis of the liver and lung pathology seen in α_1-antitrypsin deficiency?

With α_1-antitrypsin (AAT) deficiency, the cirrhosis that can result is due to polymerization and retention of AAT in the liver, its site of synthesis. The alveolar damage is due to the retention-based deficiency of AAT (a protease inhibitor) in the lung such that elastase (a protease) is unopposed.

4.3 A 7-month-old child "fell over" while crawling and now presents with a swollen leg. Imaging reveals a fracture of a bowed femur, secondary to minor trauma, and thin bones (see x-ray at right). Blue sclerae are also noted. At age 1 month, the infant had multiple fractures in various states of healing (right clavicle, right humerus, and right radius). A careful family history has ruled out nonaccidental trauma (child abuse) as a cause of the bone fractures. Which pairing of a defective (or deficient) molecule and the resulting pathology best fits this clinical description?

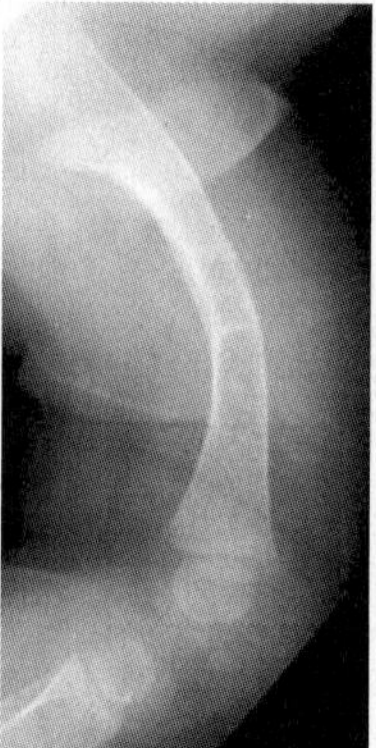

A. Elastin and emphysema
B. Fibrillin and Marfan disease
C. Type I collagen and osteogenesis imperfecta (OI)
D. Type V collagen and Ehlers-Danlos syndrome (EDS)
E. Vitamin C and scurvy

Correct answer = C. The child most likely has osteogenesis imperfecta. Most cases arise from a defect in the genes encoding type I collagen. Bones in affected patients are thin, osteoporotic, often bowed, and extremely prone to fracture. Pulmonary problems are not seen in this child. Individuals with Marfan syndrome have impaired structural integrity of the skeleton, eyes, and cardiovascular system. Defects in type V collagen cause the classic form of EDS characterized by skin extensibility and fragility and joint hypermobility. Vitamin C deficiency is characterized by capillary fragility.

4.4 How and why is proline hydroxylated in collagen?

Proline is hydroxlyated by prolyl hydroxylase, an enzyme of the rough endoplasmic reticulum that requires O_2, Fe^{2+}, and vitamin C. Hydroxylation increases interchain hydrogen bond formation, strengthening the triple helix of collagen. Vitamin C deficiency impairs hydroxylation.

Enzymes

5

I. OVERVIEW

Virtually all reactions in the body are mediated by enzymes, which are protein catalysts that increase the rate of reactions without being changed in the overall process. Among the many biologic reactions that are energetically possible, enzymes selectively channel reactants (called substrates) into useful pathways. Enzymes thus direct all metabolic events. This chapter examines the nature of these catalytic molecules and their mechanism of action.

II. NOMENCLATURE

Each enzyme is assigned two names. The first is its short, recommended name, convenient for everyday use. The second is the more complete systematic name, which is used when an enzyme must be identified without ambiguity.

A. Recommended name

Most commonly used enzyme names have the suffix "*-ase*" attached to the substrate of the reaction (for example, *glucosidase* and *urease*) or to a description of the action performed (for example, *lactate dehydrogenase* and *adenylyl cyclase*). [Note: Some enzymes retain their original trivial names, which give no hint of the associated enzymic reaction, for example, *trypsin* and *pepsin*.]

B. Systematic name

In the systematic naming system, enzymes are divided into six major classes (Figure 5.1), each with numerous subgroups. For a given enzyme, the suffix *-ase* is attached to a fairly complete description of the chemical reaction catalyzed, including the names of all the substrates, for example, *lactate:NAD$^+$ oxidoreductase*. [Note: Each enzyme is also assigned a classification number. *Lactate:NAD$^+$ oxidoreductase*, for example, is 1.1.1.27.] The systematic names are unambiguous and informative but are frequently too cumbersome to be of general use.

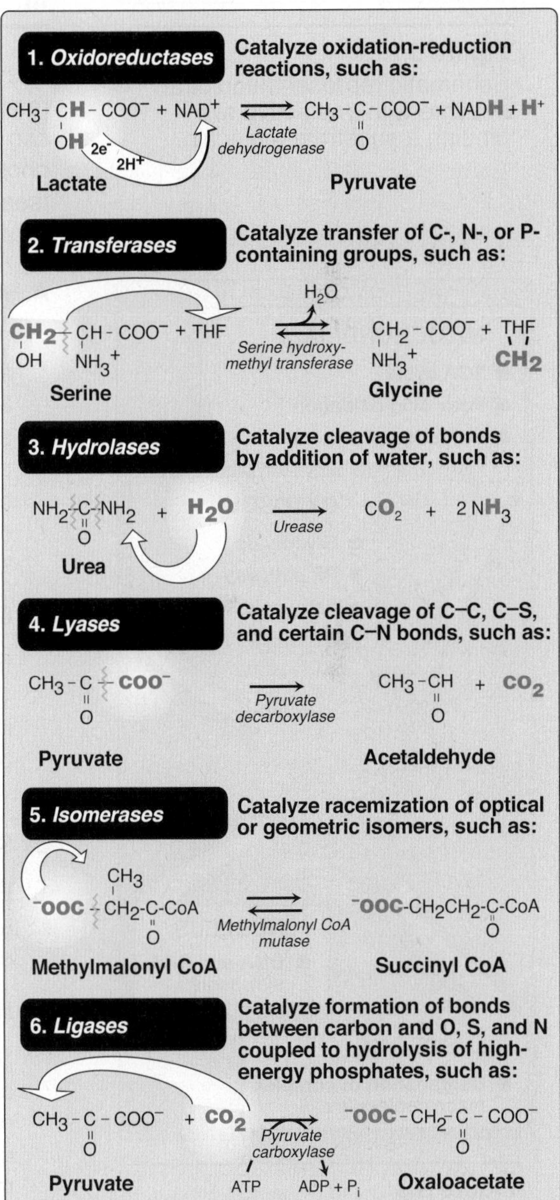

Figure 5.1
The six major classes of enzymes with examples. NAD(H) = nicotinamide adenine dinucleotide; THF = tetrahydrofolate; CoA = coenzyme A.

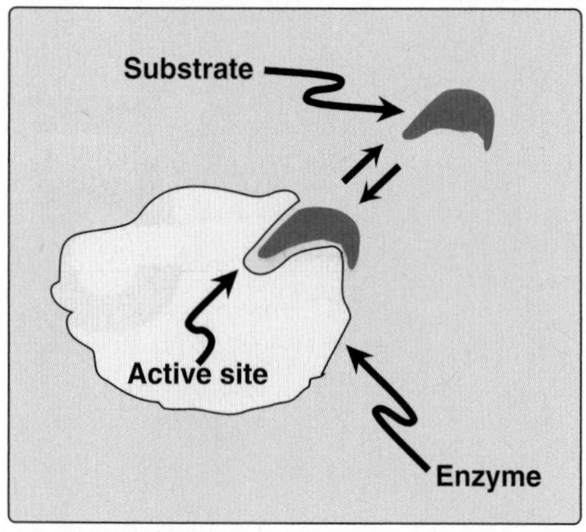

Figure 5.2
Schematic representation of an enzyme with one active site binding a substrate molecule.

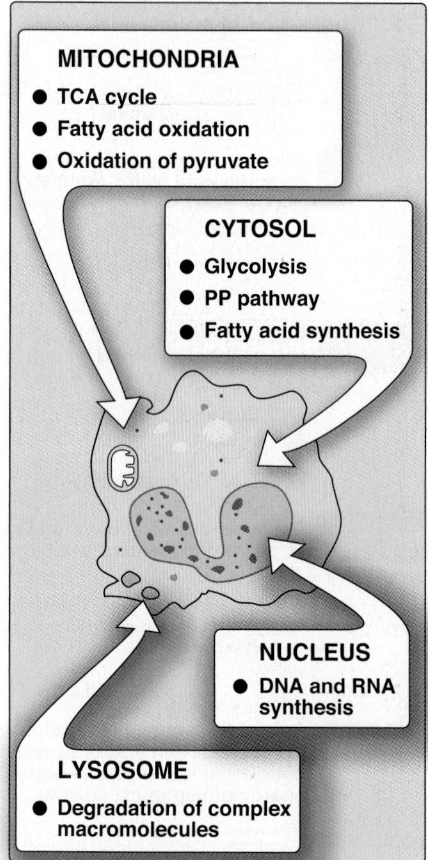

Figure 5.3
The intracellular location of some important biochemical pathways. TCA = tricarboxylic acid; PP = pentose phosphate.

> Potentially confusing enzyme nomenclature: *synthetase* (requires ATP), *synthase* (no ATP required); *phosphatase* (uses water to remove phosphoryl group), *phosphorylase* (uses P_i to break a bond and generate a phosphorylated product); *dehydrogenase* (NAD^+/FAD is an electron acceptor in a redox reaction), *oxidase* (O_2 is the acceptor, and oxygen atoms are not incorporated into substrate), *oxygenase* (one or both oxygen atoms are incorporated).

III. PROPERTIES

Enzymes are protein catalysts that increase the velocity of a chemical reaction and are not consumed during the reaction. [Note: Some RNAs can act like enzymes, usually catalyzing the cleavage and synthesis of phosphodiester bonds. RNAs with catalytic activity are called ribozymes (see p. 439) and are much less commonly encountered than protein catalysts.]

A. Active sites

Enzyme molecules contain a special pocket or cleft called the active site. The active site, formed by folding of the protein, contains amino acid side chains that participate in substrate binding and catalysis (Figure 5.2). The substrate binds the enzyme, forming an enzyme–substrate (ES) complex. Binding is thought to cause a conformational change in the enzyme (induced fit model) that allows catalysis. ES is converted to an enzyme–product (EP) complex that subsequently dissociates to enzyme and product.

B. Catalytic efficiency

Enzyme-catalyzed reactions are highly efficient, proceeding from 10^3–10^8 times faster than uncatalyzed reactions. The number of molecules of substrate converted to product per enzyme molecule per second is called the turnover number, or k_{cat}, and typically is 10^2–$10^4 s^{-1}$.

C. Specificity

Enzymes are highly specific, interacting with one or a few substrates and catalyzing only one type of chemical reaction. The set of enzymes made in a cell determines which reactions occur in that cell.

D. Holoenzymes, apoenzymes, cofactors, and coenzymes

Some enzymes require molecules other than proteins for enzymic activity. The term holoenzyme refers to the active enzyme with its nonprotein component, whereas the enzyme without its nonprotein moiety is termed an apoenzyme and is inactive. If the nonprotein moiety is a metal ion, such as Zn^{2+} or Fe^{2+}, it is called a cofactor. If it is a small organic molecule, it is termed a coenzyme. Coenzymes that only transiently associate with the enzyme are called cosubstrates. Cosubstrates dissociate from the enzyme in an altered state (NAD^+ is an example, see p. 101). If the coenzyme is permanently associated with the enzyme and returned to its original form, it is called a prosthetic group (FAD is an example, see p. 110).

Coenzymes commonly are derived from vitamins. For example, NAD^+ contains niacin, and FAD contains riboflavin (see Chapter 28).

E. Regulation

Enzyme activity can be regulated, that is, increased or decreased, so that the rate of product formation responds to cellular need.

F. Location within the cell

Many enzymes are localized in specific organelles within the cell (Figure 5.3). Such compartmentalization serves to isolate the reaction substrate or product from other competing reactions. This provides a favorable environment for the reaction and organizes the thousands of enzymes present in the cell into purposeful pathways.

IV. HOW ENZYMES WORK

The mechanism of enzyme action can be viewed from two different perspectives. The first treats catalysis in terms of energy changes that occur during the reaction. That is, enzymes provide an alternate, energetically favorable reaction pathway different from the uncatalyzed reaction. The second perspective describes how the active site chemically facilitates catalysis.

A. Energy changes occurring during the reaction

Virtually all chemical reactions have an energy barrier separating the reactants and the products. This barrier, called the free energy of activation, is the energy difference between that of the reactants and a high-energy intermediate that occurs during the formation of product. For example, Figure 5.4 shows the changes in energy during the conversion of a molecule of reactant A to product B as it proceeds through the transition state (high-energy intermediate), T*:

$$A \rightleftarrows T^* \rightleftarrows B$$

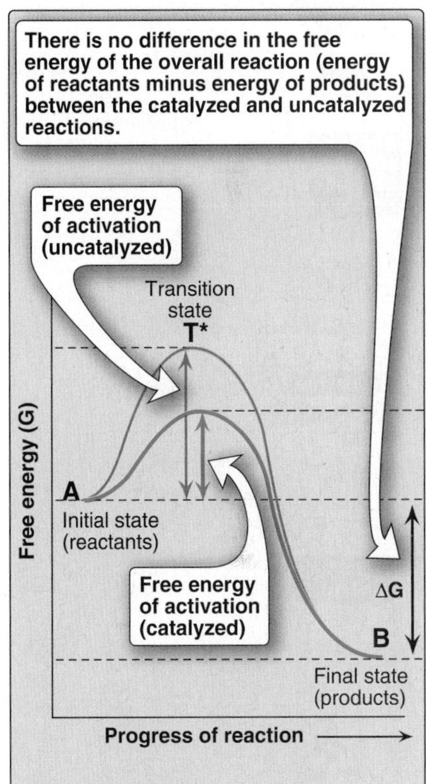

Figure 5.4
Effect of an enzyme on the activation energy of a reaction.

1. **Free energy of activation:** The peak of energy in Figure 5.4 is the difference in free energy between the reactant and T*, where the high-energy intermediate is formed during the conversion of reactant to product. Because of the high free energy of activation, the rates of uncatalyzed chemical reactions are often slow.

2. **Rate of reaction:** For molecules to react, they must contain sufficient energy to overcome the energy barrier of the transition state. In the absence of an enzyme, only a small proportion of a population of molecules may possess enough energy to achieve the transition state between reactant and product. The rate of reaction is determined by the number of such energized molecules. In general, the lower the free energy of activation, the more molecules have sufficient energy to pass through the transition state, and, therefore, the faster the rate of the reaction.

3. **Alternate reaction pathway:** An enzyme allows a reaction to proceed rapidly under conditions prevailing in the cell by providing an alternate reaction pathway with a lower free energy of activation (see Figure 5.4). The enzyme does not change the free energies of the reactants or products and, therefore, does not change the equilibrium of the reaction (see p. 70). It does, however, accelerate the rate by which equilibrium is reached.

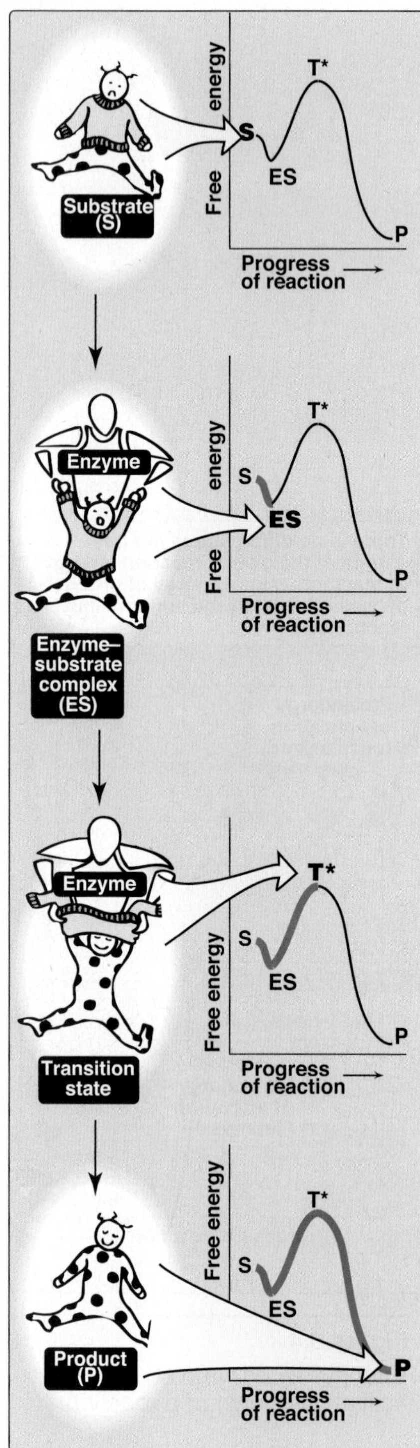

Figure 5.5
Schematic representation of energy changes accompanying formation of an enzyme–substrate complex and subsequent formation of a transition state.

B. Chemistry of the active site

The active site is not a passive receptacle for binding the substrate but, rather, is a complex molecular machine employing a diversity of chemical mechanisms to facilitate the conversion of substrate to product. A number of factors are responsible for the catalytic efficiency of enzymes, including the following examples.

1. **Transition-state stabilization:** The active site often acts as a flexible molecular template that binds the substrate and initiates its conversion to the transition state, a structure in which the bonds are not like those in the substrate or the product (see T* at the top of the curve in Figure 5.4). By stabilizing the transition state, the enzyme greatly increases the concentration of the reactive intermediate that can be converted to product and, thus, accelerates the reaction. [Note: The transition state cannot be isolated.]

2. **Other mechanisms:** The active site can provide catalytic groups that enhance the probability that the transition state is formed. In some enzymes, these groups can participate in general acid–base catalysis in which amino acid residues provide or accept protons. In other enzymes, catalysis may involve the transient formation of a covalent ES complex. [Note: The mechanism of action of *chymotrypsin*, an enzyme of protein digestion in the intestine, includes general base, general acid, and covalent catalysis. A histidine at the active site of the enzyme gains (general base) and loses (general acid) protons, mediated by the pK of histidine in proteins being close to physiologic pH. Serine at the active site forms a covalent link with the substrate.]

3. **Visualization of the transition state:** The enzyme-catalyzed conversion of substrate to product can be visualized as being similar to removing a sweater from an uncooperative infant (Figure 5.5). The process has a high energy of activation because the only reasonable strategy for removing the garment (short of ripping it off) requires that the random flailing of the baby results in both arms being fully extended over the head, an unlikely posture. However, we can envision a parent acting as an enzyme, first coming in contact with the baby (forming ES), then guiding the baby's arms into an extended, vertical position, analogous to the ES transition state. This posture (conformation) of the baby facilitates the removal of the sweater, forming the disrobed baby, which here represents product. [Note: The substrate bound to the enzyme (ES) is at a slightly lower energy than unbound substrate (S) and explains the small "dip" in the curve at ES.]

V. FACTORS AFFECTING REACTION VELOCITY

Enzymes can be isolated from cells and their properties studied in a test tube (that is, in vitro). Different enzymes show different responses to changes in substrate concentration, temperature, and pH. This section describes factors that influence the reaction velocity of enzymes. Enzymic responses to these factors give us valuable clues as to how enzymes function in living cells (that is, in vivo).

A. Substrate concentration

1. **Maximal velocity:** The rate or velocity of a reaction (v) is the number of substrate molecules converted to product per unit time. Velocity is usually expressed as µmol of product formed per minute. The rate of an enzyme-catalyzed reaction increases with substrate concentration until a maximal velocity (V_{max}) is reached (Figure 5.6). The leveling off of the reaction rate at high substrate concentrations reflects the saturation with substrate of all available binding sites on the enzyme molecules present.

2. **Hyperbolic shape of the enzyme kinetics curve:** Most enzymes show Michaelis-Menten kinetics (see p. 58), in which the plot of initial reaction velocity (v_o) against substrate concentration ([S]), is hyperbolic (similar in shape to that of the oxygen-dissociation curve of myoglobin, see p. 29). In contrast, allosteric enzymes do not follow Michaelis-Menton kinetics and show a sigmoidal curve (see p. 62) that is similar in shape to the oxygen-dissociation curve of hemoglobin (see p. 29).

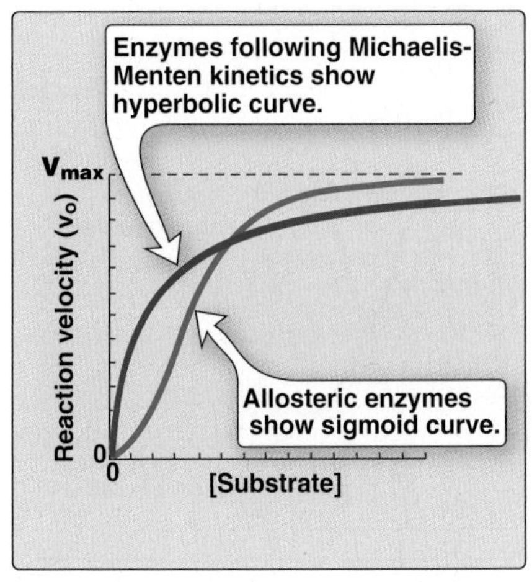

Figure 5.6
Effect of substrate concentration on reaction velocity.

B. Temperature

1. **Increase of velocity with temperature:** The reaction velocity increases with temperature until a peak velocity is reached (Figure 5.7). This increase is the result of the increased number of molecules having sufficient energy to pass over the energy barrier and form the products of the reaction.

2. **Decrease of velocity with higher temperature:** Further elevation of the temperature causes a decrease in reaction velocity as a result of temperature-induced denaturation of the enzyme (see Figure 5.7).

> The optimum temperature for most human enzymes is between 35°C and 40°C. Human enzymes start to denature at temperatures above 40°C, but thermophilic bacteria found in the hot springs have optimum temperatures of 70°C.

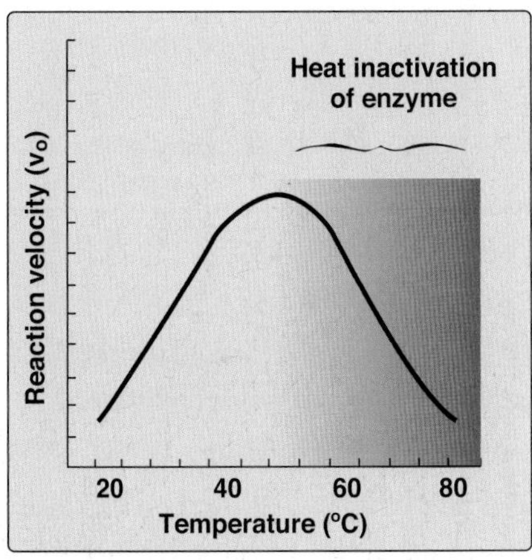

Figure 5.7
Effect of temperature on an enzyme-catalyzed reaction.

C. pH

1. **Effect of pH on the ionization of the active site:** The concentration of protons (H^+) affects reaction velocity in several ways. First, the catalytic process usually requires that the enzyme and substrate have specific chemical groups in either an ionized or un-ionized state in order to interact. For example, catalytic activity may require that an amino group of the enzyme be in the protonated form ($-NH_3^+$). At alkaline pH, this group is deprotonated, and the rate of the reaction, therefore, declines.

2. **Effect of pH on enzyme denaturation:** Extremes of pH can also lead to denaturation of the enzyme, because the structure of the catalytically active protein molecule depends on the ionic character of the amino acid side chains.

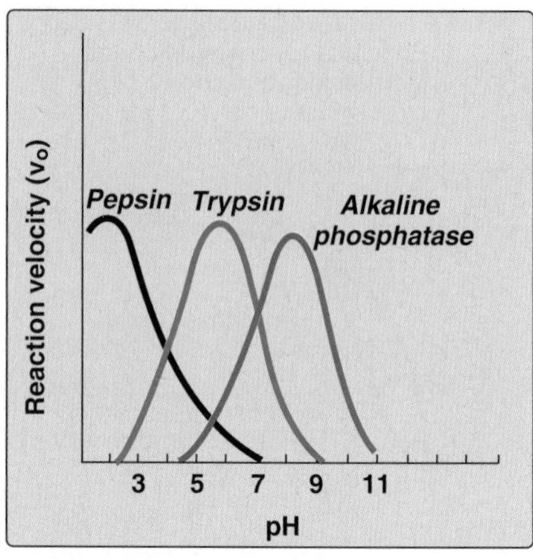

Figure 5.8
Effect of pH on enzyme-catalyzed reactions.

3. **Variable pH optimum:** The pH at which maximal enzyme activity is achieved is different for different enzymes and often reflects the [H^+] at which the enzyme functions in the body. For example, *pepsin*, a digestive enzyme in the stomach, is maximally active at pH 2, whereas other enzymes, designed to work at neutral pH, are denatured by such an acidic environment (Figure 5.8).

VI. MICHAELIS-MENTEN KINETICS

A. Reaction model

Leonor Michaelis and Maude Menten proposed a simple model that accounts for most of the features of enzyme-catalyzed reactions. In this model, the enzyme reversibly combines with its substrate to form an ES complex that subsequently yields product, regenerating the free enzyme. The model, involving one substrate molecule, is represented below:

$$E + S \underset{k_{-1}}{\overset{k_1}{\rightleftharpoons}} ES \xrightarrow{k_2} E + P$$

where S is the substrate
E is the enzyme
ES is the enzyme–substrate complex
P is the product
k_1, k_{-1}, and k_2 are rate constants

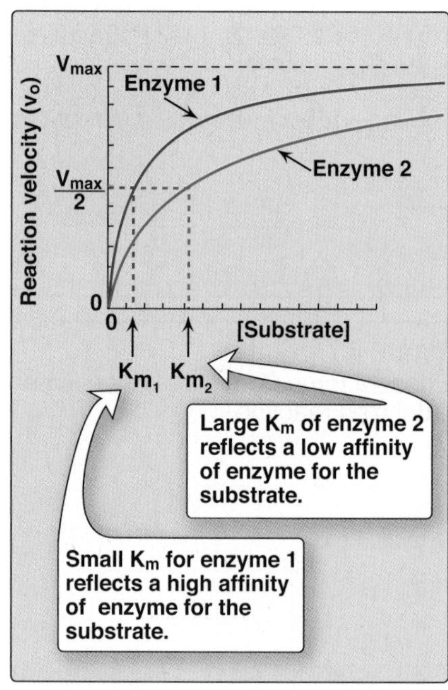

Figure 5.9
Effect of substrate concentration on reaction velocities for two enzymes: enzyme 1 with a small Michaelis constant (K_m) and enzyme 2 with a large K_m. V_{max} = maximal velocity.

B. Michaelis-Menten equation

The Michaelis-Menten equation describes how reaction velocity varies with substrate concentration:

$$v_o = \frac{V_{max}\,[S]}{K_m + [S]}$$

where V_o = initial reaction velocity
V_{max} = maximal velocity
K_m = Michaelis constant = $(k_{-1} + k_2)/k_1$
[S] = substrate concentration

The following assumptions are made in deriving the Michaelis-Menten rate equation:

1. **Relative concentrations of enzyme and substrate:** The concentration of substrate ([S]) is much greater than the concentration of enzyme ([E]), so that the percentage of total substrate bound by the enzyme at any one time is small.

2. **Steady-state assumption:** [ES] does not change with time (the steady-state assumption), that is, the rate of formation of ES is equal to that of the breakdown of ES (to E + S and to E + P). In general, an intermediate in a series of reactions is said to be in steady state when its rate of synthesis is equal to its rate of degradation.

3. **Initial velocity:** Initial reaction velocities (v_o) are used in the analysis of enzyme reactions. This means that the rate of the reaction is measured as soon as enzyme and substrate are mixed. At that time, the concentration of product is very small, and, therefore, the rate of the back reaction from product to substrate can be ignored.

C. Important conclusions

1. **Characteristics of K_m:** K_m, the Michaelis constant, is characteristic of an enzyme and its particular substrate and reflects the affinity of the enzyme for that substrate. K_m is numerically equal to the substrate concentration at which the reaction velocity is equal to $\frac{1}{2}V_{max}$. K_m does not vary with enzyme concentration.

   a. **Small K_m:** A numerically small (low) K_m reflects a high affinity of the enzyme for substrate, because a low concentration of substrate is needed to half-saturate the enzyme—that is, to reach a velocity that is $\frac{1}{2}V_{max}$ (Figure 5.9).

   b. **Large K_m:** A numerically large (high) K_m reflects a low affinity of enzyme for substrate because a high concentration of substrate is needed to half-saturate the enzyme.

2. **Relationship of velocity to enzyme concentration:** The rate of the reaction is directly proportional to the enzyme concentration at all substrate concentrations. For example, if the enzyme concentration is halved, the initial rate of the reaction (v_o), as well as that of V_{max}, are reduced to half that of the original.

3. **Order of reaction:** When [S] is much less than K_m, the velocity of the reaction is approximately proportional to the substrate concentration (Figure 5.10). The rate of reaction is then said to be first order with respect to substrate. When [S] is much greater than K_m, the velocity is constant and equal to V_{max}. The rate of reaction is then independent of substrate concentration (the enzyme is saturated with substrate) and is said to be zero order with respect to substrate concentration (see Figure 5.10).

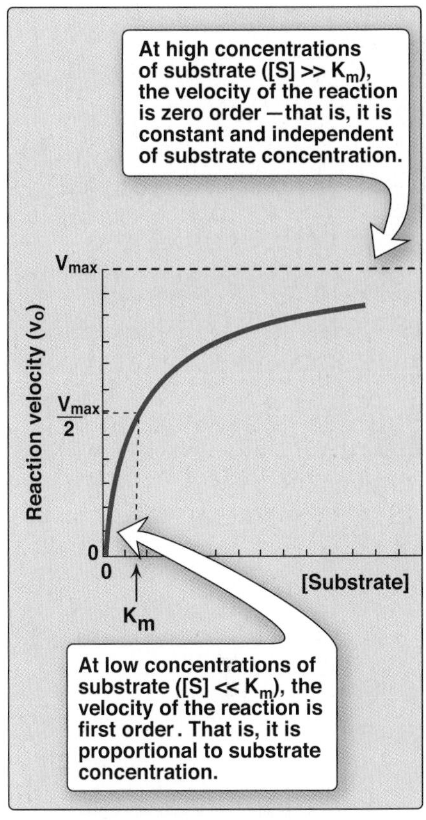

Figure 5.10
Effect of substrate concentration on reaction velocity for an enzyme-catalyzed reaction. V_{max} = maximal velocity; K_m = Michaelis constant.

D. Lineweaver-Burk plot

When v_o is plotted against [S], it is not always possible to determine when V_{max} has been achieved because of the gradual upward slope of the hyperbolic curve at high substrate concentrations. However, if $1/v_o$ is plotted versus 1/[S], a straight line is obtained (Figure 5.11). This plot, the Lineweaver-Burk plot (also called a double-reciprocal plot) can be used to calculate K_m and V_{max} as well as to determine the mechanism of action of enzyme inhibitors.

1. The equation describing the Lineweaver-Burk plot is:

$$\frac{1}{v_o} = \frac{K_m}{V_{max}[S]} + \frac{1}{V_{max}}$$

where the intercept on the x axis is equal to $-1/K_m$, and the intercept on the y axis is equal to $1/V_{max}$. [Note: The slope = K_m/V_{max}.]

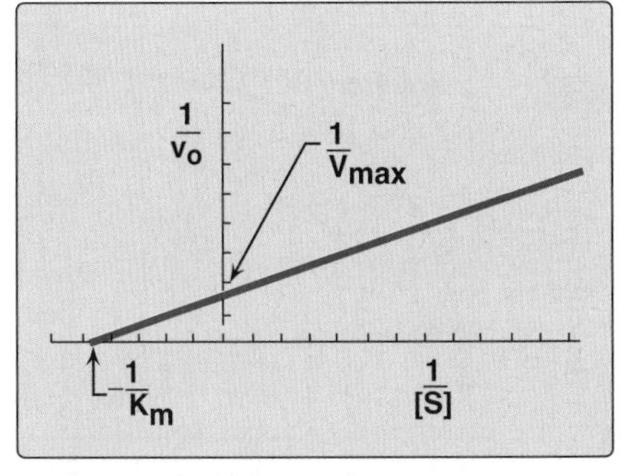

Figure 5.11
Lineweaver-Burk plot. v_o = reaction velocity; V_{max} = maximal velocity; K_m = Michaelis constant; [S] = substrate concentration.

VII. INHIBITION OF ENZYME ACTIVITY

Any substance that can decrease the velocity of an enzyme-catalyzed reaction is called an inhibitor. Inhibitors can be reversible or irreversible. Irreversible inhibitors bind to enzymes through covalent bonds. Lead, for example, forms covalent bonds with the sulfhydryl side chain of cysteine in proteins. *Ferrochelatase*, an enzyme involved in heme synthesis (see p. 279), is irreversibly inhibited by lead. [Note: An important group of irreversible inhibitors are the mechanism-based inhibitors that are converted by the enzyme itself to a form that covalently links to the enzyme, thereby inhibiting it. They also are referred to as "suicide" inhibitors.] Reversible inhibitors bind to enzymes through noncovalent bonds and, thus, dilution of the enzyme–inhibitor complex results in dissociation of the reversibly bound inhibitor and recovery of enzyme activity. The two most commonly encountered types of reversible inhibition are competitive and noncompetitive.

A. Competitive inhibition

This type of inhibition occurs when the inhibitor binds reversibly to the same site that the substrate would normally occupy and, therefore, competes with the substrate for that site.

1. **Effect on V_{max}:** The effect of a competitive inhibitor is reversed by increasing [S]. At a sufficiently high substrate concentration, the reaction velocity reaches the V_{max} observed in the absence of inhibitor (Figure 5.12).

2. **Effect on K_m:** A competitive inhibitor increases the apparent K_m for a given substrate. This means that, in the presence of a competitive inhibitor, more substrate is needed to achieve $\frac{1}{2}V_{max}$.

3. **Effect on the Lineweaver-Burk plot:** Competitive inhibition shows a characteristic Lineweaver-Burk plot in which the plots of the inhibited

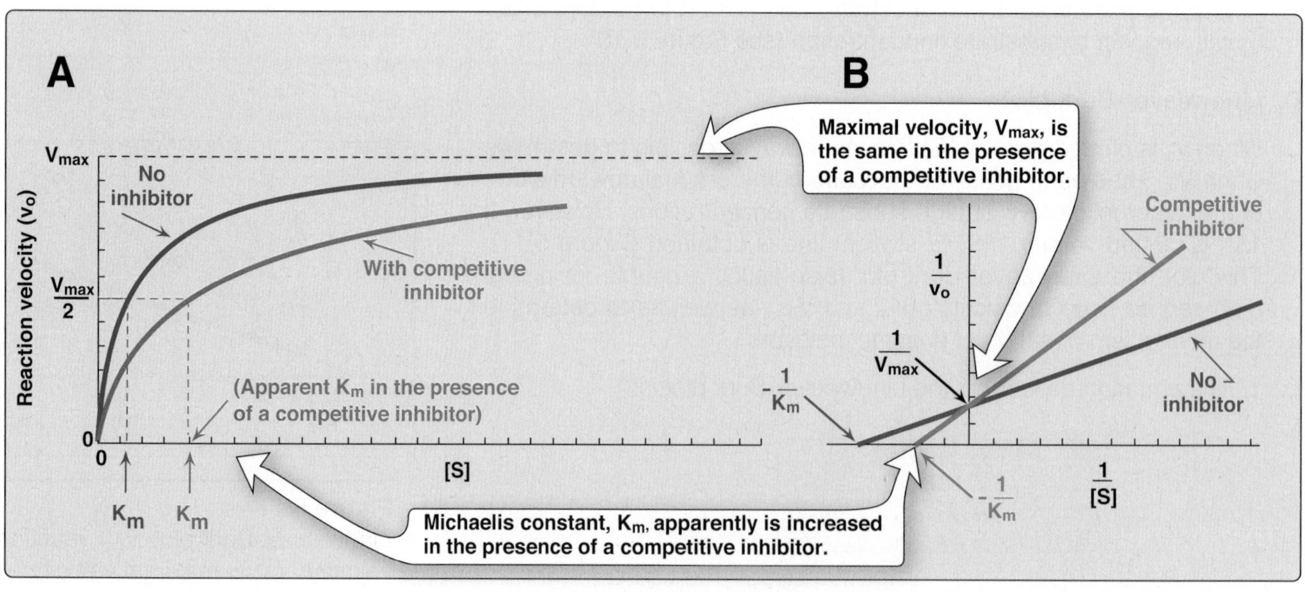

Figure 5.12
A. Effect of a competitive inhibitor on the reaction velocity versus substrate ([S]) plot. B. Lineweaver-Burk plot of competitive inhibition of an enzyme.

and uninhibited reactions intersect on the y axis at $1/V_{max}$ (V_{max} is unchanged). The inhibited and uninhibited reactions show different x-axis intercepts, indicating that the apparent K_m is increased in the presence of the competitive inhibitor because $-1/K_m$ moves closer to zero from a negative value (see Figure 5.12). [Note: An important group of competitive inhibitors are the transition state analogs, stable molecules that approximate the structure of the transition state and, therefore, bind the enzyme with a higher affinity than the substrate.]

4. **Statin drugs as examples of competitive inhibitors:** This group of antihyperlipidemic agents competitively inhibits the rate-limiting (slowest) step in cholesterol biosynthesis. This reaction is catalyzed by *hydroxymethylglutaryl–CoA reductase* (*HMG-CoA reductase*, see p. 220). Statins, such as atorvastatin (Lipitor) and pravastatin (Pravachol), are structural analogs of the natural substrate for this enzyme and compete effectively to inhibit *HMG-CoA reductase*. By doing so, they inhibit de novo cholesterol synthesis, thereby lowering plasma cholesterol levels (Figure 5.13).

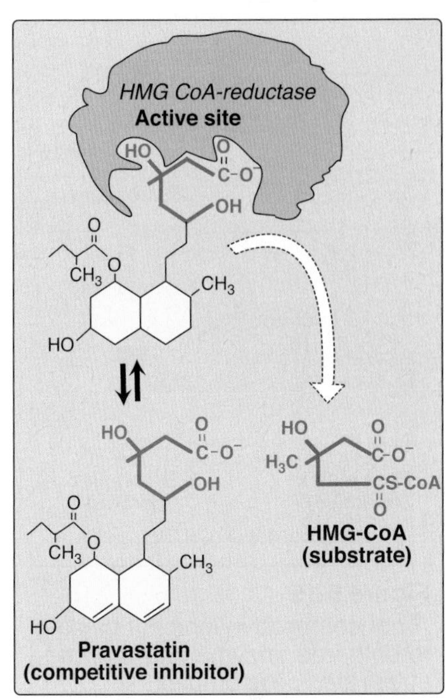

Figure 5.13
Pravastatin competes with HMG-CoA for the active site of *HMG-CoA reductase*. HMG-CoA = hydroxymethylglutaryl–coenzyme A.

B. Noncompetitive inhibition

This type of inhibition is recognized by its characteristic effect on V_{max} (Figure 5.14). Noncompetitive inhibition occurs when the inhibitor and substrate bind at different sites on the enzyme. The noncompetitive inhibitor can bind either free enzyme or the enzyme-substrate complex, thereby preventing the reaction from occurring (Figure 5.15).

1. **Effect on V_{max}:** Noncompetitive inhibition cannot be overcome by increasing the concentration of substrate. Therefore, noncompetitive inhibitors decrease the apparent V_{max} of the reaction.

2. **Effect on K_m:** Noncompetitive inhibitors do not interfere with the binding of substrate to enzyme. Therefore, the enzyme shows the same K_m in the presence or absence of the noncompetitive inhibitor.

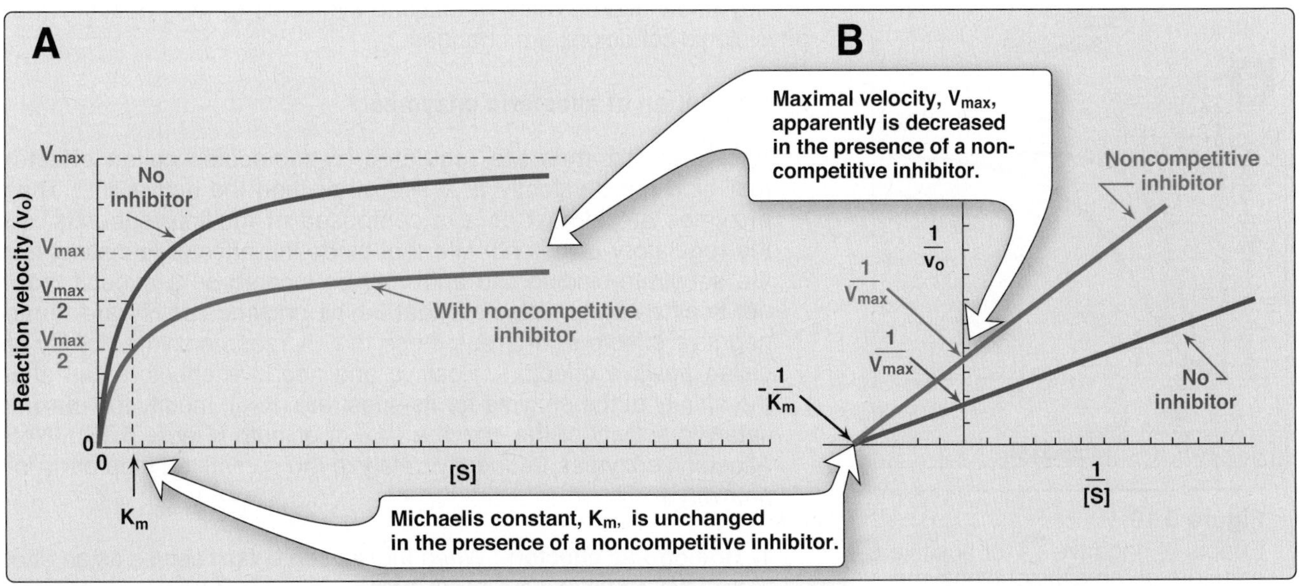

Figure 5.14
A. Effect of a noncompetitive inhibitor on the reaction velocity versus substrate ([S]) plot. B. Lineweaver-Burk plot of noncompetitive inhibition of an enzyme.

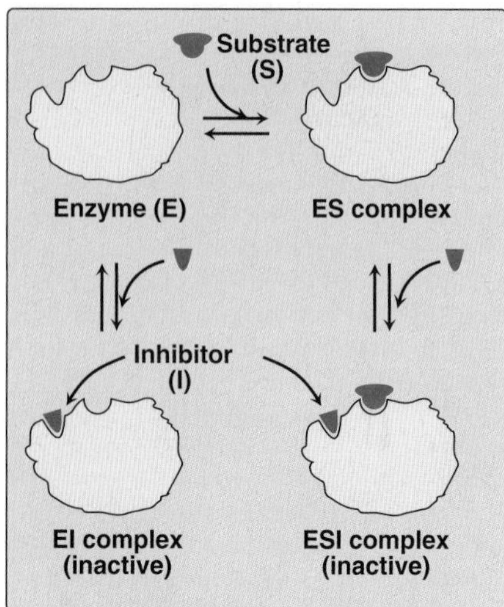

Figure 5.15
A noncompetitive inhibitor binding to both free enzyme and enzyme–substrate (ES) complex.

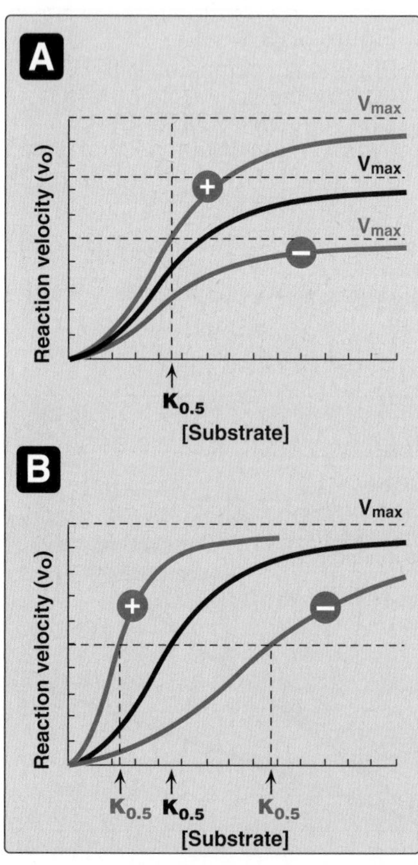

Figure 5.16
Effects of negative ⊖ or positive ⊕ effectors on an allosteric enzyme. A. V_{max} is altered. B. The substrate concentration that gives half-maximal velocity ($K_{0.5}$) is altered.

3. **Effect on Lineweaver-Burk plot:** Noncompetitive inhibition is readily differentiated from competitive inhibition by plotting $1/v_o$ versus 1/[S] and noting that the apparent V_{max} decreases in the presence of a noncompetitive inhibitor, whereas K_m is unchanged (see Figure 5.14). [Note: Oxypurinol, a metabolite of the drug allopurinol, is a noncompetitive inhibitor of *xanthine oxidase*, an enzyme of purine degradation (see p. 301).]

C. Enzyme inhibitors as drugs

At least half of the ten most commonly prescribed drugs in the United States act as enzyme inhibitors. For example, the widely prescribed β-lactam antibiotics, such as penicillin and amoxicillin, act by inhibiting enzymes involved in bacterial cell wall synthesis. Drugs may also act by inhibiting extracellular reactions. This is illustrated by *angiotensin-converting enzyme* (*ACE*) inhibitors. They lower blood pressure by blocking the enzyme that cleaves angiotensin I to form the potent vasoconstrictor, angiotensin II. These drugs, which include captopril, enalapril, and lisinopril, cause vasodilation and, therefore, a reduction in blood pressure. Aspirin, a nonprescription drug, irreversibly inhibits prostaglandin and thromboxane synthesis (see p. 214).

VIII. REGULATION OF ENZYME ACTIVITY

The regulation of the reaction velocity of enzymes is essential if an organism is to coordinate its numerous metabolic processes. The rates of most enzymes are responsive to changes in substrate concentration, because the intracellular level of many substrates is in the range of the K_m. Thus, an increase in substrate concentration prompts an increase in reaction rate, which tends to return the concentration of substrate toward normal. In addition, some enzymes with specialized regulatory functions respond to allosteric effectors and/or covalent modification or they show altered rates of enzyme synthesis (or degradation) when physiologic conditions are changed.

A. Regulation of allosteric enzymes

Allosteric enzymes are regulated by molecules called effectors that bind noncovalently at a site other than the active site. These enzymes are almost always composed of multiple subunits, and the regulatory (allosteric) site that binds the effector is distinct from the substrate-binding site and may be located on a subunit that is not itself catalytic. Effectors that inhibit enzyme activity are termed negative effectors, whereas those that increase enzyme activity are called positive effectors. Positive and negative effectors can affect the affinity of the enzyme for its substrate ($K_{0.5}$), modify the maximal catalytic activity of the enzyme (V_{max}), or both (Figure 5.16). [Note: Allosteric enzymes frequently catalyze the committed step early in a pathway.]

1. **Homotropic effectors:** When the substrate itself serves as an effector, the effect is said to be homotropic. Most often, an allosteric substrate functions as a positive effector. In such a case, the pres-

ence of a substrate molecule at one site on the enzyme enhances the catalytic properties of the other substrate-binding sites. That is, their binding sites exhibit cooperativity. These enzymes show a sigmoidal curve when reaction velocity (v_o) is plotted against substrate concentration ([S]), as shown in Figure 5.16. This contrasts with the hyperbolic curve characteristic of enzymes following Michaelis-Menten kinetics, as previously discussed. [Note: The concept of cooperativity of substrate binding is analogous to the binding of oxygen to hemoglobin (see p. 29).]

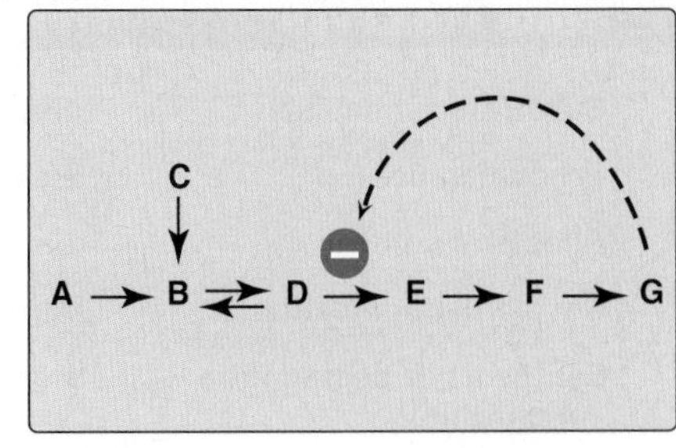

Figure 5.17
Feedback inhibition of a metabolic pathway.

2. **Heterotropic effectors:** The effector may be different from the substrate, in which case the effect is said to be heterotropic. For example, consider the feedback inhibition shown in Figure 5.17. The enzyme that converts D to E has an allosteric site that binds the endproduct, G. If the concentration of G increases (for example, because it is not used as rapidly as it is synthesized), the first irreversible step unique to the pathway is typically inhibited. Feedback inhibition provides the cell with appropriate amounts of a product it needs by regulating the flow of substrate molecules through the pathway that synthesizes that product. Heterotropic effectors are commonly encountered. For example, the glycolytic enzyme *phosphofructokinase-1* is allosterically inhibited by citrate, which is not a substrate for the enzyme (see p. 99).

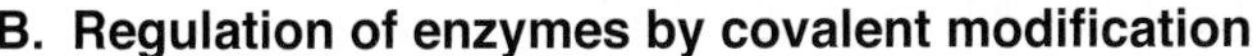

B. Regulation of enzymes by covalent modification

Many enzymes are regulated by covalent modification, most often by the addition or removal of phosphate groups from specific serine, threonine, or tyrosine residues of the enzyme. Protein phosphorylation is recognized as one of the primary ways in which cellular processes are regulated. [Note: Protein phosphorylation is mediated by hormonal signals (see p. 132).]

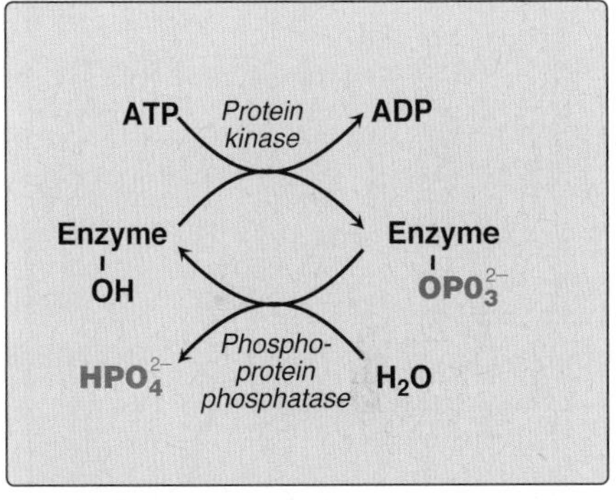

Figure 5.18
Covalent modification by the addition and removal of phosphate groups. [Note: HPO_4^{2-} may be represented as P_i.]

1. **Phosphorylation and dephosphorylation:** Phosphorylation reactions are catalyzed by a family of enzymes called *protein kinases* that use ATP as the phosphate donor. Phosphate groups are cleaved from phosphorylated enzymes by the action of *phosphoprotein phosphatases* (Figure 5.18).

2. **Response of enzyme to phosphorylation:** Depending on the specific enzyme, the phosphorylated form may be more or less active than the unphosphorylated enzyme. For example, phosphorylation of *glycogen phosphorylase* (an enzyme that degrades glycogen) increases activity, whereas phosphorylation of *glycogen synthase* (an enzyme that synthesizes glycogen) decreases activity (p. 132).

C. Induction and repression of enzyme synthesis

The regulatory mechanisms described above modify the activity of existing enzyme molecules. However, cells can also regulate the amount of enzyme present by altering the rate of enzyme degradation or, more typically, the rate of enzyme synthesis. The increase (induction) or decrease (repression) of enzyme synthesis leads to an alteration in the total population of active sites. Enzymes subject to

REGULATOR EVENT	TYPICAL EFFECTOR	RESULTS	TIME REQUIRED FOR CHANGE
Substrate availability	Substrate	Change in velocity (v_o)	Immediate
Product inhibition	Reaction product	Change in V_{max} and/or K_m	Immediate
Allosteric control	Pathway end product	Change in V_{max} and/or $K_{0.5}$	Immediate
Covalent modification	Another enzyme	Change in V_{max} and/or K_m	Immediate to minutes
Synthesis or degradation of enzyme	Hormone or metabolite	Change in the amount of enzyme	Hours to days

Figure 5.19
Mechanisms for regulating enzyme activity. [Note: Inhibition by pathway end product is also referred to as feedback inhibition.]

regulation of synthesis are often those that are needed at only one stage of development or under selected physiologic conditions. For example, elevated levels of insulin as a result of high blood glucose levels cause an increase in the synthesis of key enzymes involved in glucose metabolism (see p. 105). In contrast, enzymes that are in constant use are usually not regulated by altering the rate of enzyme synthesis. Alterations in enzyme levels as a result of induction or repression of protein synthesis are slow (hours to days), compared with allosterically or covalently regulated changes in enzyme activity, which occur in seconds to minutes. Figure 5.19 summarizes the common ways that enzyme activity is regulated.

IX. ENZYMES IN CLINICAL DIAGNOSIS

Plasma enzymes can be classified into two major groups. First, a relatively small group of enzymes are actively secreted into the blood by certain cell types. For example, the liver secretes zymogens (inactive precursors) of the enzymes involved in blood coagulation. Second, a large number of enzyme species are released from cells during normal cell turnover. These enzymes almost always function intracellularly and have no physiologic use in the plasma. In healthy individuals, the levels of these enzymes are fairly constant and represent a steady state in which the rate of release from damaged cells into the plasma is balanced by an equal rate of removal from the plasma. Increased plasma levels of these enzymes may indicate tissue damage (Figure 5.20).

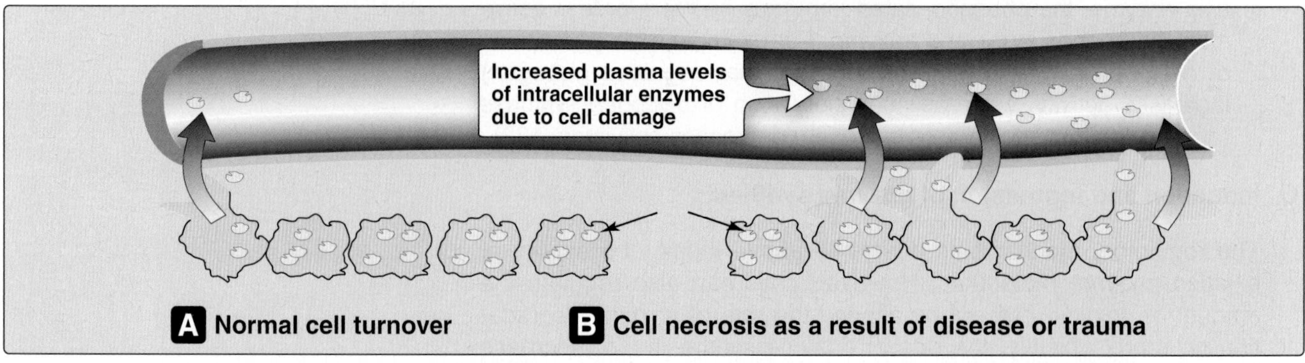

Figure 5.20
Release of enzymes from normal and diseased or traumatized cells.

> Plasma is the fluid, noncellular part of blood. Laboratory assays of enzyme activity most often use serum, which is obtained by centrifugation of whole blood after it has been allowed to coagulate. Plasma is a physiologic fluid, whereas serum is prepared in the laboratory.

A. Alteration of plasma enzyme levels in disease states

Many diseases that cause tissue damage result in an increased release of intracellular enzymes into the plasma. The activities of many of these enzymes are routinely determined for diagnostic purposes in diseases of the heart, liver, skeletal muscle, and other tissues. The level of specific enzyme activity in the plasma frequently correlates with the extent of tissue damage. Therefore, determining the degree of elevation of a particular enzyme activity in the plasma is often useful in evaluating the prognosis for the patient.

B. Plasma enzymes as diagnostic tools

Some enzymes show relatively high activity in only one or a few tissues. The presence of increased levels of these enzymes in plasma thus reflects damage to the corresponding tissue. For example, the enzyme *alanine aminotransferase* ([*ALT*] see p. 251) is abundant in the liver. The appearance of elevated levels of *ALT* in plasma signals possible damage to hepatic tissue. [Note: Measurement of *ALT* is part of the liver function test panel.] Increases in plasma levels of enzymes with a wide tissue distribution provide a less specific indication of the site of cellular injury and limits their diagnostic value.

C. Isoenzymes and diseases of the heart

Isoenzymes (also called isozymes) are enzymes that catalyze the same reaction. However, they do not necessarily have the same physical properties because of genetically determined differences in amino acid sequence. For this reason, isoenzymes may contain different numbers of charged amino acids and may, therefore, be separated from each other by electrophoresis (Figure 5.21). Different organs commonly contain characteristic proportions of different isoenzymes. The pattern of isoenzymes found in the plasma may, therefore, serve as a means of identifying the site of tissue damage. For example, the plasma levels of *creatine kinase* (*CK*) are commonly determined in the diagnosis of myocardial infarction. They are particularly useful when the electrocardiogram is difficult to interpret such as when there have been previous episodes of heart disease.

1. **Quaternary structure of isoenzymes:** Many isoenzymes contain different subunits in various combinations. For example, *CK* occurs as three isoenzymes. Each isoenzyme is a dimer composed of two polypeptides (called B and M subunits) associated in one of three combinations: *CK1* = BB, *CK2* = MB, and *CK3* = MM. Each *CK* isoenzyme shows a characteristic electrophoretic mobility (see Figure 5.21). [Note: Virtually all *CK* in the brain is the BB isoform, whereas in skeletal muscle it is MM. In cardiac muscle, about one third is MB with the rest as MM.]

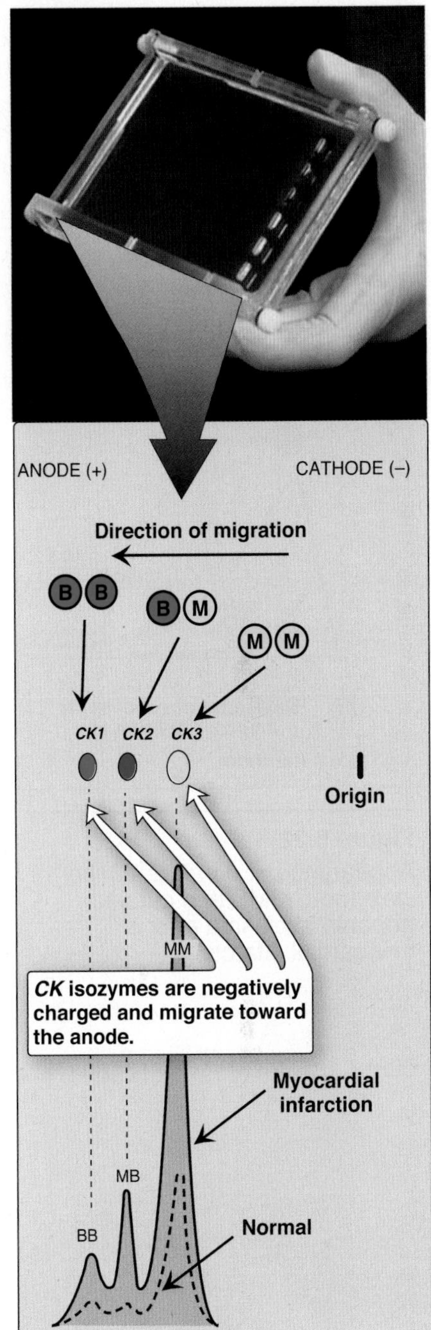

Figure 5.21
Subunit composition, electrophoretic mobility, and enzyme activity of *creatine kinase* (*CK*) isoenzymes.

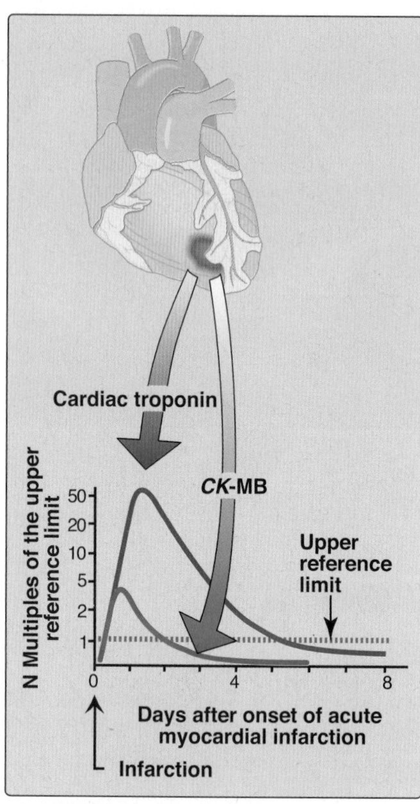

Figure 5.22
Appearance of *creatine kinase* isozyme *CK*-MB and cardiac troponin in plasma after a myocardial infarction.

2. **Diagnosis of myocardial infarction:** Measurement of blood levels of proteins with cardiac specificity (biomarkers) is used in the diagnosis of myocardial infarction (MI). Myocardial muscle is the only tissue that contains more than 5% of the total *CK* activity as the *CK2* (MB) isoenzyme. Appearance of this hybrid isoenzyme in plasma is virtually specific for infarction of the myocardium. Following an acute MI, *CK2* appears approximately 4–8 hours following onset of chest pain, reaches a peak of activity at approximately 24 hours, and returns to baseline after 48–72 hours (Figure 5.22). Troponin T and troponin I are regulatory proteins involved in myocardial contractility. They, too, are released into the plasma in response to cardiac damage. Cardiac troponin I (cTnI) is highly sensitive and specific for damage to cardiac tissue. cTnI appears in plasma within 4–6 hours after an MI, peaks in 8–28 hours, and remains elevated for 3–10 days. Elevated cTns, in combination with the clinical presentation and characteristic changes in the electrocardiogram, are currently considered the "gold standard" in the diagnosis of a MI.

X. CHAPTER SUMMARY

Enzymes are **protein catalysts** that increase the velocity of a chemical reaction by lowering the energy of the transition state (Figure 5.23). Enzymes are not consumed during the reaction they catalyze. Enzyme molecules contain a special pocket or cleft called the **active site**. The active site contains amino acid side chains that participate in substrate binding and catalysis. The active site binds the substrate, forming an **enzyme–substrate (ES) complex**. Binding is thought to cause a conformational change in the enzyme (induced fit) that allows catalysis. ES is converted to enzyme-product (EP), which subsequently dissociates to enzyme and product. An enzyme allows a reaction to proceed rapidly under conditions prevailing in the cell by providing an **alternate reaction pathway** with a **lower free energy of activation**. The enzyme does not change the free energies of the reactants or products and, therefore, does not change the equilibrium of the reaction. Most enzymes show **Michaelis-Menten kinetics**, and a plot of the **initial reaction velocity** (**v_o**) against **substrate concentration** (**[S]**) has a **hyperbolic** shape similar to the oxygen-dissociation curve of myoglobin. Any substance that can diminish the velocity of such enzyme-catalyzed reactions is called an inhibitor. The two most commonly encountered types of reversible inhibition are **competitive** (which **increases** the **apparent K_m**) and **noncompetitive** (which **decreases** the **apparent V_{max}**). In contrast, the **multisubunit allosteric enzymes** frequently show a **sigmoidal curve** similar in shape to the oxygen-dissociation curve of hemoglobin. They typically catalyze the **rate-limiting** (slowest step) of a pathway. Allosteric enzymes are regulated by molecules called **effectors** that bind noncovalently at a site other than the active site. Effectors can be either **positive** (accelerate the enzyme-catalyzed reaction) or **negative** (slow down the reaction). An allosteric effector can alter the affinity of the enzyme for its substrate, modify the maximal catalytic activity of the enzyme, or both. Enzymes can also be regulated by covalent modification and by changes in the rate of synthesis or degradation. Enzymes have diagnostic and therapeutic value in medicine.

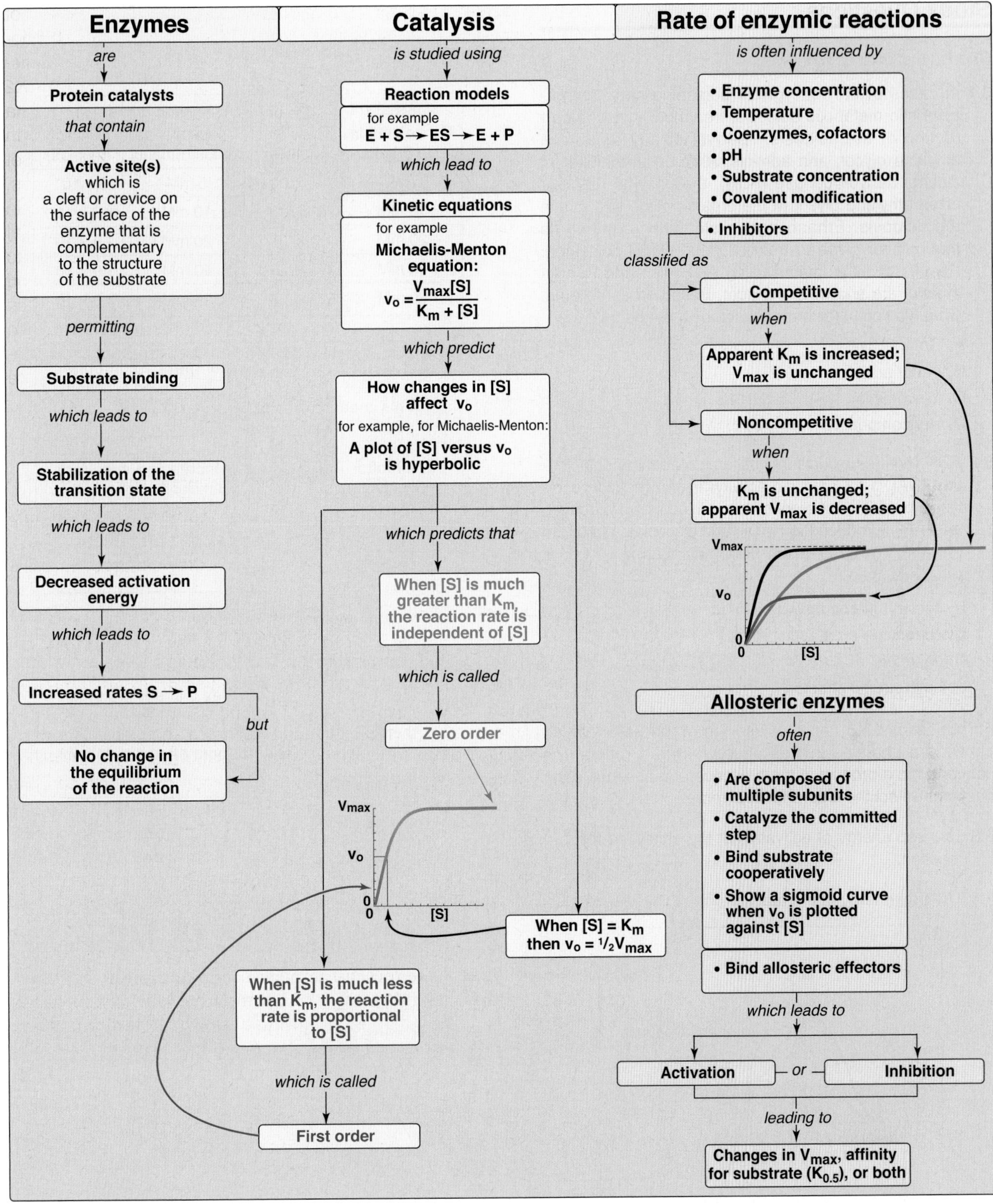

Figure 5.23
Key concept map for the enzymes. S = substrate; [S] = substrate concentration; P = product; E = enzyme; v_o = initial velocity; V_{max} = maximal velocity; K_m = Michaelis constant; $K_{0.5}$ = substrate concentration which gives half maximal velocity.

Study Questions

Choose the ONE best answer.

5.1 In cases of ethylene glycol poisoning and its characteristic metabolic acidosis, treatment involves correction of the acidosis, removal of any remaining ethylene glycol, and administration of an inhibitor of alcohol dehydrogenase (ADH), the enzyme that oxidizes ethylene glycol to the organic acids that cause the acidosis. Ethanol (grain alcohol) frequently is the inhibitor given to treat ethylene glycol poisoning. Results of experiments using ADH with and without ethanol are shown to the right. Based on these data, what type of inhibition is caused by the ethanol?

A. Competitive
B. Feedback
C. Irreversible
D. Noncompetitive

Substrate Concentration with Ethanol	Rate of Reaction (mol/L/s)	Substrate Concentration without Ethanol	Rate of Reaction (mol/L/s)
5 mM	3×10^{-7}	5 mM	8×10^{-7}
10 mM	5×10^{-7}	10 mM	1.2×10^{-6}
20 mM	1.0×10^{-6}	20 mM	1.8×10^{-6}
40 mM	1.6×10^{-6}	40 mM	1.9×10^{-6}
80 mM	2.0×10^{-6}	80 mM	2.0×10^{-6}

Correct answer = A competitive inhibitor increases the apparent K_m for a given substrate. This means that, in the presence of a competitive inhibitor, more substrate is needed to achieve $\frac{1}{2}$ V_{max}. The effect of a competitive inhibitor is reversed by increasing substrate concentration ([S]). At a sufficiently high [S], the reaction velocity reaches the V_{max} observed in the absence of inhibitor.

5.2 ADH requires oxidized nicotinamide adenine dinucleotide (NAD^+) for catalytic activity. In the reaction catalyzed by ADH, an alcohol is oxidized to an aldehyde as NAD^+ is reduced to NADH and dissociates from the enzyme. The NAD^+ is functioning as a (an):

A. apoenzyme.
B. coenzyme-cosubstrate.
C. coenzyme-prosthetic group.
D. cofactor.
E. heterotropic effector.

Correct answer = B. Coenzymes-cosubstrates are small organic molecules that associate transiently with an enzyme and leave the enzyme in a changed form. Coenzyme-prosthetic groups are small organic molecules that associate permanently with an enzyme and are returned to their original form on the enzyme. Cofactors are metal ions. Heterotropic effectors are not substrates.

For Questions 5.3 and 5.4, use the graph below which shows the changes in free energy when a reactant is converted to a product in the presence and absence of an enzyme. Select the letter that best represents:

5.3 The free energy of activation of the catalyzed forward reaction.

5.4 The free energy of the reaction.

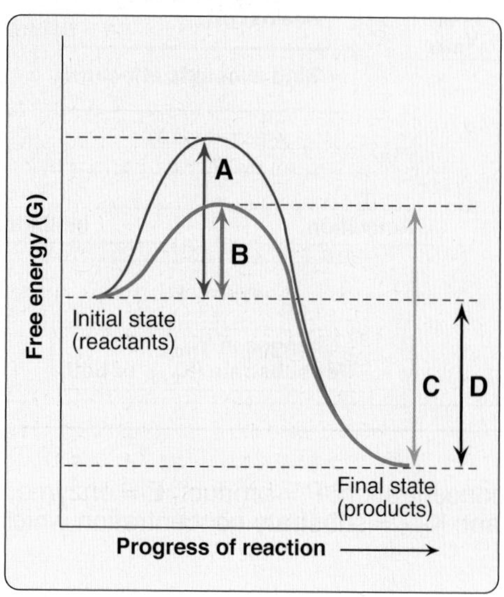

Correct answers = B; D. Enzymes (biocatalysts) provide an alternate reaction pathway with a lower free energy of activation. However, they do not change the free energy of the reactant or product. A is the free energy of the uncatalyzed reaction. C is the free energy of the catalyzed reverse reaction.

UNIT II:
Bioenergetics and Carbohydrate Metabolism

Bioenergetics and Oxidative Phosphorylation

6

I. OVERVIEW

Bioenergetics describes the transfer and utilization of energy in biologic systems. It makes use of a few basic ideas from the field of thermodynamics, particularly the concept of free energy. Changes in free energy provide a measure of the energetic feasibility of a chemical reaction and can, therefore, allow prediction of whether a reaction or process can take place. Bioenergetics concerns only the initial and final energy states of reaction components, not the mechanism or how much time is needed for the chemical change to take place (the rate). In short, bioenergetics predicts if a process is possible, whereas kinetics measures how fast the reaction occurs (see p. 54).

II. FREE ENERGY

The direction and extent to which a chemical reaction proceeds is determined by the degree to which two factors change during the reaction. These are enthalpy (ΔH, a measure of the change in heat content of the reactants and products) and entropy (ΔS, a measure of the change in randomness or disorder of reactants and products; Figure 6.1). Neither of these thermodynamic quantities by itself is sufficient to determine whether a chemical reaction will proceed spontaneously in the direction it is written. However, when combined mathematically (see Figure 6.1), enthalpy and entropy can be used to define a third quantity, free energy (G), which predicts the direction in which a reaction will spontaneously proceed.

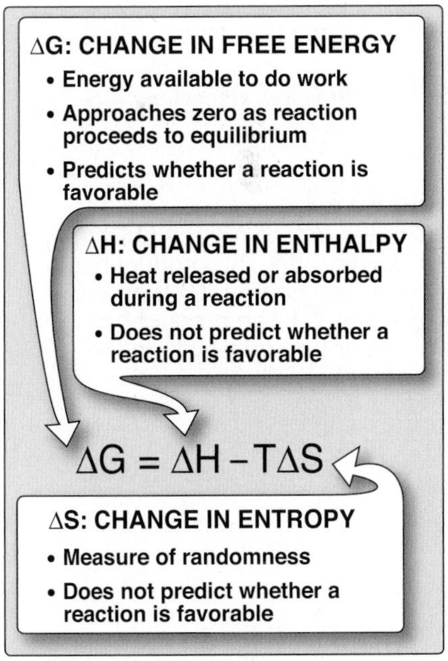

ΔG: CHANGE IN FREE ENERGY
- Energy available to do work
- Approaches zero as reaction proceeds to equilibrium
- Predicts whether a reaction is favorable

ΔH: CHANGE IN ENTHALPY
- Heat released or absorbed during a reaction
- Does not predict whether a reaction is favorable

$$\Delta G = \Delta H - T\Delta S$$

ΔS: CHANGE IN ENTROPY
- Measure of randomness
- Does not predict whether a reaction is favorable

Figure 6.1
Relationship between changes in free energy (G), enthalpy (H), and entropy (S). T is the absolute temperature in Kelvin (K): K = ^{o}C + 273.

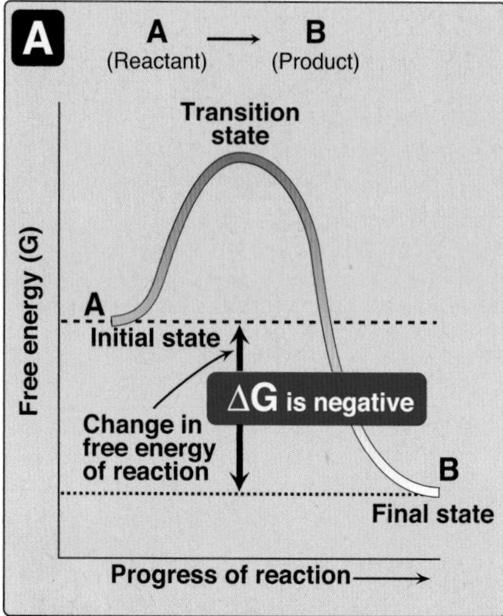

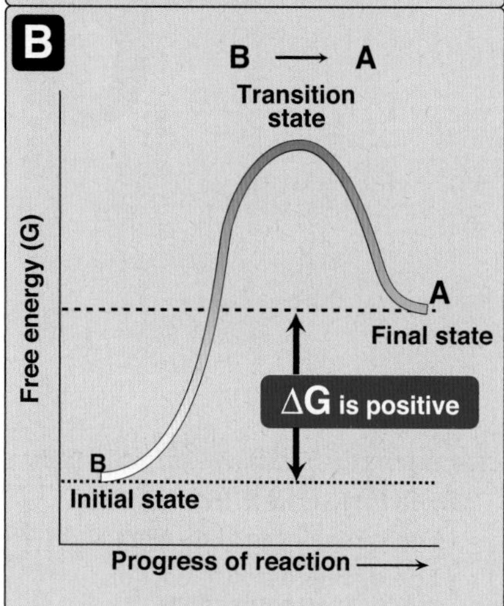

Figure 6.2
Change in free energy (ΔG) during a reaction. **A** The product has a lower free energy (G) than the reactant. **B** The product has a higher free energy than the reactant.

III. FREE ENERGY CHANGE

The change in free energy is represented in two ways, ΔG and ΔG°. The first, ΔG (without the superscript "o"), represents the change in free energy and, thus, the direction of a reaction at any specified concentration of products and reactants. ΔG, then, is a variable. This contrasts with the standard free energy change, ΔG° (with the superscript "o"), which is the energy change when reactants and products are at a concentration of 1 mol/l. [Note: The concentration of protons is assumed to be 10^{-7} mol/l (that is, pH = 7). This may be shown by a prime sign ('), for example, ΔG°'.] Although ΔG°, a constant, represents energy changes at these nonphysiologic concentrations of reactants and products, it is nonetheless useful in comparing the energy changes of different reactions. Furthermore, ΔG° can readily be determined from measurement of the equilibrium constant (see p. 72). This section outlines the uses of ΔG, and ΔG° is described on p. 71.

A. Sign of ΔG and the direction of a reaction

ΔG can be used to predict the direction of a reaction at constant temperature and pressure. Consider the reaction:

$$A \rightleftarrows B$$

1. **Negative ΔG:** If ΔG is negative, there is a net loss of energy, and the reaction goes spontaneously as written (that is, A is converted into B) as shown in Figure 6.2A. The reaction is said to be exergonic.

2. **Positive ΔG:** If ΔG is positive, there is a net gain of energy, and the reaction does not go spontaneously from B to A (see Figure 6.2B). Energy must be added to the system to make the reaction go from B to A. The reaction is said to be endergonic.

3. **ΔG is zero:** If ΔG = 0, the reactants are in equilibrium. [Note: When a reaction is proceeding spontaneously (that is, free energy is being lost) then the reaction continues until ΔG reaches zero and equilibrium is established.]

B. ΔG of the forward and back reactions

The free energy of the forward reaction (A → B) is equal in magnitude but opposite in sign to that of the back reaction (B → A). For example, if ΔG of the forward reaction is –5 kcal/mol, then that of the back reaction is +5 kcal/mol. [Note: ΔG can also be expressed in kilojoules per mole or kJ/mol (1 kcal = 4.2 kJ).]

C. ΔG and the concentration of reactants and products

The ΔG of the reaction A → B depends on the concentration of the reactant and product. At constant temperature and pressure, the following relationship can be derived:

$$\Delta G = \Delta G^o + RT \ln \frac{[B]}{[A]}$$

where ΔG^o is the standard free energy change (see below)
R is the gas constant (1.987 cal/mol K)
T is the absolute temperature (K)
[A] and [B] are the actual concentrations of the reactant and product
ln represents the natural logarithm

A reaction with a positive ΔG^o can proceed in the forward direction (have a negative overall ΔG) if the ratio of products to reactants ([B]/[A]) is sufficiently small (that is, the ratio of reactants to products is large). For example, consider the reaction:

$$\text{Glucose 6-phosphate} \rightleftarrows \text{fructose 6-phosphate}$$

Figure 6.3A shows reaction conditions in which the concentration of reactant, glucose 6-phosphate, is high compared with the concentration of product, fructose 6-phosphate. This means that the ratio of the product to reactant is small, and RT ln([fructose 6-phosphate]/[glucose 6-phosphate]) is large and negative, causing ΔG to be negative despite ΔG^o being positive. Thus, the reaction can proceed in the forward direction.

D. Standard free energy change

The standard free energy change, ΔG^o, is so called because it is equal to the free energy change, ΔG, under standard conditions (that is, when reactants and products are at 1 mol/l concentrations; see Figure 6.3B). Under these conditions, the natural logarithm of the ratio of products to reactants is zero (ln1 = 0), and, therefore, the equation shown at the bottom of the previous page becomes:

$$\Delta G = \Delta G^o + 0$$

1. **ΔG^o and the direction of a reaction:** Under standard conditions, ΔG^o can be used to predict the direction a reaction proceeds because, under these conditions, ΔG^o is equal to ΔG. However, ΔG^o cannot predict the direction of a reaction under physiologic conditions, because it is composed solely of constants (R, T, and K_{eq} [see below]) and is not, therefore, altered by changes in product or substrate concentrations.

2. **Relationship between ΔG^o and K_{eq}:** In a reaction A $\rightleftarrows$ B, a point of equilibrium is reached at which no further net chemical change takes place (that is, when A is being converted to B as fast as B is being converted to A). In this state, the ratio of [B] to [A] is constant, regardless of the actual concentrations of the two compounds:

$$K_{eq} = \frac{[B]_{eq}}{[A]_{eq}}$$

where K_{eq} is the equilibrium constant, and $[A]_{eq}$ and $[B]_{eq}$ are the concentrations of A and B at equilibrium. If the reaction A $\rightleftarrows$ B is allowed to go to equilibrium at constant temperature and pressure, then, at equilibrium, the overall ΔG is zero. Therefore,

$$\Delta G = 0 = \Delta G^o + RT \ln \frac{[B]_{eq}}{[A]_{eq}}$$

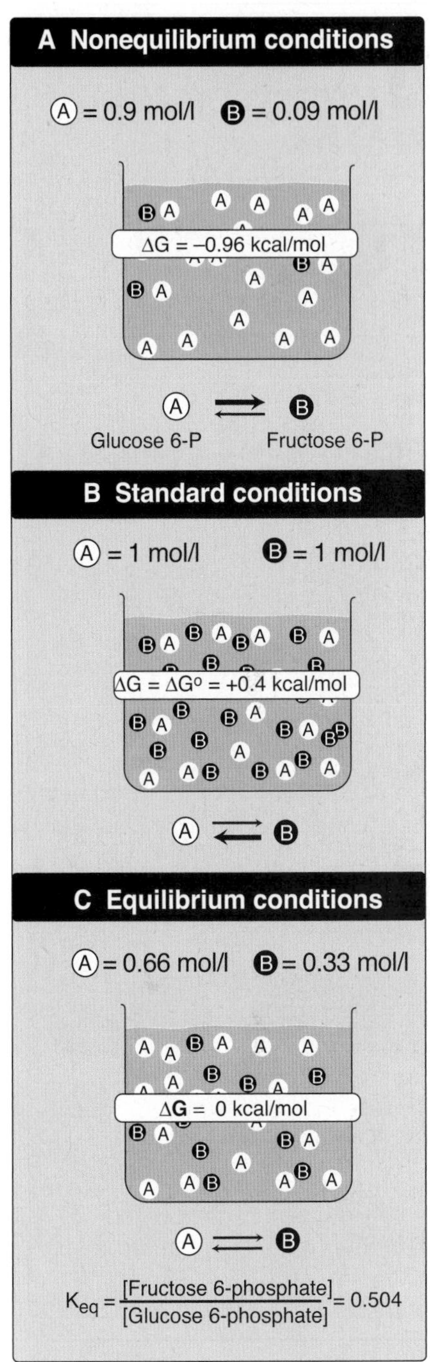

Figure 6.3
Free energy change (ΔG) of a reaction depends on the concentration of reactant Ⓐ and product Ⓑ. For the conversion of glucose 6-phosphate to fructose 6-phosphate, ΔG is negative when the ratio of reactant Ⓐ to product Ⓑ is large (top, panel A), is positive under standard conditions (middle, panel B), and is zero at equilibrium (bottom, panel C). ΔG^0 = standard free energy change.

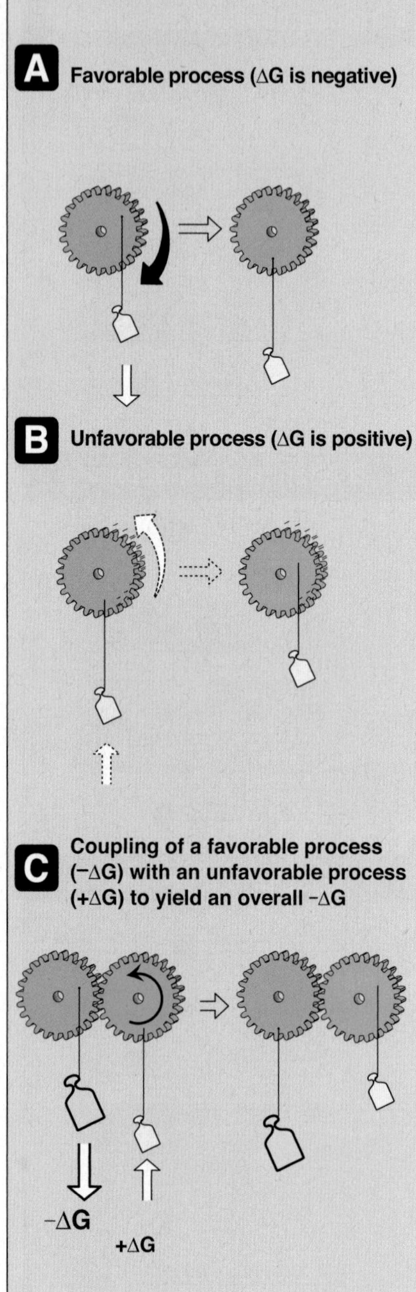

Figure 6.4
Mechanical model of coupling of favorable and unfavorable processes. **A** Gear with weight attached spontaneously turns in the direction that achieves the lowest energy state. **B** The reverse movement is energetically unfavorable (not spontaneous). **C** The energetically favorable movement can drive the unfavorable one.

where the actual concentrations of A and B are equal to the equilibrium concentrations of reactant and product $[A]_{eq}$ and $[B]_{eq}$, and their ratio is equal to the K_{eq}. Thus,

$$\Delta G^o = -RT \ln K_{eq}$$

This equation allows some simple predictions:

If $K_{eq} = 1$, then $\Delta G^o = 0$ A $\rightleftarrows$ B

If $K_{eq} > 1$, then $\Delta G^o < 0$ A $\rightarrow$ B

If $K_{eq} < 1$, then $\Delta G^o > 0$ A $\leftarrow$ B

3. **ΔG^o of two consecutive reactions:** The ΔG^os are additive in any sequence of consecutive reactions, as are the ΔGs. For example:

Glucose + ATP	→ glucose 6-phosphate + ADP	ΔG^o =	–4,000 cal/mol
Glucose 6-phosphate	→ fructose 6-phosphate	ΔG^o =	+400 cal/mol
Glucose + ATP	→ fructose 6-phosphate + ADP	ΔG^o =	–3,600 cal/mol

4. **ΔGs of a pathway:** The additive property of free energy changes is very important in biochemical pathways through which substrates must pass in a particular direction (for example, A → B → C → D →...). As long as the sum of the ΔGs of the individual reactions is negative, the pathway can potentially proceed as written, even if some of the individual reactions of the pathway have a positive ΔG. The actual rate of the reactions does, of course, depend on the lowering of activation energies by the enzymes that catalyze the reactions (see p. 55).

IV. ADENOSINE TRIPHOSPHATE AS AN ENERGY CARRIER

Reactions or processes that have a large positive ΔG, such as moving ions against a concentration gradient across a cell membrane, are made possible by coupling the endergonic movement of ions with a second, spontaneous process with a large negative ΔG such as the exergonic hydrolysis of adenosine triphosphate (ATP). [Note: In the absence of enzymes, ATP is a stable molecule because its hydrolysis has a high activation energy (see p. 55).] Figure 6.4 shows a mechanical model of energy coupling. The simplest example of energy coupling in biologic reactions occurs when the energy-requiring and the energy-yielding reactions share a common intermediate.

A. Common intermediates

Two chemical reactions have a common intermediate when they occur sequentially so that the product of the first reaction is a substrate for the second. For example, given the reactions

$$A + B \rightarrow C + D$$
$$D + X \rightarrow Y + Z$$

D is the common intermediate and can serve as a carrier of chemical energy between the two reactions. Many coupled reactions use ATP to generate a common intermediate. These reactions may involve the transfer of a phosphate group from ATP to another molecule. Other reactions involve the transfer of phosphate from an energy-rich intermediate to adenosine diphosphate (ADP), forming ATP.

B. Energy carried by adenosine triphosphate

ATP consists of a molecule of adenosine (adenine + ribose) to which three phosphate groups are attached (Figure 6.5). If one phosphate is removed, ADP is produced. If two phosphates are removed, adenosine monophosphate (AMP) results. The standard free energy of hydrolysis of ATP, ΔG^o, is approximately –7.3 kcal/mol for each of the two terminal phosphate groups. Because of this large negative ΔG^o, ATP is called a high-energy phosphate compound.

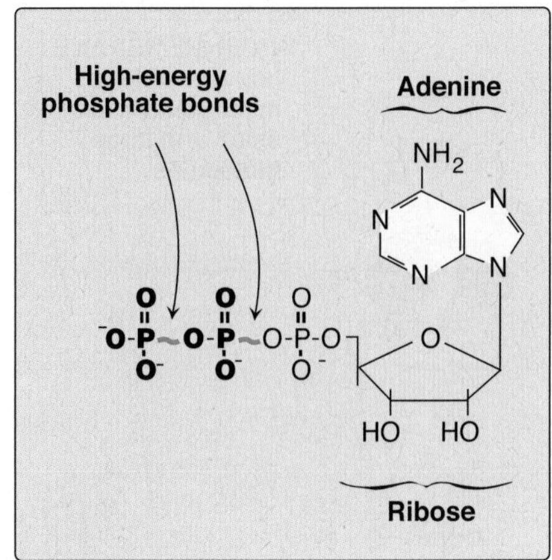

Figure 6.5
Adenosine triphosphate.

V. ELECTRON TRANSPORT CHAIN

Energy-rich molecules, such as glucose, are metabolized by a series of oxidation reactions ultimately yielding CO_2 and water (Figure 6.6). The metabolic intermediates of these reactions donate electrons to specific coenzymes, nicotinamide adenine dinucleotide (NAD^+) and flavin adenine dinucleotide (FAD), to form the energy-rich reduced forms, NADH and $FADH_2$. These reduced coenzymes can, in turn, each donate a pair of electrons to a specialized set of electron carriers, collectively called the electron transport chain (ETC), described in this section. As electrons are passed down the ETC, they lose much of their free energy. This energy is used to move protons across the inner mitochondrial membrane, creating a proton gradient that drives the production of ATP from ADP and inorganic phosphate (P_i), described on p. 77. The coupling of electron transport with ATP synthesis is called oxidative phosphorylation, often denoted as OXPHOS. It proceeds continuously in all tissues that contain mitochondria. [Note: The remainder of the free energy not trapped as ATP is used to drive ancillary reactions such as calcium transport into mitochondria (see p. 133) and to generate heat.]

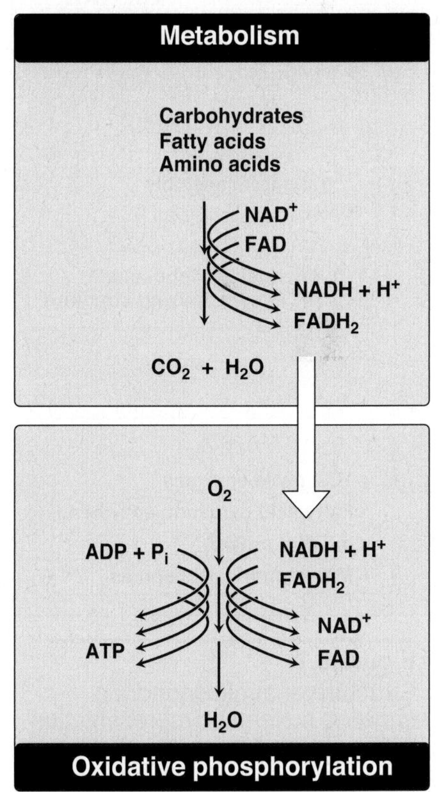

Figure 6.6
The metabolic breakdown of energy-yielding molecules. NAD(H) = nicotinamide adenine dinucleotide; $FAD(H_2)$= flavin adenine dinucleotide; ADP = adenosine diphosphate; ATP = adenosine triphosphate; P_i = inorganic phosphate.

A. The electron transport chain of the mitochondrion

The ETC (except for cytochrome c; see p. 75) is located in the inner mitochondrial membrane and is the final common pathway by which electrons derived from different fuels of the body flow to oxygen (O_2).

1. **Membranes of the mitochondrion:** The mitochondrion contains an outer and an inner membrane separated by the intermembrane space. Although the outer membrane contains special channels (formed by the protein porin), making it freely permeable to most ions and small molecules, the inner membrane is a specialized structure that is impermeable to most small ions, including protons and small molecules such as ATP, ADP, pyruvate, and other metabolites important to mitochondrial function (Figure 6.7). Specialized carriers or transport systems are required to move ions or molecules across this membrane. The inner mitochondrial membrane is unusually rich in protein, over half of which is directly involved in oxidative phosphorylation. It also is highly convoluted. The convolutions, called cristae, serve to greatly increase the surface area of the inner membrane.

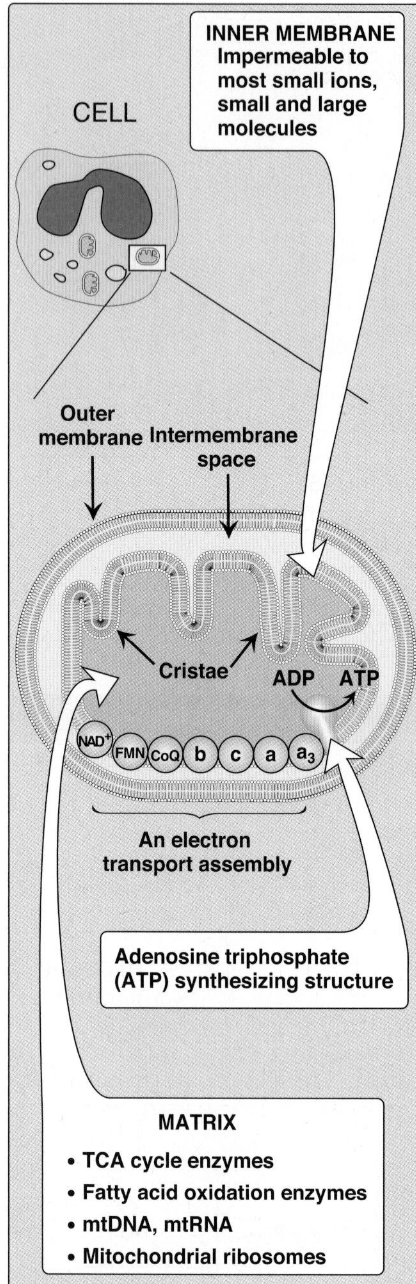

Figure 6.7
Structure of a mitochondrion showing schematic representation of the electron transport chain and the ATP synthesizing structure on the inner membrane. [Note: In contrast to the inner membrane, the outer membrane is highly permeable, and the milieu of the intermembrane space is like that of the cytosol.] mtDNA = mitochondrial DNA; mtRNA = mitochondrial RNA; TCA = tricarboxylic acid.

2. **Matrix of the mitochondrion:** This gel-like solution in the interior of mitochondria is also rich in protein. These molecules include the enzymes responsible for the oxidation of pyruvate, amino acids, and fatty acids (by β-oxidation) as well as those of the tricarboxylic acid (TCA) cycle. The synthesis of glucose, urea, and heme occurs partially in the matrix of mitochondria. In addition, the matrix contains NAD^+ and FAD (the oxidized forms of the two coenzymes that are required as hydrogen acceptors), and ADP and P_i, which are used to produce ATP. [Note: The matrix also contains mitochondrial DNA (mtDNA) and RNA (mtRNA) and ribosomes.]

B. Organization of the electron transport chain

The inner mitochondrial membrane contains five separate protein complexes, called Complexes I, II, III, IV, and V. Complexes I–IV each contain part of the ETC (Figure 6.8). These complexes accept or donate electrons to the relatively mobile electron carriers, coenzyme Q and cytochrome c. Each carrier in the ETC can receive electrons from an electron donor and can subsequently donate electrons to the next acceptor in the chain. The electrons ultimately combine with O_2 and protons to form water. This requirement for O_2 makes the electron transport process the respiratory chain, which accounts for the greatest portion of the body's use of O_2. Complex V is described on p. 78.

C. Reactions of the electron transport chain

With the exception of coenzyme Q, which is a lipid-soluble quinone, all members of this chain are proteins. These may function as enzymes as is the case with the flavin-containing *dehydrogenases*, may contain iron as part of an iron-sulfur center, may contain iron as part of the porphyrin prosthetic group of heme as in the cytochromes, or may contain copper as does the cytochrome a + a_3 complex.

1. **Formation of NADH:** NAD^+ is reduced to NADH by *dehydrogenases* that remove two hydrogen atoms from their substrate. (For examples of these reactions, see the discussion of the *dehydrogenases* of the TCA cycle, p. 112.) Both electrons but only one proton (that is, a hydride ion [$:H^-$]) are transferred to the NAD^+, forming NADH plus a free proton.

2. **NADH dehydrogenase:** The free proton plus the hydride ion carried by NADH are transferred to *NADH dehydrogenase*, a protein complex (Complex I) embedded in the inner mitochondrial membrane. Complex I has a tightly bound molecule of flavin mononucleotide (FMN), a coenzyme structurally related to FAD (see Figure 28.15, p. 380) that accepts the two hydrogen atoms ($2e^- + 2H^+$), becoming $FMNH_2$. *NADH dehydrogenase* also contains peptide subunits with iron-sulfur centers (Figure 6.9). At Complex I, electrons move from NADH to FMN to the iron of the iron-sulfur centers and then to coenzyme Q. As electrons flow, they lose energy. This energy is used to pump protons across the inner mitochondrial membrane, from the matrix to the intermembrane space.

3. **Succinate dehydrogenase:** At Complex II, electrons from the *succinate dehydrogenase*–catalyzed oxidation of succinate to fumarate move from the coenzyme, $FADH_2$, to an iron-sulfur protein,

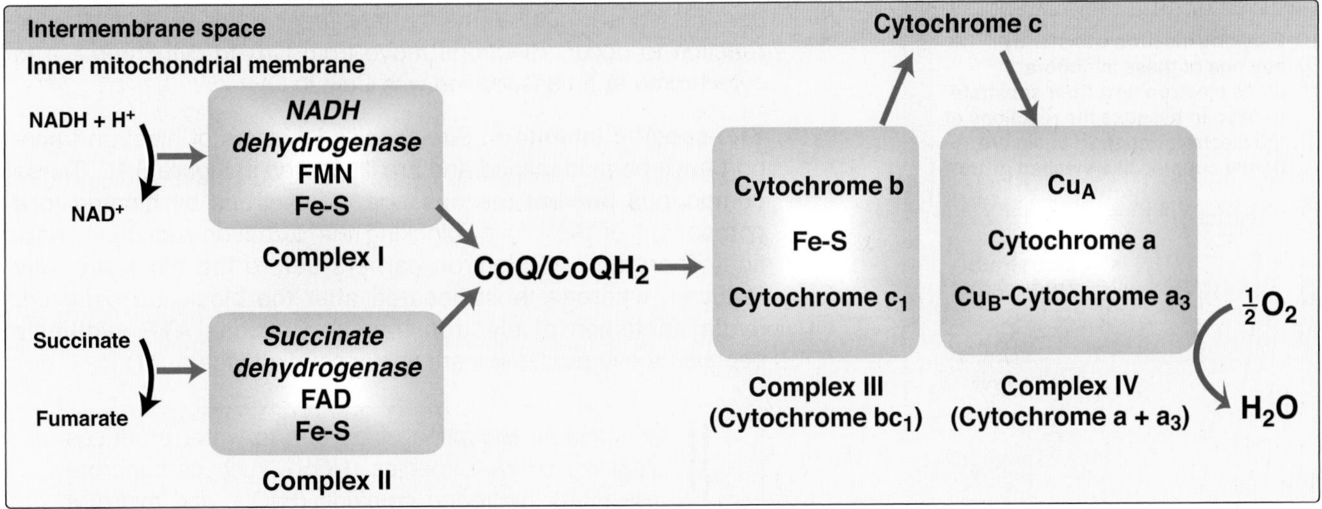

Figure 6.8
Electron transport chain. The flow of electrons is shown by the magenta arrows. NAD(H) = nicotinamide adenine dinucleotide; FMN = flavin mononucleotide; FAD = flavin adenine dinucleotide; Fe-S = iron-sulfur center; CoQ = coenzyme Q.

and then to coenzyme Q. [Note: No energy is lost in this process, and, therefore, no protons are pumped at Complex II.]

4. **Coenzyme Q:** Coenzyme Q (CoQ) is a quinone derivative with a long, hydrophobic isoprenoid tail. It is also called ubiquinone because it is ubiquitous in biologic systems. CoQ is a mobile electron carrier and can accept hydrogen atoms from *NADH dehydrogenase* (Complex I), from *succinate dehydrogenase* (Complex II), and from other mitochondrial *dehydrogenases*: *glycerophosphate dehydrogenase* (see p. 79) and *acyl CoA dehydrogenase* (see p. 192). CoQ transfers electrons to Complex III (cytochrome bc_1). CoQ, then, links the flavoprotein *dehydrogenases* to the cytochromes.

5. **Cytochromes:** The remaining members of the ETC are cytochrome proteins. Each contains a heme group (a porphyrin ring plus iron). Unlike the heme groups of hemoglobin, the cytochrome iron is reversibly converted from its ferric (Fe^{3+}) to its ferrous (Fe^{2+}) form as a normal part of its function as an acceptor and donor of electrons. Electrons are passed along the chain from cytochrome bc_1 (Complex III), to cytochrome c, and then to cytochromes a + a_3 (Complex IV; see Figure 6.8). As electrons flow, protons are pumped across the inner mitochondrial membrane at Complexes III and IV. [Note: Cytochrome c is located in the intermembrane space, loosely associated with the outer face of the inner membrane. As seen with CoQ, cytochrome c is a mobile carrier of electrons.]

6. **Cytochrome a + a_3:** This cytochrome complex (Complex IV) is the only electron carrier in which the heme iron has an available coordination site that can react directly with O_2 and so also is called *cytochrome oxidase*. At Complex IV, the transported electrons, O_2, and free protons are brought together, and O_2 is reduced to water (see Figure 6.8). [Note: Four electrons are required to reduce one molecule of O_2 to two molecules of water.] *Cytochrome oxidase*

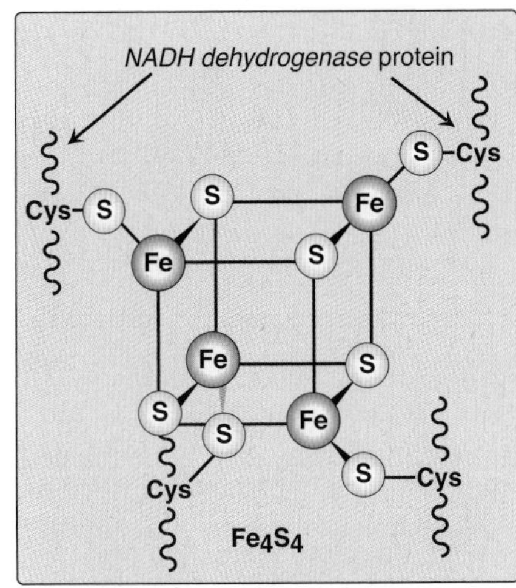

Figure 6.9
Iron-sulfur (Fe-S) center of Complex I. [Note: Complexes II and III also contain iron-sulfur centers.] NADH = nicotinamide adenine dinucleotide;Cys = cysteine.

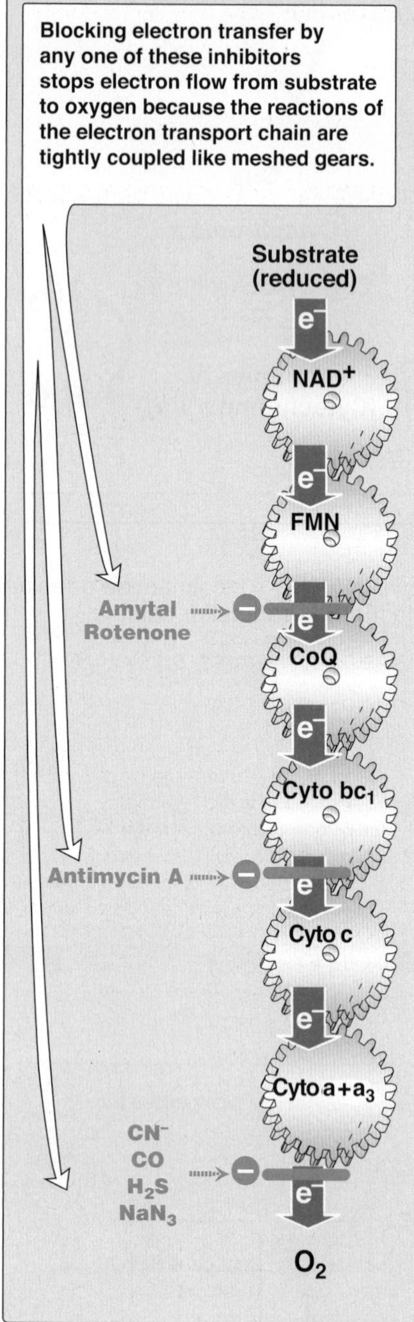

Figure 6.10
Site-specific inhibitors of electron transport shown using a mechanical model for the coupling of oxidation-reduction reactions. [Note: Figure illustrates normal direction of electron flow.] CN^- = cyanide; CO = carbon monoxide; H_2S = hydrogen sulfide; NaN_3 = sodium azide; FMN = flavin mononucleotide; FAD = flavin adenine dinucleotide; CoQ = coenzyme Q; Cyto = cytochrome.

contains copper (Cu) atoms that are required for this complicated reaction to occur. Electrons move from Cu_A to cytochrome a to cytochrome a_3 (in association with Cu_B) to O_2.

7. **Site-specific inhibitors:** Site-specific inhibitors of electron transport have been identified and are illustrated in Figure 6.10. These compounds prevent the passage of electrons by binding to a component of the chain, blocking the oxidation-reduction reaction. Therefore, all electron carriers before the block are fully reduced, whereas those located after the block are oxidized. [Note: Inhibition of electron transport inhibits ATP synthesis because these processes are tightly coupled (see p. 77).]

> Incomplete reduction of oxygen to water produces reactive oxygen species (ROS), such as superoxide ($O_2^{\cdot-}$), hydrogen peroxide (H_2O_2), and hydroxyl radicals (OH•). ROS damage DNA and proteins and cause lipid peroxidation. Enzymes such as *superoxide dismutase* (*SOD*), *catalase*, and *glutathione peroxidase* are cellular defenses against ROS.

D. Release of free energy during electron transport

The free energy released as electrons are transferred along the ETC from an electron donor (reducing agent or reductant) to an electron acceptor (oxidizing agent or oxidant) is used to pump protons at Complexes I, III, and IV. [Note: The electrons can be transferred as hydride ions ($:H^-$) to NAD^+; as hydrogen atoms (•H) to FMN, CoQ, and FAD; or as electrons (e^-) to cytochromes.]

1. **Redox pairs:** Oxidation (loss of electrons) of one substance is always accompanied by reduction (gain of electrons) of a second. For example, Figure 6.11 shows the oxidation of NADH to NAD^+ by *NADH dehydrogenase* at Complex I, accompanied by the reduction of FMN, the prosthetic group, to $FMNH_2$. Such oxidation-reduction reactions can be written as the sum of two separate half-reactions, one an oxidation and the other a reduction (see Figure 6.11). NAD^+ and NADH form a redox pair, as do FMN and $FMNH_2$. Redox pairs differ in their tendency to lose electrons. This tendency is a characteristic of a particular redox pair and can be quantitatively specified by a constant, E_o (the standard reduction potential), with units in volts.

2. **Standard reduction potential:** The E_o of various redox pairs can be ordered from the most negative E_o to the most positive. The more negative the E_o of a redox pair, the greater the tendency of the reductant member of that pair to lose electrons. The more positive the E_o, the greater the tendency of the oxidant member of that pair to accept electrons. Therefore, electrons flow from the pair with the more negative E_o to that with the more positive E_o. The E_o values for some members of the ETC are shown in Figure 6.12. [Note: The components of the chain are arranged in order of increasingly positive E_o values.]

3. **Relationship of ΔG^o to ΔE_o:** The ΔG^o is related directly to the magnitude of the change in E_o:

$$\Delta G^o = -\, n\, F\, \Delta E_o$$

where n = number of electrons transferred (1 for a cytochrome, 2 for NADH, $FADH_2$, and coenzyme Q)

F = Faraday constant (23.1 kcal/volt mol)

ΔE_0 = E_0 of the electron-accepting pair minus the E_0 of the electron-donating pair

ΔG^o = change in the standard free energy

4. **ΔG° of ATP:** The ΔG^o for the phosphorylation of ADP to ATP is +7.3 kcal/mol. The transport of a pair of electrons from NADH to O_2 through the ETC releases 52.58 kcal. Therefore, more than sufficient energy is available to produce 3 ATP from 3 ADP and 3 P_i (3 x 7.3 = 21.9 kcal/mol), sometimes expressed as a P:O ratio (ATP made per O atom reduced) of 3:1. The remaining calories are used for ancillary reactions or released as heat. [Note: The P:O for $FADH_2$ is 2:1 because Complex I is bypassed.]

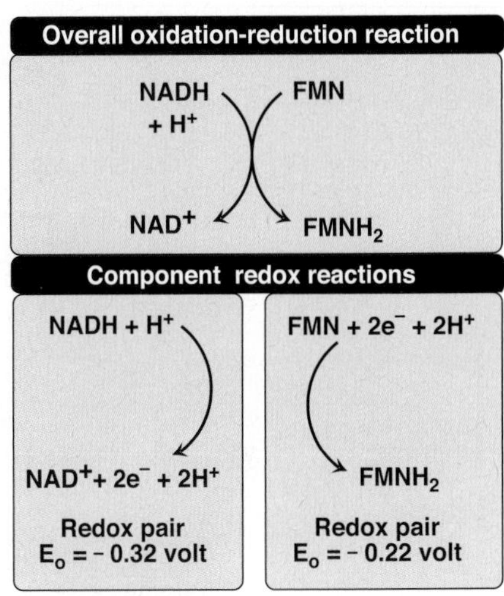

Figure 6.11
Oxidation of NADH by FMN, separated into two component half-reactions. NAD(H) = nicotinamide adenine dinucleotide; $FMN(H_2)$ = flavin mononucleotide.

VI. PHOSPHORYLATION OF ADP TO ATP

The transfer of electrons down the ETC is energetically favored because NADH is a strong electron donor and O_2 is an avid electron acceptor. However, the flow of electrons does not directly result in ATP synthesis.

A. Chemiosmotic hypothesis

The chemiosmotic hypothesis (also known as the Mitchell hypothesis) explains how the free energy generated by the transport of electrons by the ETC is used to produce ATP from ADP + P_i.

1. **Proton pump:** Electron transport is coupled to the phosphorylation of ADP by the pumping of protons across the inner mitochondrial membrane, from the matrix to the intermembrane space, at Complexes I, III, and IV. This process creates an electrical gradient (with more positive charges on the outside of the membrane than on the inside) and a pH gradient (the outside of the membrane is at a lower pH than the inside) as shown in Figure 6.13. The energy generated by this proton gradient is sufficient to drive ATP synthesis. Thus, the proton gradient serves as the common intermediate that couples oxidation to phosphorylation.

2. **ATP synthase:** The multisubunit enzyme *ATP synthase* (Complex V; see Figure 6.14) synthesizes ATP using the energy of the proton gradient. It contains a domain (F_o) that spans the inner mitochondrial membrane, and an extramembranous domain (F_1) that appears as a sphere that protrudes into the mitochondrial matrix (see Figure 6.13). The chemiosmotic hypothesis proposes that after protons have been pumped to the cytosolic side of the inner mitochondrial membrane, they reenter the matrix by passing through a proton channel in the F_o domain, driving rotation of the c ring of F_o and, at the same time, dissipating the pH and electrical gradients. F_o rotation causes conformational changes in the β subunits of the F_1 domain that allow them to bind ADP + P_i, phosphorylate ADP to ATP, and release ATP. [Note: *ATP synthase* is also called *F_1/F_o-ATPase* because the isolated enzyme can catalyze the hydrolysis of ATP to ADP and P_i.]

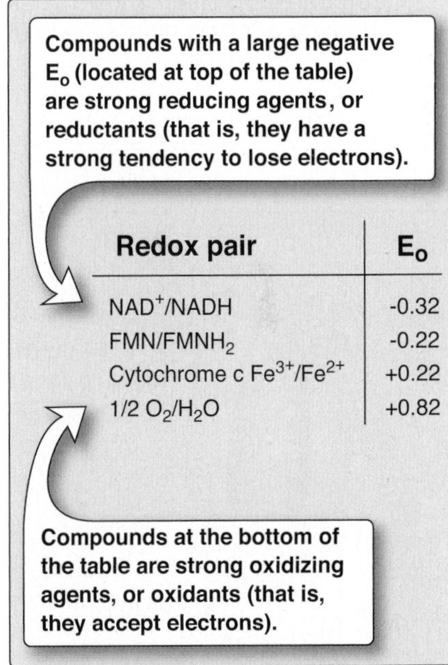

Redox pair	E_o
$NAD^+/NADH$	-0.32
$FMN/FMNH_2$	-0.22
Cytochrome c Fe^{3+}/Fe^{2+}	+0.22
1/2 O_2/H_2O	+0.82

Figure 6.12
Standard reduction potentials (E_o) of some reactions. NAD(H) = nicotinamide adenine dinucleotide; $FMN(H_2)$ = flavin mononucleotide.

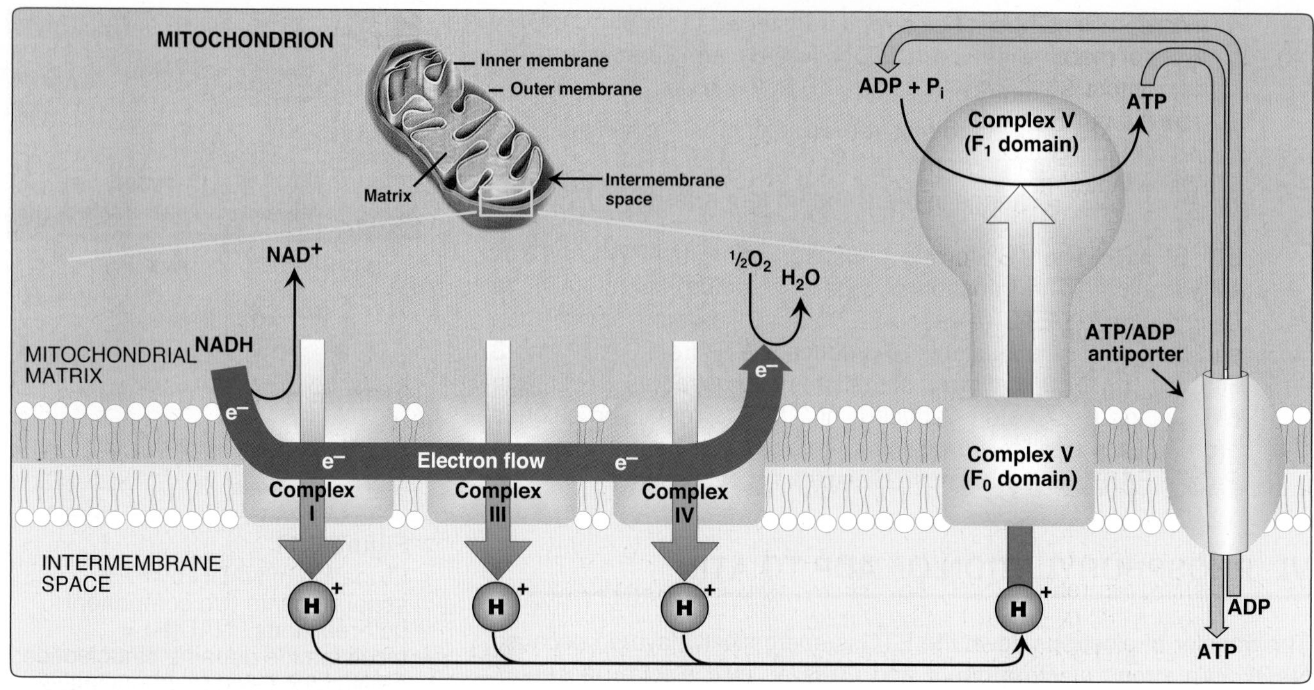

Figure 6.13
Electron transport chain shown in association with the transport of protons (H^+). A total of ten H^+ are pumped for each nicotinamide adenine dinucleotide (NADH) oxidized. [Note: H^+ are not pumped at Complex II.]

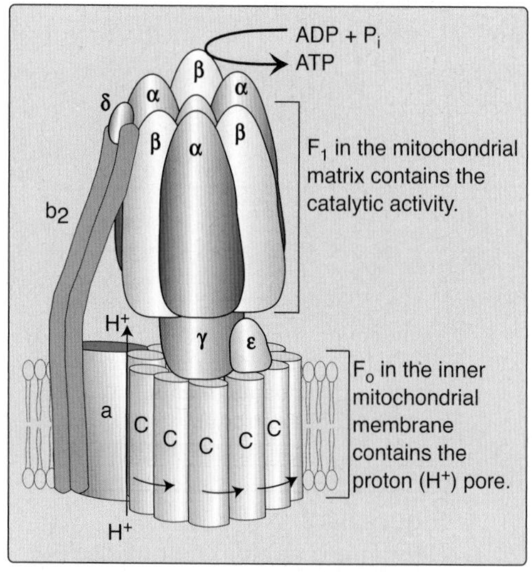

Figure 6.14
ATP synthase (*F_1F_O–ATPase*). [Note: The rotation of the ring of c subunits in the F_O domain results in conformational changes in the β subunits of the F_1 domain that allow phosphorylation of adenosine diphosphate (ADP) to adenosine triphosphate (ATP). P_i = inorganic phosphate.

a. **Coupling in oxidative phosphorylation:** In normal mitochondria, ATP synthesis is coupled to electron transport through the proton gradient. Increasing (or decreasing) one process has the same effect on the other. For example, hydrolysis of ATP to ADP and P_i in energy-requiring reactions increases the availability of substrates for *ATP synthase* and, thus, increases proton flow through the enzyme. Electron transport and proton pumping by the ETC increase to maintain the proton gradient. [Note: Increased oxidation of NADH at Complex I and, consequently, an increase in NADH-producing pathways of metabolism, such as the TCA cycle, results.]

b. **Oligomycin:** This drug binds to the F_o (hence the letter "o") domain of *ATP synthase,* closing the proton channel and preventing reentry of protons into the matrix, thereby preventing phosphorylation of ADP to ATP. Because the pH and electrical gradients cannot be dissipated in the presence of this drug, electron transport stops because of the difficulty of pumping any more protons against the steep gradients. This dependency of cellular respiration on the ability to phosphorylate ADP to ATP is known as respiratory control and is the consequence of the tight coupling of these processes.

c. **Uncoupling proteins:** Uncoupling proteins (UCPs) occur in the inner mitochondrial membrane of mammals, including humans. These proteins form channels that allow protons to reenter the mitochondrial matrix without energy being captured as ATP (Figure 6.15). The energy is released as heat, and the process is called nonshivering thermogenesis. UCP1, also called thermogenin, is responsible for heat production in the brown adipocytes of mammals. In brown fat, unlike the more abundant white fat, almost 90% of its respiratory energy is used for thermogenesis in response to cold in the neonate and during arousal in hibernating animals. However, humans appear to have few concentrated deposits of brown fat (except in the newborn), and UCP1 does not appear to play a major role in energy balance. [Note: Uncoupling proteins UCP2–UCP5 have been found in other tissues, but their full significance remains unclear.]

d. **Synthetic uncouplers:** Electron transport and phosphorylation can also be uncoupled by compounds that pick up protons in the intermembrane space and release them in the matrix, dissipating the gradient. The classic example is 2,4-dinitrophenol, a lipophilic proton carrier that readily diffuses through the mitochondrial membrane. This uncoupler causes electron transport to proceed at a rapid rate without establishing a proton gradient, much as do the UCPs (see Figure 6.15). Again, energy is released as heat rather than being used to synthesize ATP. [Note: In high doses, aspirin and other salicylates uncouple oxidative phosphorylation. This explains the fever that accompanies toxic overdoses of these drugs.]

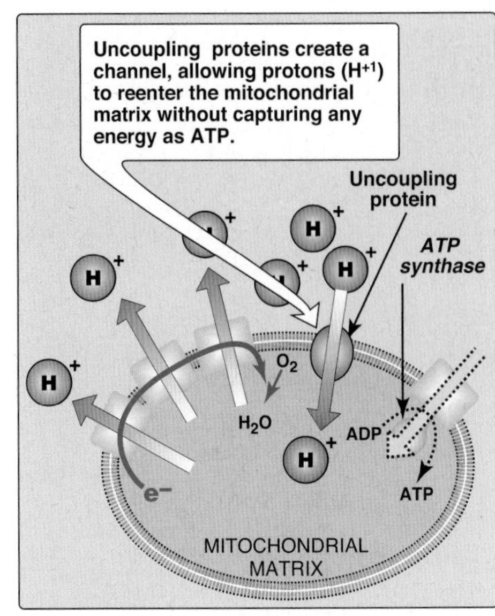

Figure 6.15
Transport of protons across the mitochondrial membrane by an uncoupling protein. ADP = adenosine diphosphate; ATP = adenosine triphosphate.

B. Membrane transport systems

The inner mitochondrial membrane is impermeable to most charged or hydrophilic substances. However, it contains numerous transport proteins that permit passage of specific molecules from the cytosol (or more correctly, the intermembrane space) to the mitochondrial matrix.

1. **ATP and ADP transport:** The inner membrane requires specialized carriers to transport ADP and P_i from the cytosol (where ATP is hydrolyzed to ADP in many energy-requiring reactions) into mitochondria, where ATP can be resynthesized. An adenine nucleotide antiporter imports one ADP from the cytosol into the matrix, while exporting one ATP from the matrix into the cytosol (see Figure 6.13). A transporter moves P_i from the cytosol into mitochondria.

2. **Transport of reducing equivalents:** The inner mitochondrial membrane lacks an NADH transporter, and NADH produced in the cytosol (for example, in glycolysis; see p. 101) cannot directly enter the mitochondrial matrix. However, two electrons (reducing equivalents) of NADH are transported from the cytosol into the matrix using substrate shuttles. In the glycerophosphate shuttle (Figure 6.16A), two electrons are transferred from NADH to dihydroxyacetone phosphate by cytosolic *glycerophosphate dehydrogenase*. The glycerol 3-phosphate produced is oxidized by the mitochondrial isozyme as FAD is reduced to $FADH_2$. CoQ of the ETC oxidizes the $FADH_2$. The glycerophosphate shuttle, therefore, results in the synthesis of two ATPs for each cytosolic NADH oxidized. This contrasts with the malate-aspartate shuttle (Figure 6.16B), which produces NADH (rather than $FADH_2$) in the mitochondrial matrix and, therefore, yields three ATPs for each cytosolic NADH oxidized by *malate dehydrogenase* as oxaloacetate is reduced to malate. A transport protein moves malate into the matrix.

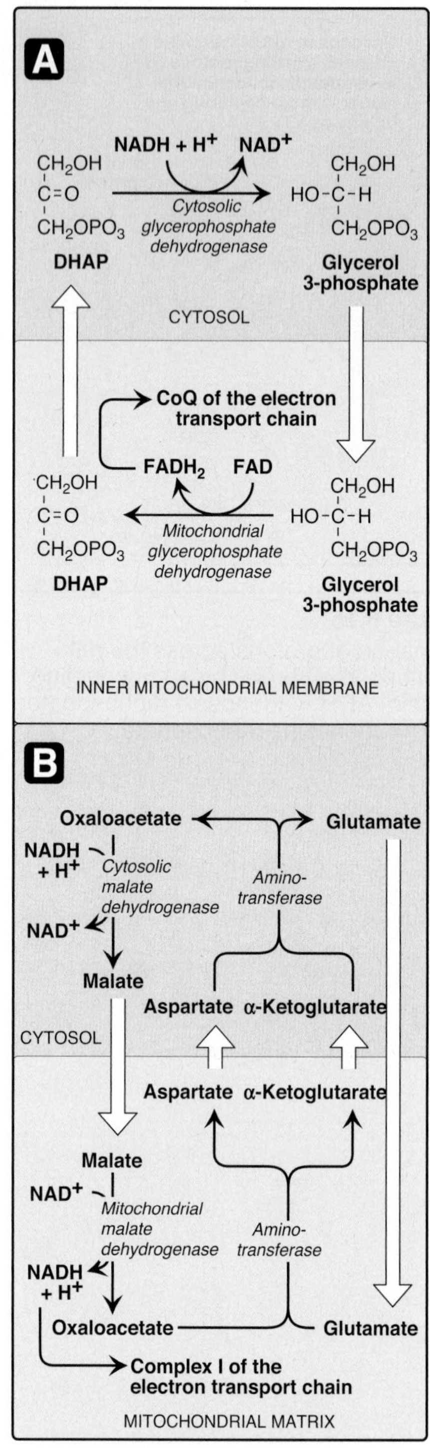

Figure 6.16
Substrate shuttles for the transport of electrons across the inner mitochondrial membrane.
A. Glycerophosphate shuttle.
B. Malate-aspartate shuttle.
DHAP = dihydroxyacetone phosphate; NAD(H) = nicotinamide adenine dinucleotide; FAD(H_2) = flavin adenine dinucleotide; CoQ = coenzyme Q.

C. Inherited defects in oxidative phosphorylation

Thirteen of the approximately 90 polypeptides required for oxidative phosphorylation are coded for by mtDNA and synthesized in mitochondria, whereas the remaining proteins are coded for by nuclear DNA, synthesized in the cytosol, and transported into mitochondria posttranslationally. Defects in oxidative phosphorylation are more likely a result of alterations in mtDNA, which has a mutation rate about 10 times greater than that of nuclear DNA. Tissues with the greatest ATP requirement (for example, central nervous system, skeletal and heart muscle, and liver) are most affected by defects in oxidative phosphorylation. Mutations in mtDNA are responsible for several diseases, including some cases of mitochondrial myopathies, and Leber hereditary optic neuropathy, a disease in which bilateral loss of central vision occurs as a result of neuroretinal degeneration, including damage to the optic nerve. [Note: mtDNA is maternally inherited because mitochondria from the sperm cell do not enter the fertilized egg.]

D. Mitochondria and apoptosis

The process of apoptosis, or programmed cell death, may be initiated through the intrinsic (mitochondrial-mediated) pathway by the formation of pores in the outer mitochondrial membrane. These pores allow cytochrome c to leave the intermembrane space and enter the cytosol. There, cytochrome c, in association with pro-apoptotic factors, activates a family of proteolytic enzymes (the *caspases*), causing cleavage of key proteins and resulting in the morphologic and biochemical changes characteristic of apoptosis.

VII. CHAPTER SUMMARY

The change in **free energy** (**ΔG**) occurring during a reaction predicts the direction in which that reaction will spontaneously proceed. If ΔG is **negative** (that is, the product has a lower free energy than the substrate), the **reaction goes spontaneously**. If **ΔG** is **positive**, the reaction **does not go spontaneously**. If **$\Delta G = 0$**, the reactions are in **equilibrium**. The **ΔG** of the forward reaction is equal in magnitude but opposite in sign to that of the back reaction. The **ΔGs** are **additive** in any sequence of consecutive reactions, as are the standard free energy changes (**ΔG^os**). Therefore, reactions or processes that have a large, positive ΔG are made possible by **coupling** with those that have a large, negative ΔG such as hydrolysis of **adenosine triphosphate** (**ATP**). The reduced coenzymes **nicotinamide adenine dinucleotide** (**NADH**) and **flavin adenine dinucleotide** (**$FADH_2$**) each donate a pair of electrons to a specialized set of electron carriers, consisting of **flavin mononucleotide** (**FMN**), **iron-sulfur centers**, **coenzyme Q**, and a series of **cytochromes**, collectively called the **electron transport chain**. This pathway is present in the **inner mitochondrial membrane** (impermeable to most substances) and is the final common pathway by which electrons derived from different fuels of the body flow to O_2, reducing it to water. The terminal cytochrome, *cytochrome oxidase*, is the only cytochrome able to bind O_2. **Electron transport** results in the **pumping of protons** across the inner mitochondrial membrane from

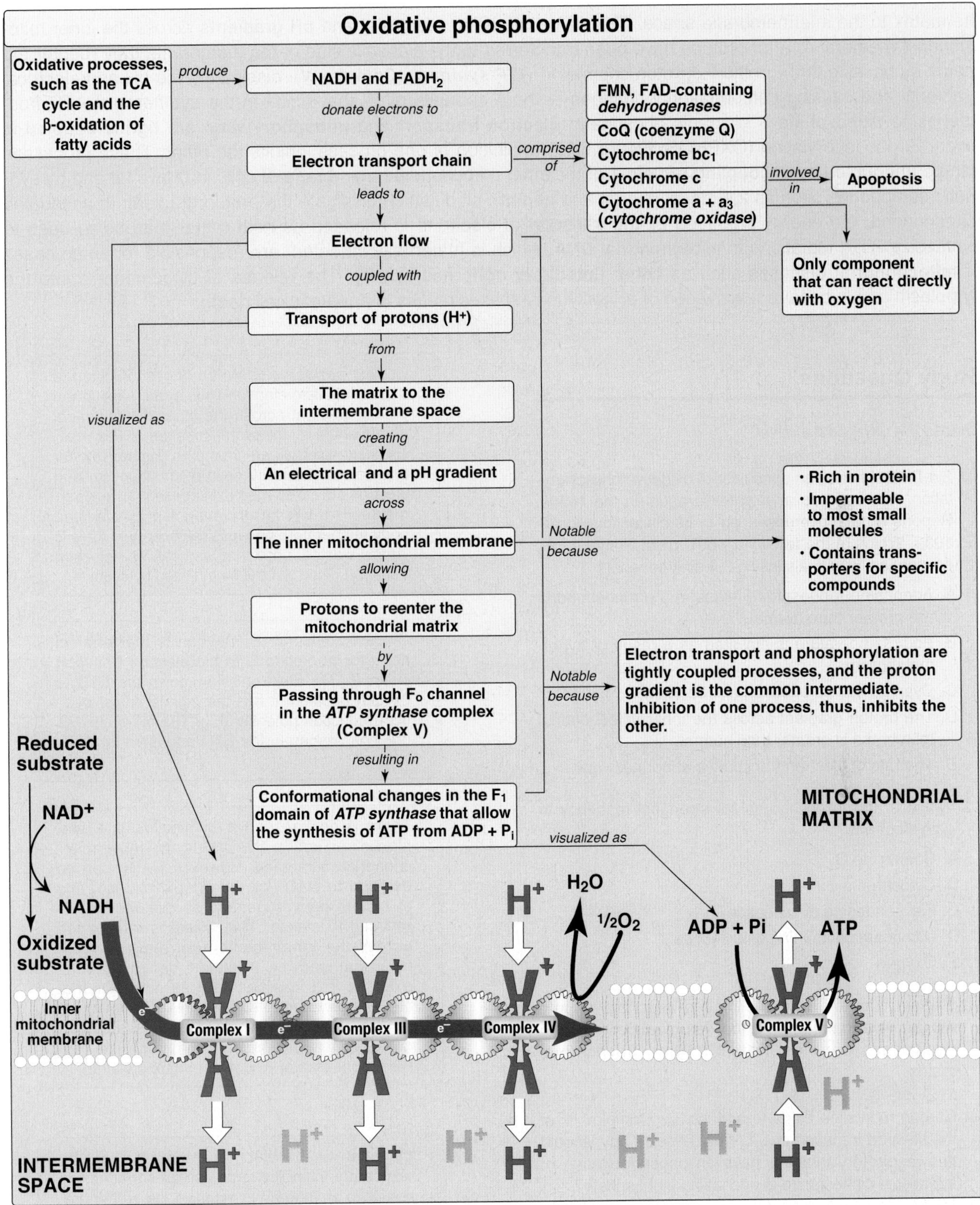

Figure 6.17

Key concept map for oxidative phosphorylation (OXPHOS). [Note: Electron (e^-) flow and ATP synthesis are envisioned as sets of interlocking gears to emphasize the idea of coupling.] TCA = tricarboxylic acid; NAD(H) = nicotinamide adenine dinucleotide; FAD(H_2) = flavin adenine dinucleotide; FMN = flavin mononucleotide.

the matrix to the intermembrane space. This process creates **electrical** and **pH gradients** across the inner mitochondrial membrane. After protons have been transferred to the cytosolic side of the membrane, they reenter the matrix by passing through the F_o proton channel in ***ATP synthase*** (**Complex V**), dissipating the pH and electrical gradients and causing conformational changes in the β subunits of F_1 that result in the synthesis of ATP from adenosine diphosphate + inorganic phosphate. **Electron transport** and **phosphorylation** are **tightly coupled** in oxidative phosphorylation (OXPHOS, Figure 6.17). Inhibition of one process inhibits the other. These processes can be **uncoupled** by **uncoupling protein-1** of the inner mitochondrial membrane of cells in brown fat and by synthetic compounds such as **2,4-dinitrophenol** and **aspirin**, all of which dissipate the proton gradient. In uncoupled mitochondria, the energy produced by the transport of electrons is released as **heat** rather than being used to synthesize ATP. Mutations in **mitochondrial DNA**, which is maternally inherited, are responsible for some cases of **mitochondrial diseases** such as **Leber hereditary optic neuropathy**. The release of cytochrome c into the cytoplasm and subsequent activation of proteolytic *caspases* results in apoptotic cell death.

Study Questions

Choose the ONE best answer.

6.1 2,4-Dinitrophenol, an uncoupler of oxidative phosphorylation, was used as a weight-loss agent in the 1930s. Reports of fatal overdoses led to its discontinuation in 1939. Which of the following would most likely be true concerning individuals taking 2,4-dinitrophenol?

A. Adenosine triphosphate levels in the mitochondria are greater than normal.
B. Body temperature is elevated as a result of hypermetabolism.
C. Cyanide has no effect on electron flow.
D. The proton gradient across the inner mitochondrial membrane is greater than normal.
E. The rate of electron transport is abnormally low.

Correct answer = B. When phosphorylation is uncoupled from electron flow, a decrease in the proton gradient across the inner mitochondrial membrane and, therefore, impaired ATP synthesis is expected. In an attempt to compensate for this defect in energy capture, metabolism and electron flow to oxygen is increased. This hypermetabolism will be accompanied by elevated body temperature because the energy in fuels is largely wasted, appearing as heat. The electron transport chain will still be inhibited by cyanide.

6.2 Which of the following has the strongest tendency to gain electrons?

A. Coenzyme Q
B. Cytochrome c
C. Flavin adenine dinucleotide
D. Nicotinamide adenine dinucleotide
E. Oxygen

Correct answer = E. Oxygen is the terminal acceptor of electrons in the electron transport chain (ETC). Electrons flow down the ETC to oxygen because it has the highest (most positive) reduction potential (E_0). The other choices precede oxygen in the ETC and have lower E_0 values.

6.3 Explain why and how the malate-aspartate shuttle moves nicotinamide adenine dinucleotide reducing equivalents from the cytosol to the mitochondrial matrix.

There is no transporter for nicotinamide adenine dinucleotide (NADH) in the inner mitochondrial membrane. However, NADH can be oxidized to NAD^+ by the cytoplasmic isozyme of malate dehydrogenase as oxaloacetate is reduced to malate. The malate is transported across the inner membrane, and the mitochondrial isozyme of malate dehydrogenase oxidizes it to oxaloacetate as mitochondrial NAD^+ is reduced to NADH. This NADH can be oxidized by Complex I of the electron transport chain, generating three ATP through the coupled processes of oxidative phosphorylation.

6.4 Carbon monoxide binds to and inhibits Complex IV of the electron transport chain. What effect, if any, should this respiratory inhibitor have on phosphorylation of adenosine diphosphate to adenosine triphosphate?

Inhibition of the electron transport chain by respiratory inhibitors such as carbon monoxide results in an inability to maintain the proton gradient. Phosphorylation of ADP to ATP is, therefore, inhibited, as are ancillary reactions such as calcium uptake by mitochondria, because they also require the proton gradient.

Introduction to Carbohydrates

7

I. OVERVIEW

Carbohydrates (saccharides) are the most abundant organic molecules in nature. They have a wide range of functions, including providing a significant fraction of the dietary calories for most organisms, acting as a storage form of energy in the body, and serving as cell membrane components that mediate some forms of intercellular communication. Carbohydrates also serve as a structural component of many organisms, including the cell walls of bacteria, the exoskeleton of many insects, and the fibrous cellulose of plants. The empiric formula for many of the simpler carbohydrates is $(CH_2O)_n$, where $n \geq 3$, hence the name "hydrate of carbon."

II. CLASSIFICATION AND STRUCTURE

Monosaccharides (simple sugars) can be classified according to the number of carbon atoms they contain. Examples of some monosaccharides commonly found in humans are listed in Figure 7.1. They can also be classified by the type of carbonyl group they contain. Carbohydrates with an aldehyde as their carbonyl group are called aldoses, whereas those with a keto as their carbonyl group are called ketoses (Figure 7.2). For example, glyceraldehyde is an aldose, whereas dihydroxyacetone is a ketose. Carbohydrates that have a free carbonyl group have the suffix –ose. [Note: Ketoses have an additional "ul" in their suffix such as xyulose. There are exceptions, such as fructose, to this rule.] Monosaccharides can be linked by glycosidic bonds to create larger structures (Figure 7.3). Disaccharides contain two monosaccharide units, oligosaccharides contain three to ten monosaccharide units, and polysaccharides contain more than ten monosaccharide units and can be hundreds of sugar units in length.

Generic names	Examples
3 Carbons: trioses	Glyceraldehyde
4 Carbons: tetroses	Erythrose
5 Carbons: pentoses	Ribose
6 Carbons: hexoses	Glucose
7 Carbons: heptoses	Sedoheptulose
9 Carbons: nonoses	Neuraminic acid

Figure 7.1
Examples of monosaccharides found in humans, classified according to the number of carbons they contain.

A. Isomers and epimers

Compounds that have the same chemical formula but have different structures are called isomers. For example, fructose, glucose, mannose, and galactose are all isomers of each other, having the same chemical formula, $C_6H_{12}O_6$. Carbohydrate isomers that differ in configuration around only one specific carbon atom (with the exception of the carbonyl carbon; see "anomers" below) are defined as epimers of each other. For example, glucose and galactose are

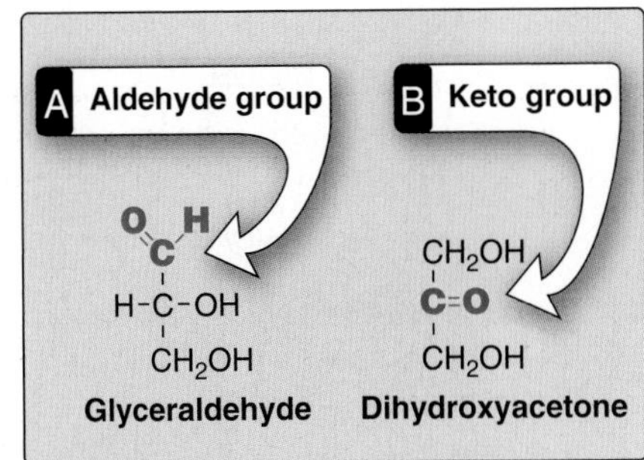

Figure 7.2
Examples of an aldose (A) and a ketose (B) sugar.

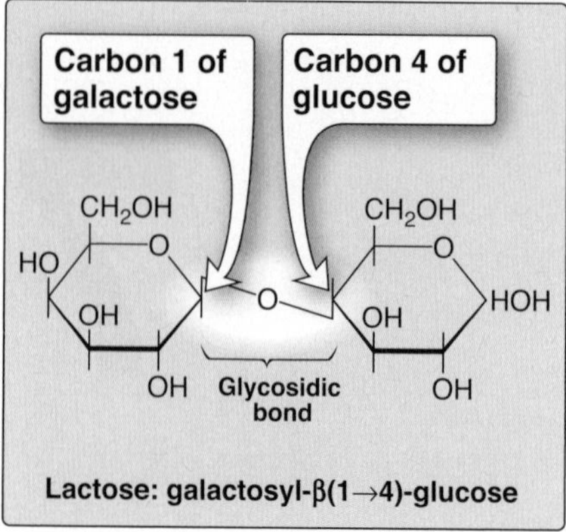

Figure 7.3
A glycosidic bond between two hexoses producing a disaccharide.

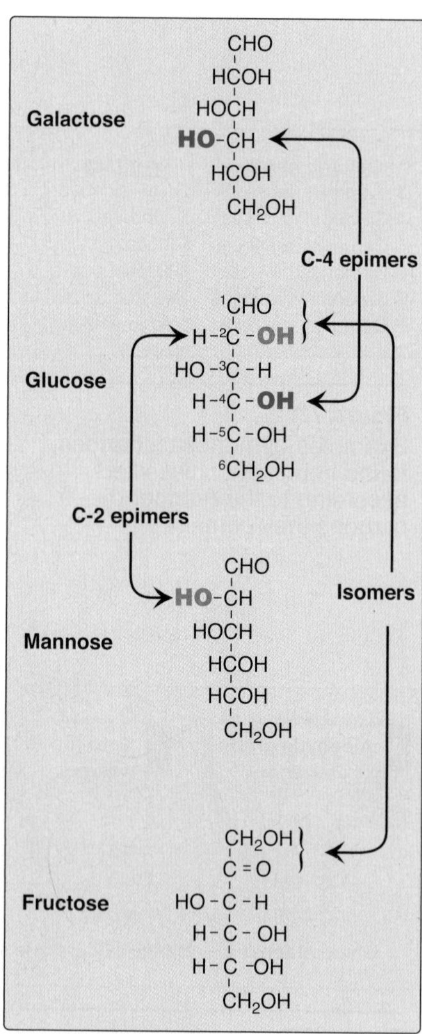

Figure 7.4
C-2 and C-4 epimers and an isomer of glucose.

C-4 epimers because their structures differ only in the position of the –OH group at carbon 4. [Note: The carbons in sugars are numbered beginning at the end that contains the carbonyl carbon (that is, the aldehyde or keto group) as shown in Figure 7.4.] Glucose and mannose are C-2 epimers. However, because galactose and mannose differ in the position of –OH groups at two carbons (carbons 2 and 4), they are isomers rather than epimers (see Figure 7.4).

B. Enantiomers

A special type of isomerism is found in the pairs of structures that are mirror images of each other. These mirror images are called enantiomers, and the two members of the pair are designated as a D- and an L-sugar (Figure 7.5). The vast majority of the sugars in humans are D-sugars. In the D isomeric form, the –OH group on the asymmetric carbon (a carbon linked to four different atoms or groups) farthest from the carbonyl carbon is on the right, whereas in the L-isomer, it is on the left. Most enzymes are specific for either the D or the L form, but enzymes known as *racemases* are able to interconvert D- and L-isomers.

C. Cyclization of monosaccharides

Less than 1% of each of the monosaccharides with five or more carbons exists in the open-chain (acyclic) form in solution. Rather, they are predominantly found in a ring (cyclic) form, in which the aldehyde (or keto) group has reacted with an alcohol group on the same sugar, making the carbonyl carbon (carbon 1 for an aldose, carbon 2 for a ketose) asymmetric. This asymmetric carbon is referred to as the anomeric carbon.

1. **Anomers:** Creation of an anomeric carbon (the former carbonyl carbon), generates a new pair of isomers, the α and β configurations of the sugar (for example, α-D-glucopyranose and β-D-glucopyranose; see Figure 7.6), that are anomers of each other. [Note: In the α configuration, the –OH group on the anomeric carbon projects to the same side as the ring in a modified Fischer projection formula (Figure 7.6A) and is trans to the CH_2OH group in a Haworth projection formula (Figure 7.6B). The α and β forms are not mirror images, and they are referred to as diastereomers.] Enzymes are able to distinguish between these two structures and use one or the other preferentially. For example, glycogen is synthesized from α-D-glucopyranose, whereas cellulose is synthesized from β-D-glucopyranose. The cyclic α and β anomers of a sugar in solution spontaneously (but slowly) form an equilibrium mixture, a process known as mutarotation (see Figure 7.6). [Note: For glucose, the α form makes up 36% of the mixture.]

2. **Reducing sugars:** If the hydroxyl group on the anomeric carbon of a cyclized sugar is not linked to another compound by a glycosidic bond, the ring can open. The sugar can act as a reducing agent and is termed a reducing sugar. Such sugars can react with chromogenic agents (for example, the Benedict reagent) causing the reagent to be reduced and colored, with the aldehyde group of the acyclic sugar becoming oxidized. All monosaccharides, but not all disaccharides, are reducing sugars. [Note:

Glucose can have its terminal hydroxyl group oxidized to a carboxyl group, forming glucuronic acid (see p. 161), or its aldehyde group oxidized to a hydroxyl group, forming a sugar alcohol.]

> A colorimetric test can detect a reducing sugar in urine. A positive result is indicative of an underlying pathology, because sugars are not normally present in urine, and can be followed up by more specific tests to identify the reducing sugar.

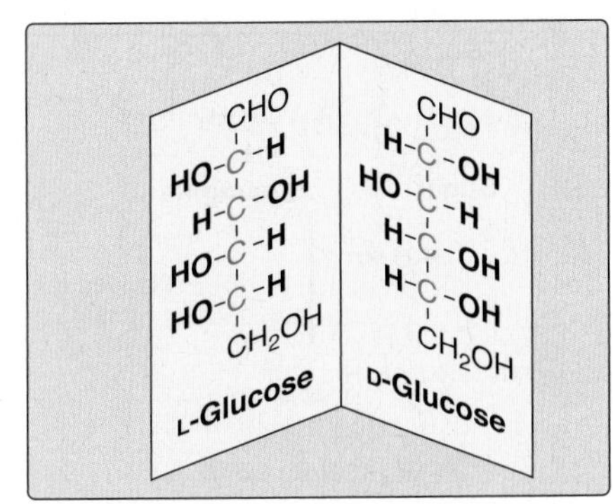

Figure 7.5
Enantiomers (mirror images) of glucose. Designation of D and L is by comparison to the triose, glyceraldehyde. [Note: The asymmetric carbons are shown in green.]

D. Joining of monosaccharides

Monosaccharides can be joined to form disaccharides, oligosaccharides, and polysaccharides. Important disaccharides include lactose (galactose + glucose), sucrose (glucose + fructose), and maltose (glucose + glucose). Important polysaccharides include branched glycogen (from animal sources) and starch (plant sources) and unbranched cellulose (plant sources). Each is a polymer of glucose. The bonds that link sugars are called glycosidic bonds. These are formed by enzymes known as *glycosyltransferases* that use nucleotide sugars such as uridine diphosphate glucose as substrates.

1. **Naming glycosidic bonds:** Glycosidic bonds between sugars are named according to the numbers of the connected carbons and with regard to the position of the anomeric hydroxyl group of the sugar involved in the bond. If this anomeric hydroxyl is in the α configuration, the linkage is an α-bond. If it is in the β configuration, the linkage is a β-bond. Lactose, for example, is synthesized by forming a glycosidic bond between carbon 1 of β-galactose and carbon 4 of glucose. The linkage is, therefore, a $\beta(1\rightarrow4)$ glycosidic bond (see Figure 7.3). [Note: Because the anomeric end of the glucose residue is not involved in the glycosidic linkage, it (and, therefore, lactose) remains a reducing sugar.]

E. Complex carbohydrates

Carbohydrates can be attached by glycosidic bonds to noncarbohydrate structures, including purine and pyrimidine bases (found in

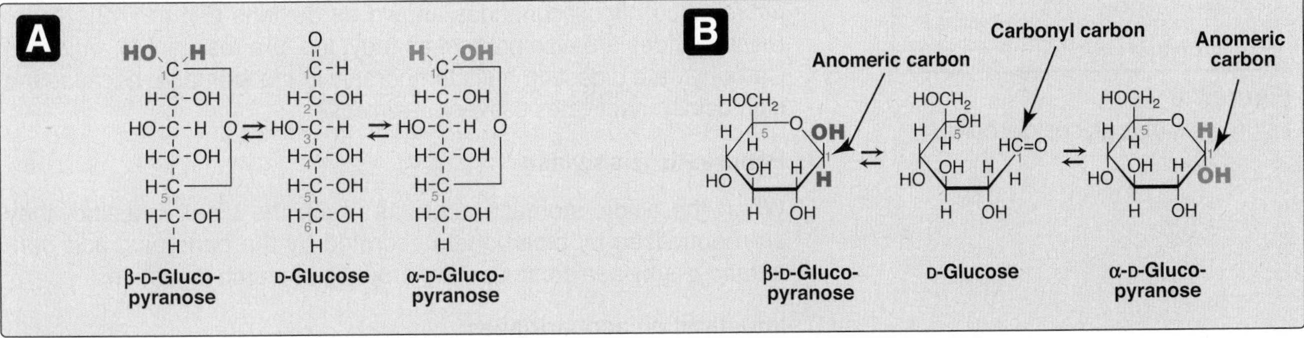

Figure 7.6
A The interconversion (mutarotation) of the α and β anomeric forms of glucose shown as modified Fischer projection formulas. B. The interconversion shown as Haworth projection formulas. [Note: A sugar with a six-membered ring (5C + 1O) is termed a pyranose, whereas one with a five-membered ring (4C + 1O) is a furanose. Virtually all glucose in solution is in the pyranose form.]

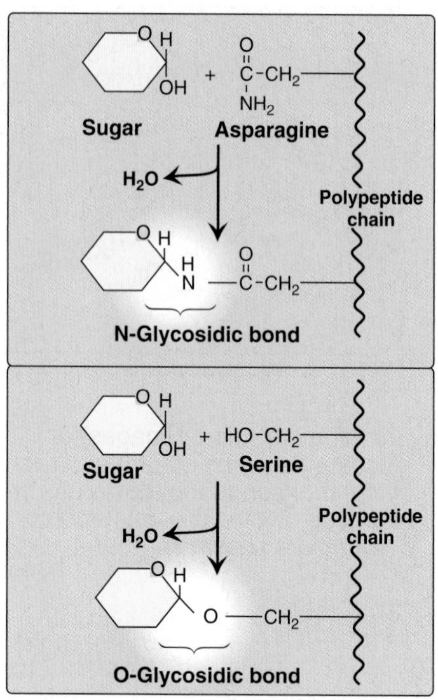

Figure 7.7
Glycosides: examples of N- and O-glycosidic bonds.

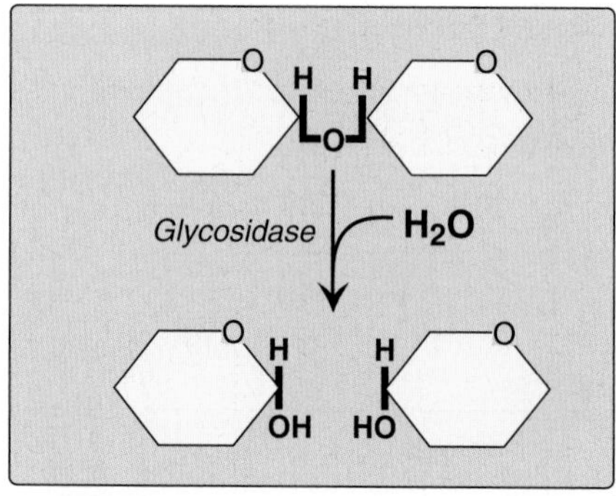

Figure 7.8
Hydrolysis of a glycosidic bond.

nucleic acids), aromatic rings (such as those found in steroids and bilirubin), proteins (found in glycoproteins and proteoglycans), and lipids (found in glycolipids), to form glycosides.

1. **N- and O-glycosides:** If the group on the noncarbohydrate molecule to which the sugar is attached is an $-NH_2$ group, the structure is an N-glycoside, and the bond is called an N-glycosidic link. If the group is an –OH, the structure is an O-glycoside, and the bond is an O-glycosidic link (Figure 7.7). [Note: All sugar–sugar glycosidic bonds are O-type linkages.]

III. DIGESTION OF DIETARY CARBOHYDRATES

The principal sites of dietary carbohydrate digestion are the mouth and intestinal lumen. This digestion is rapid and is catalyzed by enzymes known as *glycoside hydrolases* (*glycosidases*) that hydrolyze glycosidic bonds (Figure 7.8). Because there is little monosaccharide present in diets of mixed animal and plant origin, the enzymes are primarily *endoglycosidases* that hydrolyze polysaccharides and oliosaccharides, and *disaccharidases* that hydrolyse tri- and disaccharides into their reducing sugar components. *Glycosidases* are usually specific for the structure and configuration of the glycosyl residue to be removed as well as for the type of bond to be broken. The final products of carbohydrate digestion are the monosaccharides, glucose, galactose, and fructose that are absorbed by cells of the small intestine.

A. Salivary α-amylase

The major dietary polysaccharides are of plant (starch, composed of amylose and amylopectin) and animal (glycogen) origin. During mastication, *salivary α-amylase* acts briefly on dietary starch and glycogen, hydrolyzing random α(1→4) bonds. [Note: There are both *α(1→4)-* and *β(1→4)-endoglucosidases* in nature, but humans do not produce the latter. Therefore, we are unable to digest cellulose, a carbohydrate of plant origin containing β(1→4) glycosidic bonds between glucose residues.] Because branched amylopectin and glycogen also contain α(1→6) bonds, which *α-amylase* cannot hydrolyze, the digest resulting from its action contains a mixture of short, branched and unbranched oligosaccharides known as dextrins (Figure 7.9). [Note: Disaccharides are also present as they, too, are resistant to *amylase*.] Carbohydrate digestion halts temporarily in the stomach, because the high acidity inactivates salivary *α-amylase*.

B. Pancreatic α-amylase

When the acidic stomach contents reach the small intestine, they are neutralized by bicarbonate secreted by the pancreas, and *pancreatic α-amylase* continues the process of starch digestion.

C. Intestinal disaccharidases

The final digestive processes occur primarily at the mucosal lining of the upper jejunum and include the action of several *disaccharidases* (see Figure 7.9). For example, *isomaltase* cleaves the α(1→6) bond in isomaltose, and *maltase* cleaves the α(1→4) bond in maltose and maltotriose, each producing glucose. *Sucrase* cleaves the α(1→2) bond in sucrose, producing glucose and fructose, and *lactase* (*β-galactosidase*) cleaves the β(1→4) bond in lactose, producing galactose and glucose. [Note: The substrates for *isomaltase* are broader than its name suggests, and it hydrolyzes the majority of maltose.] Trehalose, an α(1→1) disaccharide of glucose found in mushrooms and other fungi is cleaved by *trehalase*. These enzymes are transmembrane proteins of the brush border on the luminal surface of the intestinal mucosal cells.

Sucrase and *isomaltase* are enzymic activities of a single protein (*SI*) which is cleaved into two functional subunits that remain associated in the cell membrane, forming the *sucrase-isomaltase* complex. In contrast, *maltase* is one of two enzymic activities of a single membrane protein *maltase-glucoamylase* (*MGA*) that does not get cleaved. Its second enzymic activity, *glucoamylase*, cleaves α(1→4) glycosidic bonds in dextrins.

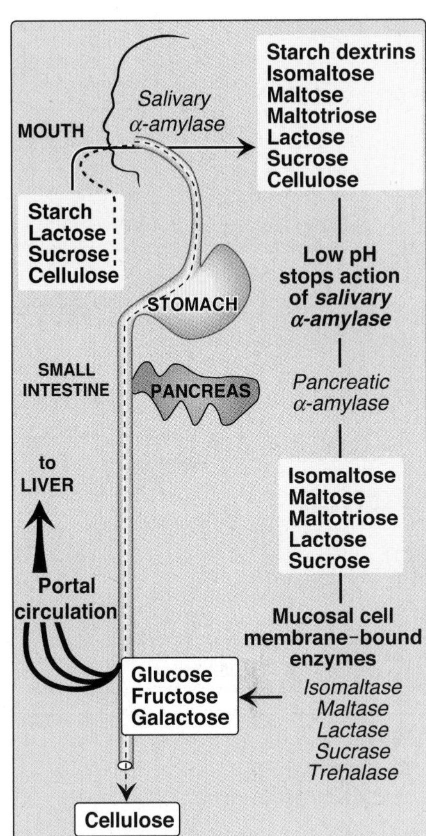

Figure 7.9
Digestion of carbohydrates. [Note: Indigestible cellulose enters the colon and is excreted.]

D. Intestinal absorption of monosaccharides

The duodenum and upper jejunum absorb the bulk of the monosaccharide products of digestion. However, different sugars have different mechanisms of absorption (Figure 7.10). For example, galactose and glucose are transported into the mucosal cells by an active, energy-dependent process that requires a concurrent uptake of sodium ions, and the transport protein is the sodium-dependent glucose cotransporter 1 (SGLT-1). Fructose utilizes an energy- and sodium-independent monosaccharide transporter (GLUT-5) for its absorption. All three monosaccharides are transported from the intestinal mucosal cell into the portal circulation by yet another transporter, GLUT-2. (See p. 97 for a discussion of these transporters.)

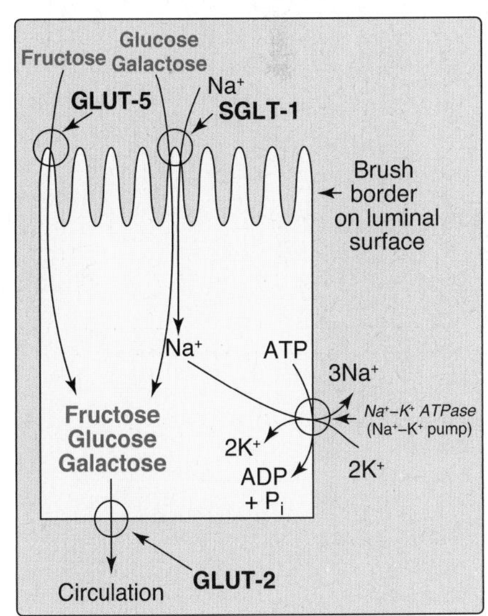

Figure 7.10
Absorption by intestinal mucosal cells of the monosaccharide products of carbohydrate digestion. SGLT-1 = sodium-dependent glucose transporter.

E. Abnormal degradation of disaccharides

The overall process of carbohydrate digestion and absorption is so efficient in healthy individuals that ordinarily all digestible dietary carbohydrate is absorbed by the time the ingested material reaches the lower jejunum. However, because only monosaccharides are absorbed, any deficiency (genetic or acquired) in a specific *disaccharidase* activity of the intestinal mucosa causes the passage of undigested carbohydrate into the large intestine. As a consequence of the presence of this osmotically active material, water is drawn from the mucosa into the large intestine, causing osmotic diarrhea. This is reinforced by the bacterial fermentation of the remaining carbohydrate to two- and three-carbon compounds (which are also osmotically active) plus large volumes of CO_2 and H_2 gas, causing abdominal cramps, diarrhea, and flatulence.

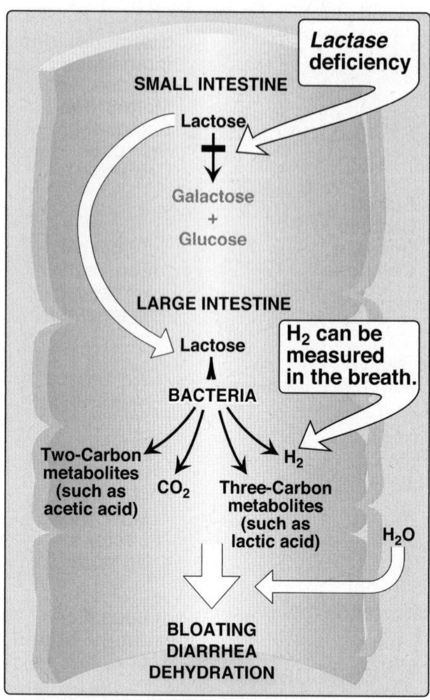

Figure 7.11
Abnormal lactose metabolism. H_2 = hydrogen gas.

1. **Digestive enzyme deficiencies:** Genetic deficiencies of the individual *disaccharidases* result in disaccharide intolerance. Alterations in disaccharide degradation can also be caused by a variety of intestinal diseases, malnutrition, and drugs that injure the mucosa of the small intestine. For example, brush border enzymes are rapidly lost in normal individuals with severe diarrhea, causing a temporary, acquired enzyme deficiency. Therefore, patients suffering or recovering from such a disorder cannot drink or eat significant amounts of dairy products or sucrose without exacerbating the diarrhea.

2. **Lactose intolerance:** More than 70% of the world's adults are lactose intolerant (Figure 7.11). This is particularly manifested in certain populations. For example, up to 90% of adults of African or Asian descent are *lactase*-deficient and, therefore, are less able to metabolize lactose than individuals of Northern European origin. The age-dependent loss of *lactase* activity represents a reduction in the amount of enzyme produced. It is thought to be caused by small variations in the DNA sequence of a region on chromosome 2 that controls expression of the gene for *lactase*, also on chromosome 2. Treatment for this disorder is to reduce consumption of milk and eat yogurts and some cheeses (bacterial action and aging process decrease lactose content) as well as green vegetables, such as broccoli, to ensure adequate calcium intake; to use *lactase*-treated products; or to take *lactase* in pill form prior to eating. [Note: Because the loss of *lactase* is the norm for most of the world's adults, use of the term "adult hypolactasia" for lactose intolerance is becoming more common.] Rare cases of congenital *lactase* deficiency are known.

3. **Congenital sucrase-isomaltase deficiency:** This autosomal recessive disorder results in an intolerance of ingested sucrose. Congenital *sucrase-isomaltase* deficiency has a prevalence of 0.02% in individuals of European descent and appears to be much more common in the Inuit people of Greenland and Canada. Treatment includes the dietary restriction of sucrose and enzyme replacement therapy.

4. **Diagnosis:** Identification of a specific enzyme deficiency can be obtained by performing oral tolerance tests with the individual disaccharides. Measurement of hydrogen gas in the breath is a reliable test for determining the amount of ingested carbohydrate not absorbed by the body, but which is metabolized instead by the intestinal flora (see Figure 7.11).

IV. CHAPTER SUMMARY

Monosaccharides (Figure 7.12) containing an aldehyde group are called **aldoses**, and those with a keto group are called **ketoses**. **Disaccharides**, **oligosaccharides**, and **polysaccharides** consist of monosaccharides linked by **glycosidic bonds**. Compounds with the same chemical formula but different structures are called **isomers**. If two monosaccharide isomers differ in configuration around one specific carbon atom (with the exception of the carbonyl carbon), they are defined as **epimers** of each other. If a pair of sugars are mirror images (**enantiomers**), the two members of the pair are designated as **D-** and **L-sugars**. If the aldehyde group on an acyclic sugar gets oxidized as a chromogenic agent gets reduced, that sugar is a reducing sugar. When a sugar cyclizes, an **anomeric carbon** is created from the aldehyde group of an aldose or keto group of a ketose. The sugar can have two configurations, **α** or **β**. A sugar with its anomeric carbon linked to another structure forms a **glycoside**. Sugars can be attached either to an $-NH_2$ or an –OH group, producing **N-** and **O-glycosides**. ***Salivary α-amylase*** acts on **dietary polysaccharides** (starch, glycogen), producing oligosaccharides. ***Pancreatic α-amylase*** continues the process of carbohydrate digestion.The final digestive processes occur at the **mucosal lining** of the **small intestine**. Several *disaccharidases* (for example, ***lactase*** [***β-galactosidase***], ***sucrase***, ***isomaltase***, and ***maltase***) produce monosaccharides (glucose, galactose, and fructose). These enzymes are **transmembrane proteins** of the luminal **brush border** of **intestinal mucosal cells**. Absorption of the monosaccharides requires specific transporters. If carbohydrate degradation is deficient (as a result of heredity, disease, or drugs that injure the intestinal mucosa), undigested carbohydrate will pass into the large intestine, where it can cause **osmotic diarrhea**. Bacterial fermentation of the material produces large volumes of CO_2 and H_2, causing abdominal cramps, diarrhea, and flatulence. **Lactose intolerance**, primarily caused by the age-dependent loss of ***lactase*** (**adult hypolactasia**), is by far the most common of these deficiencies.

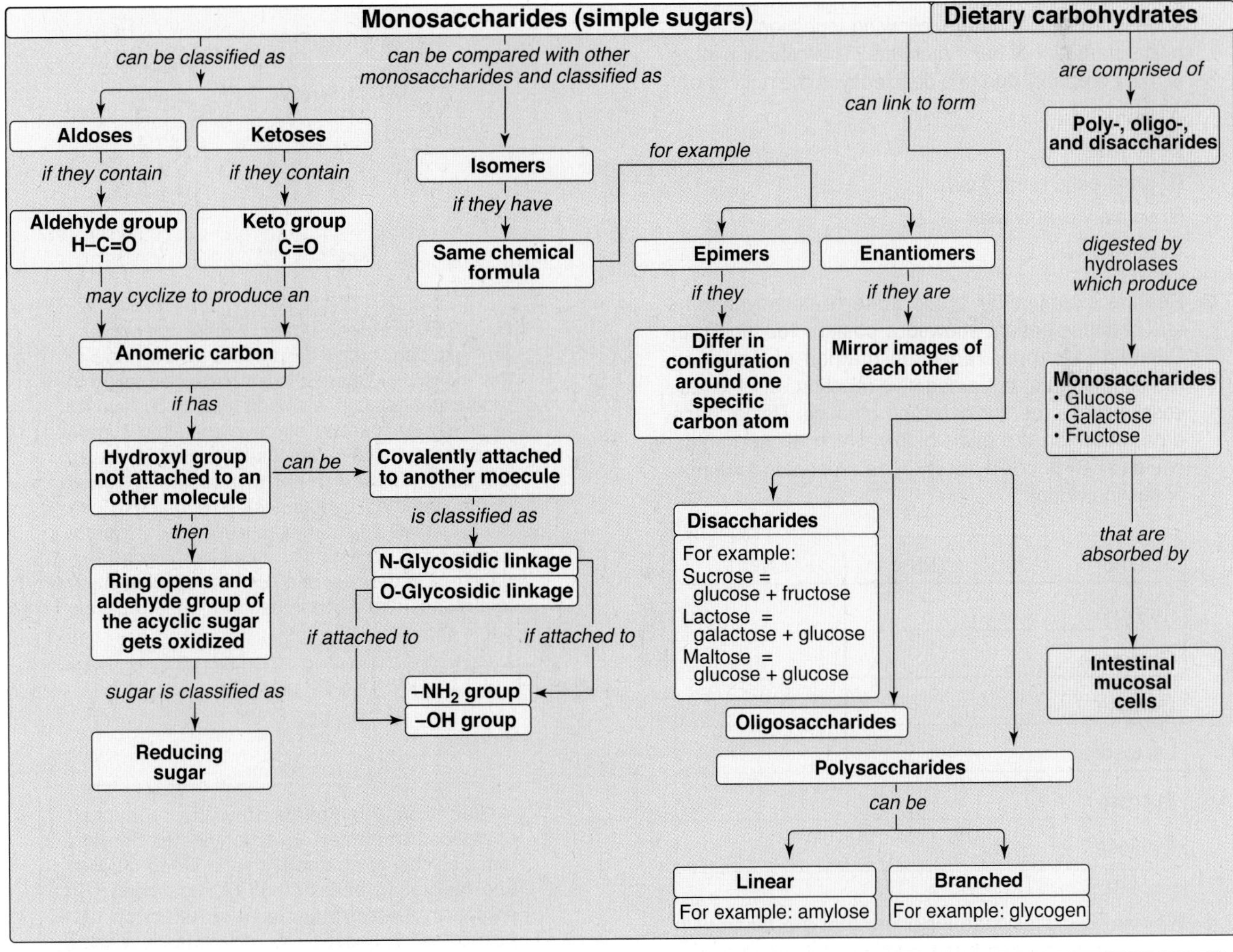

Figure 7.12
Key concept map for the classification and structure of monosaccharides and the digestion of dietary carbohydrates.

Study Question

Choose the ONE best answer.

7.1 Which of the following statements best describes glucose?

A. It is a C-4 epimer of galactose.

B. It is a ketose and usually exists as a furanose ring in solution.

C. It is produced from dietary starch by the action of α-amylase.

D. It is utilized in biological systems only in the L-isomeric form.

Correct answer = A. Glucose and galactose differ only in configuration around carbon 4 and so are C-4 epimers that are interconvertible by the action of an epimerase. Glucose is an aldose sugar that typically exists as a pyranose ring in solution. Fructose, however, is a ketose with a furanose ring. α-Amylase does not produce monosaccharides. The D-isomeric form of carbohydrates is most typically the form found in biologic systems, in contrast to amino acids.

7.2 A young man entered his physician's office complaining of bloating and diarrhea. His eyes were sunken, and the physician noted additional signs of dehydration. The patient's temperature was normal. He explained that the episode had occurred following a birthday party at which he had participated in an ice cream–eating contest. The patient reported prior episodes of a similar nature following ingestion of a significant amount of dairy products. This clinical picture is most probably due to a deficiency in the activity of:

A. isomaltase.

B. lactase.

C. pancreatic α-amylase.

D. salivary α-amylase.

E. sucrase.

Correct answer = B. The physical symptoms suggest a deficiency in an enzyme responsible for carbohydrate degradation. The symptoms observed following the ingestion of dairy products suggest that the patient is deficient in lactase.

7.3 Routine examination of the urine of an asymptomatic pediatric patient showed a positive reaction with Clinitest (a copper reduction method of detecting reducing sugars) but a negative reaction with the glucose oxidase test for detecting glucose. Using these data, show on the chart below which of the sugars could (YES) or could not (NO) be present in the urine of this individual.

SUGAR	YES	NO
Fructose		
Galactose		
Glucose		
Lactose		
Sucrose		
Xylulose		

Each of the listed sugars, except for sucrose and glucose, could be present in the urine of this individual. Clinitest is a nonspecific test that produces a change in color if urine is positive for reducing substances such as reducing sugars (fructose, galactose, glucose, lactose, xylulose). Because sucrose is not a reducing sugar, it is not detected by Clinitest. The glucose oxidase test will detect only glucose, and it cannot detect other sugars. The negative glucose oxidase test in the face of a positive reducing sugar test means that glucose cannot be the reducing sugar in the patient's urine.

7.4 Why are α-glucosidase inhibitors that are taken with meals, such as acarbose and miglitol, used in the treatment of diabetes? What effect should these drugs have on the digestion of lactose?

α-Glucosidase inhibitors slow the production of glucose from dietary carbohydrates, thereby reducing the postprandial rise in blood glucose and facilitating better blood glucose control in diabetics. These drugs have no effect on lactose digestion because the disaccharide lactose contains a β-glycosidic bond, not an α-glycosidic bond.

Introduction to Metabolism and Glycolysis

8

I. INTRODUCTION TO METABOLISM

In Chapter 5, individual enzymic reactions were analyzed in an effort to explain the mechanisms of catalysis. However, in cells, these reactions rarely occur in isolation but, rather, are organized into multistep sequences called pathways, such as that of glycolysis (Figure 8.1). In a pathway, the product of one reaction serves as the substrate of the subsequent reaction. Different pathways can also intersect, forming an integrated and purposeful network of chemical reactions. These are collectively called metabolism, which is the sum of all the chemical changes occurring in a cell, a tissue, or the body. Most pathways can be classified as either catabolic (degradative) or anabolic (synthetic). Catabolic reactions break down complex molecules, such as proteins, polysaccharides, and lipids, to a few simple molecules (for example, CO_2, NH_3 [ammonia], and H_2O). Anabolic pathways form complex end products from simple precursors, for example, the synthesis of the polysaccharide, glycogen, from glucose. [Note: Pathways that regenerate a component are called cycles.] In the following chapters, this text focuses on the central metabolic pathways that are involved in synthesizing and degrading carbohydrates, lipids, and amino acids.

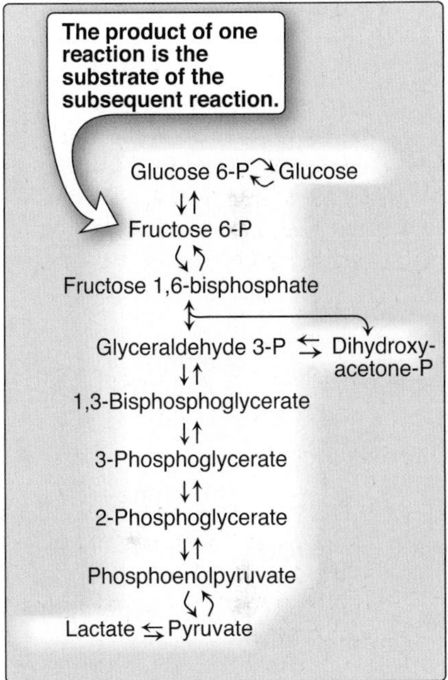

Figure 8.1
Glycolysis, an example of a metabolic pathway. [Note: Pyruvate to phosphoenolpyruvate requires two reactions.] Curved reaction arrows (⟲) indicate forward and reverse reactions that are catalyzed by different enzymes.P = phosphate.

A. Metabolic map

It is convenient to investigate metabolism by examining its component pathways. Each pathway is composed of multienzyme sequences, and each enzyme, in turn, may exhibit important catalytic or regulatory features. To provide the reader with the "big picture," a metabolic map containing the important central pathways of energy metabolism is presented in Figure 8.2. This map is useful in tracing connections between pathways, visualizing the purposeful "movement" of metabolic intermediates, and depicting the effect on the flow of intermediates if a pathway is blocked (for example, by a drug or an inherited deficiency of an enzyme). Throughout the next three units of this book, each pathway under discussion will be repeatedly featured as part of the major metabolic map shown in Figure 8.2.

B. Catabolic pathways

Catabolic reactions serve to capture chemical energy in the form of adenosine triphosphate (ATP) from the degradation of energy-rich fuel molecules. Catabolism also allows molecules in the diet (or nutrient molecules stored in cells) to be converted into building blocks needed for the synthesis of complex molecules. Energy generation by

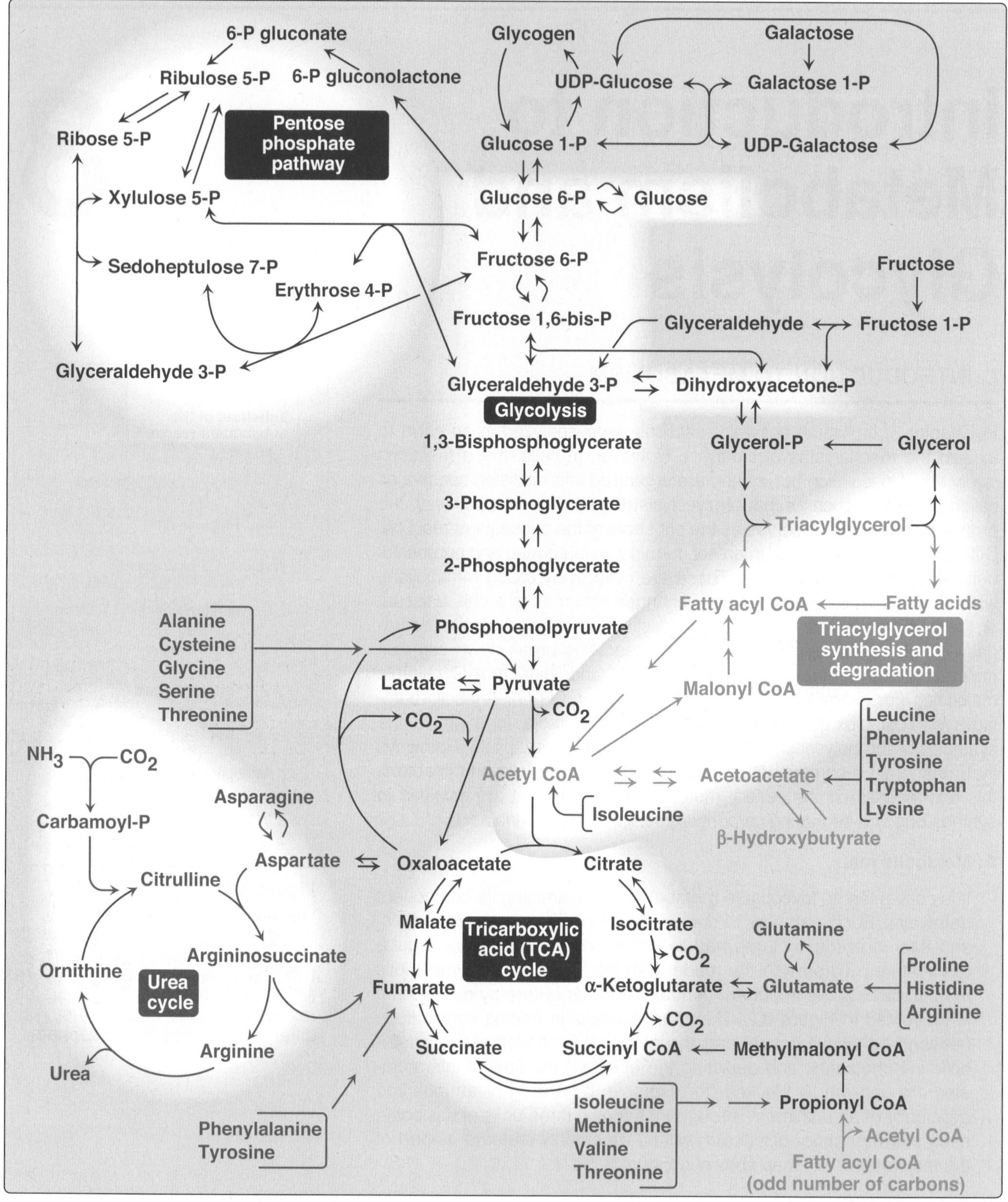

Figure 8.2

Important reactions of intermediary metabolism. Several important pathways to be discussed in later chapters are highlighted. Curved reaction arrows (⥁) indicate forward and reverse reactions that are catalyzed by different enzymes. The straight arrows (⇆) indicate forward and reverse reactions that are catalyzed by the same enzyme. **Blue text** = intermediates of carbohydrate metabolism; **brown text** = intermediates of lipid metabolism; **green text** = intermediates of protein metabolism. UDP = uridine diphosphate; P = phosphate; CoA = coenzyme A.

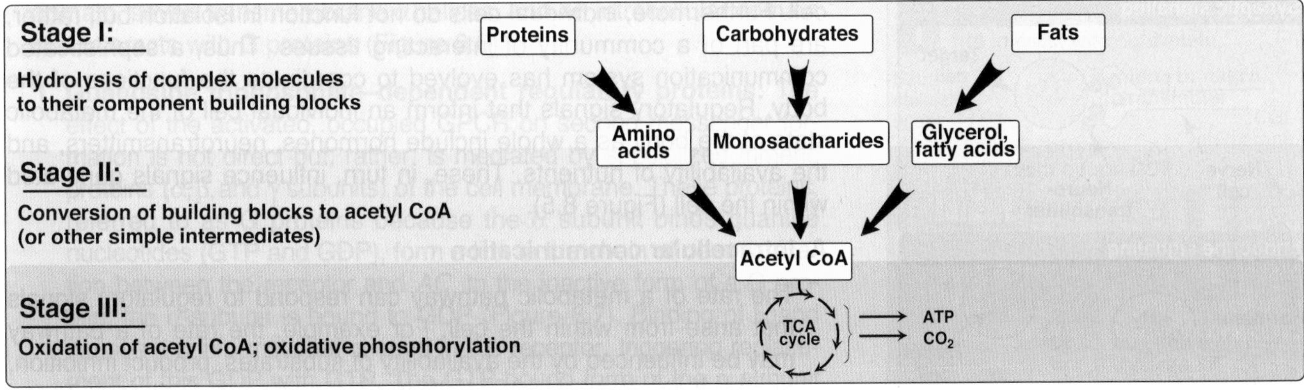

Figure 8.3
Three stages of catabolism. CoA = coenzyme A; TCA = tricarboxylic acid.

degradation of complex molecules occurs in three stages as shown in Figure 8.3. [Note: Catabolic pathways are typically oxidative, and require oxidized coenzymes such as nicotinamide adenine dinucleotide (NAD^+).]

1. **Hydrolysis of complex molecules:** In the first stage, complex molecules are broken down into their component building blocks. For example, proteins are degraded to amino acids, polysaccharides to monosaccharides, and fats (triacylglycerols) to free fatty acids and glycerol.

2. **Conversion of building blocks to simple intermediates:** In the second stage, these diverse building blocks are further degraded to acetyl coenzyme A (CoA) and a few other simple molecules. Some energy is captured as ATP, but the amount is small compared with the energy produced during the third stage of catabolism.

3. **Oxidation of acetyl coenzyme A:** The tricarboxylic acid (TCA) cycle (see p. 109) is the final common pathway in the oxidation of fuel molecules that produce acetyl CoA. Oxidation of acetyl CoA generates large amounts of ATP via oxidative phosphorylation as electrons flow from NADH and flavin adenine dinucleotide ($FADH_2$) to oxygen (see p. 73).

C. Anabolic pathways

Anabolic reactions combine small molecules, such as amino acids, to form complex molecules such as proteins (Figure 8.4). Anabolic reactions require energy (are endergonic), which is generally provided by the hydrolysis of ATP to adenosine diphosphate (ADP) and inorganic phosphate (P_i). Anabolic reactions often involve chemical reductions in which the reducing power is most frequently provided by the electron donor NADPH (see p. 147). Note that catabolism is a convergent process (that is, a wide variety of molecules are transformed into a few common end products). By contrast, anabolism is a divergent process in which a few biosynthetic precursors form a wide variety of polymeric, or complex, products.

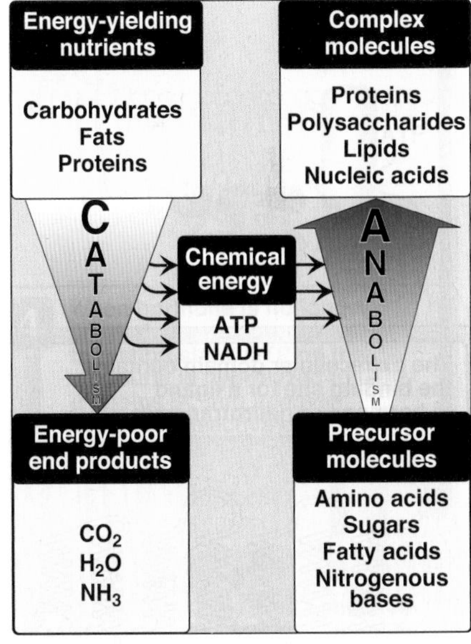

Figure 8.4
Comparison of catabolic and anabolic pathways. ATP = adenosine triphosphate; NADH = nicotinamide adenine dinucleotide.

II. REGULATION OF METABOLISM

The pathways of metabolism must be coordinated so that the production of energy or the synthesis of end products meets the needs of the

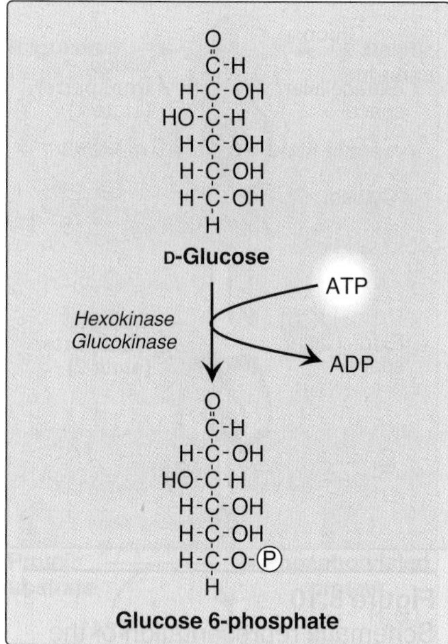

Figure 8.12
Energy-investment phase: phosphorylation of glucose. [Note: *Kinases* utilize ATP complexed with a divalent metal ion, most typically Mg^{2+}.]

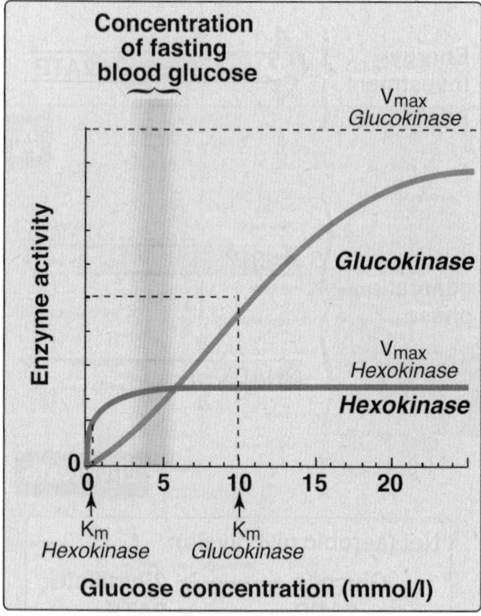

Figure 8.13
Effect of glucose concentration on the rate of phosphorylation catalyzed by *hexokinase* and *glucokinase*. K_m = Michaelis constant; V_{max} = maximal velocity.

A. Phosphorylation of glucose

Phosphorylated sugar molecules do not readily penetrate cell membranes because there are no specific transmembrane carriers for these compounds and because they are too polar to diffuse through the lipid core of membranes. The irreversible phosphorylation of glucose (Figure 8.12), therefore, effectively traps the sugar as cytosolic glucose 6-phosphate, thereby committing it to further metabolism in the cell. Mammals have four (I–IV) isozymes of the enzyme *hexokinase* that catalyze the phosphorylation of glucose to glucose 6-phosphate.

1. **Hexokinases I–III:** In most tissues, phosphorylation of glucose is catalyzed by one of these isozymes of *hexokinase*, which is one of three regulatory enzymes of glycolysis (see also *phosphofructokinase* and *pyruvate kinase*). These isozymes have broad substrate specificity and are able to phosphorylate several hexoses in addition to glucose. They are inhibited by the reaction product, glucose 6-phosphate, which accumulates when further metabolism of this hexose phosphate is reduced. *Hexokinases I-III* have a low Michaelis constant (K_m) (and, therefore, a high affinity; see p. 59) for glucose. This permits the efficient phosphorylation and subsequent metabolism of glucose even when tissue concentrations of glucose are low (Figure 8.13). These isozymes, however, have a low maximal velocity ([V_{max}] see p. 59) for glucose and, therefore, do not sequester (trap) cellular phosphate in the form of phosphorylated hexoses, or phosphorylate more sugars than the cell can use.

2. **Hexokinase IV (or, glucokinase):** In liver parenchymal cells and β cells of the pancreas, *glucokinase* (the *hexokinase IV* isozyme) is the predominant enzyme responsible for the phosphorylation of glucose. In β cells, *glucokinase* functions as a glucose sensor, determining the threshold for insulin secretion (see p. 309). [Note: *Hexokinase IV* also serves as a glucose sensor in neurons of the hypothalamus, playing a key role in the adrenergic response to hypoglycemia (see p. 315.] In the liver, the enzyme facilitates glucose phosphorylation during hyperglycemia. Despite the popular but misleading name *glucokinase*, the sugar specificity of the enzyme is similar to that of other *hexokinase* isozymes.

   a. **Kinetics:** *Glucokinase* differs from *hexokinases I–III* in several important properties. For example, it has a much higher K_m, requiring a higher glucose concentration for half-saturation (see Figure 8.13). Thus, *glucokinase* functions only when the intracellular concentration of glucose in the hepatocyte is elevated such as during the brief period following consumption of a carbohydrate-rich meal, when high levels of glucose are delivered to the liver via the portal vein. *Glucokinase* has a high V_{max}, allowing the liver to effectively remove the flood of glucose delivered by the portal blood. This prevents large amounts of glucose from entering the systemic circulation following such a meal thereby minimizing hyperglycemia during the absorptive period. [Note: GLUT-2 insures that blood glucose equilibrates rapidly across the membrane of the hepatocyte.]

   b. **Regulation by fructose 6-phosphate and glucose:** *Glucokinase* activity is not directly inhibited by glucose 6-phosphate as are the other *hexokinases* but, rather, is indirectly inhibited by fructose 6-phosphate (which is in equilibrium with glucose

6-phosphate, a product of *glucokinase*) and is indirectly stimulated by glucose (a substrate of *glucokinase*) via the following mechanism. Glucokinase regulatory protein (GKRP) in the liver regulates the activity of *glucokinase* through reversible binding. In the presence of fructose 6-phosphate, *glucokinase* is translocated into the nucleus and binds tightly to the regulatory protein, thereby rendering the enzyme inactive (Figure 8.14). When glucose levels in the blood (and also in the hepatocyte, as a result of GLUT-2) increase, *glucokinase* is released from the regulatory protein, and the enzyme reenters the cytosol where it phosphorylates glucose to glucose 6-phosphate. [Note: Fructose 1-phosphate inhibits formation of the *glucokinase*–GKRP complex.]

> *Glucokinase* functions as a glucose sensor in the maintenance of blood glucose homeostasis. Inactivating mutations of *glucokinase* are the cause of a rare form of diabetes, maturity onset diabetes of the young type 2 (MODY 2) that is characterized by impaired insulin secretion.

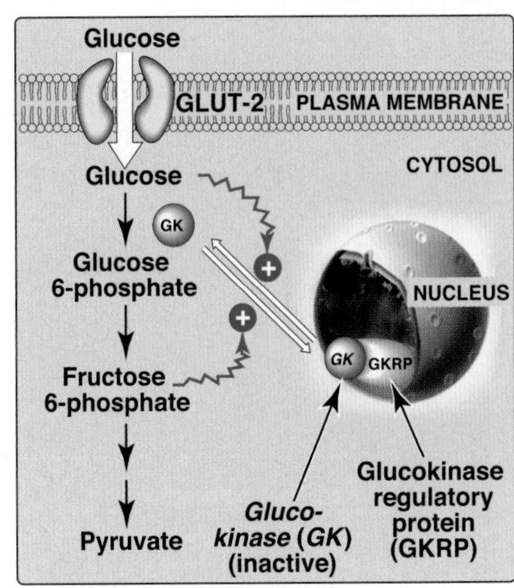

Figure 8.14
Regulation of *glucokinase* activity by glucokinase regulatory protein. GLUT = glucose transporter.

B. Isomerization of glucose 6-phosphate

The isomerization of glucose 6-phosphate to fructose 6-phosphate is catalyzed by *phosphoglucose isomerase* (Figure 8.15). The reaction is readily reversible and is not a rate-limiting or regulated step.

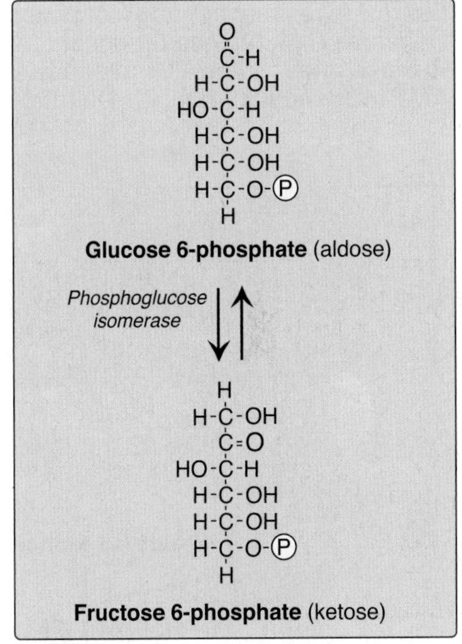

Figure 8.15
Aldose-ketose isomerization of glucose 6-phosphate to fructose 6-phosphate. P = phosphate.

C. Phosphorylation of fructose 6-phosphate

The irreversible phosphorylation reaction catalyzed by *phosphofructokinase-1* (*PFK-1*) is the most important control point and the rate-limiting and committed step of glycolysis (Figure 8.16). *PFK-1* is controlled by the available concentrations of the substrates ATP and fructose 6-phosphate as well as by regulatory substances described below.

1. **Regulation by energy levels within the cell:** *PFK-1* is inhibited allosterically by elevated levels of ATP, which act as an "energy-rich" signal indicating an abundance of high-energy compounds. Elevated levels of citrate, an intermediate in the TCA cycle (see p. 109), also inhibit *PFK-1*. [Note: Inhibition by citrate favors the use of glucose for glycogen synthesis (see p. 125).] Conversely, *PFK-1* is activated allosterically by high concentrations of AMP, which signal that the cell's energy stores are depleted.

2. **Regulation by fructose 2,6-bisphosphate:** Fructose 2,6-bisphosphate is the most potent activator of *PFK-1* (see Figure 8.16) and is able to activate the enzyme even when ATP levels are high. Fructose 2,6-bisphosphate is formed from fructose 6-phosphate by *phosphofructokinase-2* (*PFK-2*), an enzyme different than *PFK-1*. *PFK-2* is a bifunctional protein that has both the *kinase* activity that produces fructose 2,6-bisphosphate and the *phosphatase* activity that dephosphorylates fructose 2,6-bisphosphate back to fructose 6-phosphate. In the liver, the *kinase* domain is active if dephosphorylated and is inactive if phosphorylated (Figure 8.17). [Note: Fructose 2,6-bisphosphate is an inhibitor

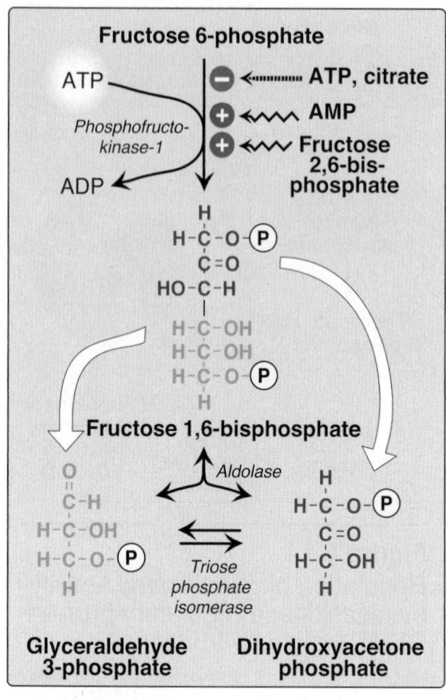

Figure 8.16
Energy–investment phase (continued): Conversion of fructose 6-phosphate to triose phosphates. P = phosphate; AMP = adenosine monophosphate.

of *fructose 1,6-bisphosphatase*, an enzyme of gluconeogenesis (see p. 120). The reciprocal actions of fructose 2,6-bisphosphate on glycolysis (activation) and gluconeogenesis (inhibition) ensure that both pathways are not fully active at the same time, preventing a futile cycle in which glucose would be converted to pyruvate followed by resynthesis of glucose from pyruvate.]

a. **During the well-fed state:** Decreased levels of glucagon and elevated levels of insulin, such as occur following a carbohydrate-rich meal, cause an increase in fructose 2,6-bisphosphate and, thus, in the rate of glycolysis in the liver (see Figure 8.17). Fructose 2,6-bisphosphate, therefore, acts as an intracellular signal, indicating that glucose is abundant.

b. **During fasting:** Elevated levels of glucagon and low levels of insulin, such as occur during fasting (see p. 327), decrease the intracellular concentration of hepatic fructose 2,6-bisphosphate. This results in inhibition of glycolysis and activation of gluconeogenesis.

D. Cleavage of fructose 1,6-bisphosphate

Aldolase cleaves fructose 1,6-bisphosphate to dihydroxyacetone phosphate and glyceraldehyde 3-phosphate (see Figure 8.16). The reaction is reversible and not regulated. [Note: *Aldolase B*, the isoform found primarily in the liver, also cleaves fructose 1-phosphate and functions in the metabolism of dietary fructose (see p. 138).]

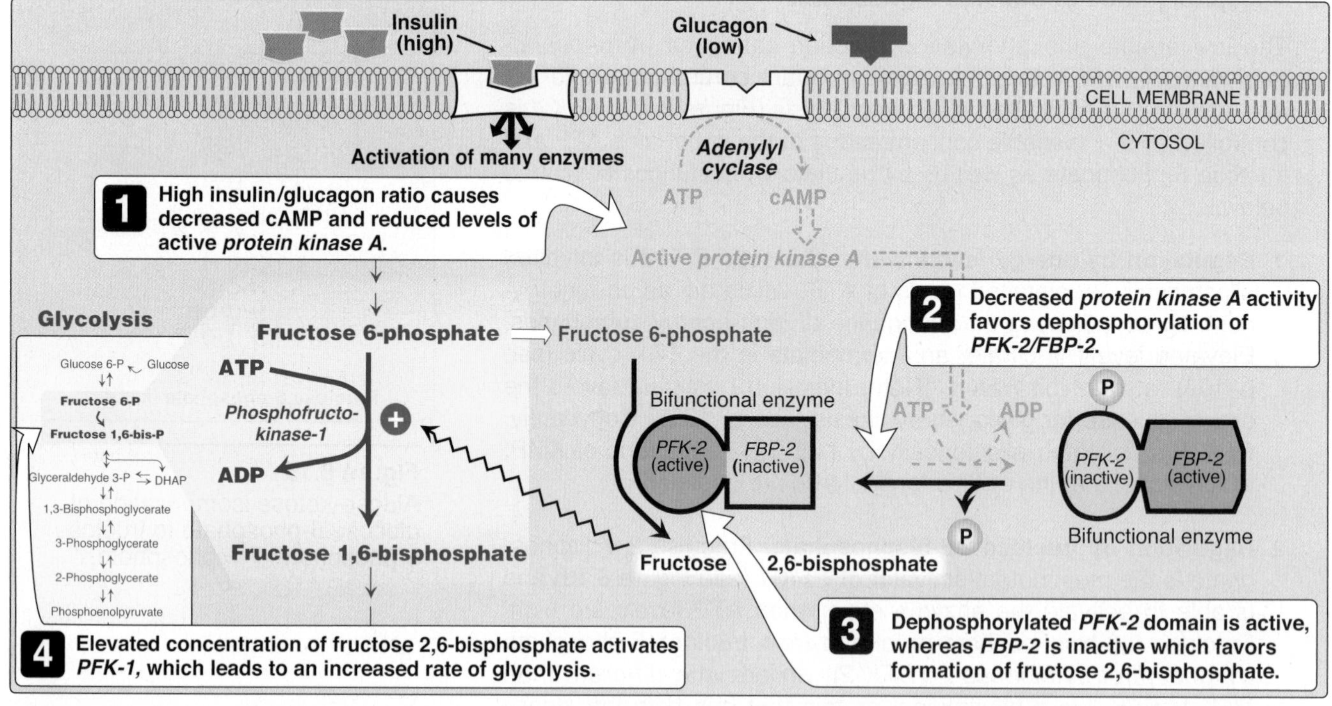

Figure 8.17
Effect of elevated insulin concentration on the intracellular concentration of fructose 2,6-bisphosphate in liver. *PFK-2 = phosphofructokinase-2*; *FBP-2 = fructose 2,6-bisphosphatase;* cAMP = cyclic AMP; P = phosphate.

E. Isomerization of dihydroxyacetone phosphate

Triose phosphate isomerase interconverts dihydroxyacetone phosphate (DHAP) and glyceraldehyde 3-phosphate (see Figure 8.16). DHAP must be isomerized to glyceraldehyde 3-phosphate for further metabolism by the glycolytic pathway. This isomerization results in the net production of two molecules of glyceraldehyde 3-phosphate from the cleavage products of fructose 1,6-bisphosphate. [Note: DHAP is utilized in triacylglycerol synthesis (see p. 188).]

F. Oxidation of glyceraldehyde 3-phosphate

The conversion of glyceraldehyde 3-phosphate to 1,3-bisphosphoglycerate (1,3-BPG) by *glyceraldehyde 3-phosphate dehydrogenase* is the first oxidation-reduction reaction of glycolysis (Figure 8.18). [Note: Because there is only a limited amount of NAD^+ in the cell, the NADH formed by this reaction must be reoxidized to NAD^+ for glycolysis to continue. Two major mechanisms for oxidizing NADH are 1) the NADH-linked conversion of pyruvate to lactate (anaerobic; see p. 96) and 2) oxidation of NADH via the respiratory chain (aerobic; see p. 74). The latter requires the malate-aspartate and glycerol 3-phosphate substrate shuttles (see p. 79.]

1. **Synthesis of 1,3-bisphosphoglycerate:** The oxidation of the aldehyde group of glyceraldehyde 3-phosphate to a carboxyl group is coupled to the attachment of P_i to the carboxyl group. The high-energy phosphate group at carbon 1 of 1,3-BPG conserves much of the free energy produced by the oxidation of glyceraldehyde 3-phosphate. The energy of this high-energy phosphate drives the synthesis of ATP in the next reaction of glycolysis.

2. **Mechanism of arsenic poisoning:** The toxicity of arsenic is due primarily to the inhibition by trivalent arsenic (arsenite) of enzymes such as the *pyruvate dehydrogenase complex*, which require lipoic acid as a coenzyme (see p. 110). However, pentavalent arsenic (arsenate) can prevent net ATP and NADH production by glycolysis without inhibiting the pathway itself. It does so by competing with P_i as a substrate for *glyceraldehyde 3-phosphate dehydrogenase*, forming a complex that spontaneously hydrolyzes to form 3-phosphoglycerate (see Figure 8.18). By bypassing the synthesis of and phosphate transfer from 1,3-BPG, the cell is deprived of energy usually obtained from the glycolytic pathway. [Note: Arsenate also competes with P_i on the F_1 domain of *ATP synthase* (see p. 77), resulting in formation of ADP-arsenate that is rapidly hydrolyzed.]

3. **Synthesis of 2,3-bisphosphoglycerate in red blood cells:** Some of the 1,3-BPG is converted to 2,3-BPG by the action of *bisphosphoglycerate mutase* (see Figure 8.18). 2,3-BPG, which is found in only trace amounts in most cells, is present at high concentration in red blood cells (RBCs) and serves to increase O_2 delivery (see p. 31). 2,3-BPG is hydrolyzed by a *phosphatase* to 3-phosphoglycerate, which is also an intermediate in glycolysis (see Figure 8.18). In the RBC, glycolysis is modified by inclusion of these “shunt” reactions.

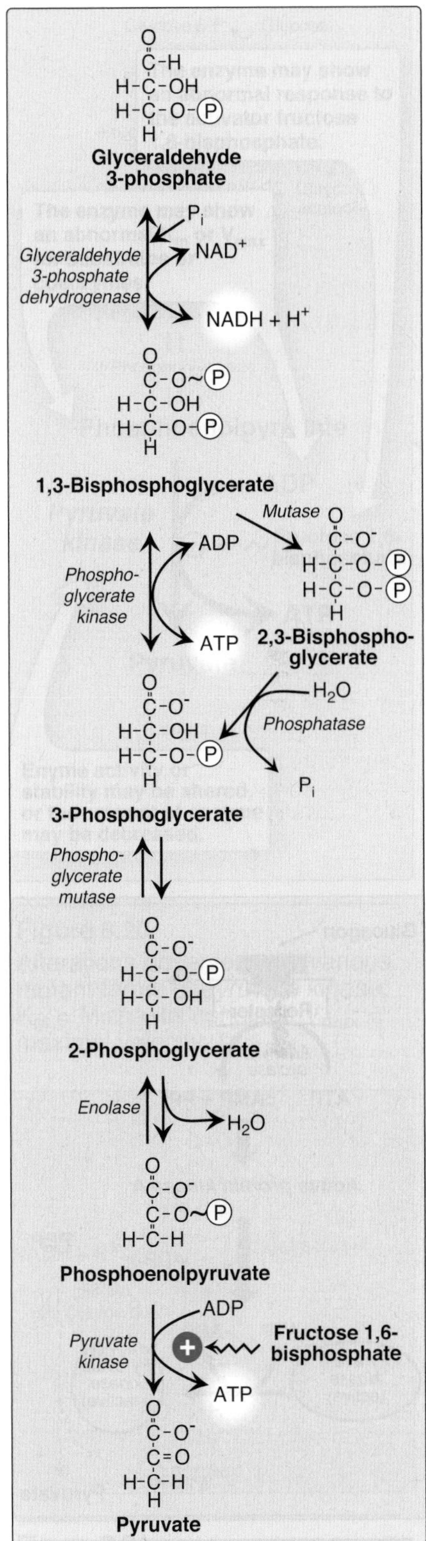

Figure 8.18
Energy–generating phase: conversion of glyceraldehyde 3-phosphate to pyruvate. NAD(H) = nicotinamide adenine dinucleotide P = phosphate; P_i = inorganic phosphate.

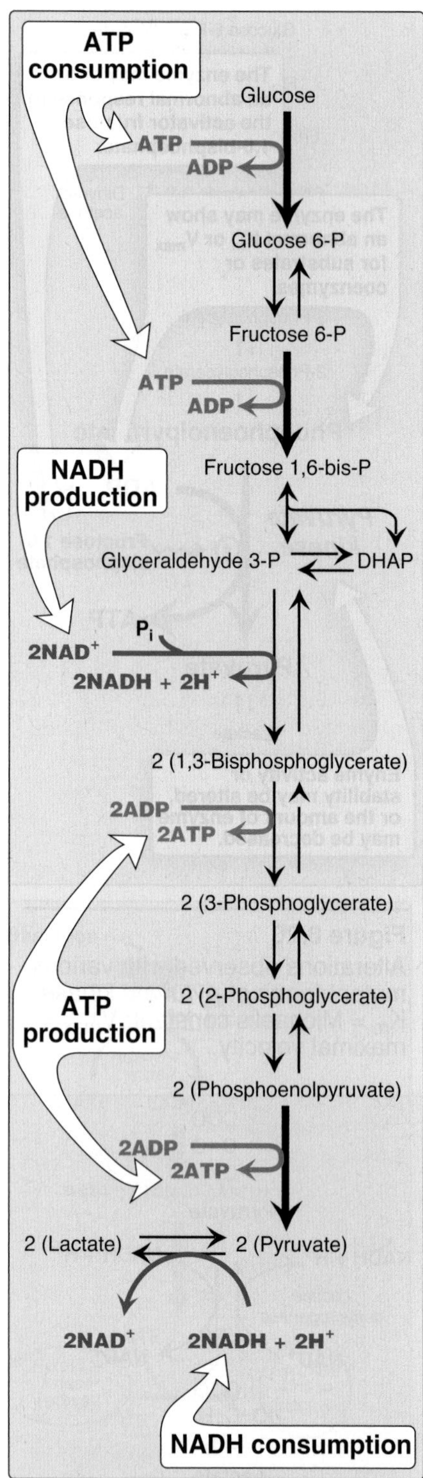

Figure 8.22
Summary of anaerobic glycolysis. Reactions involving the production or consumption of ATP or NADH are indicated. The three irreversible reactions of glycolysis are shown with thick arrows. DHAP = dihydroxyacetone phosphate; NAD(H) = nicotinamide adenine dinucleotide; P = phosphate.

3. **Lactic acidosis:** Elevated concentrations of lactate in the plasma, termed lactic acidosis (a type of metabolic acidosis), occur when there is a collapse of the circulatory system, such as in myocardial infarction, pulmonary embolism, and uncontrolled hemorrhage, or when an individual is in shock. The failure to bring adequate amounts of oxygen to the tissues results in impaired oxidative phosphorylation and decreased ATP synthesis. To survive, the cells rely on anaerobic glycolysis for generating ATP, producing lactic acid as the end product. [Note: Production of even meager amounts of ATP may be life-saving during the period required to reestablish adequate blood flow to the tissues.] The excess oxygen required to recover from a period when the availability of oxygen has been inadequate is termed the "oxygen debt."

> The oxygen debt is often related to patient morbidity or mortality. In many clinical situations, measuring the blood levels of lactic acid allows the rapid, early detection of oxygen debt in patients and the monitoring of their recovery.

L. Energy yield from glycolysis

Despite the production of some ATP during glycolysis, the end product, pyruvate or lactate, still contains most of the energy originally contained in glucose. The TCA cycle is required to release that energy completely (see p. 109).

1. **Anaerobic glycolysis:** Two molecules of ATP are generated for each molecule of glucose converted to two molecules of lactate (Figure 8.22). There is no net production or consumption of NADH.

2. **Aerobic glycolysis:** The direct consumption and formation of ATP is the same as in anaerobic glycolysis (that is, a net gain of two ATP per molecule of glucose). Two molecules of NADH are also produced per molecule of glucose. Ongoing aerobic glycolysis requires the oxidation of most of this NADH by the electron transport chain, producing approximately three ATP for each NADH molecule entering the chain (see p. 77). [Note: NADH cannot cross the inner mitochondrial membrane, and substrate shuttles are required (see p. 79).]

VI. HORMONAL REGULATION OF GLYCOLYSIS

The regulation of glycolysis by allosteric activation or inhibition, or the covalent phosphorylation/dephosphorylation of rate-limiting enzymes, is short-term (that is, they influence glucose consumption over periods of minutes or hours). Superimposed on these moment-to-moment effects are slower, and often more profound, hormonal influences on gene expression, or the amount of enzyme protein synthesized. These effects can result in 10-fold to 20-fold increases in enzyme activity that typically occur over hours to days. Although the current focus is on glycolysis, reciprocal changes occur in the rate-limiting enzymes of gluconeogenesis, which are described in Chapter 10 (see p. 117). Regular consumption of meals rich in carbohydrate or administration of insulin initiates an increase in the amount of *glucokinase*, *phosphofructokinase*, and *PK* in the liver (Figure 8.23). These changes reflect an increase in gene transcription, resulting in increased enzyme synthesis. High activity of these three enzymes favors the conversion of glucose to pyruvate, a characteristic of the absorptive state (see p. 321). Conversely, gene transcription and synthesis of *glucokinase, phosphofructokinase,* and *PK* are decreased when plasma glucagon is high and insulin is low (for example, as seen in fasting or diabetes).

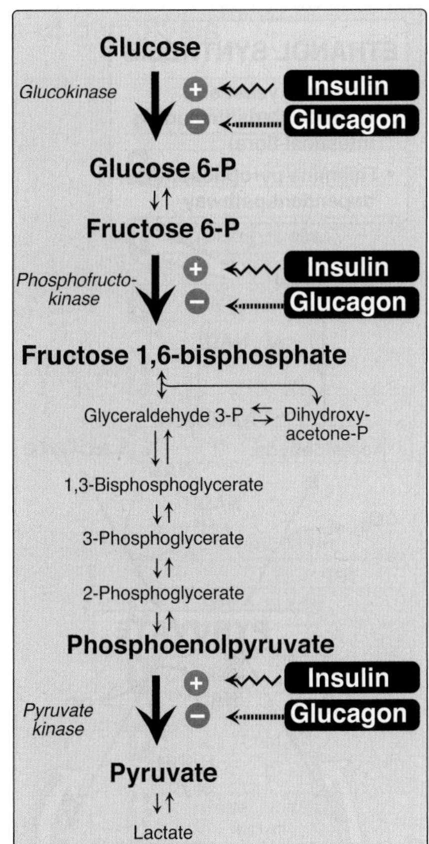

Figure 8.23
Effect of insulin and glucagon on the synthesis of key enzymes of glycolysis in liver. P = phosphate.

VII. ALTERNATE FATES OF PYRUVATE

A. Oxidative decarboxylation of pyruvate

Oxidative decarboxylation of pyruvate by the *pyruvate dehydrogenase complex* is an important pathway in tissues with a high oxidative capacity such as cardiac muscle (Figure 8.24). *Pyruvate dehydrogenase* irreversibly converts pyruvate, the end product of glycolysis, into acetyl CoA, a major fuel for the TCA cycle (see p. 109) and the building block for fatty acid synthesis (see p. 183).

B. Carboxylation of pyruvate to oxaloacetate

Carboxylation of pyruvate to oxaloacetate by *pyruvate carboxylase* is a biotin-dependent reaction (see Figure 8.24). This reaction is important because it replenishes the TCA cycle intermediates and provides substrate for gluconeogenesis (see p. 118).

C. Reduction of pyruvate to ethanol (microorganisms)

The conversion of pyruvate to ethanol occurs by the two reactions summarized in Figure 8.24. The decarboxylation of pyruvate by *pyruvate decarboxylase* occurs in yeast and certain other microorganisms but not in humans. The enzyme requires thiamine pyrophosphate as a coenzyme and catalyzes a reaction similar to that described for *pyruvate dehydrogenase* (see p. 110).

VIII. CHAPTER SUMMARY

Most pathways can be classified as either **catabolic** (**degrade** complex molecules to a few simple products) or **anabolic** (**synthesize** complex end products from simple precursors). **Catabolic reactions** also **capture chemical energy** in the form of **ATP** from the degradation of energy-rich molecules. **Anabolic reactions require energy**, which is generally provided by the hydrolysis of ATP. The rate of a metabolic pathway can respond to **regulatory signals** such as **allosteric activators** or **inhibitors** that arise from **within the cell**. Signaling **between cells** provides for the integration of metabolism. The most important route of this communication is **chemical signaling** (for example, by **hormones** or **neurotransmitters**). **Second messenger molecules** transduce a chemical signal (hormone or neurotransmitter) to appropriate intracellular responders.

Study Questions

Choose the ONE best answer.

8.1 Which of the following best describes the activity level and phosphorylation state of the listed hepatic enzymes in an individual who consumed a carbohydrate-rich meal about an hour ago? PFK-1 = phosphofructokinase-1; PFK-2 = phosphofructokinase-2; P = phosphorylated.

Choice	PFK-1		PFK-2		Pyruvate Kinase	
	Activity	P	Activity	P	Activity	P
A.	Low	No	Low	No	Low	No
B.	High	Yes	Low	Yes	Low	Yes
C.	High	No	High	No	High	No
D.	High	Yes	High	Yes	High	Yes

Correct answer = C. In the period immediately following a meal, blood glucose levels and hepatic uptake of glucose increase. The glucose is phosphorylated to glucose 6-phosphate and used in glycolysis. In response to the rise in blood glucose, the insulin-to-glucagon ratio increases. As a result, the kinase domain of PFK-2 is dephosphorylated and active. Its product, fructose 2,6-bisphosphate, allosterically activates PFK-1. (PFK-1 is not covalently regulated.) Active PFK-1 produces fructose 1,6-bisphosphate that is a feedforward activator of pyruvate kinase. Hepatic pyruvate kinase is covalently regulated, and the rise in insulin favors dephosphorylation.

8.2 Which of the following statements is true for anabolic pathways only?

A. Their irreversible (nonequilibrium) reactions are regulated.
B. They are called cycles if they regenerate an intermediate.
C. They are convergent and generate a few simple products.
D. They are synthetic and require energy.
E. They typically require oxidized coenzymes.

Correct answer = D. Anabolic processes are synthetic and energy requiring (endergonic). Statements A and B apply to both anabolic and catabolic processes, whereas C and E apply only to catabolic processes.

8.3 Compared with the resting state, vigorously contracting skeletal muscle shows:

A. decreased AMP/ATP ratio.
B. decreased levels of fructose 2,6-bisphosphate.
C. decreased NADH/NAD^+ ratio.
D. increased oxygen availability.
E. increased reduction of pyruvate to lactate.

Correct answer = E. Vigorously contracting muscle shows an increase in the reduction of pyruvate to lactate compared with resting skeletal muscle. The levels of adenosine monophosphate (AMP) and reduced nicotinamide adenine dinucleotide (NADH) increase, whereas change in the concentration of fructose 2,6-bisphosphate is not a key regulatory factor in skeletal muscle. The rise in the NADH to NAD^+ ratio exceeds the oxidative capacity of the respiratory chain.

8.4 Glucose uptake by:

A. liver cells is through facilitated diffusion involving a glucose transporter.
B. intestinal mucosal cells requires insulin.
C. brain cells is through energy-requiring (active) transport.
D. most cells is through simple diffusion up a concentration gradient.

Correct answer = A. Glucose uptake in the liver, brain, muscle, and adipose tissue is down a concentration gradient, and the diffusion is facilitated by tissue-specific glucose transporters (GLUTs). In adipose and muscle, insulin is required for glucose uptake. Moving glucose against a concentration gradient requires energy, and is seen with sodium-dependent glucose transporter-1 (SGLT-1) of intestinal mucosal cells.

8.5 Given that the K_m of glucokinase for glucose is 10 mM whereas that of hexokinase is 0.1 mM, which isozyme will more closely approach V_{max} at the normal blood glucose concentration of 5 mM?

Correct answer = Hexokinase. K_m is that substrate concentration that gives $\frac{1}{2}$ V_{max}. When blood glucose concentration is 5 mM, hexokinase (K_m = 0.1 mM) will be saturated, but glucokinase (K_m = 10 mM) will not.

8.6 In patients with whooping cough, $G\alpha_i$ is inhibited. How does this lead to a rise in cyclic AMP?

Liganded G proteins of the $G\alpha_i$ type inhibit adenylyl cyclase. If $G\alpha_i$ is inhibited by toxin, adenylyl cyclase production of cyclic adenosine monophosphate (cAMP) is inappropriately activated.

Tricarboxylic Acid Cycle and Pyruvate Dehydrogenase Complex

9

I. OVERVIEW

The tricarboxylic acid cycle ([TCA cycle] also called the citric acid cycle or the Krebs cycle) plays several roles in metabolism. It is the final pathway where the oxidative catabolism of carbohydrates, amino acids, and fatty acids converge, their carbon skeletons being converted to CO_2 (Figure 9.1). This oxidation provides energy for the production of the majority of adenosine triphosphate (ATP) in most animals, including humans. The TCA cycle occurs totally in the mitochondria and is, therefore, in close proximity to the reactions of electron transport (see p. 73), which oxidize the reduced coenzymes (NADH and $FADH_2$) produced by the cycle. The TCA cycle is an aerobic pathway, because O_2 is required as the final electron acceptor. Reactions such as the catabolism of some amino acids generate intermediates of the cycle and are called anaplerotic ("filling up") reactions. The TCA cycle also supplies intermediates for a number of important synthetic reactions. For example, the cycle functions in the formation of glucose from the carbon skeletons of some amino acids, and it provides building blocks for the synthesis of some amino acids (see p. 267) and heme (see p. 278). Therefore, this cycle should not be viewed as a closed circle but, instead, as a traffic circle with compounds entering and leaving as required.

II. REACTIONS OF THE CYCLE

In the TCA cycle, oxaloacetate is first condensed with an acetyl group from acetyl coenzyme A (CoA) and then is regenerated as the cycle is completed (Figure 9.1). Therefore, the entry of one acetyl CoA into one round of the TCA cycle does not lead to the net production or consumption of intermediates. [Note: Two carbons entering the cycle as acetyl CoA are balanced by two CO_2 exiting.]

A. Oxidative decarboxylation of pyruvate

The major source of acetyl CoA, the two-carbon substrate for the TCA cycle, is the oxidative decarboxylation of pyruvate. Pyruvate, the end product of aerobic glycolysis, must be transported from the cytosol into the mitochondrion. This is accomplished by a specific transporter that facilitates movement of pyruvate across the inner mitochondrial membrane. Once in the mitochondrial matrix, pyruvate

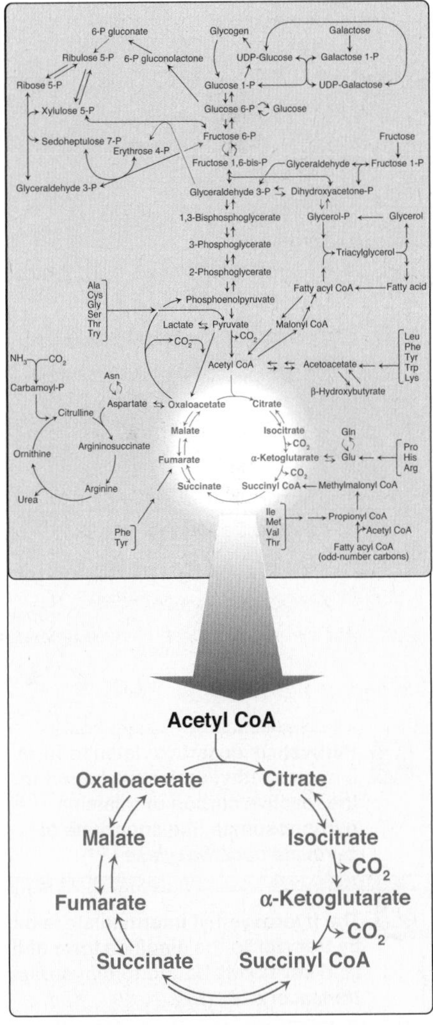

Figure 9.1
The tricarboxylic acid cycle shown as a part of the essential pathways of energy metabolism. (See Figure 8.2, p. 92 for a more detailed view of the metabolic map.) CoA = coenzyme A.

is converted to acetyl CoA by the *pyruvate dehydrogenase complex* (*PDH complex*), which is a multienzyme complex. [Note: Strictly speaking, the *PDH complex* is not part of the TCA cycle, but it supplies substrate for the cycle.]

1. **Component enzymes:** The *PDH complex* is a protein aggregate of multiple copies of three enzymes, *pyruvate carboxylase* (*E1*, sometimes called *pyruvate dehydrogenase*), *dihydrolipoyl transacetylase* (*E2*), and *dihydrolipoyl dehydrogenase* (*E3*). Each catalyzes a part of the overall reaction (Figure 9.2). Their physical association links the reactions in proper sequence without the release of intermediates. In addition to the enzymes participating in the conversion of pyruvate to acetyl CoA, the complex also contains two tightly bound regulatory enzymes, *pyruvate dehydrogenase kinase* (*PDH kinase*) and *pyruvate dehydrogenase phosphatase* (*PDH phosphatase*).

2. **Coenzymes:** The *PDH complex* contains five coenzymes that act as carriers or oxidants for the intermediates of the reactions shown in Figure 9.2. *E1* requires thiamine pyrophosphate (TPP), *E2* requires lipoic acid and CoA, and *E3* requires flavin adenine dinucleotide (FAD) and nicotinamide adenine dinucleotide (NAD^+). [Note: TPP, lipoic acid, and FAD are tightly bound to the enzymes and function as coenzymes-prosthetic groups (see p. 54).]

Deficiencies of thiamine or niacin can cause serious central nervous system problems. This is because brain cells are unable to produce sufficient ATP (via the TCA cycle) if the *PDH complex* is inactive. Wernicke-Korsakoff, an encephalopathy-psychosis syndrome due to thiamine deficiency, may be seen with alcohol abuse.

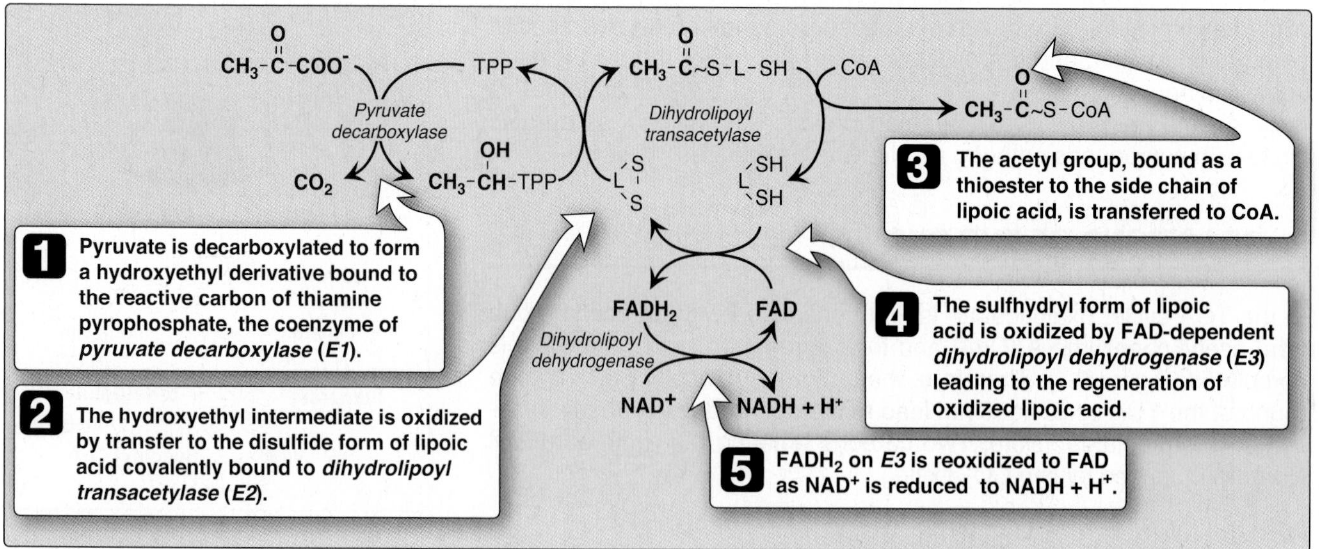

Figure 9.2
Mechanism of action of the *pyruvate dehydrogenase complex.* [Note: All the coenzymes of the complex, except for lipoic acid, are derived from vitamins. TPP is from thiamine, FAD from riboflavin, NAD from niacin, and CoA from pantothenic acid.] TPP = thiamine pyrophosphate; L = lipoic acid; CoA = coenzyme A; FAD(H_2) = flavin adenine dinucleotide; NAD(H) = nicotinamide adenine dinucleotide.

3. **Regulation of the pyruvate dehydrogenase complex:** Covalent modifications by the two regulatory enzymes that are part of the complex alternately activate and inactivate *E1*. The cyclic AMP–independent *PDH kinase* phosphorylates and, thereby, inactivates *E1*, whereas *PDH phosphatase* dephosphorylates and activates *E1* (Figure 9.3). The *kinase* itself is allosterically activated by ATP, acetyl CoA, and NADH. Therefore, in the presence of these high-energy signals, the *PDH complex* is turned off. [Note: It is actually the rise in the ATP/ADP, NADH/NAD$^+$, or acetyl CoA/CoA ratios that affects enzymic activity.] Pyruvate is a potent inhibitor of *PDH kinase*. Thus, if pyruvate concentrations are elevated, *E1* will be maximally active. Calcium (Ca^{2+}) is a strong activator of *PDH phosphatase*, stimulating *E1* activity. This is particularly important in skeletal muscle, where release of Ca^{2+} during contraction stimulates the *PDH complex* and, thereby, energy production. [Note: Although covalent regulation by the *kinase* and *phosphatase* is primary, the complex is also subject to product (NADH and acetyl CoA) inhibition.]

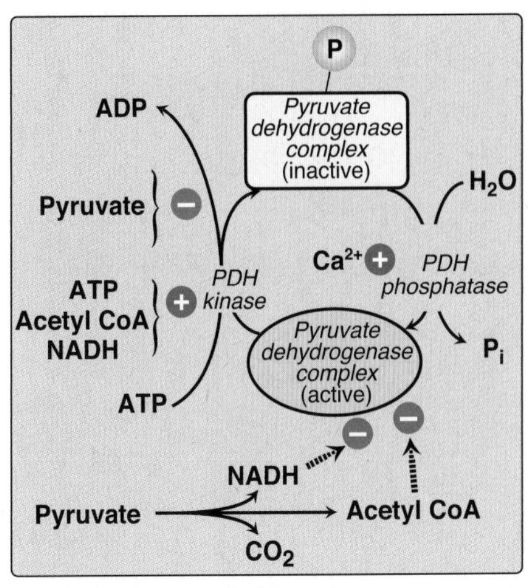

Figure 9.3
Regulation of *pyruvate dehydrogenase (PDH) complex.* [⋯⋯> denotes product inhibition.]

4. **Pyruvate dehydrogenase complex deficiency:** A deficiency in the activity of the α subunit of the dimeric *E1* component of the *PDH complex,* although rare, is the most common biochemical cause of congenital lactic acidosis. This enzyme deficiency results in an inability to convert pyruvate to acetyl CoA, causing pyruvate to be shunted to lactate via *lactate dehydrogenase* (see p. 103). This creates particular problems for the brain, which relies on the TCA cycle for most of its energy and is particularly sensitive to acidosis. Symptoms are variable and include neurodegeneration; muscle spasticity; and, in the neonatal onset form, early death. The gene for the α subunit is X linked, and, because both males and females may be affected, the deficiency is classified as X-linked dominant. Although there is no proven treatment for *PDH complex* deficiency, dietary restriction of carbohydrate and supplementation with thiamine may reduce symptoms in select patients.

> Leigh syndrome (subacute necrotizing encephalomyelopathy) is a rare, progressive, neurodegenerative disorder caused by defects in mitochondrial ATP production, primarily as a result of mutations in genes that code for proteins of the *PDH complex*, the electron transport chain, or *ATP synthase*. Both nuclear and mitochondrial DNA can be affected.

5. **Mechanism of arsenic poisoning:** As previously described (see p. 101), pentavalent arsenic (arsenate) can interfere with glycolysis at the *glyceraldehyde 3-phosphate* step, thereby decreasing ATP production. "Arsenic poisoning" is, however, due primarily to inhibition of enzymes that require lipoic acid as a coenzyme, including *E2* of the *PDH complex*, *α-ketoglutarate dehydrogenase* (see below), and *branched-chain α-keto acid dehydrogenase* (see p. 266). Arsenite (the trivalent form of arsenic) forms a stable complex with the thiol (–SH) groups of lipoic acid, making that compound unavailable to serve as a coenzyme. When it binds to lipoic acid in the *PDH complex*, pyruvate (and, consequently, lactate)

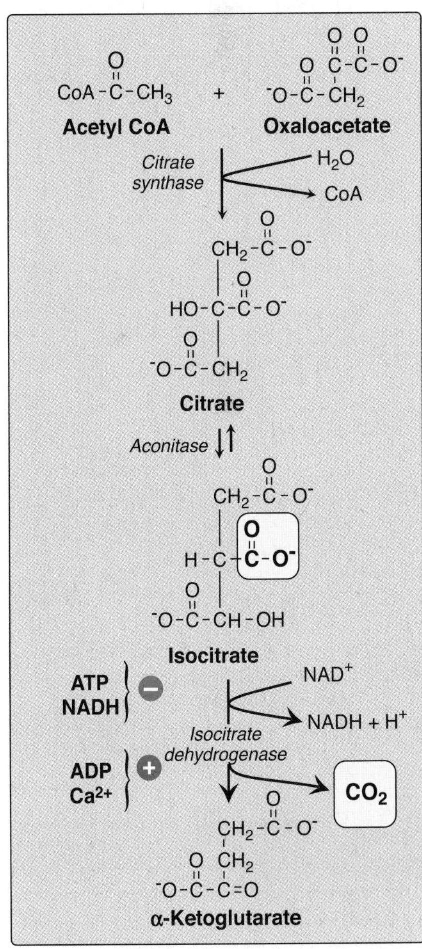

Figure 9.4
Formation of α-ketoglutarate from acetyl coenzyme A (CoA) and oxaloacetate. NAD(H) = nicotinamide adenine dinucleotide

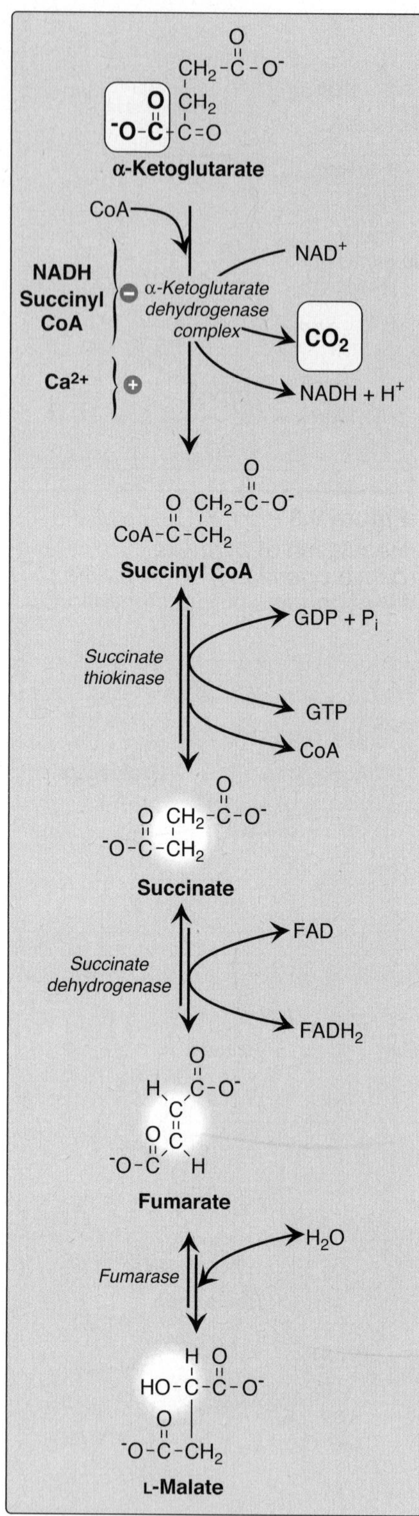

Figure 9.5
Formation of malate from α-ketoglutarate. NAD(H) = nicotinamide adenine dinucleotide; GDP = guanosine diphosphate; P = phosphate; CoA = coenzyme A; FAD(H_2) = flavin adenine dinucleotide.

accumulates. As with *PDH complex* deficiency, this particularly affects the brain, causing neurologic disturbances and death.

B. Synthesis of citrate from acetyl coenzyme A and oxaloacetate

The condensation of acetyl CoA and oxaloacetate (OAA) to form citrate (a tricarboxylic acid) is catalyzed by *citrate synthase* (Figure 9.4). This aldol condensation has an equilibrium far in the direction of citrate synthesis. In humans, *citrate synthase* is not an allosteric enzyme. It is inhibited by its product, citrate. Substrate availability is another means of regulation for *citrate synthase*. The binding of OAA causes a conformational change in the enzyme that generates a binding site for acetyl CoA. [Note: Citrate, in addition to being an intermediate in the TCA cycle, provides a source of acetyl CoA for the cytosolic synthesis of fatty acids (see p. 183). Citrate also inhibits *phosphofructokinase-1 (PFK-1)*, the rate-limiting enzyme of glycolysis (see p. 99), and activates *acetyl CoA carboxylase* (the rate-limiting enzyme of fatty acid synthesis; see p. 183).]

C. Isomerization of citrate

Citrate is isomerized to isocitrate by *aconitase* (*aconitate hydratase*), an Fe-S protein (see Figure 9.4). [Note: *Aconitase* is inhibited by fluoroacetate, a plant toxin that is used as a pesticide. Fluoroacetate is converted to fluoroacetyl CoA, which condenses with OAA to form fluorocitrate (a potent inhibitor of *aconitase*), resulting in citrate accumulation.]

D. Oxidative decarboxylation of isocitrate

Isocitrate dehydrogenase catalyzes the irreversible oxidative decarboxylation of isocitrate, yielding the first of three NADH molecules produced by the cycle and the first release of CO_2 (see Figure 9.4). This is one of the rate-limiting steps of the TCA cycle. The enzyme is allosterically activated by ADP (a low-energy signal) and Ca^{2+} and is inhibited by ATP and NADH, levels of which are elevated when the cell has abundant energy stores.

E. Oxidative decarboxylation of α-ketoglutarate

The conversion of α-ketoglutarate to succinyl CoA is catalyzed by the *α-ketoglutarate dehydrogenase complex*, a protein aggregate of multiple copies of three enzymes (Figure 9.5). The mechanism of this oxidative decarboxylation is very similar to that used for the conversion of pyruvate to acetyl CoA by the *PDH complex*. The reaction releases the second CO_2 and produces the second NADH of the cycle. The coenzymes required are TPP, lipoic acid, FAD, NAD$^+$, and CoA. Each functions as part of the catalytic mechanism in a way analogous to that described for the *PDH complex* (see p. 110). The equilibrium of the reaction is far in the direction of succinyl CoA, a high-energy thioester similar to acetyl CoA. *α-Ketoglutarate dehydrogenase complex* is inhibited by its products, NADH and succinyl CoA, and activated by Ca^{2+}. However, it is not regulated by phosphorylation/dephosphorylation reactions as described for *PDH complex*. [Note: α-Ketoglutarate is also produced by the oxidative deamination (see p. 252) and transamination of the amino acid glutamate (see p. 250).]

F. Cleavage of succinyl coenzyme A

Succinate thiokinase (also called *succinyl CoA synthetase*, named for the reverse reaction) cleaves the high-energy thioester bond of succinyl CoA (see Figure 9.5). This reaction is coupled to phosphorylation of guanosine diphosphate (GDP) to guanosine triphosphate (GTP). GTP and ATP are energetically interconvertible by the *nucleoside diphosphate kinase* reaction:

$$\text{GTP} + \text{ADP} \rightleftarrows \text{GDP} + \text{ATP}$$

The generation of GTP by *succinate thiokinase* is another example of substrate-level phosphorylation (see p. 102). [Note: Succinyl CoA is also produced from propionyl CoA derived from the metabolism of fatty acids with an odd number of carbon atoms (see p. 193), and from the metabolism of several amino acids (see pp. 265–266).]

G. Oxidation of succinate

Succinate is oxidized to fumarate by *succinate dehydrogenase*, as FAD (its coenzyme) is reduced to $FADH_2$ (see Figure 9.5). *Succinate dehydrogenase* is the only enzyme of the TCA cycle that is embedded in the inner mitochondrial membrane. As such, it functions as Complex II of the electron transport chain (see p. 75). [Note: FAD, rather than NAD^+, is the electron acceptor because the reducing power of succinate is not sufficient to reduce NAD^+.]

H. Hydration of fumarate

Fumarate is hydrated to malate in a freely reversible reaction catalyzed by *fumarase* (*fumarate hydratase*; see Figure 9.5). [Note: Fumarate is also produced by the urea cycle (see p. 255), in purine synthesis (see p. 294), and during catabolism of the amino acids phenylalanine and tyrosine (see p. 263).]

I. Oxidation of malate

Malate is oxidized to oxaloacetate by *malate dehydrogenase* (Figure 9.6). This reaction produces the third and final NADH of the cycle. The standard free energy change (ΔG^0; see p. 70) of the reaction is positive, but the reaction is driven in the direction of OAA by the highly exergonic *citrate synthase* reaction. [Note: OAA is also produced by the transamination of the amino acid aspartic acid (see p. 250).]

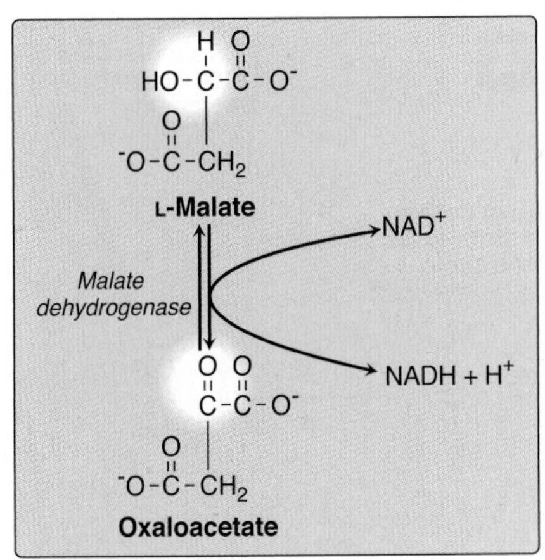

Figure 9.6
Formation (regeneration) of oxaloacetate from malate. NAD(H) = nicotinamide adenine dinucleotide.

III. ENERGY PRODUCED BY THE CYCLE

Two carbon atoms enter the cycle as acetyl CoA and leave as CO_2. The cycle does not involve net consumption or production of OAA or of any other intermediate. Four pairs of electrons are transferred during one turn of the cycle: three pairs of electrons reducing three NAD^+ to NADH and one pair reducing FAD to $FADH_2$. Oxidation of one NADH by the electron transport chain leads to formation of approximately three ATP, whereas oxidation of $FADH_2$ yields approximately two ATP (see p. 77). The total yield of ATP from the oxidation of one acetyl CoA is shown in Figure 9.7. Figure 9.8 summarizes the reactions of the TCA cycle.

Energy-producing reaction	Number of ATP produced
3 NADH ⟶ 3 NAD^+	9
$FADH_2$ ⟶ FAD	2
GDP + P_i ⟶ GTP	1
	12 ATP/acetyl CoA oxidized

Figure 9.7
Number of ATP molecules produced from the oxidation of one molecule of acetyl coenzyme A (CoA) using both substrate-level and oxidative phosphorylation.

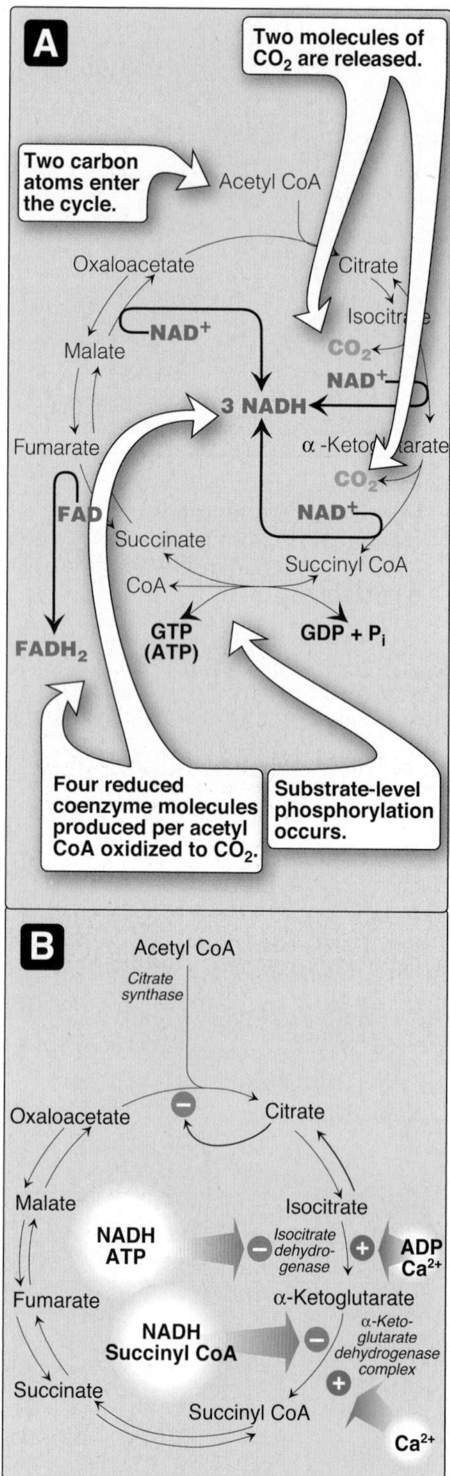

Figure 9.8
A. [Note: GTP and ATP are interconverted by *nucleoside diphosphate kinase*.] Production of reduced coenzymes, ATP, and CO_2 in the citric acid cycle. B. Inhibitors and activators of the cycle.

IV. REGULATION OF THE CYCLE

In contrast to glycolysis, which is regulated primarily by *PFK-1,* the TCA cycle is controlled by the regulation of several enzymes (see Figure 9.8). The most important of these regulated enzymes are those that catalyze reactions with highly negative ΔG^0: *citrate synthase, isocitrate dehydrogenase*, and *α-ketoglutarate dehydrogenase complex*. Reducing equivalents needed for oxidative phosphorylation are generated by the *PDH complex* and the TCA cycle, and both processes are upregulated in response to a decrease in the ratio of ATP to ADP.

V. CHAPTER SUMMARY

Pyruvate is **oxidatively decarboxylated** by ***pyruvate dehydrogenase*** (***PDH***) ***complex***, producing **acetyl coenzyme A** (**CoA**), which is the major fuel for the tricarboxylic acid cycle ([TCA cycle] Figure 9.9). This multienzyme complex requires five coenzymes: **thiamine pyrophosphate**, **lipoic acid**, **flavin adenine dinucleotide** (**FAD**), **nicotinamide adenine dinucleotide** (**NAD⁺**), and **CoA**. *PDH complex* is regulated by covalent modification of *E1* (*pyruvate decarboxylase*) by *PDH kinase* and *PDH phosphatase*: phosphorylation inhibits *E1*. *PDH kinase* is allosterically activated by ATP, acetyl CoA, and NADH and inhibited by pyruvate. The *phosphatase* is activated by Ca^{2+}. ***PDH complex*** **deficiency** is the most common biochemical cause of **congenital lactic acidosis**. The central nervous system is particularly affected in this **X-linked dominant** disorder. **Arsenic poisoning** causes inactivation of the *PDH complex* by binding to lipoic acid. **Citrate** is synthesized from **oxaloacetate** and **acetyl CoA** by ***citrate synthase***. This enzyme is subject to product inhibition by citrate. Citrate is isomerized to **isocitrate** by ***aconitase*** (***aconitate hydratase***). **Isocitrate** is oxidatively decarboxylated by ***isocitrate dehydrogenase*** to **α-ketoglutarate**, producing CO_2 and **NADH**. The enzyme is inhibited by ATP and NADH, and activated by ADP and Ca^{2+}. **α-Ketoglutarate** is oxidatively decarboxylated to **succinyl CoA** by the ***α-ketoglutarate dehydrogenase complex***, producing CO_2 and **NADH**. The enzyme is very similar to the *PDH complex* and uses the same coenzymes. *α-Ketoglutarate dehydrogenase complex* is activated by Ca^{+2} and inhibited by NADH and succinyl CoA but is not covalently regulated. **Succinyl CoA** is cleaved by ***succinate thiokinase*** (also called ***succinyl CoA synthetase***), producing **succinate** and **GTP**. This is an example of **substrate-level phosphorylation**. **Succinate** is oxidized to **fumarate** by ***succinate dehydrogenase***, producing $FADH_2$. **Fumarate** is hydrated to **malate** by ***fumarase*** (***fumarate hydratase***), and **malate** is oxidized to **oxaloacetate** by ***malate dehydrogenase***, producing **NADH**. **Three NADH**, **one** $FADH_2$, and **one GTP** (whose terminal phosphate can be transferred to ADP by *nucleoside diphosphate kinase*, producing ATP) are produced by one round of the TCA cycle. The generation of acetyl CoA by the oxidation of pyruvate via the *PDH complex* also produces an NADH. Oxidation of the NADH and $FADH_2$ by the electron transport chain yields 14 ATP. An additional ATP (GTP) comes from substrate level phosphorylation in the TCA cycle. Therefore, a total of 15 ATP are produced from the complete mitochondrial oxidation of pyruvate to CO_2.

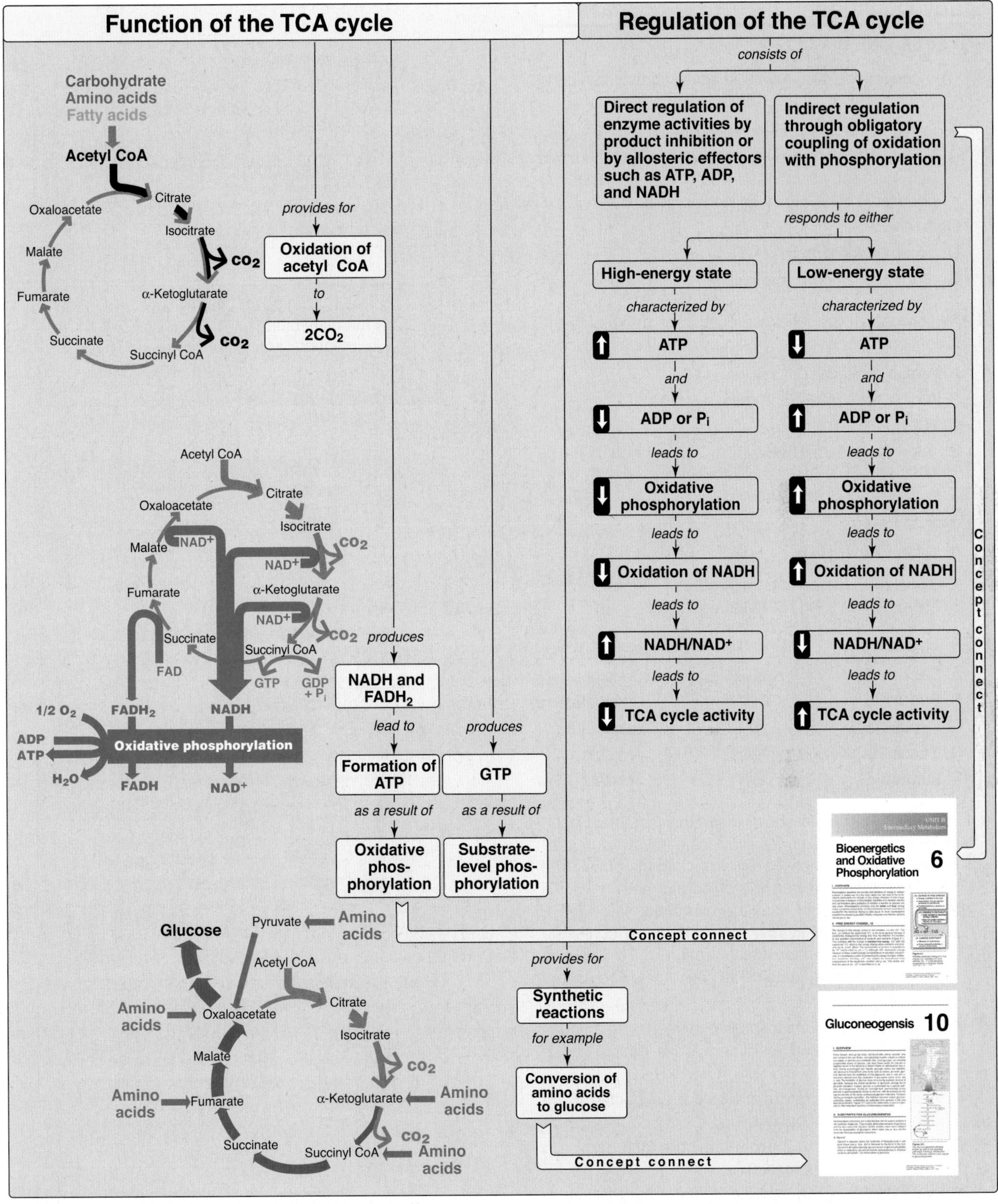

Figure 9.9
Key concept map for the tricarboxylic acid (TCA) cycle. CoA = coenzyme A; NAD(H) = nicotinamide adenine dinucleotide; FAD(H_2) = flavin adenine dinucleotide; GDP = guanosine diphosphate; GTP = guanosine triphosphate; ADP = adenosine diphosphate; P_i = inorganic phosphate.

Study Questions

Choose the ONE best answer.

9.1 The conversion of pyruvate to acetyl coenzyme A and CO_2:

A. involves the participation of lipoic acid.
B. is activated when pyruvate decarboxylase of the pyruvate dehydrogenase (PDH) complex is phosphorylated by PDH kinase in the presence of ATP.
C. is reversible.
D. occurs in the cytosol.
E. requires the coenzyme biotin.

Correct answer = A. Lipoic acid is an intermediate acceptor of the acetyl group formed in the reaction. Pyruvate dehydrogenase complex catalyzes an irreversible reaction that is inhibited when the decarboxylase component is phosphorylated. The enzyme complex is located in the mitochondrial matrix. Biotin is utilized by carboxylases, not decarboxylases.

9.2 Which one of the following conditions decreases the oxidation of acetyl coenzyme A by the citric acid cycle?

A. A high availability of calcium
B. A high acetyl CoA/CoA ratio
C. A low ATP/ADP ratio
D. A low NAD^+/NADH ratio

Correct answer = D. A low NAD^+/NADH ratio limits the rates of the NAD^+-requiring dehydrogenases. High availability of calcium and substrate (acetyl CoA), and a low ATP/ADP ratio stimulates the cycle.

9.3 The following is the sum of three steps in the citric acid cycle.

$$A + B + FAD + H_2O \rightarrow C + FADH_2 + NADH$$

Choose the lettered answer that corresponds to the missing "A," "B," and "C" in the equation.

Reactant A	Reactant B	Reactant C
A. Succinyl CoA	GDP	Succinate
B. Succinate	NAD^+	Oxaloacetate
C. Fumarate	NAD^+	Oxaloacetate
D. Succinate	NAD^+	Malate
E. Fumarate	GTP	Malate

Correct answer = B. Succinate + NAD^+ + FAD + H_2O $\rightarrow$ oxaloacetate + NADH + $FADH_2$

9.4 A 1-month-old male shows neurologic problems and lactic acidosis. Enzyme assay for pyruvate dehydrogenase (PDH) complex activity on extracts of cultured skin fibroblasts showed 5% of normal activity with a low concentration of thiamine pyrophosphate (TPP), but 80% of normal activity when the assay contained a thousand-fold higher concentration of TPP. Which one of the following statements concerning this patient is correct?

A. Administration of thiamine is expected to reduce his serum lactate level and improve his clinical symptoms.
B. A high carbohydrate diet would be expected to be beneficial for this patient.
C. Citrate production from aerobic glycolysis is expected to be increased.
D. PDH kinase, a regulatory enzyme of the PDH complex, is expected to be active.

Correct answer = A. The patient appears to have a thiamine-responsive pyruvate dehydrogenase (PDH) complex deficiency. The pyruvate decarboxylase (E1) component of the PDH complex fails to bind thiamine pyrophosphate at low concentration, but shows significant activity at a high concentration of the coenzyme. This mutation, which affects the K_m of the enzyme for the coenzyme, is present in some, but not all, cases of PDH complex deficiency. Because the PDH complex is an integral part of carbohydrate metabolism, a diet low in carbohydrates would be expected to blunt the effects of the enzyme deficiency. Aerobic glycolysis generates pyruvate, the substrate of the PDH complex. Decreased activity of the complex decreases production of acetyl coenzyme A, a substrate for citrate synthase. PDH kinase is allosterically inhibited by pyruvate and, therefore, is inactive.

9.5 Which coenzyme-cosubstrate is used by the dehydrogenases of both glycolysis and the tricarboxylic acid cycle?

Oxidized nicotinamide adenine dinucleotide (NAD^+) is used by glyceraldehyde 3-phosphate dehydrogenase of glycolysis and by isocitrate dehydrogenase, α-ketoglutarate dehydrogenase, and malate dehydrogenase of the tricarboxylic acid cycle.

Gluconeogenesis 10

I. OVERVIEW

Some tissues, such as the brain, red blood cells (RBCs), kidney medulla, lens and cornea of the eye, testes, and exercising muscle, require a continuous supply of glucose as a metabolic fuel. Liver glycogen, an essential postprandial source of glucose, can meet these needs for only 10–18 hours in the absence of dietary intake of carbohydrate (see p. 329). During a prolonged fast, however, hepatic glycogen stores are depleted, and glucose is formed from noncarbohydrate precursors such as lactate, pyruvate, glycerol (derived from the backbone of triacylglycerols; see p. 190), and α-keto acids (derived from the catabolism of glucogenic amino acids; see p. 261). The formation of glucose does not occur by a simple reversal of glycolysis, because the overall equilibrium of glycolysis strongly favors pyruvate formation. Instead, glucose is synthesized by a special pathway, gluconeogenesis, which requires both mitochondrial and cytosolic enzymes. During an overnight fast, approximately 90% of gluconeogenesis occurs in the liver, with the remaining 10% occurring in the kidneys. However, during prolonged fasting, the kidneys become major glucose-producing organs, contributing an estimated 40% of the total glucose production. Figure 10.1 shows the relationship of gluconeogenesis to other essential pathways of energy metabolism.

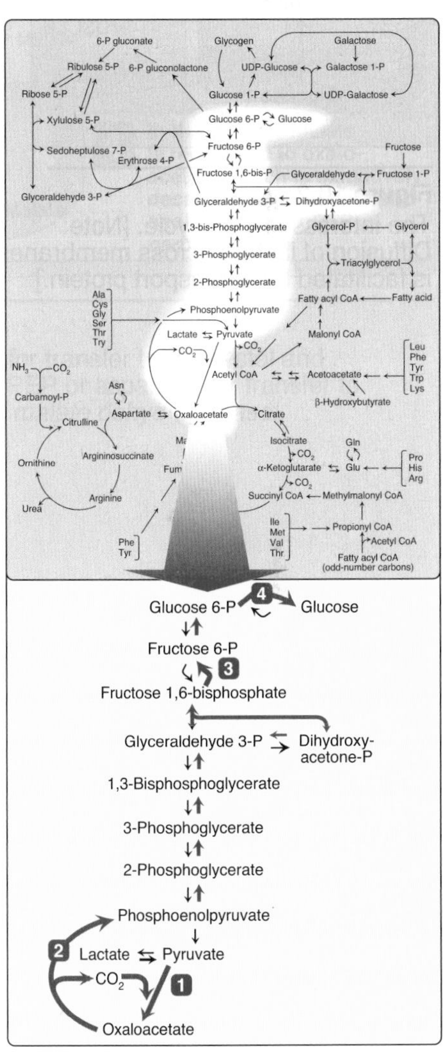

Figure 10.1
The gluconeogenesis pathway shown as one of the essential pathways of energy metabolism. The numbered reactions are unique to gluconeogenesis. (See Figure 8.2, p. 92, for a more detailed map of metabolism.) P = phosphate.

II. SUBSTRATES FOR GLUCONEOGENESIS

Gluconeogenic precursors are molecules that can be used to produce a net synthesis of glucose. The most important gluconeogenic prescurors are glycerol, lactate, and the α-keto acids obtained from the metabolism of glucogenic amino acids. [Note: Alanine, which directly gives rise to pyruvate, is an important example of a glucogenic amino acid.]

A. Glycerol

Glycerol is released during the hydrolysis of triacylglycerols in adipose tissue (see p. 190) and is delivered by the blood to the liver. Glycerol is phosphorylated by *glycerol kinase* to glycerol phosphate, which is oxidized by *glycerol phosphate dehydrogenase* to dihydroxyacetone phosphate, an intermediate of glycolysis. [Note: Adipocytes cannot phosphorylate glycerol because they essentially lack *glycerol kinase*.]

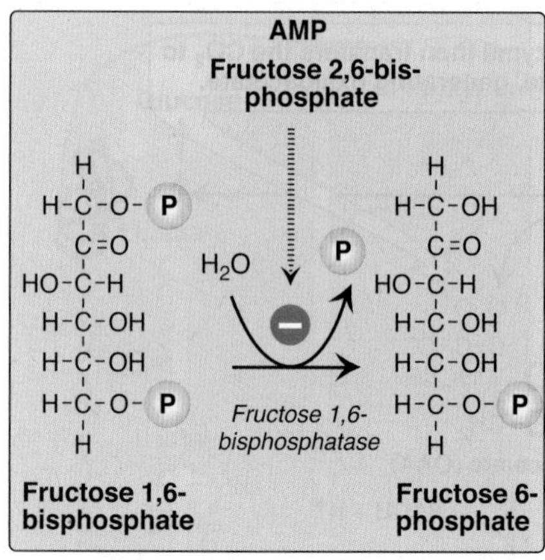

Figure 10.4
Dephosphorylation of fructose 1,6-bisphosphate. AMP = adenosine monophosphate; P = phosphate.

C. Decarboxylation of cytosolic oxaloacetate

OAA is decarboxylated and phosphorylated to PEP in the cytosol by *PEP-carboxykinase* (also referred to as *PEPCK*). The reaction is driven by hydrolysis of guanosine triphosphate ([GTP] see Figure 10.3). The combined actions of *pyruvate carboxylase* and *PEP-carboxykinase* provide an energetically favorable pathway from pyruvate to PEP. PEP is then acted on by the reactions of glycolysis running in the reverse direction until it becomes fructose 1,6-bisphosphate.

> The pairing of carboxylation with decarboxylation, as seen in gluconeogenesis, drives reactions that would otherwise be energetically unfavorable. A similar strategy is used in fatty acid synthesis (see pp. 183–184).

D. Dephosphorylation of fructose 1,6-bisphosphate

Hydrolysis of fructose 1,6-bisphosphate by *fructose 1,6-bisphosphatase*, found in liver and kidney, bypasses the irreversible *phosphofructokinase-1 (PFK-1)* reaction, and provides an energetically favorable pathway for the formation of fructose 6-phosphate (Figure 10.4). This reaction is an important regulatory site of gluconeogenesis.

1. **Regulation by energy levels within the cell:** *Fructose 1,6-bisphosphatase* is inhibited by elevated levels of adenosine monophos-

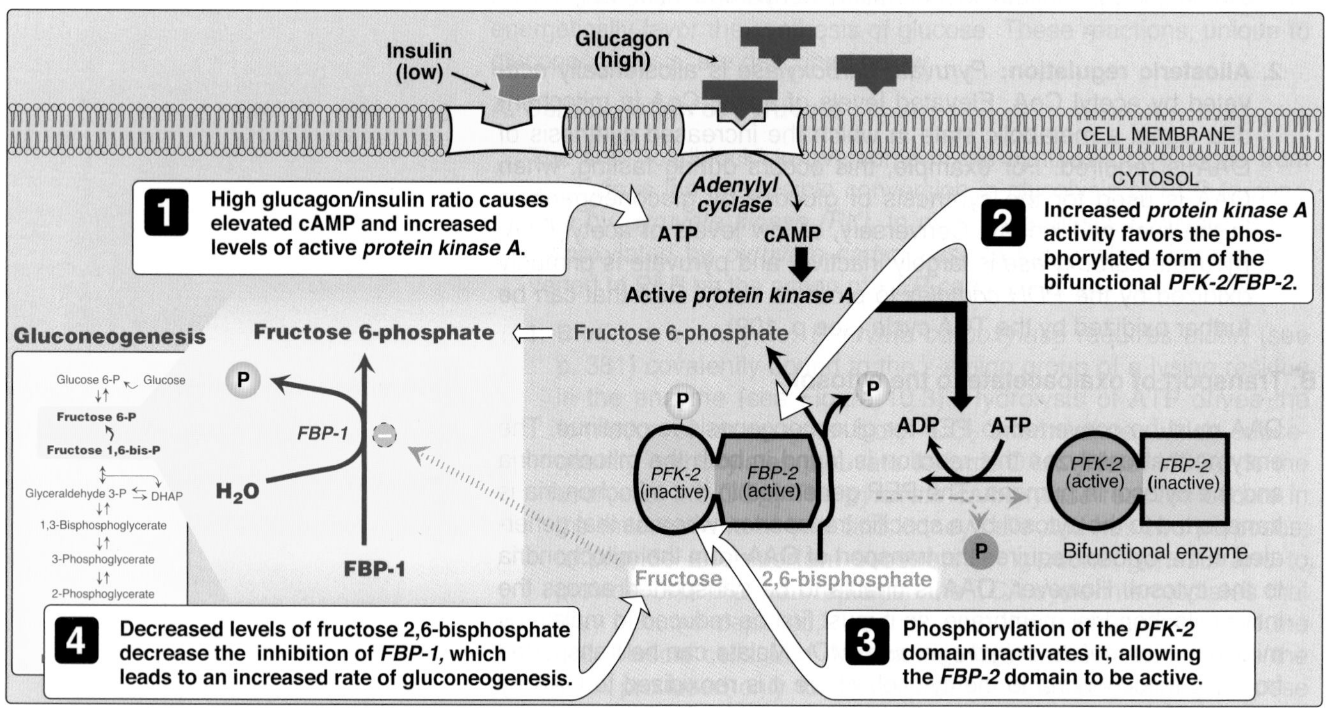

Figure 10.5
Effect of elevated glucagon on the intracellular concentration of fructose 2,6-bisphosphate in the liver. cAMP = cyclic AMP; *PFK-2 = phosphofructokinase-2*; *FBP-2 = fructose 2,6-bisphosphatase; FBP-1 = fructose 1,6-bisphosphatase;* P = phosphate.

phate (AMP), which signal an "energy-poor" state in the cell. Conversely, high levels of ATP and low concentrations of AMP stimulate gluconeogenesis, an energy-requiring pathway.

2. **Regulation by fructose 2,6-bisphosphate:** *Fructose 1,6-bisphosphatase* is inhibited by fructose 2,6-bisphosphate, an allosteric effector whose concentration is influenced by the insulin to glucagon ratio: when glucagon is high, the effector is not made and, thus, the *phosphatase* is active. (Figure 10.5). [Note: The signals that inhibit (low energy, high fructose 2,6-bisphosphate) or activate (high energy, low fructose 2,6-bisphosphate) gluconeogenesis have the opposite effect on glycolysis, providing reciprocal control of the pathways that synthesize and oxidize glucose (see p. 100).]

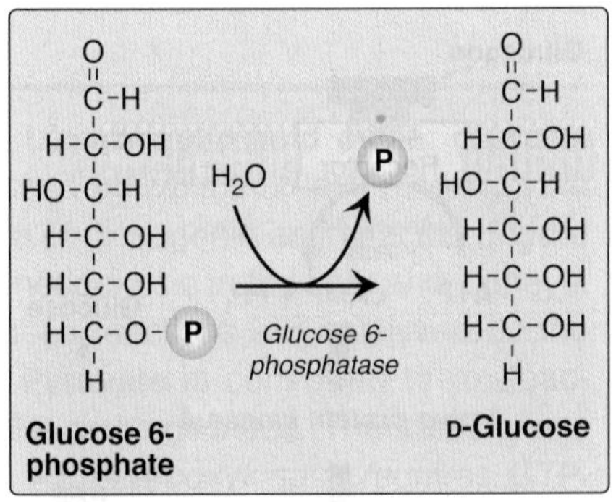

Figure 10.6
Dephosphorylation of glucose 6-phosphate allows release of free glucose from the liver and kidney into blood. P = phosphate.

E. Dephosphorylation of glucose 6-phosphate

Hydrolysis of glucose 6-phosphate by *glucose 6-phosphatase* bypasses the irreversible *hexokinase/glucokinase* reaction and provides an energetically favorable pathway for the formation of free glucose (Figure 10.6). Liver and kidney are the only organs that release free glucose from glucose 6-phosphate. This process actually requires a complex of two proteins: glucose 6-phosphate translocase, which transports glucose 6-phosphate across the endoplasmic reticular (ER) membrane, and the enzyme *glucose 6-phosphatase* (found only in gluconeogenic cells), which removes the phosphate, producing free glucose (see Figure 10.6). [Note: These ER-membrane proteins are also required for the final step of glycogen degradation (see p. 130). Type Ia and Ib glycogen storage disease, caused by deficiencies in the *phosphatase* and the transferase, respectively, are characterized by severe fasting hypoglycemia, because free glucose is unable to be produced from either gluconeogenesis or glycogenolysis.] Specific glucose transporters (GLUTs) are responsible for moving free glucose into the cytosol and then into blood. [Note: Glucose 6-phosphate translocase moves inorganic phosphate out of the ER as it moves glucose 6-phosphate in.]

F. Summary of the reactions of glycolysis and gluconeogenesis

Of the 11 reactions required to convert pyruvate to free glucose, 7 are catalyzed by reversible glycolytic enzymes (Figure 10.7). The irreversible reactions of glycolysis catalyzed by *hexokinase/glucokinase*, *PFK-1*, and *PK* are circumvented by *glucose 6-phosphatase*, *fructose 1,6-bisphosphatase*, and *pyruvate carboxylase/PEP-carboxykinase*. In gluconeogenesis, the equilibria of the 7 reversible reactions of glycolysis are pushed in favor of glucose synthesis as a result of the essentially irreversible formation of PEP, fructose 6-phosphate, and glucose catalyzed by the gluconeogenic enzymes. [Note: The stoichiometry of gluconeogenesis from pyruvate couples the cleavage of six high-energy phosphate bonds and the oxidation of two NADH with the formation of each molecule of glucose (see Figure 10.7).]

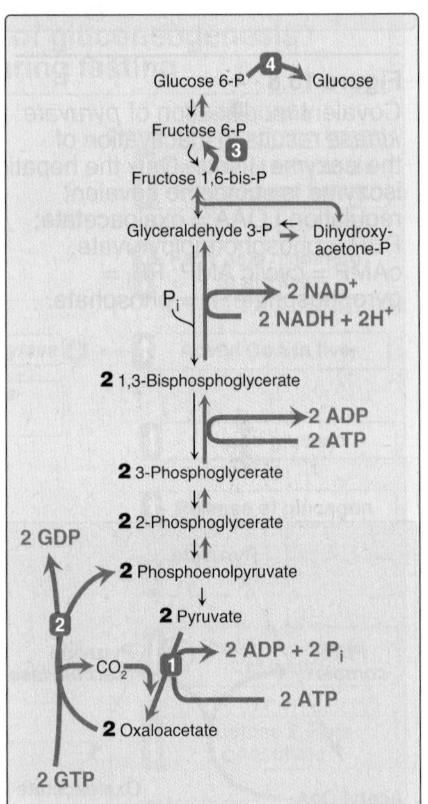

Figure 10.7
Summary of the reactions of glycolysis and gluconeogenesis, showing the energy requirements of gluconeogenesis. The numbered reactions are unique to gluconeogenesis. P = phosphate; GDP = guanosine diphosphate; GTP = guanosine triphosphate; NAD(H) = nicotinamide adenine dinucleotide.

IV. REGULATION OF GLUCONEOGENESIS

The moment-to-moment regulation of gluconeogenesis is determined primarily by the circulating level of glucagon and by the availability of gluconeogenic substrates. In addition, slow adaptive changes in

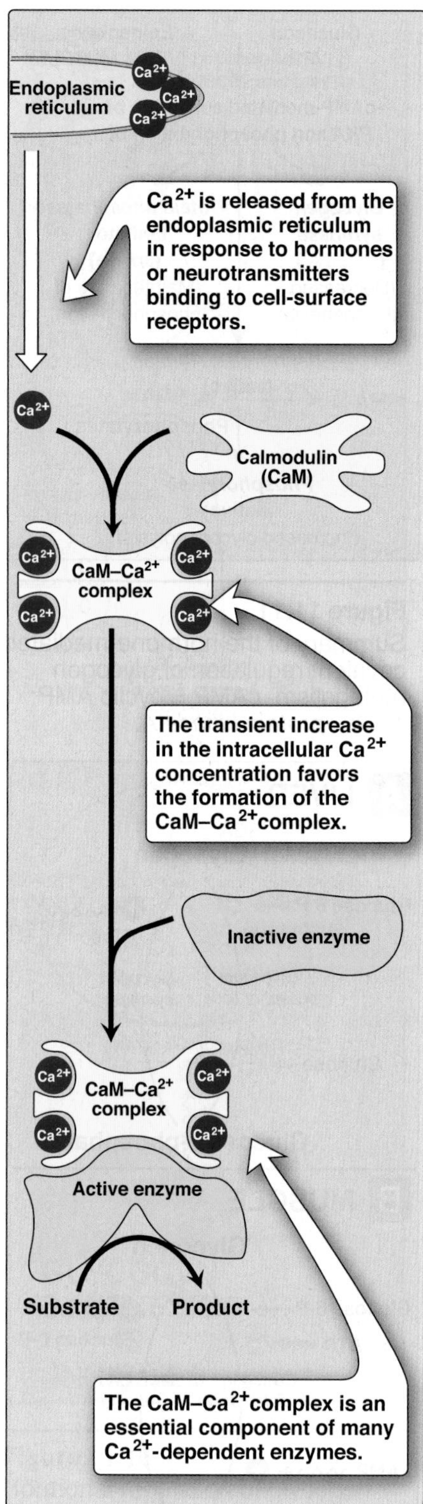

Figure 11.13
Calmodulin mediates many effects of intracellular Ca^{2+}.

b. **Calcium activation of liver phosphorylase kinase:** During physiologic stress, epinephrine is released from the adrenal medulla and signals the need for blood glucose. This glucose initially comes from hepatic glycogenolysis. Binding of epinephrine to hepatocyte α-adrenergic GPCRs activates a phospholipid-dependent cascade (see p. 205) that results in movement of Ca^{2+} from the ER into the cytoplasm. A Ca^{2+}–CaM complex forms and activates hepatic *phosphorylase kinase b*. [Note: The released Ca^{2+} also helps to activate *protein kinase C* that can phosphorylate (therefore, inactivate) *glycogen synthase a*.]

3. **Activation of glycogen degradation in muscle:** Muscle *glycogen phosphorylase* is active in the presence of the high adenosine monophosphate (AMP) concentrations that occur under extreme conditions of anoxia and ATP depletion. AMP binds to *glycogen phosphorylase b*, causing its activation without phosphorylation (see Figure 11.9). [Note: Recall that AMP also activates *phosphofructokinase-1* of glycolysis (see p. 99), allowing glucose from glycogenolysis to be oxidized.]

VI. GLYCOGEN STORAGE DISEASES

These are a group of genetic diseases that are caused by defects in enzymes required for glycogen degradation or, more rarely, glycogen synthesis. They result either in formation of glycogen that has an abnormal structure or in the accumulation of excessive amounts of normal glycogen in specific tissues as a result of impaired degradation. A particular enzyme may be defective in a single tissue, such as liver (resulting in hypoglycemia) or muscle (causing muscle weakness), or the defect may be more generalized, affecting a variety of tissues. The severity of the GSDs ranges from fatal in early childhood to mild disorders that are not life threatening. Some of the more prevalent GSDs are illustrated in Figure 11.8. [Note: Only one GSD is lysosomal because glycogen metabolism occurs primarily in the cytosol.]

VII. CHAPTER SUMMARY

The **main stores** of glycogen in the body are found in **skeletal muscle**, where they serve as a **fuel reserve** for the synthesis of ATP during **muscle contraction**, and in the **liver**, where they are used to **maintain the blood glucose** concentration, particularly during the **early stages of a fast**. Glycogen is a **highly branched** polymer of **α-D-glucose**. The primary glycosidic bond is an **α(1→4) linkage**. After about eight to ten glucosyl residues, there is a **branch** containing an **α(1→6) linkage**. **Uridine diphosphate (UDP)-glucose**, the **building block** of glycogen, is synthesized from **glucose 1-phosphate** and **UTP** by ***UDP-glucose pyrophosphorylase*** (Figure 11.14). Glucose from UDP-glucose is transferred to the nonreducing ends of glycogen chains by primer-requiring ***glycogen synthase***, which makes **α(1→4) linkages**. The primer is made by *glycogenin*. **Branches** are formed by ***amylo-α(1→4)→α(1→6)-transglucosidase*** (common name, ***glucosyl 4:6 transferase***), which transfers a set of six to eight glucosyl residues from the nonreducing end of the glycogen chain (**breaking** an **α(1→4) linkage**), and attaches it with an **α(1→6) linkage** to another residue in the chain. Pyridoxal phosphate–requiring ***glycogen phosphorylase*** cleaves the **α(1→4) bonds** between glucosyl residues at the **nonreducing ends** of the glycogen chains, producing **glucose 1-phosphate**. This sequential degradation continues until four glucosyl units remain before a branch point. The resulting structure is called a **limit dextrin** that is degraded by the bifunctional debranching enzyme. ***Oligo-α(1→4)→α(1→4)-glucantransferase*** (common name, ***glucosyl 4:4 transferase***) removes the outer three of the four glucosyl residues at a branch and transfers them to the nonreducing end of another chain, where they can be converted to glucose 1-phosphate by *glycogen phosphorylase*. The remaining single glucose residue attached in an **α(1→6) linkage** is removed hydrolytically by the ***amylo-(1→6) glucosidase*** activity of *debranching enzyme*, releasing **free glucose**. **Glucose 1-phosphate** is converted to **glucose 6-phosphate** by ***phosphoglucomutase***. In the **muscle**, glucose 6-phosphate enters glycolysis. In the **liver**, the phosphate is removed by ***glucose 6-phosphatase***, releasing **free glucose** that can be used to maintain blood glucose levels at the beginning of a fast. A **deficiency** of the ***phosphatase*** causes **glycogen storage disease Type 1a** (**Von Gierke disease**). This disease results in an inability of the liver to provide free glucose to the body during a fast. It affects both glycogen degradation and gluconeogenesis. Glycogen synthesis and degradation are reciprocally regulated to meet whole-body needs by the same hormonal signals (namely, an **elevated insulin** level results in overall **increased glycogenesis** and **decreased glycogenolysis**, whereas an **elevated glucagon**, or **epinephrine**, level causes **increased glycogenolysis** and **decreased glycogenesis**). Key enzymes are phosphorylated by a family of ***protein kinases***, some of which are **cyclic adenosine monophosphate dependent** (a compound increased by glucagon and epinephrine). Phosphate groups are removed by *protein phosphatase-1* (active when its inhibitor is inactive in response to elevated insulin levels). ***Glycogen synthase***, ***phosphorylase kinase***, and ***phosphorylase*** are also **allosterically regulated** to meet tissues needs. In the well-fed state, ***glycogen synthase*** is **activated** by **glucose 6-phosphate**, but ***glycogen phosphorylase*** is inhibited by **glucose 6-phosphate** as well as by **ATP**. In the liver, glucose also serves an an allosteric inhibitor of *glycogen phosphorylase*. The Ca^{2+} released from the endoplasmic reticulum in muscle during exercise and in liver in response to epinephrine **activates *phosphorylase kinase*** by binding to the enzyme's **calmodulin** subunit. This allows the enzyme to activate ***glycogen phosphorylase***, thereby causing glycogen degradation. **AMP** activates *glycogen phosphorylase* in muscle.

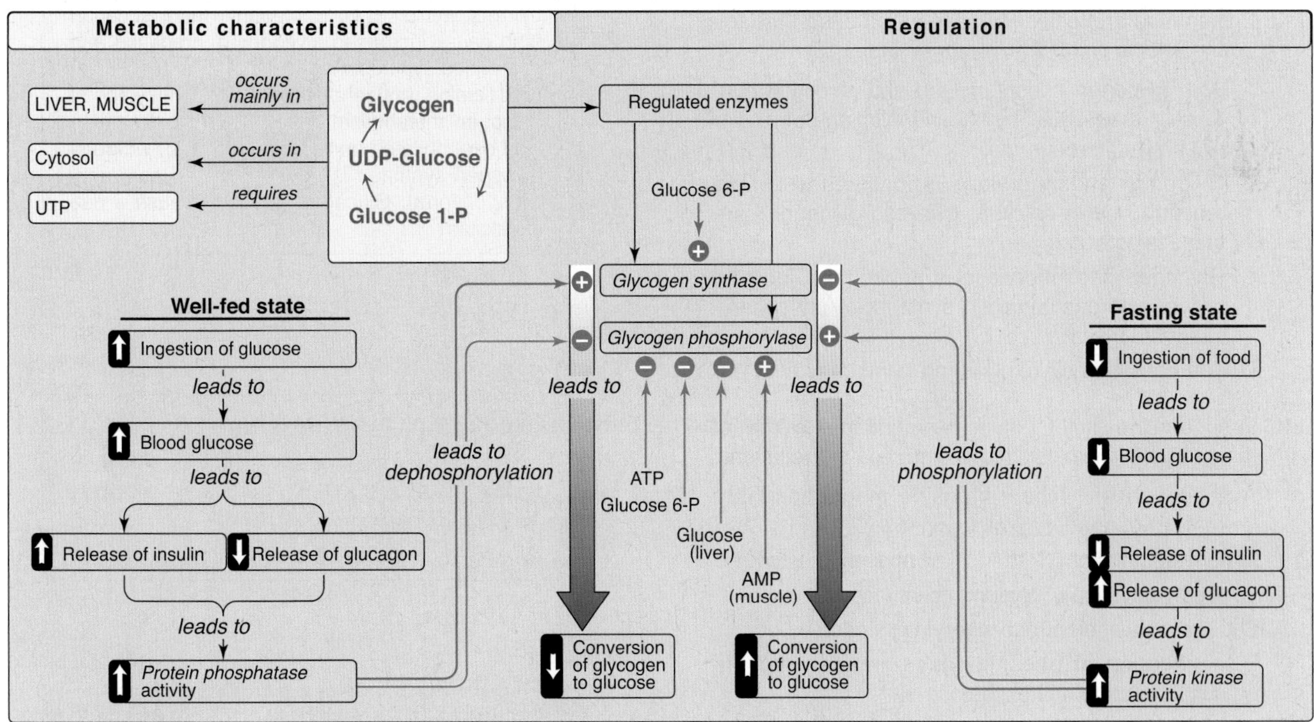

Figure 11.14
Key concept map for glycogen metabolism in the liver. [Note: *Glycogen phosphorylase* is phosphorylated by *phosphorylase kinase*, the "b" form of which can be activated by calcium.] UDP = uridine diphosphate; UTP = uridine triphosphate; P = phosphate.

Study Questions

Choose the ONE best answer.

For Questions 11.1–11.4, match the deficient enzyme to the clinical finding in selected glycogen storage diseases (GSDs).

CHOICE	GSD	DEFICIENT ENZYME
A	Type Ia	Glucose 6-phosphatase
B	Type II	Acid maltase
C	Type III	4:4 Transferase
D	Type IV	4:6 Transferase
E	Type V	Myophosphorylase
F	Type VI	Liver phosphorylase

11.1 Exercise intolerance, with no rise in blood lactate during exercise

11.2 Fatal, progressive cirrhosis and glycogen with longer-than-normal outer chains

11.3 Generalized accumulation of glycogen, severe hypotonia, and death from heart failure

11.4 Severe fasting hypoglycemia, lacticacidemia, hyperuricemia, and hyperlipidemia

Correct answer = E. Myophosphorylase deficiency prevents glycogen degradation in muscle, depriving muscle of glycogen-derived glucose, resulting in decreased glycolysis and its anaerobic product, lactate.

Correct Answer = D. 4:6 Transferase (branching enzyme) deficiency, a defect in glycogen synthesis, results in formation of glycogen with fewer branches and decreased solubility.

Correct answer = B. Acid maltase [α(1→4)-glucosidase] deficiency prevents degradation of any glycogen brought into lysosomes. A variety of tissues are affected, with the most severe pathology resulting from heart damage.

Correct answer = A. Glucose 6-phosphatase deficiency prevents the liver from releasing free glucose into the blood, causing severe fasting hypoglycemia, lacticacidemia, hyperuricemia, and hyperlipidemia.

11.5 Epinephrine and glucagon have which one of the following effects on hepatic glycogen metabolism?

A. Both glycogen phosphorylase and glycogen synthase are activated by phosphorylation but at significantly different rates.

B. Glycogen phosphorylase is inactivated by the resuting rise in calcium, whereas glycogen synthase is activated.

C. Glycogen phosphorylase is phosphorylated and active, whereas glycogen synthase is phosphorylated and inactive.

D. The net synthesis of glycogen is increased.

Correct answer = C. Epinephrine and glucagon both cause increased glycogen degradation and decreased synthesis in the liver through covalent modification (phosphorylation) of key enzymes of glycogen metabolism. Glycogen phosphorylase is phosphorylated and active ("a" form), whereas glycogen synthase is phosphorylated and inactive ("b" form). Glucagon does not cause a rise in calcium.

11.6 In contracting skeletal muscle, a sudden elevation of the sarcoplasmic calcium concentration will result in:

A. activation of cyclic adenosine monophosphate (cAMP)-dependent protein kinase A.

B. conversion of cAMP to AMP by phosphodiesterase.

C. direct activation of glycogen synthase b.

D. direct activation of phosphorylase kinase b.

E. inactivation of phosphorylase kinase a by the action of protein phosphatase-1.

Correct answer = D. Ca^{2+} released from the sarcoplasmic reticulum during exercise binds to the calmodulin subunit of phosphorylase kinase, thereby allosterically activating the "b" form of this enzyme. The other choices are not caused by an elevation of cytosolic calcium.

11.7 Explain why the hypoglycemia seen with Type Ia glycogen storage disease (glucose 6-phosphatase deficiency) is severe, whereas that seen with Type VI (liver phosphorylase deficiency) is mild.

With Type Ia, the liver is unable to generate free glucose either from glycogenolysis or gluconeogenesis because both processes produce glucose 6-phosphate. With Type VI, the liver is still able to produce free glucose from gluconeogenesis, but glycogenolysis is inhibited.

Metabolism of Monosaccharides and Disaccharides

12

I. OVERVIEW

Glucose is the most common monosaccharide consumed by humans, and its metabolism has already been discussed. However, two other monosaccharides, fructose and galactose, occur in significant amounts in the diet (primarily in disaccharides) and make important contributions to energy metabolism. In addition, galactose is an important component of structural carbohydrates. Figure 12.1 shows the metabolism of fructose and galactose as part of the essential pathways of energy metabolism.

II. FRUCTOSE METABOLISM

About 10% of the calories comprising the Western diet are supplied by fructose (approximately 55 g/day). The major source of fructose is the disaccharide sucrose, which, when cleaved in the intestine, releases equimolar amounts of fructose and glucose. Fructose is also found as a free monosaccharide in many fruits, in honey, and in high-fructose corn syrup (typically, 55% fructose/45% glucose), which is used to sweeten soft drinks and many foods. Fructose transport into cells is not insulin dependent (unlike that of glucose into certain tissues; see p. 97), and, in contrast to glucose, fructose does not promote the secretion of insulin.

A. Phosphorylation of fructose

For fructose to enter the pathways of intermediary metabolism, it must first be phosphorylated (Figure 12.2). This can be accomplished by either *hexokinase* or *fructokinase*. *Hexokinase* phosphorylates glucose in most cells of the body (see p. 98), and several additional hexoses can serve as substrates for this enzyme. However, it has a low affinity (that is, a high Michaelis constant [K_m]; see p. 59) for fructose. Therefore, unless the intracellular concentration of fructose becomes unusually high, the normal presence of saturating concentrations of glucose means that little fructose is phosphorylated by *hexokinase*. *Fructokinase* provides the primary mechanism for fructose phosphorylation (see Figure 12.2). The enzyme has a low K_m for fructose and a high V_{max} (or, maximal velocity; see p. 59). It is found in the liver (which processes most of the dietary fructose), kidney, and the small intestinal mucosa and converts fructose to fructose 1-phosphate, using adenosine triphosphate (ATP) as the phosphate donor. [Note: These three tissues also contain *aldolase B*, discussed in section B.]

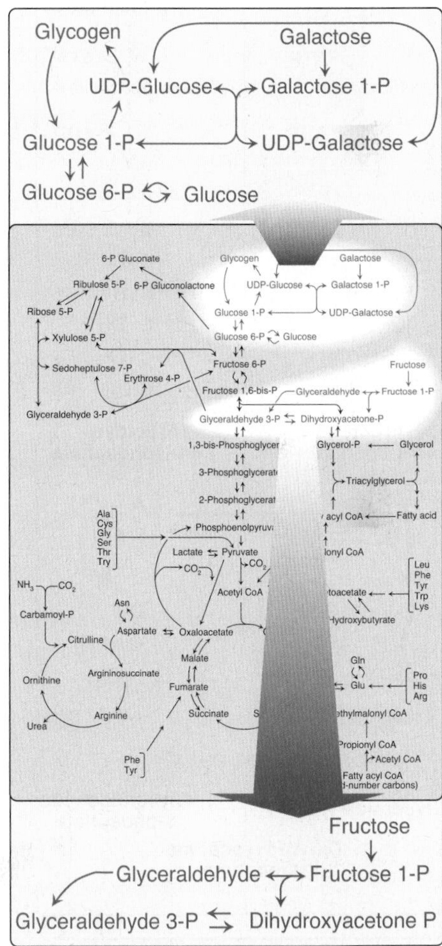

Figure 12.1
Galactose and fructose metabolism as part of the essential pathways of energy metabolism (see Figure 8.2, p. 92, for a more detailed view of the overall reactions of metabolism). UDP = uridine diphosphate; P = phosphate.

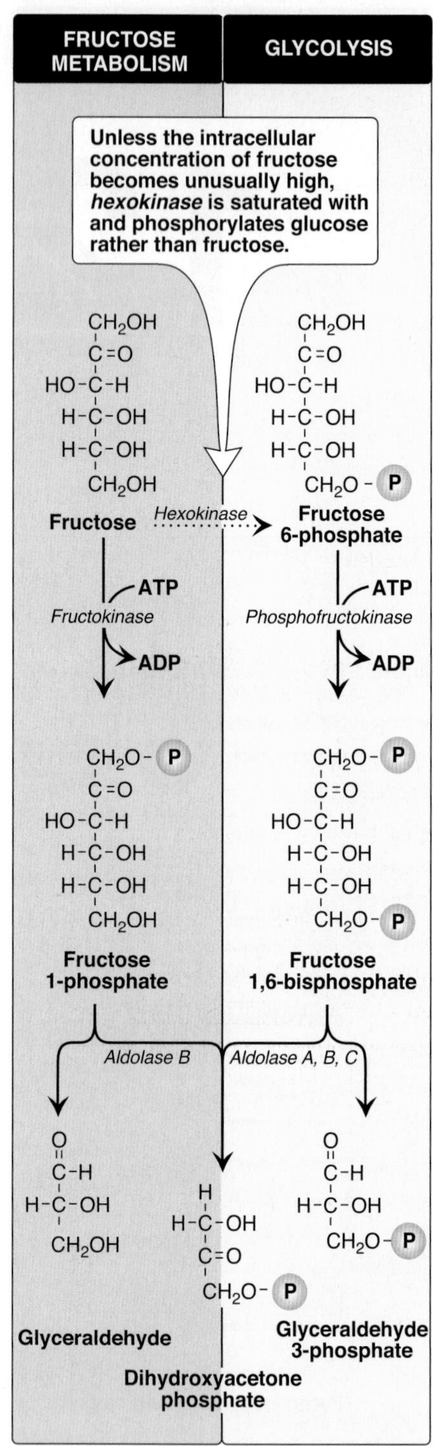

Figure 12.2
Phosphorylation products of fructose and their cleavage. P = phosphate; ADP = adenosine diphosphate.

B. Cleavage of fructose 1-phosphate

Fructose 1-phosphate is not phosphorylated to fructose 1,6-bisphosphate as is fructose 6-phosphate (see p. 99) but is cleaved by *aldolase B* (also called *fructose 1-phosphate aldolase*) to dihydroxyacetone phosphate (DHAP) and glyceraldehyde. [Note: Humans express three *aldolases*, *A*, *B* and *C*, the products of three different genes. *Aldolase A* (found in most tissues), *aldolase B* (in liver, kidney, and small intestine), and *aldolase C* (in brain) all cleave fructose 1,6-bisphosphate produced during glycolysis to DHAP and glyceraldehyde 3-phosphate (see p. 100), but only *aldolase B* cleaves fructose 1-phosphate.] DHAP can directly enter glycolysis or gluconeogenesis, whereas glyceraldehyde can be metabolized by a number of pathways, as illustrated in Figure 12.3.

C. Kinetics of fructose metabolism

The rate of fructose metabolism is more rapid than that of glucose because the trioses formed from fructose 1-phosphate bypass *phosphofructokinase-1,* the major rate-limiting step in glycolysis (see p. 99).

D. Disorders of fructose metabolism

A deficiency of one of the key enzymes required for the entry of fructose into metabolic pathways can result in either a benign condition as a result of *fructokinase* deficiency (essential fructosuria) or a severe disturbance of liver and kidney metabolism as a result of *aldolase B* deficiency (hereditary fructose intolerance [HFI]), which is estimated to occur in 1:20,000 live births (see Figure 12.3). The first symptoms of HFI appear when a baby is weaned from milk (see p. 142) and begins to be fed food containing sucrose or fructose. Fructose 1-phosphate accumulates, resulting in a drop in the level of inorganic phosphate (P_i) and, therefore, of ATP production. As ATP falls, adenosine monophosphate (AMP) rises. The AMP is degraded, causing hyperuricemia (and lactic acidosis; see p. 299). The decreased availability of hepatic ATP affects gluconeogenesis (causing hypoglycemia with vomiting) and protein synthesis (causing a decrease in blood clotting factors and other essential proteins). Kidney function may also be affected. [Note: The drop in P_i also inhibits glycogenolysis (see p. 128).] Diagnosis of HFI can be made on the basis of fructose in the urine, enzyme assay using liver cells, or by DNA-based testing (see Chapter 33). *Aldolase B* deficiency is part of the newborn screening panel. With HFI, sucrose, as well as fructose, must be removed from the diet to prevent liver failure and possible death. Individuals with HFI display an aversion to sweets and, consequently, have an absence of dental caries.

E. Conversion of mannose to fructose 6-phosphate

Mannose, the C-2 epimer of glucose (see p. 84), is an important component of glycoproteins (see p. 166). *Hexokinase* phosphorylates mannose, producing mannose 6-phosphate, which, in turn, is reversibly isomerized to fructose 6-phosphate by *phosphomannose isomerase*. [Note: There is little mannose in dietary carbohydrates. Most intracellular mannose is synthesized from fructose or is preexisting mannose produced by the degradation of structural carbohydrates and salvaged by *hexokinase*.]

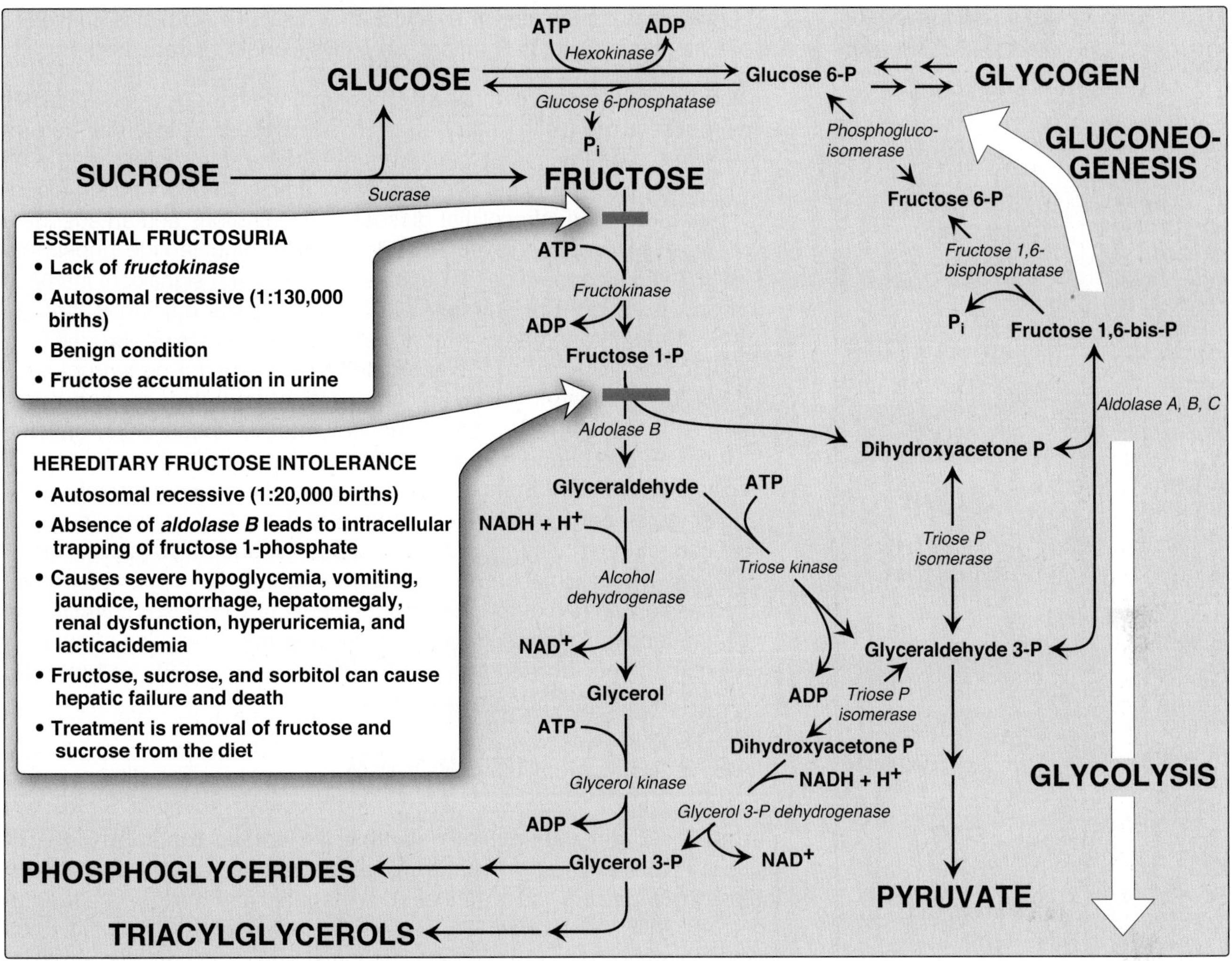

Figure 12.3
Summary of fructose metabolism. P = phosphate; P_i = inorganic phosphate; NAD(H) = nicotinamide adenine dinucleotide; ADP = adenosine diphosphate.

F. Conversion of glucose to fructose via sorbitol

Most sugars are rapidly phosphorylated following their entry into cells. Therefore, they are trapped within the cells, because organic phosphates cannot freely cross membranes without specific transporters. An alternate mechanism for metabolizing a monosaccharide is to convert it to a polyol (sugar alcohol) by the reduction of an aldehyde group, thereby producing an additional hydroxyl group.

1. **Synthesis of sorbitol:** *Aldose reductase* reduces glucose, producing sorbitol (glucitol; Figure 12.4). This enzyme is found in many tissues, including the lens, retina, Schwann cells of peripheral nerves, liver, kidney, placenta, red blood cells, and cells of the ovaries and seminal vesicles. In cells of the liver, ovaries, and seminal vesicles, there is a second enzyme, *sorbitol dehydrogenase,* which can oxidize the sorbitol to produce fructose (see Figure 12.4). The two-reaction pathway from glucose to fructose in the seminal vesicles benefits sperm cells, which use fructose as a major carbohydrate energy source. The pathway from sorbitol to fructose in the liver

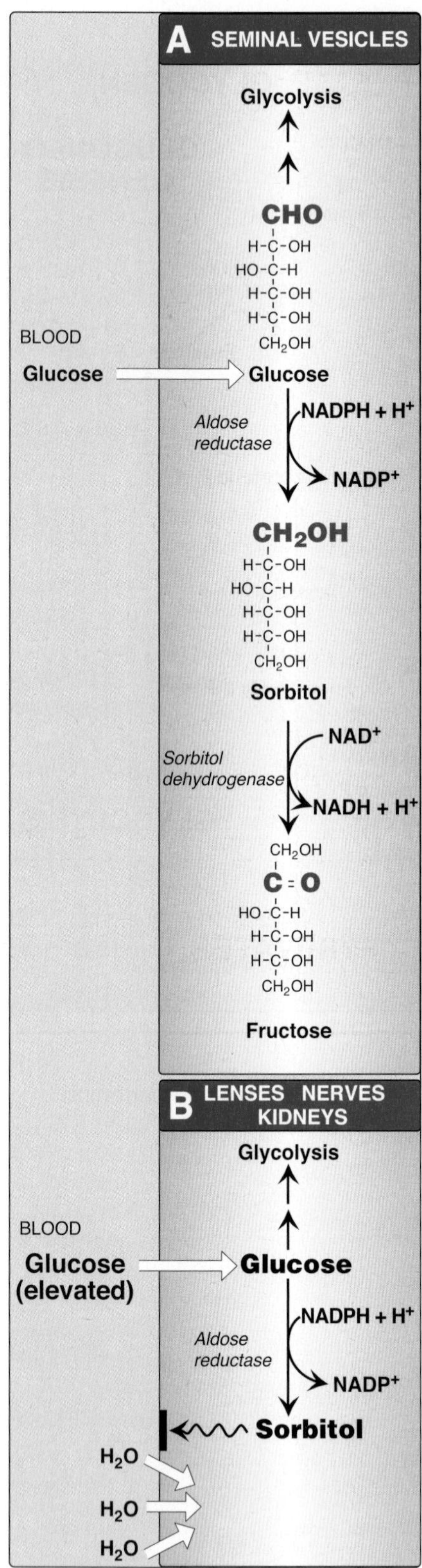

Figure 12.4
Sorbitol metabolism. NAD(H) = nicotinamide adenine dinucleotide; NADP(H) = nicotinamide adenine dinucleotide phosphate.

provides a mechanism by which any available sorbitol is converted into a substrate that can enter glycolysis or gluconeogenesis.

2. **Effect of hyperglycemia on sorbitol metabolism:** Because insulin is not required for the entry of glucose into the cells listed in the previous paragraph, large amounts of glucose may enter these cells during times of hyperglycemia (for example, in uncontrolled diabetes). Elevated intracellular glucose concentrations and an adequate supply of reduced nicotinamide adenine dinucleotide phosphate (NADPH) cause *aldose reductase* to produce a significant increase in the amount of sorbitol, which cannot pass efficiently through cell membranes and, in turn, remains trapped inside the cell (see Figure 12.4). This is exacerbated when *sorbitol dehydrogenase* is low or absent (for example, in retina, lens, kidney, and nerve cells). As a result, sorbitol accumulates in these cells, causing strong osmotic effects and, therefore, cell swelling as a result of water retention. Some of the pathologic alterations associated with diabetes can be attributed, in part, to this phenomenon, including cataract formation, peripheral neuropathy, and microvascular problems leading to nephropathy and retinopathy. (See p. 344 for a discussion of the complications of diabetes.) [Note: Use of NADPH in the *aldose reductase* reaction decreases the generation of reduced glutathione, an important antioxidant (see p. 148), and may be related to diabetic complications.]

III. GALACTOSE METABOLISM

The major dietary source of galactose is lactose (galactosyl β-1,4-glucose) obtained from milk and milk products. [Note: The digestion of lactose by *β-galactosidase* (*lactase*) of the intestinal mucosal cell membrane was discussed on p. 87.] Some galactose can also be obtained by lysosomal degradation of complex carbohydrates, such as glycoproteins and glycolipids, which are important membrane components. Like fructose, the transport of galactose into cells is not insulin dependent.

A. Phosphorylation of galactose

Like fructose, galactose must be phosphorylated before it can be further metabolized. Most tissues have a specific enzyme for this purpose, *galactokinase*, which produces galactose 1-phosphate (Figure 12.5). As with other *kinases*, ATP is the phosphate donor.

B. Formation of uridine diphosphate-galactose

Galactose 1-phosphate cannot enter the glycolytic pathway unless it is first converted to uridine diphosphate (UDP)-galactose (Figure 12.6). This occurs in an exchange reaction, in which UDP-glucose reacts with galactose 1-phosphate, producing UDP-galactose and glucose 1-phosphate (see Figure 12.5). The enzyme that catalyzes this reaction is *galactose 1-phosphate uridylyltransferase* (*GALT*).

C. Use of uridine diphosphate-galactose as a carbon source for glycolysis or gluconeogenesis

For UDP-galactose to enter the mainstream of glucose metabolism, it must first be converted to its C-4 epimer, UDP-glucose, by *UDP-*

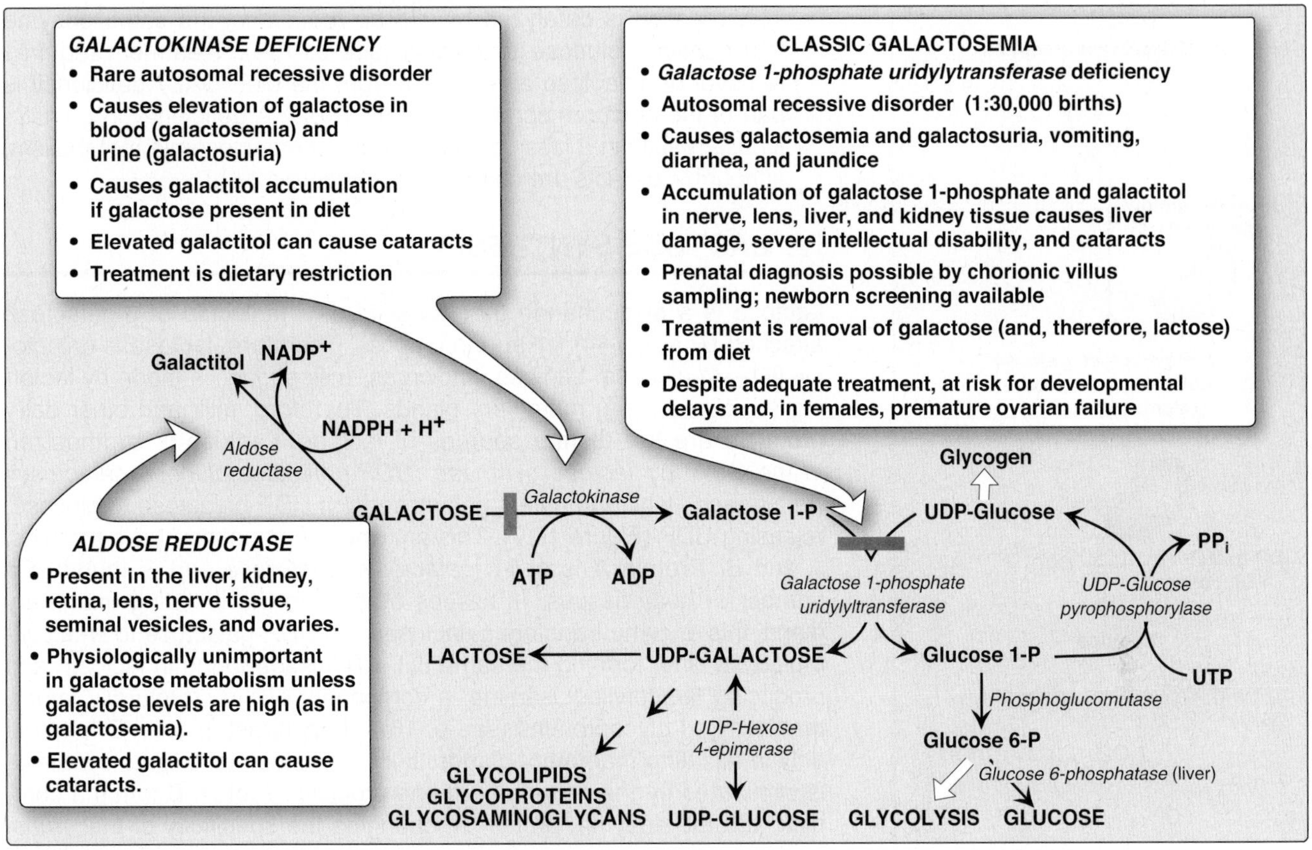

GALACTOKINASE DEFICIENCY

- Rare autosomal recessive disorder
- Causes elevation of galactose in blood (galactosemia) and urine (galactosuria)
- Causes galactitol accumulation if galactose present in diet
- Elevated galactitol can cause cataracts
- Treatment is dietary restriction

CLASSIC GALACTOSEMIA

- *Galactose 1-phosphate uridylytransferase* deficiency
- Autosomal recessive disorder (1:30,000 births)
- Causes galactosemia and galactosuria, vomiting, diarrhea, and jaundice
- Accumulation of galactose 1-phosphate and galactitol in nerve, lens, liver, and kidney tissue causes liver damage, severe intellectual disability, and cataracts
- Prenatal diagnosis possible by chorionic villus sampling; newborn screening available
- Treatment is removal of galactose (and, therefore, lactose) from diet
- Despite adequate treatment, at risk for developmental delays and, in females, premature ovarian failure

ALDOSE REDUCTASE

- Present in the liver, kidney, retina, lens, nerve tissue, seminal vesicles, and ovaries.
- Physiologically unimportant in galactose metabolism unless galactose levels are high (as in galactosemia).
- Elevated galactitol can cause cataracts.

Figure 12.5
Metabolism of galactose. UDP = uridine diphosphate; UTP = uridine triphosphate; P = phosphate; PP_i = pyrophosphate; NADP(H) = nicotinamide adenine dinucleotide phosphate; ADP = adenosine diphosphate.

hexose 4-epimerase. This "new" UDP-glucose (produced from the original UDP-galactose) can then participate in many biosynthetic reactions as well as being used in the *GALT* reaction described above. (See Figure 12.5 for a summary of this interconversion.)

D. Role of uridine diphosphate-galactose in biosynthetic reactions

UDP-galactose can serve as the donor of galactose units in a number of synthetic pathways, including synthesis of lactose (see below), glycoproteins (see p. 166), glycolipids (see p. 210), and glycosaminoglycans (see p. 158). [Note: If galactose is not provided by the diet (for example, when it cannot be released from lactose as a result of a lack of *β-galactosidase* in people who are lactose intolerant), all tissue requirements for UDP-galactose can be met by the action of *UDP-hexose 4-epimerase* on UDP-glucose, which is efficiently produced from glucose 1-phosphate (see Figure 12.5).]

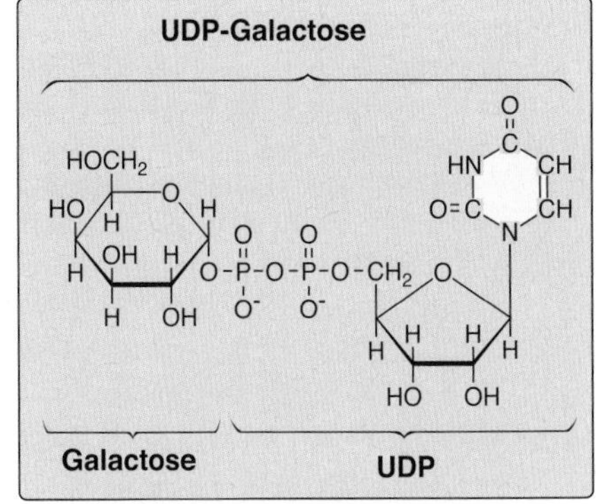

Figure 12.6
Structure of UDP-galactose. UDP = uridine diphosphate.

E. Disorders of galactose metabolism

GALT is deficient in individuals with classic galactosemia (see Figure 12.5). In this disorder, galactose 1-phosphate and, therefore, galactose accumulate. Physiologic consequences are similar to those found in hereditary fructose intolerance (see p. 138), but a broader spectrum of tissues is affected. The accumulated galactose is shunted into side pathways such as that of galactitol production.

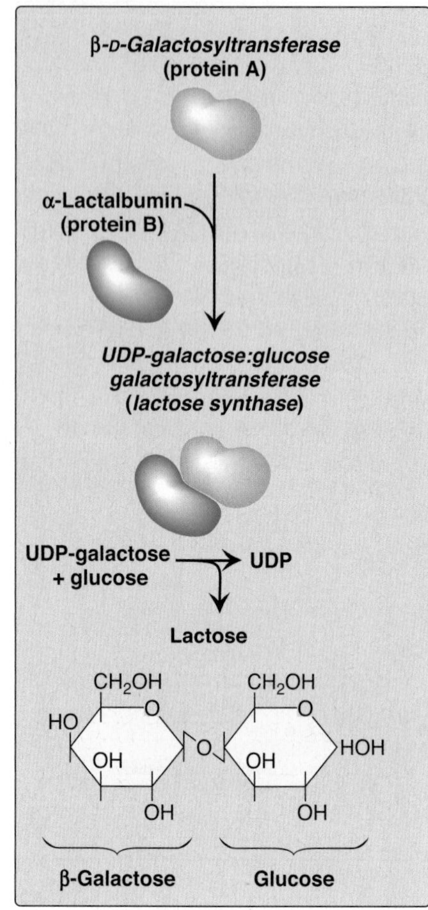

Figure 12.7
Lactose synthesis. UDP = uridine diphosphate.

This reaction is catalyzed by *aldose reductase,* the same enzyme that converts glucose to sorbitol (see p. 139). Treatment requires removal of galactose and lactose from the diet. *GALT* deficiency is part of the newborn screening panel. [Note: A deficiency in *galactokinase* results in a less severe disorder of galactosemia metabolism, although cataracts are common (see Figure 12.5).]

IV. LACTOSE SYNTHESIS

Lactose is a disaccharide that consists of a molecule of β-galactose attached by a β(1→4) linkage to glucose. Therefore, lactose is galactosyl β(1→4)-glucose. Lactose, known as "milk sugar," is made by lactating (milk-producing) mammary glands. Therefore, milk and other dairy products are the dietary sources of lactose. Lactose is synthesized in the Golgi by *lactose synthase (UDP-galactose:glucose galactosyltransferase),* which transfers galactose from UDP-galactose to glucose, releasing UDP (Figure 12.7). This enzyme is composed of two proteins, A and B. Protein A is a *β-D-galactosyltransferase* and is found in a number of body tissues. In tissues other than the lactating mammary gland, this enzyme transfers galactose from UDP-galactose to N-acetyl-D-glucosamine, forming the same β(1→4) linkage found in lactose, and producing N-acetyllactosamine, a component of the structurally important N-linked glycoproteins (see p. 167). In contrast, protein B is found only in lactating mammary glands. It is α-lactalbumin, and its synthesis is stimulated by the peptide hormone prolactin. Protein B forms a complex with the enzyme, protein A, changing the specificity of that *transferase* so that lactose, rather than N-acetyllactosamine, is produced (see Figure 12.7).

V. CHAPTER SUMMARY

The major source of fructose is **sucrose**, which, when cleaved, releases equimolar amounts of fructose and glucose (Figure 12.8). Transport of fructose into cells is **insulin independent**. Fructose is first phosphorylated to **fructose 1-phosphate** by ***fructokinase*** and then cleaved by ***aldolase B*** to **dihydroxyacetone phosphate** and **glyceraldehyde**. These enzymes are found in the **liver**, **kidney**, and **small intestinal mucosa**. A **deficiency** of ***fructokinase*** causes a benign condition (**essential fructosuria**), but a **deficiency** of ***aldolase B*** causes **hereditary fructose intolerance (HFI)**, in which **severe hypoglycemia** and **liver failure** lead to **death** if fructose (and sucrose) in the diet is not eliminated. **Mannose**, an important component of **glycoproteins**, is phosphorylated by ***hexokinase*** to **mannose 6-phosphate**, which is reversibly isomerized to **fructose 6-phosphate** by ***phosphomannose isomerase***. **Glucose** can be reduced to **sorbitol (glucitol)** by ***aldose reductase*** in many tissues, including the **lens, retina, Schwann cells, liver, kidney, ovaries**, and **seminal vesicles**. In cells of the **liver, ovaries**, and **seminal vesicles**, a second enzyme, ***sorbitol dehydrogenase***, can oxidize sorbitol to produce **fructose**. **Hyperglycemia** results in the accumulation of sorbitol in those cells lacking *sorbitol dehydrogenase*. The resulting **osmotic events** cause cell swelling and may contribute to the **cataract formation**, **peripheral neuropathy**, **nephropathy**, and **retinopathy** seen in **diabetes**. The major dietary source of galactose is **lactose**. The transport of galactose into cells is not insulin dependent. Galactose is first phosphorylated by ***galactokinase*** (a deficiency results in cataracts) to **galactose 1-phosphate**. This compound is converted to **uridine diphosphate (UDP)-galactose** by ***galactose 1-phosphate uridyltransferase*** **(*GALT*)**, with the nucleotide supplied by UDP-glucose. A **deficiency** of this enzyme causes **classic galactosemia**. Galactose 1-phosphate accumulates, and excess galactose is converted to **galactitol** by ***aldose reductase***. This causes **liver damage**, **severe intellectual disability**, and **cataracts**. Treatment requires removal of galactose (and lactose) from the diet. For UDP-galactose to enter the mainstream of glucose metabolism, it must first be converted to UDP-glucose by ***UDP-hexose 4-epimerase***. This enzyme can also be used to produce UDP-galactose from UDP-glucose when the former is required for the synthesis of structural carbohydrates. **Lactose** is a disaccharide that consists of **galactose** and **glucose**. Milk and other dairy products are the dietary sources of lactose. Lactose is synthesized by ***lactose synthase*** from **UDP-galactose** and **glucose** in the **lactating mammary gland**. The enzyme has two subunits, **protein A** (which is a ***galactosyltransferase*** found in most cells where it synthesizes **N-acetyllactosamine**) and **protein B** (**α-lactalbumin**, which is found only in the lactating mammary glands, and whose synthesis is stimulated by the peptide hormone **prolactin**). When both subunits are present, the *transferase* produces lactose.

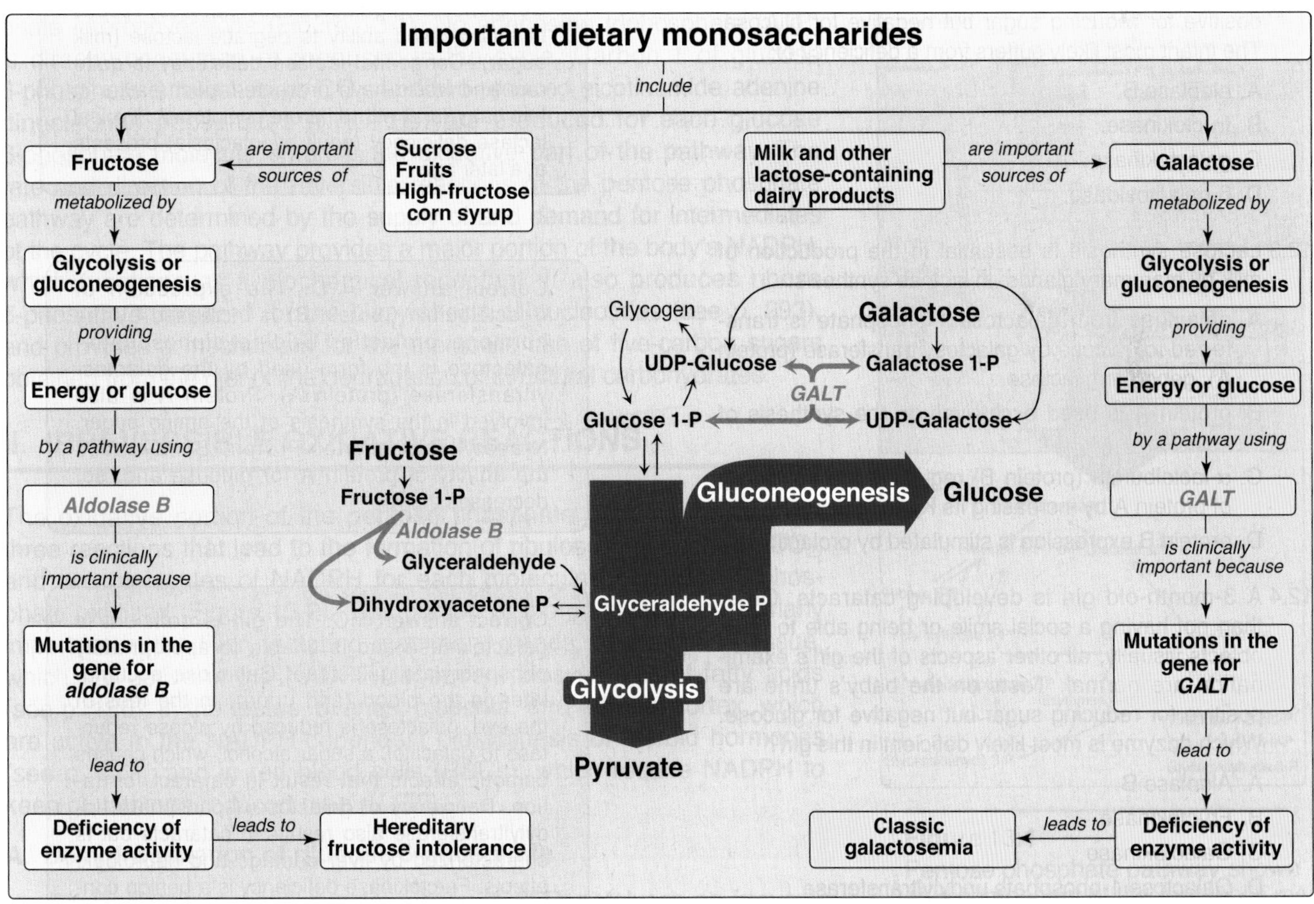

Figure 12.8
Key concept map for metabolism of fructose and galactose. *GALT* = *galactose 1-phosphate uridylyltransferase*; UDP = uridine diphosphate; P = phosphate.

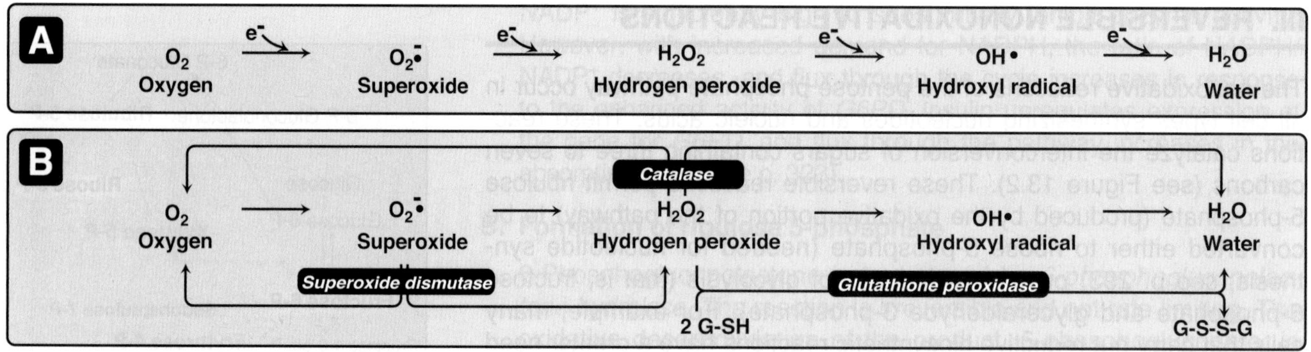

Figure 13.5
A. Formation of reactive intermediates from molecular oxygen. e− = electrons. B. Actions of antioxidant enzymes. G-SH = reduced glutathione; G-S-S-G = oxidized glutathione. (See Figure 13.6B for the regeneration of G-SH.)

B. Reduction of hydrogen peroxide

Hydrogen peroxide (H_2O_2) is one of a family of reactive oxygen species (ROS) that are formed from the partial reduction of molecular oxygen (Figure 13.5A). These compounds are formed continuously as byproducts of aerobic metabolism, through reactions with drugs and environmental toxins, or when the level of antioxidants is diminished, all creating the condition of oxidative stress. The highly reactive oxygen intermediates can cause serious chemical damage to DNA, proteins, and unsaturated lipids and can lead to cell death. ROS have been implicated in a number of pathologic processes, including reperfusion injury, cancer, inflammatory disease, and aging. The cell has several protective mechanisms that minimize the toxic potential of these compounds.

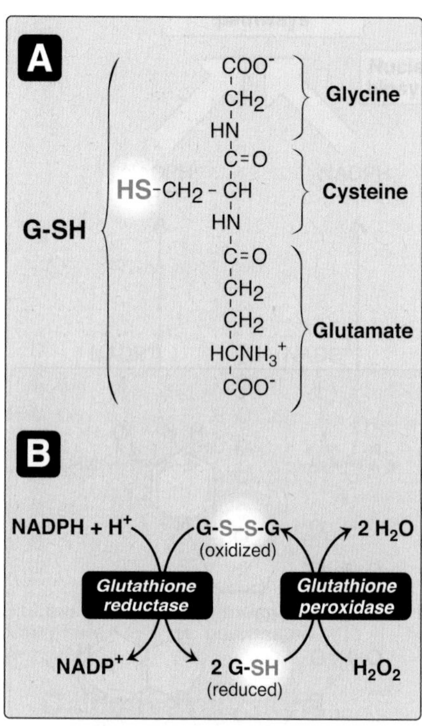

Figure 13.6
A. Structure of reduced glutathione (G-SH). [Note: Glutamate is linked to cysteine through a γ-carboxyl, rather than an α-carboxyl.]
B. Glutathione-mediated reduction of hydrogen peroxide (H_2O_2) by reduced nicotinamide adenine dinucleotide phosphate (NADPH). G-S-S-G = oxidized glutathione.

1. **Enzymes that catalyze antioxidant reactions:** Reduced glutathione (G-SH), a tripeptide-thiol (γ-glutamylcysteinylglycine) present in most cells, can chemically detoxify H_2O_2 (Figure 13.5B). This reaction, catalyzed by the selenium-containing *glutathione peroxidase*, forms oxidized glutathione (G-S-S-G), which no longer has protective properties. The cell regenerates G-SH in a reaction catalyzed by *glutathione reductase,* using NADPH as a source of reducing equivalents. Thus, NADPH indirectly provides electrons for the reduction of H_2O_2 (Figure 13.6). [Note: RBCs are totally dependent on the pentose phosphate pathway for their supply of NADPH because, unlike other cell types, RBCs do not have an alternate source for this essential coenzyme.] Additional enzymes, such as *superoxide dismutase* and *catalase*, catalyze the conversion of other reactive oxygen intermediates to harmless products (see Figure 13.5B). As a group, these enzymes serve as a defense system to guard against the toxic effects of ROS.

2. **Antioxidant chemicals:** A number of intracellular reducing agents, such as ascorbate (see p. 377), vitamin E (see p. 391), and β-carotene (see p. 382), are able to reduce and, thereby, detoxify reactive oxygen intermediates in the laboratory. Consumption of foods rich in these antioxidant compounds has been correlated with a reduced risk for certain types of cancers as well as decreased frequency of certain other chronic health

problems. Therefore, it is tempting to speculate that the effects of these compounds are, in part, an expression of their ability to quench the toxic effect of ROS. However, clinical trials with antioxidants as dietary supplements have failed to show clear beneficial effects. In the case of dietary supplementation with β-carotene, the rate of lung cancer in smokers increased rather than decreased. Thus, the health-promoting effects of dietary fruits and vegetables likely reflect a complex interaction among many naturally occurring compounds, which has not been duplicated by consumption of isolated antioxidant compounds.

C. Cytochrome P450 monooxygenase system

Monooxygenases (*mixed-function oxidases*) incorporate one atom from molecular oxygen into a substrate (creating a hydroxyl group), with the other atom being reduced to water. In the *cytochrome P450 monooxygenase* system, NADPH provides the reducing equivalents required by this series of reactions (Figure 13.7). This system performs different functions in two separate locations in cells. The overall reaction catalyzed by a *cytochrome P450* enzyme is:

$$R\text{-}H + O_2 + NADPH + H^+ \rightarrow R\text{-}OH + H_2O + NADP^+$$

where R may be a steroid, drug, or other chemical. [Note: *Cytochrome P450* (*CYP*) enzymes are actually a superfamily of related, heme-containing *monooxygenases* that participate in a broad variety of reactions. The P450 in the name reflects the absorbance at 450 nm by the protein.]

1. **Mitochondrial system:** An important function of the *cytochrome P450 monooxygenase* system found associated with the inner mitochondrial membrane is the biosynthesis of steroid hormones. In steroidogenic tissues, such as the placenta, ovaries, testes, and adrenal cortex, it is used to hydroxylate intermediates in the conversion of cholesterol to steroid hormones, a process that makes these hydrophobic compounds more water soluble (see p. 237). The liver uses this same system in bile acid synthesis (see p. 224) and the hydroxylation of cholecalciferol to 25-hydroxycholecalciferol (vitamin D_3; see p. 386), and the kidney uses it to hydroxylate vitamin D_3 to its biologically active 1,25-dihydroxylated form.

2. **Microsomal system:** An extremely important function of the microsomal *cytochrome P450 monooxygenase* system found associated with the membrane of the smooth endoplasmic reticulum (particularly in the liver) is the detoxification of foreign compounds (xenobiotics). These include numerous drugs and such varied pollutants as petroleum products and pesticides. *CYP* enzymes of the microsomal system (for example, *CYP3A4*), can be used to hydroxylate these toxins. The purpose of these modifications is two-fold. First, it may itself activate or inactivate a drug and second, make a toxic compound more soluble, thereby facilitating its excretion in the urine or feces. Frequently, however, the new hydroxyl group will serve as a site for conjugation with a polar molecule, such as glucuronic acid (see p. 161), which will significantly increase the compound's solubility. [Note: Polymorphisms (see p.473) in the genes for *CYP* enzymes can lead to differences in drug metabolism.]

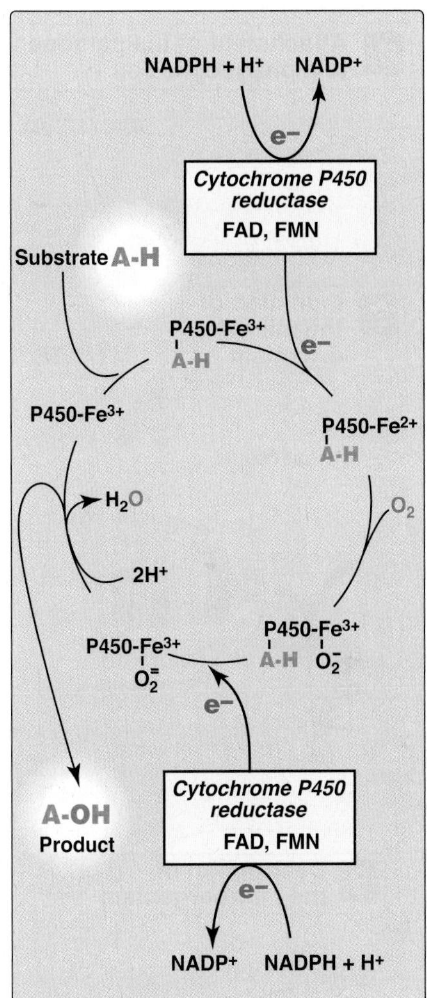

Figure 13.7
Cytochrome P450 monooxygenase cycle (simplified). Electrons (e⁻) move from NADPH to FAD to FMN of the *reductase* and then to the heme iron (Fe) of the *P450* enzyme. [Note: In the mitochondrial system, electrons move from FAD to an iron-sulfur protein and then to the *P450* enzyme.] FAD = flavin adenine dinucleotide; FMN = flavin mononucleotide; NADPH = reduced nicotinamide adenine dinucleotide phosphate.

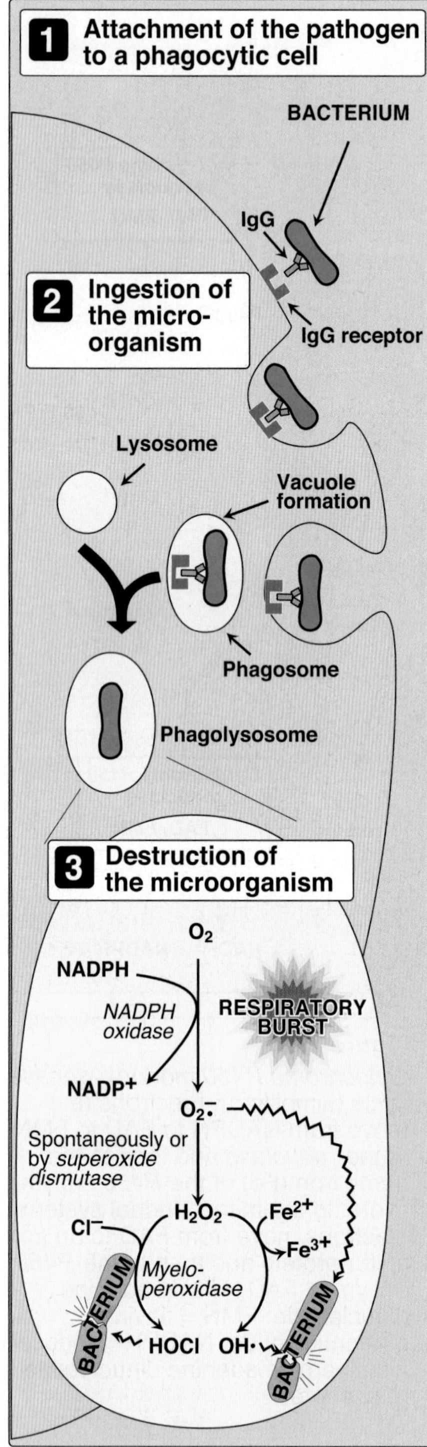

Figure 13.8
Phagocytosis and the oxygen-dependent pathway of microbial killing. IgG = the antibody immunoglobulin G; NADPH = reduced nicotinamide adenine dinucleotide phosphate; $O_2^{\bullet-}$ = superoxide; HOCl = hypochlorous acid; OH• = hydroxyl radical.

D. Phagocytosis by white blood cells

Phagocytosis is the ingestion by receptor-mediated endocytosis of microorganisms, foreign particles, and cellular debris by cells such as neutrophils and macrophages (monocytes). It is an important defense mechanism, particularly in bacterial infections. Neutrophils and monocytes are armed with both oxygen-independent and oxygen-dependent mechanisms for killing bacteria.

1. **Oxygen-independent mechanism:** Oxygen-independent mechanisms use pH changes in phagolysosomes and lysosomal enzymes to destroy pathogens.

2. **Oxygen-dependent system:** Oxygen-dependent mechanisms include the enzymes *NADPH oxidase* and *myeloperoxidase* (*MPO*) that work together in killing bacteria (Figure 13.8). Overall, the *MPO* system is the most potent of the bactericidal mechanisms. An invading bacterium is recognized by the immune system and attacked by antibodies that bind it to a receptor on a phagocytic cell. After internalization of the microorganism has occurred, *NADPH oxidase*, located in the leukocyte cell membrane, is activated and reduces O_2 from the surrounding tissue to superoxide ($O_2^{\bullet-}$), a free radical, as NADPH is oxidized. The rapid consumption of O_2 that accompanies formation of $O_2^{\bullet-}$ is referred to as the "respiratory burst." [Note: Active *NADPH oxidase* is a membrane-associated complex containing a flavocytochrome plus additional peptides that translocate from the cytoplasm upon activation of the leukocyte. Electrons move from NADPH to O_2 via flavin adenine nucleotide (FAD) and heme, generating $O_2^{\bullet-}$. Rare genetic deficiencies in *NADPH oxidase* cause chronic granulomatous disease (CGD) characterized by severe, persistent infections and the formation of granulomas (nodular areas of inflammation) that sequester the bacteria that were not destroyed.] Next, $O_2^{\bullet-}$ is converted to H_2O_2 (a ROS), either spontaneously or catalyzed by *superoxide dismutase*. In the presence of *MPO*, a heme-containing lysosomal enzyme present within the phagolysosome, peroxide plus chloride ions are converted to hypochlorous acid ([HOCl] the major component of household bleach), which kills the bacteria. The peroxide can also be partially reduced to the hydroxyl radical (OH•), a ROS, or be fully reduced to water by *catalase* or *glutathione peroxidase*. [Note: Deficiencies in *MPO* do not confer increased susceptibility to infection because peroxide from *NADPH oxidase* is bactericidal.]

E. Synthesis of nitric oxide

Nitric oxide (NO) is recognized as a mediator in a broad array of biologic systems. NO is the endothelium-derived relaxing factor, which causes vasodilation by relaxing vascular smooth muscle. NO also acts as a neurotransmitter, prevents platelet aggregation, and plays an essential role in macrophage function. NO has a very short half-life in tissues (3–10 seconds) because it reacts with oxygen and superoxide and then is converted into nitrates and nitrites including peroxynitrite ($O{=}NOO^-$), a reactive nitrogen species (RNS). [Note: NO is a free radical gas that is often confused with nitrous oxide (N_2O), the "laughing gas" that is used as an anesthetic and is chemically stable.]

1. **Nitric oxide synthase:** Arginine, O_2, and NADPH are substrates for cytosolic *NO synthase* ([*NOS*] Figure 13.9). Flavin mononucleotide (FMN), FAD, heme, and tetrahydrobiopterin (see p. 268) are coenzymes, and NO and citrulline are products of the reaction. Three *NOS*, each the product of a different gene, have been identified. Two are constitutive (synthesized at a constant rate), Ca^{2+}–calmodulin-dependent enzymes (see p. 133). They are found primarily in endothelium (*eNOS*) and neural tissue (*nNOS*) and constantly produce very low levels of NO for vasodilation and neurotransmission. An inducible, Ca^{2+}-independent enzyme (*iNOS*) can be expressed in many cells, including macrophages and neutrophils, as an early defense against pathogens. The specific inducers for *iNOS* vary with cell type, and include proinflammatory cytokines, such as tumor necrosis factor-α (TNF-α) and interferon-γ (IFN-γ), and bacterial endotoxins such as lipopolysaccharide (LPS). These compounds promote synthesis of *iNOS*, which can result in large amounts of NO being produced over hours or even days.

2. **Actions of nitric oxide on vascular endothelium:** NO is an important mediator in the control of vascular smooth muscle tone. NO is synthesized by *eNOS* in endothelial cells and diffuses to vascular smooth muscle, where it activates the cytosolic form of *guanylate cyclase* (also known as *guanylyl cyclase*) to form cyclic guanosine monophosphate (cGMP). [Note: This reaction is analogous to the formation of cyclic AMP by *adenylate cyclase* (see p. 94), except that this *guanylate cyclase* is not membrane associated.] The resultant rise in cGMP causes activation of *protein kinase G*, which phosphorylates Ca^{2+} channels, causing decreased entry of Ca^{2+} into smooth muscle cells. This decreases the calcium–calmodulin activation of *myosin light-chain kinase*, thereby decreasing smooth muscle contraction and favoring relaxation. Vasodilator nitrates, such as nitroglycerin, are metabolized to NO, which causes relaxation of vascular smooth muscle and, therefore, lowers blood pressure. Thus, NO can be envisioned as an endogenous nitrovasodilator. [Note: NO is involved in penile erection. Sildenafil citrate, used in the treatment of erectile dysfunction, inhibits the *phosphodiesterase* that inactivates cGMP.]

3. **Role of nitric oxide in macrophage bactericidal activity:** In macrophages, *iNOS* activity is normally low, but synthesis of the enzyme is significantly stimulated by bacterial LPS and by release of IFN-γ and TNF-α in response to the infection. Activated macrophages form $O_2^{\bar{\cdot}}$ radicals (see p. 150) that combine with NO to form intermediates that decompose, producing the highly bactericidal OH• radical.

4. **Other functions of nitric oxide:** NO is a potent inhibitor of platelet adhesion and aggregation (by activating the cGMP pathway). It is also characterized as a neurotransmitter in the central and peripheral nervous systems.

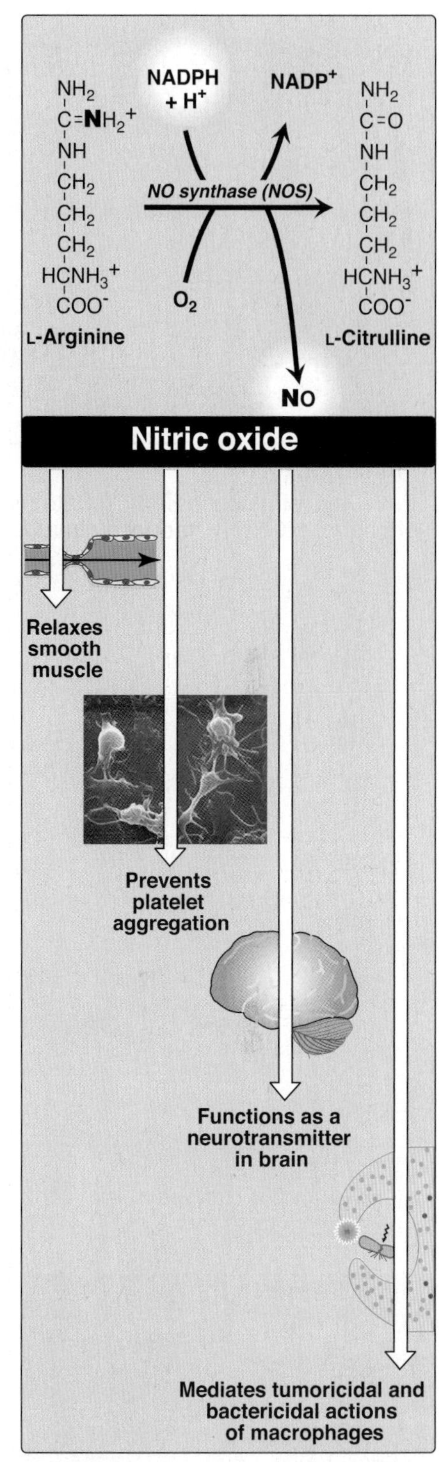

Figure 13.9
Synthesis and some of the actions of nitric oxide (NO). NADPH = reduced nicotinamide adenine dinucleotide phosphate. [Note: Flavin mononucleotide, flavin adenine dinucleotide, heme, and tetrahydrobiopterin are additional coenzymes required by *NOS*.]

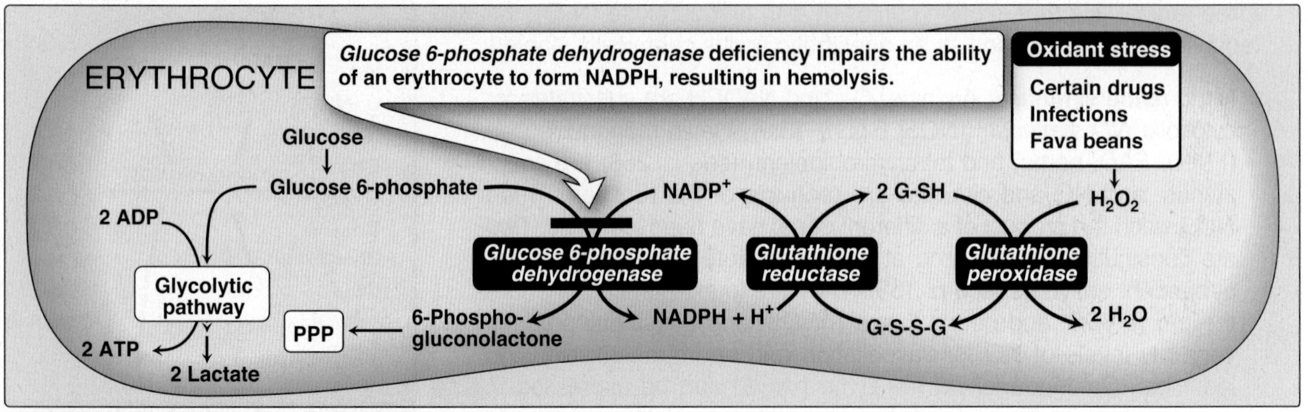

Figure 13.10
Pathways of glucose 6-phosphate metabolism in the erythrocyte. NADP(H) = nicotinamide adenine dinucleotide phosphate; G-SH = reduced glutathionine; G-S-S-G = oxidized glutathionine; PPP = pentose phosphate pathway.

V. GLUCOSE 6-PHOSPHATE DEHYDROGENASE DEFICIENCY

G6PD deficiency is a hereditary disease characterized by hemolytic anemia caused by the inability to detoxify oxidizing agents. *G6PD* deficiency is the most common disease-producing enzyme abnormality in humans, affecting more than 400 million individuals worldwide. This deficiency has the highest prevalence in the Middle East, tropical Africa and Asia, and parts of the Mediterranean. *G6PD* deficiency is X linked and is, in fact, a family of deficiencies caused by a number of different mutations in the gene coding for *G6PD*. Only some of the resulting protein variants cause clinical symptoms. [Note: In addition to hemolytic anemia, a clinical manifestation of *G6PD* deficiency is neonatal jaundice appearing 1–4 days after birth. The jaundice, which may be severe, typically results from increased production of unconjugated bilirubin (see p. 285).] The life span of individuals with a severe form of *G6PD* deficiency may be somewhat shortened as a result of complications arising from chronic hemolysis. This negative effect of *G6PD* deficiency has been balanced in evolution by an advantage in survival—an increased resistance to Plasmodium falciparum malaria. [Note: Sickle cell trait and β-thalassemia minor also confer resistance to malaria.]

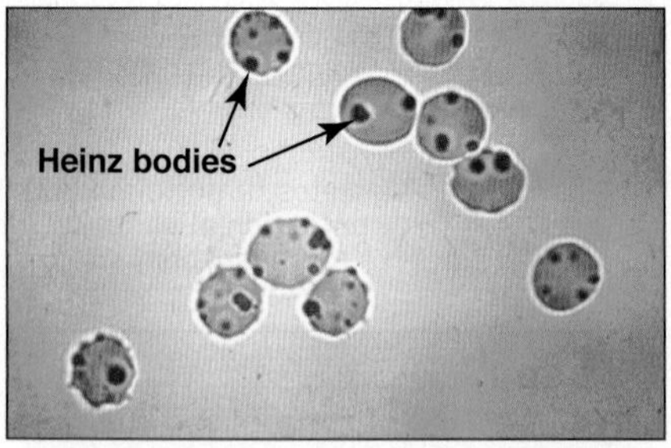

Figure 13.11
Heinz bodies in erythrocytes of a patient with *glucose 6-phosphate dehydrogenase* deficiency.

A. Role of glucose 6-phosphate dehydrogenase in red blood cells

Diminished *G6PD* activity impairs the ability of the cell to form the NADPH that is essential for the maintenance of the G-SH pool. This results in a decrease in the cellular detoxification of free radicals and peroxides formed within the cell (Figure 13.10). G-SH also helps maintain the reduced states of sulfhydryl groups in proteins, including hemoglobin. Oxidation of those sulfhydryl groups leads to the formation of denatured proteins that form insoluble masses (called Heinz bodies) that attach to RBC membranes (Figure 13.11). Additional oxidation of membrane proteins causes RBCs to be rigid (less deformable), and they are removed from the circulation by macrophages in the spleen and liver. Although *G6PD* deficiency occurs in all cells of the affected individual, it is most severe in RBCs, where the pentose phosphate pathway provides the only means of generating NADPH.

Other tissues have alternative sources for NADPH production (such as *$NADP^+$-dependent malate dehydrogenase* [*malic enzyme*]; see p. 186) that can keep G-SH reduced. The RBC has no nucleus or ribosomes and cannot renew its supply of the enzyme. Thus, RBCs are particularly vulnerable to enzyme variants with diminished stability.

B. Precipitating factors in glucose 6-phosphate dehydrogenase deficiency

Most individuals who have inherited one of the *G6PD* mutations do not show clinical manifestations (that is, they are asymptomatic). However, some patients with *G6PD* deficiency develop hemolytic anemia if they are treated with an oxidant drug, ingest fava beans, or contract a severe infection.

1. **Oxidant drugs:** Commonly used drugs that produce hemolytic anemia in patients with *G6PD* deficiency are best remembered from the mnemonic AAA: antibiotics (for example, sulfamethoxazole and chloramphenicol), antimalarials (for example, primaquine but not chloroquine or quinine), and antipyretics (for example, acetanilid but not acetaminophen).

2. **Favism:** Some forms of *G6PD* deficiency, for example the Mediterranean variant, are particularly susceptible to the hemolytic effect of the fava (broad) bean, a dietary staple in the Mediterranean region. Favism, the hemolytic effect of ingesting fava beans, is not observed in all individuals with *G6PD* deficiency, but all patients with favism have *G6PD* deficiency.

3. **Infection:** Infection is the most common precipitating factor of hemolysis in *G6PD* deficiency. The inflammatory response to infection results in the generation of free radicals in macrophages, which can diffuse into the RBC and cause oxidative damage.

C. Properties of the variant enzymes

Almost all *G6PD* variants are caused by point mutations (see p. 433) in the gene for *G6PD.* Some mutations do not disrupt the structure of the enzyme's active site and, therefore, do not affect enzymic activity. However, many mutant enzymes show altered kinetic properties. For example, variant enzymes may show decreased catalytic activity, decreased stability, or an alteration of binding affinity for $NADP^+$, NADPH, or glucose 6-phosphate. The severity of the disease usually correlates with the amount of residual enzyme activity in the patient's RBC. For example, variants can be classified as shown in Figure 13.12. *G6PD A^-* is the prototype of the moderate (Class III) form of the disease. The RBCs contain an unstable but kinetically normal *G6PD,* with most of the enzyme activity present in the reticulocytes and younger RBCs (Figure 13.13). The oldest RBCs, therefore, have the lowest level of enzyme activity and are preferentially removed in a hemolytic episode. *G6PD Mediterranean* is the prototype of a more severe (Class II) deficiency in which the enzyme has decreased stability resulting in decreased enzymic activity. Class I mutations (rare) are the most severe and are associated with chronic nonspherocytic hemolytic anemia, which occurs even in the absence of oxidative stress.

Class	Clinical symptoms	Residual enzyme activity
I	Very severe (chronic hemolytic anemia)	<10%
II	Severe (episodic hemolytic anemia)	<10%
III	Moderate	10%–60%
IV	None	>60%

Figure 13.12
Classification of *glucose 6-phosphate dehydrogenase* (*G6PD*) deficiency variants. Note: Class V variants (not shown in table) result in overproduction of *G6PD.*

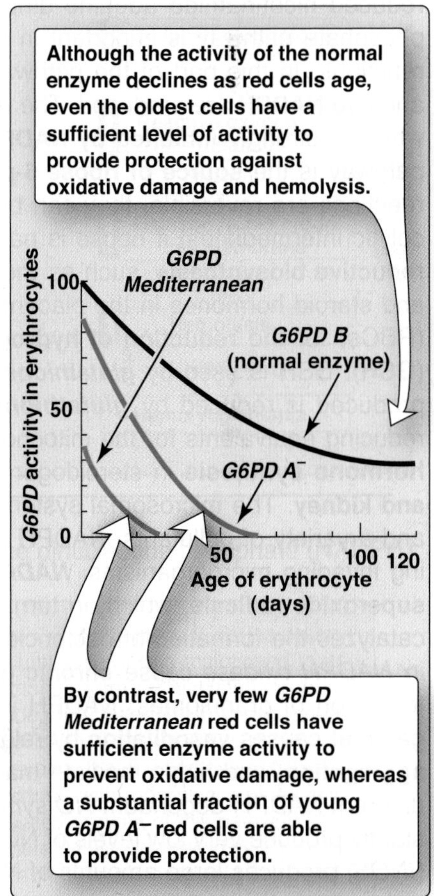

Figure 13.13
Decline of erythrocyte *glucose 6-phosphate dehydrogenase* (*G6PD*) activity with cell age for the three most commonly encountered forms of the enzyme.

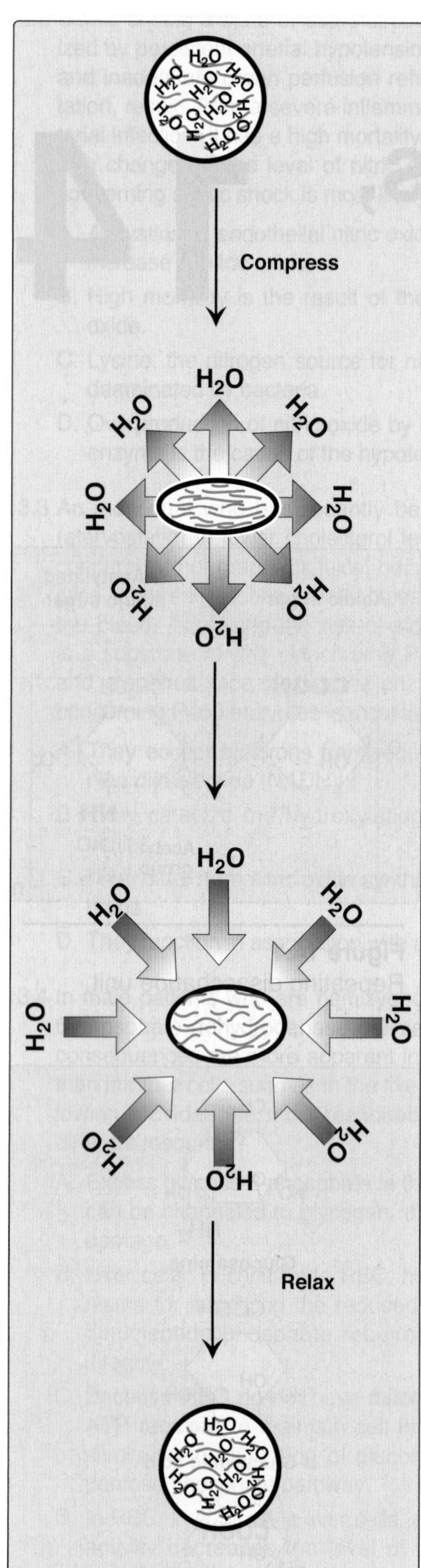

Figure 14.3
Resilience of glycosaminoglycans.

the "slippery" consistency of mucous secretions and synovial fluid. When a solution of GAGs is compressed, the water is "squeezed out," and the GAGs are forced to occupy a smaller volume. When the compression is released, the GAGs spring back to their original, hydrated volume because of the repulsion of their negative charges. This property contributes to the resilience of synovial fluid and the vitreous humor of the eye (Figure 14.3).

B. Classification of the glycosaminoglycans

The six major types of glycosaminoglycans are divided according to monomeric composition, type of glycosidic linkages, and degree and location of sulfate units. The structure of the GAGs and their distribution in the body is illustrated in Figure 14.4. All GAGs, except for hyaluronic acid, are sulfated and are found covalently attached to protein, forming proteoglycan monomers.

C. Proteoglycans

Proteoglycans are found in the ECM and on the outer surface of cells.

1. **Structure of proteoglycan monomers:** A proteoglycan monomer found in cartilage consists of a core protein to which up to 100 linear chains of GAGs are covalently attached. These chains, which may each be composed of up to 200 disaccharide units, extend out from the core protein and remain separated from each other because of charge repulsion. The resulting structure resembles a "bottle brush" (Figure 14.5). In cartilage proteoglycan, the species of GAGs include chondroitin sulfate and keratan sulfate. [Note: Proteoglycans are grouped into gene families that encode core proteins with common structural features. The aggrecan family (aggrecan, versecan, neurocan, and brevican), abundant in cartilage, is an example.]

2. **Linkage between the carbohydrate chain and the protein:** This linkage is most commonly through a trihexoside (galactose-galactose-xylose) and a serine residue, respectively. An O-glycosidic bond is formed between the xylose and the hydroxyl group of the serine (Figure 14.6).

3. **Proteoglycan aggregates:** The proteoglycan monomers associate with a molecule of hyaluronic acid to form proteoglycan aggregates.The association is not covalent but occurs primarily through ionic interactions between the core protein and the hyaluronic acid. The association is stabilized by additional small proteins called link proteins (Figure 14.7).

III. SYNTHESIS OF GLYCOSAMINOGLYCANS

The heteropolysaccharide chains are elongated by the sequential addition of alternating acidic and amino sugars donated by their uridine diphosphate (UDP)-derivatives. The reactions are catalyzed by a family of specific *glycosyltransferases*. The synthesis of GAGs is analogous to that of glycogen (see p. 126) except that GAGs are produced for export from the cell. Their synthesis occurs, therefore, primarily in the Golgi, rather than in the cytosol.

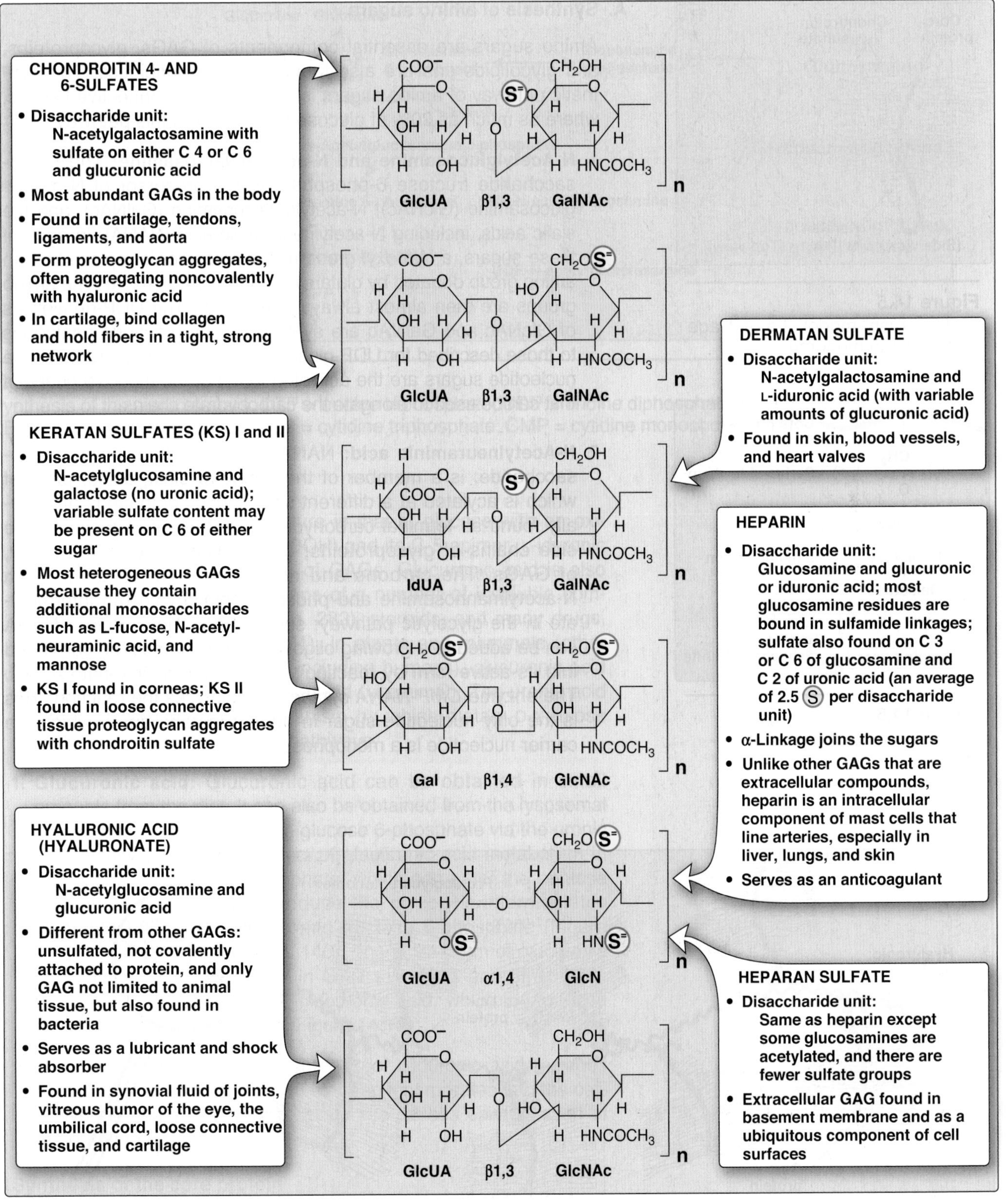

Figure 14.4
Structure and distribution of glycosaminoglycans (GAGs). Sulfate groups (Ⓢ) are shown in all possible positions. GlcUA = glucuronic acid; IdUA = iduronic acid; GalNAc = N-acetylgalactosamine; GlcNAc = N-acetylglucosamine; GlcN = glucosamine; Gal = galactose.

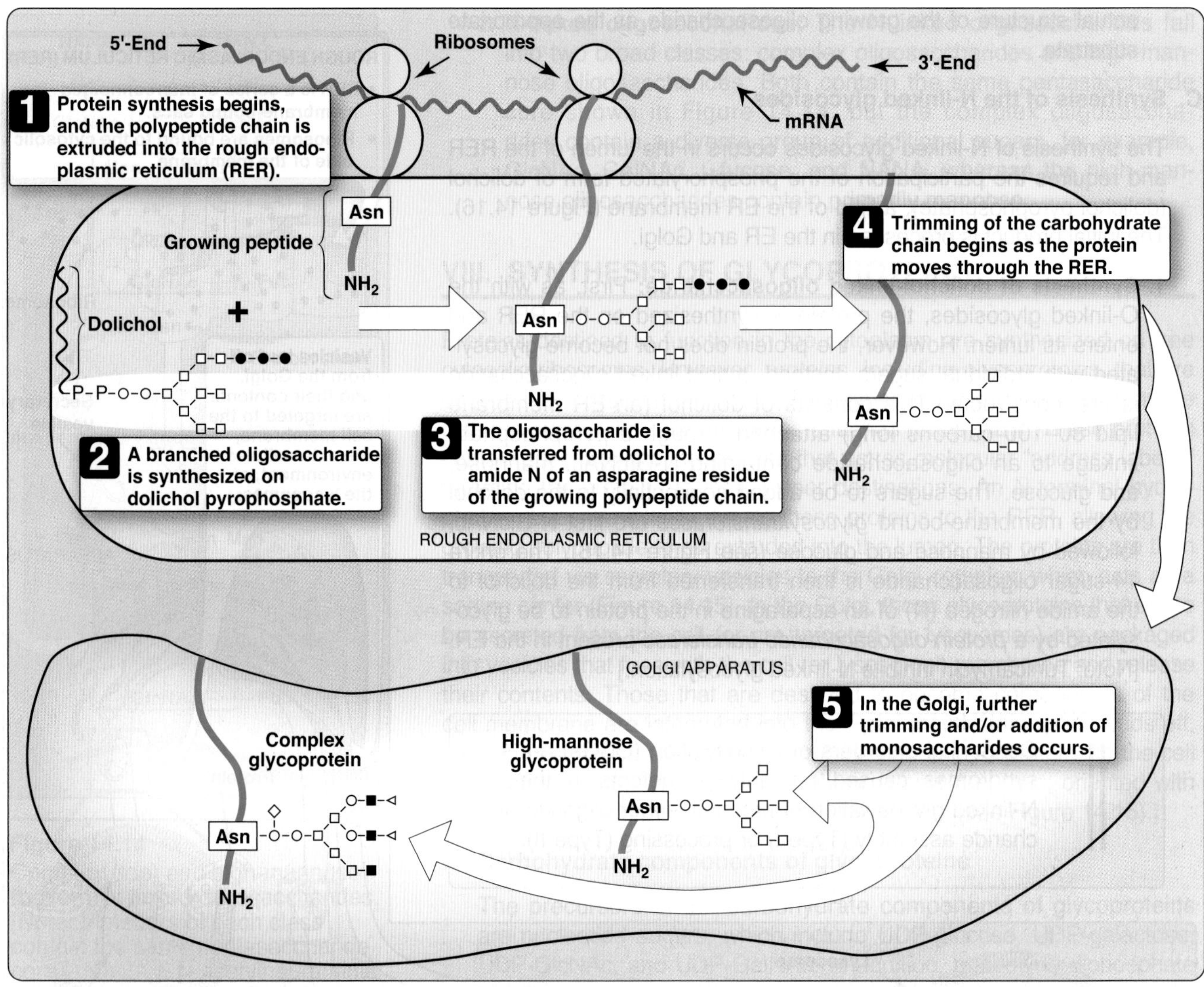

Figure 14.16
Synthesis of N-linked glycoproteins. ○ = N-acetylglucosamine; □ = mannose; ● = glucose; ■ = N-acetylgalactosamine; ◇ or ◁ = terminal group (fucose or N-acetylneuraminic acid); mRNA = messenger RNA; Asn = asparagine.

2. **Final processing of N-linked oligosaccharides:** After incorporation into the protein, the N-linked oligosaccharide is processed by the removal of specific mannosyl and glucosyl residues as the glycoprotein moves through the RER. Finally, the oligosaccharide chains are completed in the Golgi by addition of a variety of sugars (for example, N-GlcNAc, N-GalNAc, and additional mannoses, and then fucose or NANA as terminal groups) to produce a complex glycoprotein. Alternatively, they are not processed further, leaving branched, mannose-containing chains in a high-mannose glycoprotein (see Figure 14.16). The ultimate fate of N-linked glycoproteins is the same as that of the O-glycoproteins linked (for example, they can be released by the cell or become part of a cell membrane). In addition, N-linked glycoproteins can be targeted to the lysosomes. [Note: Nonenzymatic glycosylation of proteins is known as glycation (see p. 345).]

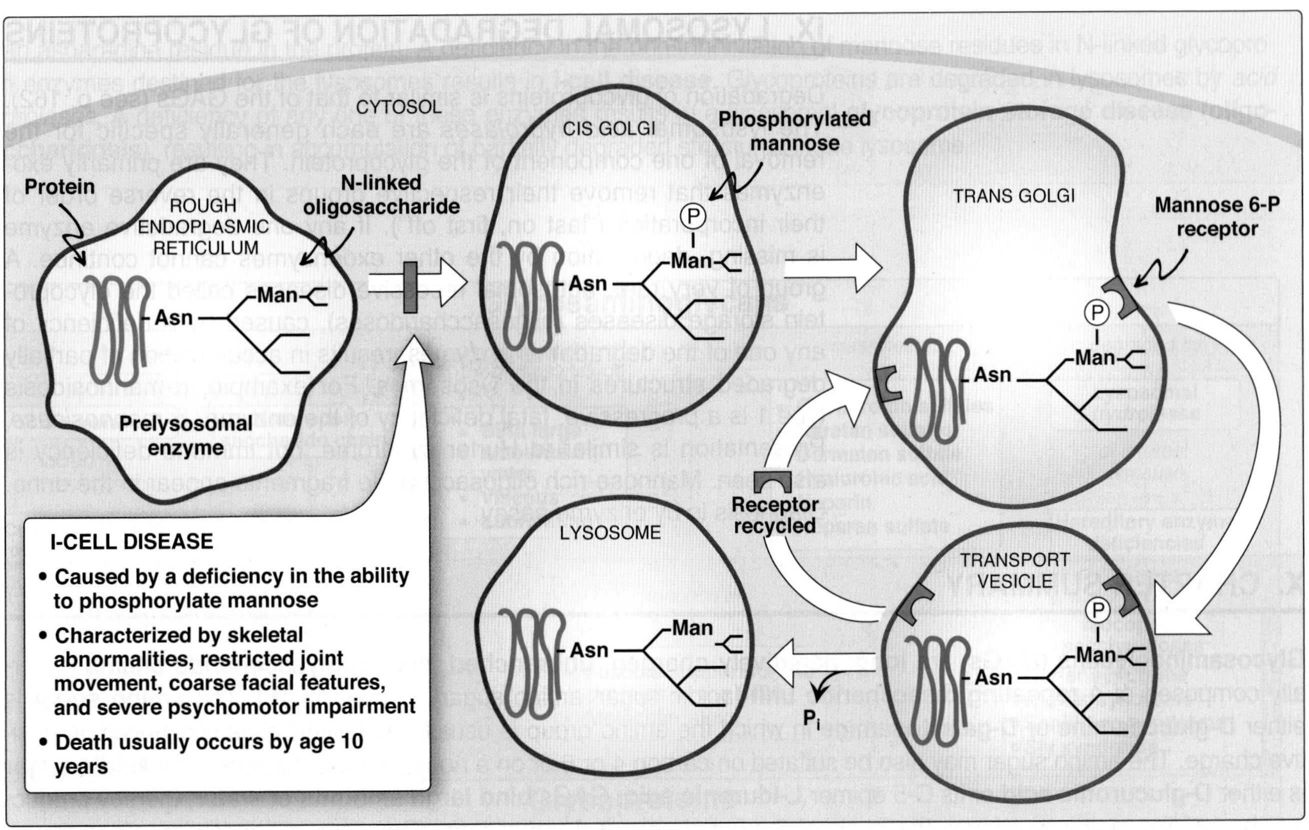

Figure 14.17
Mechanism for transport of N-linked glycoproteins to the lysosomes. Asn = asparagine; Man = mannose; P = phosphate; P_i = inorganic phosphate.

3. **Enzymes destined for lysosomes:** N-linked glycoproteins being processed through the Golgi can be phosphorylated on carbon 6 of one or more specific mannosyl residues. Mannose 6-phosphate receptors, located in the Golgi apparatus, bind the mannose 6-phosphate residues of these targeted enzymes, which are then packaged into vesicles and sent to the lysosomes. I-cell disease is a rare lysosomal storage disease in which the *acid hydrolases* normally found in lysosomes are absent, resulting in an accumulation of substrates normally degraded by these enzymes. [Note: I-cell disease is so-named because of the large inclusion bodies seen in cells of patients with this disease.] In addition, high amounts of lysosomal enzymes are found in the patient's plasma and urine, indicating that the targeting process to lysosomes (rather than the synthetic pathway of these enzymes) is deficient. Individuals with I-cell disease are lacking the *phosphotransferase* needed to phosphorylate the mannose residues of potential lysosomal enzymes, causing the enzymes to be secreted (by default), rather than being targeted to lysosomal vesicles (Figure 14.17). I-cell disease is characterized by skeletal abnormalities, restricted joint movement, coarse (dysmorphic) facial features, and severe psychomotor impairment. [Note: Because I-cell disease has features in common with the mucopolysaccharidoses and sphingolipidoses (see p. 211), it is termed a mucolipidosis.] Currently, there is no cure, and death from cardiopulmonary complications usually occurs by age 10 years.

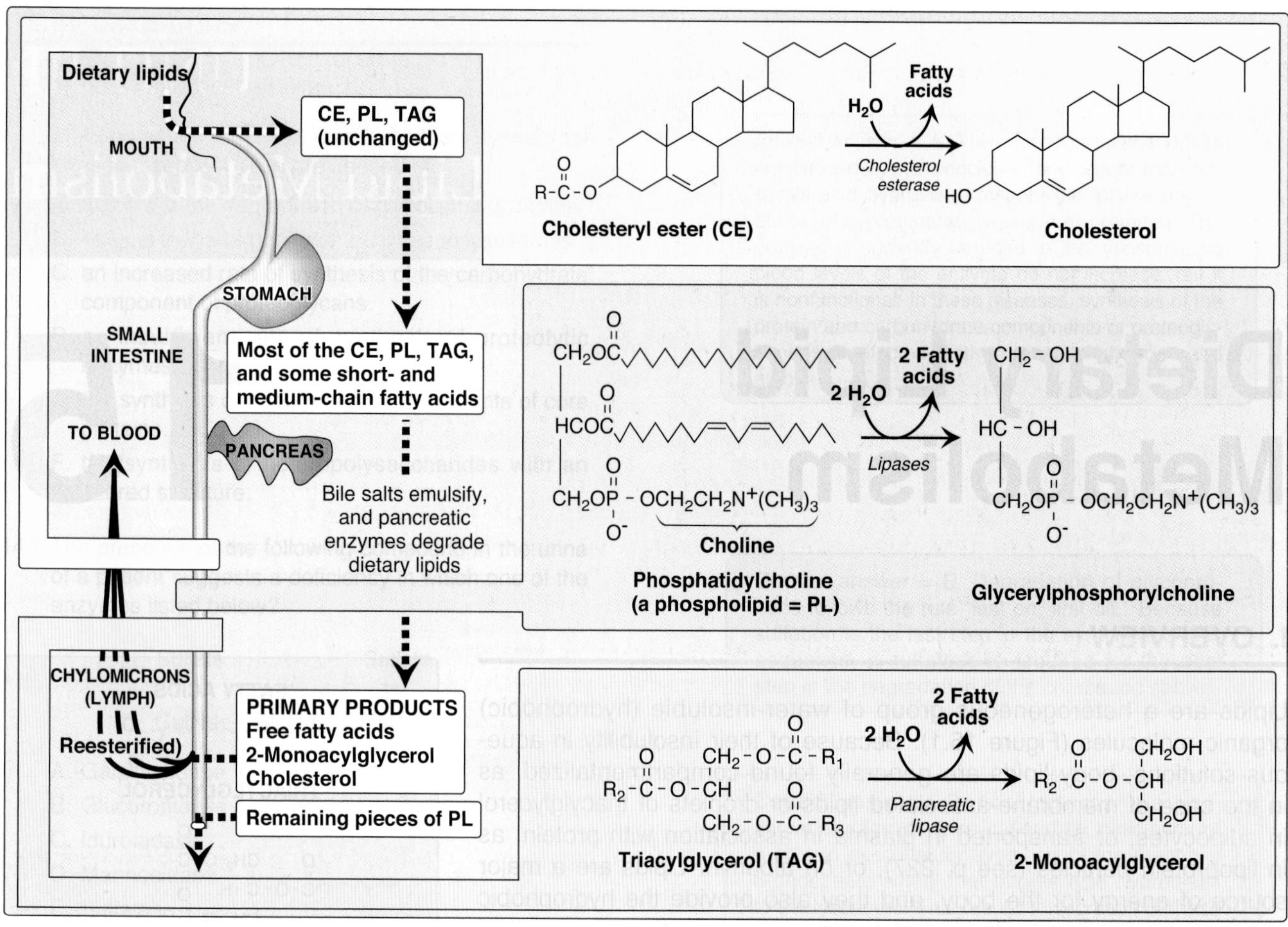

Figure 15.2
Overview of lipid digestion.

acid stable, with pH optimums of pH 4 to pH 6. These "*acid lipases*" play a particularly important role in lipid digestion in neonates, for whom milk fat is the primary source of calories. They also become important digestive enzymes in individuals with pancreatic insufficiency such as those with cystic fibrosis (CF). *Lingual* and *gastric lipases* aid these patients in degrading TAG molecules (especially those with short- to medium-chain length fatty acids) despite a near or complete absence of *pancreatic lipase* (see below).

1. **Cystic fibrosis:** CF is the most common lethal genetic disease in Caucasians of Northern European ancestry and has a prevalence of about 1:3,300 births in the United States. CF is an autosomal recessive disorder caused by mutations to the gene for the CF transmembrane conductance regulator (CFTR) protein that functions as a chloride channel on epithelium in the pancreas, lungs, testes, and sweat gands. Defective CFTR results in decreased secretion of chloride and increased uptake of sodium and water. In the pancreas, the depletion of water on the cell surface results in thickened secretions that clog the pancreatic ducts, preventing pancreatic enzymes from reaching the intestine, thereby leading to pancreatic insufficiency. Treatment includes replacement of these enzymes and supplementation with fat-soluble vitamins. [Note: CF also causes chronic lung infections with progressive pulmonary disease and male infertility.]

B. Emulsification of dietary lipid in the small intestine

The critical process of emulsification of dietary lipids occurs in the duodenum. Emulsification increases the surface area of the hydrophobic lipid droplets so that the digestive enzymes, which work at the interface of the droplet and the surrounding aqueous solution, can act effectively. Emulsification is accomplished by two complementary mechanisms, namely, use of the detergent properties of the conjugated bile salts and mechanical mixing due to peristalsis. Bile salts, made in the liver and stored in the gallbladder, are amphipathic derivatives of cholesterol (see p. 224). Conjugated bile salts consist of a hydroxylated sterol ring structure with a side chain to which a molecule of glycine or taurine is covalently attached by an amide linkage (Figure 15.3). These emulsifying agents interact with the dietary lipid particles and the aqueous duodenal contents, thereby stabilizing the particles as they become smaller from peristalsis and preventing them from coalescing. A more complete discussion of bile salt metabolism is given on p. 225.

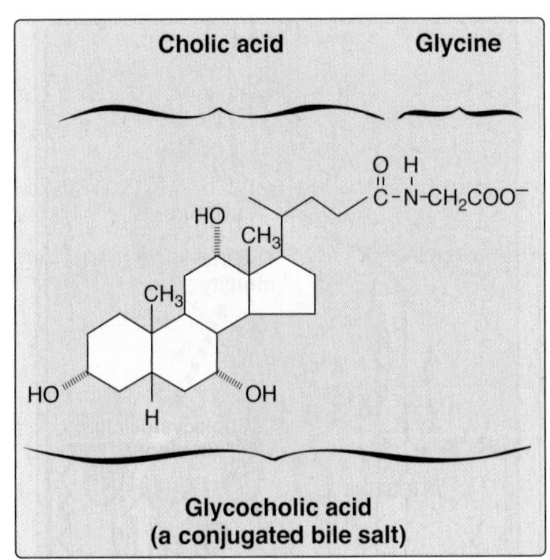

Figure 15.3
Structure of glycocholic acid.

C. Degradation of dietary lipids by pancreatic enzymes

The dietary TAG, cholesteryl esters, and phospholipids are enzymically degraded ("digested") by pancreatic enzymes, whose secretion is hormonally controlled.

1. **Triacylglycerol degradation:** TAG molecules are too large to be taken up efficiently by the mucosal cells of the intestinal villi. They are, therefore, acted upon by an *esterase*, *pancreatic lipase*, which preferentially removes the fatty acids at carbons 1 and 3. The primary products of hydrolysis are, thus, a mixture of 2-monoacylglycerol and free fatty acids (see Figure 15.2). [Note: This enzyme is found in high concentrations in pancreatic secretions (2%–3% of the total protein present), and it is highly efficient catalytically, thus insuring that only severe pancreatic deficiency, such as that seen in CF, results in significant malabsorption of fat.] A second protein, *colipase*, also secreted by the pancreas, binds the *lipase* at a ratio of 1:1 and anchors it at the lipid–aqueous interface. *Colipase* restores activity to *lipase* in the presence of inhibitory substances like bile salts that bind the micelles. [Note: *Colipase* is secreted as the zymogen, procolipase, which is activated in the intestine by *trypsin*.] Orlistat, an antiobesity drug, inhibits *gastric* and *pancreatic lipases,* thereby decreasing fat absorption, resulting in weight loss.

2. **Cholesteryl ester degradation:** Most dietary cholesterol is present in the free (nonesterified) form, with 10%–15% present in the esterified form. Cholesteryl esters are hydrolyzed by pancreatic *cholesteryl ester hydrolase* (*cholesterol esterase*), which produces cholesterol plus free fatty acids (see Figure 15.2). Activity of this enzyme is greatly increased in the presence of bile salts.

3. **Phospholipid degradation:** Pancreatic juice is rich in the proenzyme of *phospholipase* A_2 that, like procolipase, is activated by *trypsin* and, like *cholesteryl ester hydrolase*, requires bile salts for optimum activity. *Phospholipase* A_2 removes one fatty acid from carbon 2 of a phospholipid, leaving a lysophospholipid. For example, phosphatidylcholine (the predominant phospholipid of

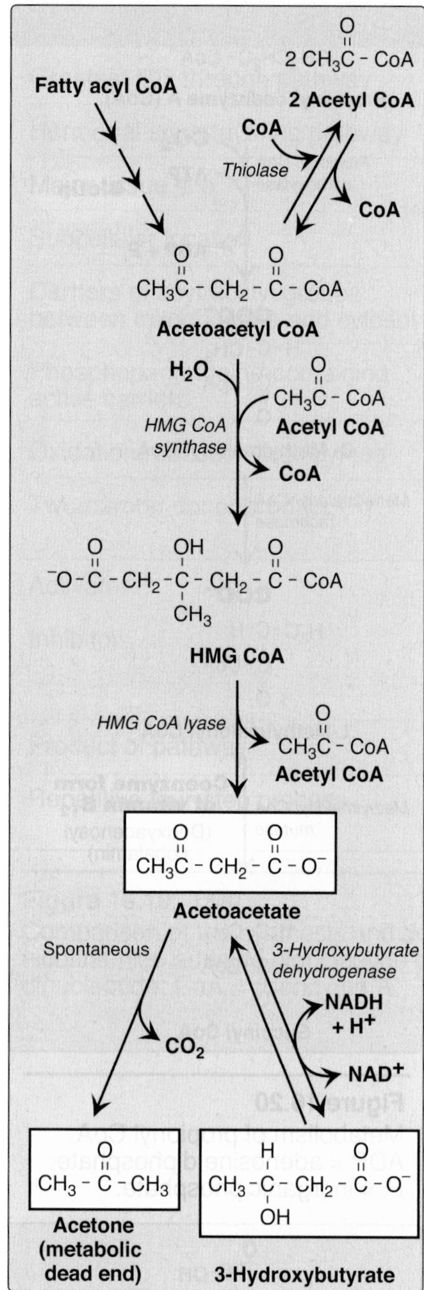

Figure 16.22
Synthesis of ketone bodies. [Note: The release of CoA in ketogenesis supports continued fatty acid oxidation.] CoA = coenzyme A; HMG = hydroxymethylglutarate; NAD(H) = nicotinamide adenine dinucleotide.

which can be oxidized by the TCA cycle. Ketone bodies are important sources of energy for the peripheral tissues because 1) they are soluble in aqueous solution and, therefore, do not need to be incorporated into lipoproteins or carried by albumin as do the other lipids; 2) they are produced in the liver during periods when the amount of acetyl CoA present exceeds the oxidative capacity of the liver; and 3) they are used in proportion to their concentration in the blood by extrahepatic tissues, such as the skeletal and cardiac muscle, intestinal mucosa, and renal cortex. Even the brain can use ketone bodies to help meet its energy needs if the blood levels rise sufficiently. Thus, ketone bodies spare glucose, which is particularly important during prolonged periods of fasting (see p. 332). [Note: Disorders of fatty acid oxidation present with the general picture of hypoketosis (due to decreased availability of acetyl CoA) and hypoglycemia (due to increased reliance on glucose for energy.]

A. Synthesis of ketone bodies by the liver: ketogenesis

During a fast, the liver is flooded with fatty acids mobilized from adipose tissue. The resulting elevated hepatic acetyl CoA produced by fatty acid oxidation inhibits *pyruvate dehydrogenase* (see p. 111), and activates *pyruvate carboxylase* (see p. 119). The OAA produced is used by the liver for gluconeogenesis rather than for the TCA cycle. Therefore, acetyl CoA is channeled into ketone body synthesis. Additionally, fatty acid oxidation decreases the NAD^+ to NADH ratio, and the rise in NADH shifts OAA to malate (see p. 113). This also pushes acetyl CoA into ketogenesis (Figure 16.24).] [Note: Acetyl CoA for ketogenesis is also generated by the catabolism of ketogenic amino acids (see p. 262).]

1. **Synthesis of 3-hydroxy-3-methylglutaryl coenzyme A:** The first step, formation of acetoacetyl CoA, occurs by reversal of the *thiolase* reaction of fatty acid oxidation (see Figure 16.17). Mitochondrial 3-hydroxy-3-methylglutaryl (*HMG*) *CoA synthase* combines a third molecule of acetyl CoA with acetoacetyl CoA to produce HMG CoA. *HMG CoA synthase* is the rate-limiting step in the synthesis of ketone bodies and is present in significant quantities only in the liver. [Note: HMG CoA is also an intermediate in cytosolic cholesterol synthesis (see p. 220). The two pathways are separated by location in, and conditions of, the cell.]

2. **Synthesis of the ketone bodies:** HMG CoA is cleaved by *HMG CoA lyase* to produce acetoacetate and acetyl CoA, as shown in Figure 16.22. Acetoacetate can be reduced to form 3-hydroxybutyrate with NADH as the hydrogen donor. Acetoacetate can also spontaneously decarboxylate in the blood to form acetone, a volatile, biologically nonmetabolized compound that can be released in the breath. The equilibrium between acetoacetate and 3-hydroxybutyrate is determined by the NAD^+/NADH ratio. Because this ratio is low during fatty acid oxidation, 3-hydroxybutyrate synthesis is favored. [Note: The generation of free CoA during ketogenesis allows fatty acid oxidation to continue.]

B. Use of ketone bodies by the peripheral tissues: ketolysis

Although the liver constantly synthesizes low levels of ketone bodies, their production becomes much more significant during fasting when ketone bodies are needed to provide energy to the periph-

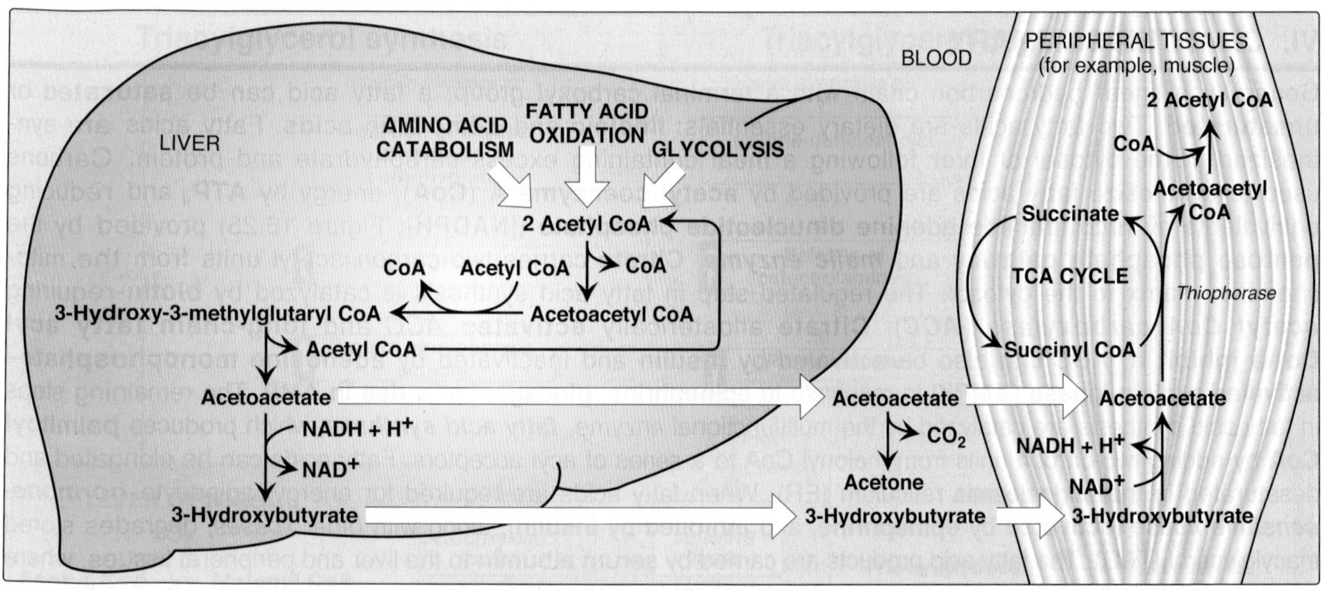

Figure 16.23
Ketone body synthesis in the liver and use in peripheral tissues. Liver and red blood cells cannot use ketone bodies. [Note: *Thiophorase* is also known as *succinyl CoA:acetoacetate CoA transferase*.] CoA = coenzyme A; NAD(H) = nicotinamide adenine dinucleotide; TCA = tricarboxylic acid.

eral tissues. 3-Hydroxybutyrate is oxidized to acetoacetate by *3-hydroxybutyrate dehydrogenase*, producing NADH (Figure 16.23). Acetoacetate is then provided with a CoA molecule taken from succinyl CoA by *succinyl CoA:acetoacetate CoA transferase* (*thiophorase*). This reaction is reversible, but the product, acetoacetyl CoA, is actively removed by its conversion to two acetyl CoAs. This pulls the reaction forward. Extrahepatic tissues, including the brain but excluding cells lacking mitochondria (for example, RBCs), efficiently oxidize acetoacetate and 3-hydroxybutyrate in this manner. In contrast, although the liver actively produces ketone bodies, it lacks *thiophorase* and, therefore, is unable to use ketone bodies as fuel.

C. Excessive production of ketone bodies in diabetes mellitus

When the rate of formation of ketone bodies is greater than the rate of their use, their levels begin to rise in the blood (ketonemia) and, eventually, in the urine (ketonuria). This is seen most often in cases of uncontrolled type 1 diabetes mellitus. In diabetic individuals with severe ketosis, urinary excretion of the ketone bodies may be as high as 5,000 mg/24 hr, and the blood concentration may reach 90 mg/dl (versus less than 3 mg/dl in normal individuals). A frequent symptom of diabetic ketoacidosis (DKA) is a fruity odor on the breath, which results from increased production of acetone. An elevation of the ketone body concentration in the blood results in acidemia. [Note: The carboxyl group of a ketone body has a pK_a of about 4. Therefore, each ketone body loses a proton (H^+) as it circulates in the blood, which lowers the pH. Also, in DKA, urinary loss of glucose and ketone bodies results in dehydration. Therefore, the increased number of H^+ circulating in a decreased volume of plasma can cause severe acidosis (ketoacidosis).] Ketoacidosis may also be seen in cases of prolonged fasting (see p. 330) and excessive ethanol consumption (see p. 318).

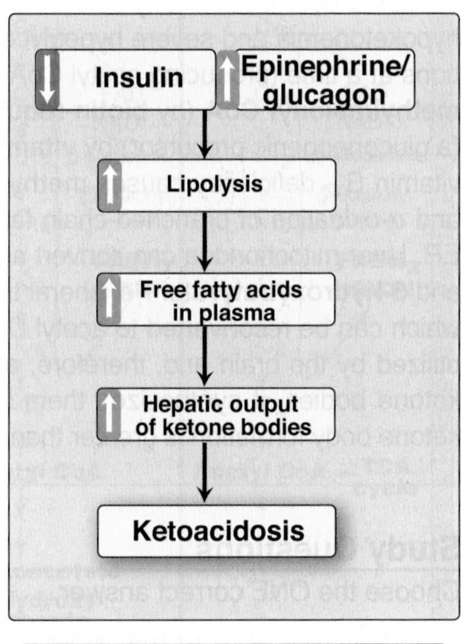

Figure 16.24
Mechanism of diabetic ketoacidosis seen in type 1 diabetes.

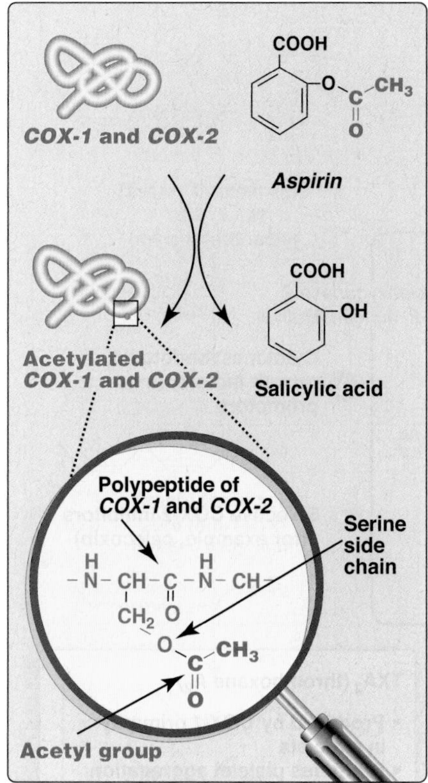

Figure 17.24
Irreversible acetylation of *cyclooxygenase* (*COX*)-*1* and *COX-2* by aspirin.

IX. CHAPTER SUMMARY

Phospholipids are **polar**, **ionic** compounds composed of an **alcohol** (for example, **choline** or **ethanolamine**) attached by a phosphodiester bond to either **diacylglycerol** (DAG), producing **phosphatidylcholine** or **phosphatidylethanolamine**, or to the amino alcohol **sphingosine** (Figure 17.25). Addition of a long-chain fatty acid to sphingosine produces a **ceramide**. Addition of a **phosphorylcholine** produces the phospholipid **sphingomyelin**. Phospholipids are the predominant lipids of **cell membranes**. Nonmembrane phospholipids serve as components of **lung surfactant** and **bile**. **Dipalmitoylphosphatidylcholine**, also called **dipalmitoyl lecithin**, is the major lipid component of **lung surfactant**. Insufficient surfactant production causes **respiratory distress syndrome**. **Phosphatidylinositol** (**PI**) serves as a reservoir for **arachidonic acid** in membranes. The phosphorylation of membrane-bound PI produces **phosphatidylinositol 4,5-bisphosphate** (**PIP_2**). This compound is degraded by ***phospholipase C*** in response to the binding of a variety of neurotransmitters, hormones, and growth factors to membrane G protein–coupled receptors. The products of this degradation, **inositol 1,4,5-trisphosphate** (**IP_3**) and **DAG** mediate the mobilization of intracellular **calcium** and the activation of ***protein kinase C***, which act synergistically to evoke cellular responses. Specific proteins can be covalently attached via a carbohydrate bridge to membrane-bound phosphatidylinositol (**glycosyl phosphatidylinositol**, or **GPI**), forming a GPI anchor. A deficiency in the synthesis of GPI in hematopoietic cells results in a hemolytic disease, **paroxysmal nocturnal hemoglobinuria**. The **degradation** of phosphoglycerides is performed by ***phospholipases*** found in all tissues and pancreatic juice. **Sphingomyelin** is degraded to a ceramide plus phosphorylcholine by the lysosomal enzyme ***sphingomyelinase***, a deficiency of which causes **Niemann-Pick (A + B) disease**. Glycosphingolipids are derivatives of **ceramides** to which carbohydrates have been attached. When one sugar molecule is added to the ceramide, a **cerebroside** is produced. If an oligosaccharide is added, a **globoside** is produced. If an acidic N-acetylneuraminic acid molecule is added, a **ganglioside** is produced. Glycosphingolipids are found predominantly in cell membranes of the **brain** and **peripheral nervous tissue**, with high concentrations in the **myelin sheath**. They are **antigenic**. Glycolipids are degraded in the **lysosomes** by ***acid hydrolases***. A deficiency of any one of these enzymes produces a **sphingolipidosis**, in which a characteristic sphingolipid accumulates. **Prostaglandins** (**PGs**), **thromboxanes** (**TXs**), and **leukotrienes** (**LTs**) are produced in very small amounts in almost all tissues, act locally, and have an extremely short half-life. **They serve as mediators of the inflammatory response. Arachidonic acid** is the immediate precursor of the predominant class of PGs in humans (those with two double bonds). It is derived by the elongation and desaturation of the essential fatty acid linoleic acid and is stored in the membrane as a component of a phospholipid, generally PI. Arachidonic acid is released from the phospholipid by ***phospholipase A_2*** (inhibited by cortisol). Synthesis of the **PGs** and **TXs** begins with the oxidative cyclization of free arachidonic acid to yield PGH_2 by ***prostaglandin endoperoxide synthase*** (*PGH synthase*), an endoplasmic reticulum membrane protein that has two catalytic activities: ***fatty acid cyclooxygenase*** (***COX***) and ***peroxidase***. There are two isozymes of *PGH synthase*: ***COX-1*** (constitutive) and ***COX-2*** (nonconstitutive). Aspirin irreversibly inhibits both. Opposing effects of PGI_2 and TXA_2 limit clot formation. **LTs** are linear molecules produced from arachidonic acid by the ***5-lipoxygenase*** pathway. They mediate allergic response and are not inhibited by aspirin or other NSAIDs.

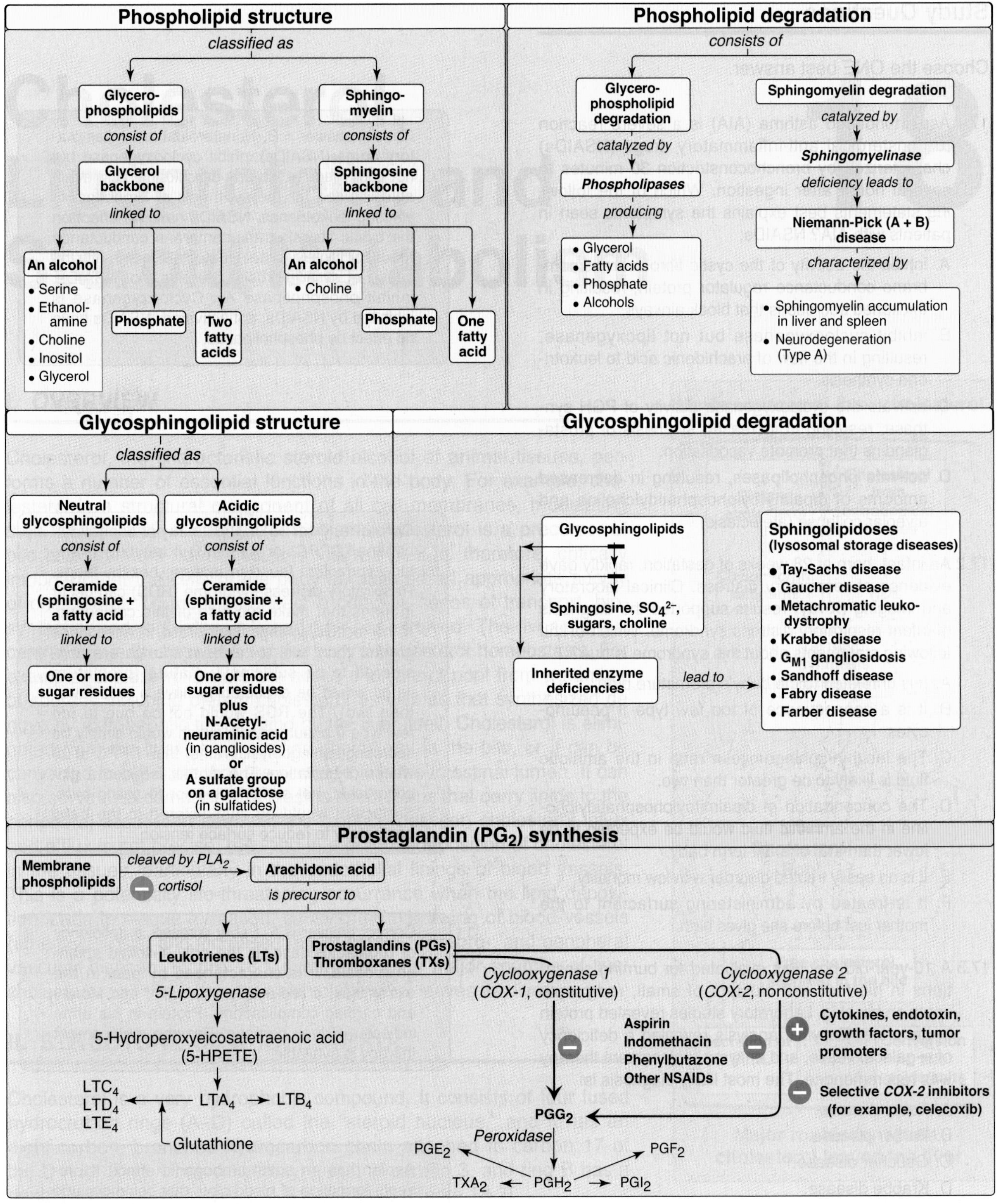

Figure 17.25
Key concept map for complex lipids. *PLA_2 = phospholipase A_2*; SO_4^{2-} = sulfate ion; NSAIDs = nonsteroidal anti-inflammatory drugs.

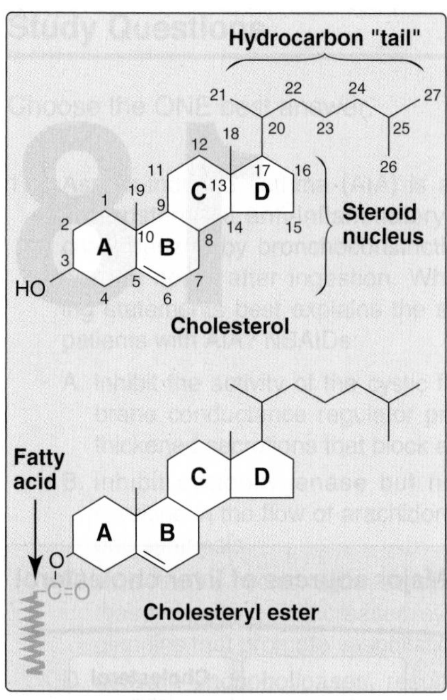

Figure 18.2
Structure of cholesterol and its ester.

Cholesterol is the major sterol in animal tissues. It arises from de novo synthesis and absorption of dietary cholesterol. [Note: Intestinal uptake of cholesterol is mediated, at least in part, by the protein Niemann-Pick C1-like 1 protein (NPC1-L1), the target of the drug ezetimibe that reduces absorption of dietary cholesterol (see p. 176). Plant sterols (phytosterols), such as β-sitosterol, are poorly absorbed by humans (5% absorbed as compared to 40% for cholesterol). After entering the enterocytes, they are actively transported back into the intestinal lumen. Defects in the transporter result in the rare condition of sitosterolemia. Because some cholesterol is transported back as well, plant sterols reduce the absorption of dietary cholesterol. Daily ingestion of plant sterol esters supplied, for example, in spreads or juices, is one of a number of dietary strategies to reduce plasma cholesterol levels (see p. 363).]

B. Cholesteryl esters

Most plasma cholesterol is in an esterified form (with a fatty acid attached at carbon 3, as shown in Figure 18.2), which makes the structure even more hydrophobic than free (unesterified) cholesterol. Cholesteryl esters are not found in membranes and are normally present only in low levels in most cells. Because of their hydrophobicity, cholesterol and its esters must be transported in association with protein as a component of a lipoprotein particle (see p. 227) or be solubilized by phospholipids and bile salts in the bile (see p. 226).

III. SYNTHESIS OF CHOLESTEROL

Cholesterol is synthesized by virtually all tissues in humans, although liver, intestine, adrenal cortex, and reproductive tissues, including ovaries, testes, and placenta, make the largest contributions to the body's cholesterol pool. As with fatty acids, all the carbon atoms in cholesterol are provided by acetyl coenzyme A (CoA), and nicotinamide adenine dinucleotide phosphate (NADPH) provides the reducing equivalents. The pathway is endergonic, being driven by hydrolysis of the high-energy thioester bond of acetyl CoA and the terminal phosphate bond of adenosine triphosphate (ATP). Synthesis requires enzymes in both the cytosol and the membrane of the smooth endoplasmic reticulum (ER). The pathway is responsive to changes in cholesterol concentration, and regulatory mechanisms exist to balance the rate of cholesterol synthesis within the body against the rate of cholesterol excretion. An imbalance in this regulation can lead to an elevation in circulating levels of plasma cholesterol, with the potential for vascular disease.

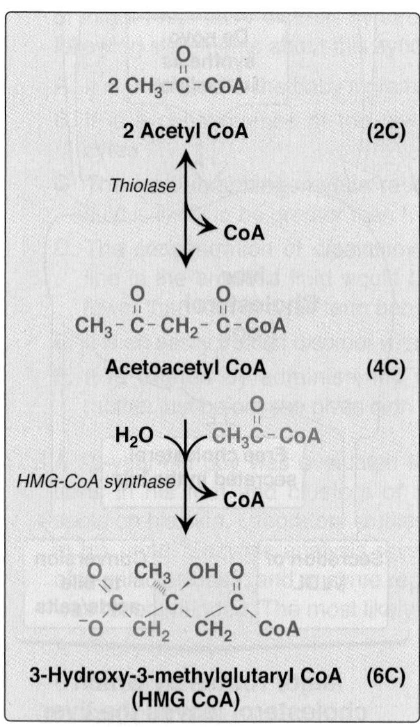

Figure 18.3
Synthesis of HMG CoA. CoA = coenzyme A.

A. Synthesis of 3-hydroxy-3-methylglutaryl coenzyme A

The first two reactions in the cholesterol synthetic pathway are similar to those in the pathway that produces ketone bodies (see Figure 16.22, p. 196). They result in the production of 3-hydroxy-3-methylglutaryl CoA ([HMG CoA] Figure 18.3). First, two acetyl CoA molecules condense to form acetoacetyl CoA. Next, a third molecule of acetyl CoA is added by *HMG CoA synthase*, producing HMG CoA, a six-carbon compound. [Note: Liver parenchymal cells contain two isoenzymes of the *synthase*. The cytosolic enzyme participates in cholesterol synthesis, whereas the mitochondrial enzyme functions in the pathway for ketone body synthesis.]

B. Synthesis of mevalonate

The next step, the reduction of HMG CoA to mevalonate, is catalyzed by *HMG CoA reductase* and is the rate-limiting and key regulated step in cholesterol synthesis. It occurs in the cytosol, uses two molecules of NADPH as the reducing agent, and releases CoA, making the reaction irreversible (Figure 18.4). [Note: *HMG CoA reductase* is an integral membrane protein of the ER, with its catalytic domain projecting into the cytosol.] Regulation of *reductase* activity is discussed below.

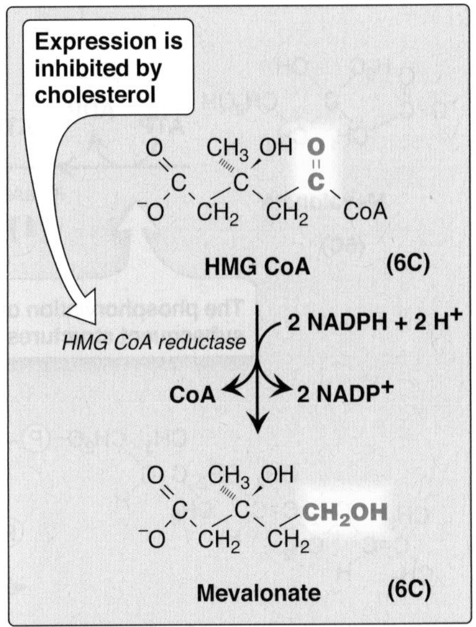

Figure 18.4
Synthesis of mevalonate. HMG CoA = hydroxymethylglutaryl coenzyme A; NADP(H) = nicotinamide adenine dinucleotide phosphate.

C. Synthesis of cholesterol

The reactions and enzymes involved in the synthesis of cholesterol from mevalonate are illustrated in Figure 18.5. [Note: The numbers shown in brackets below correspond to numbered reactions shown in this figure.]

[1] Mevalonate is converted to 5-pyrophosphomevalonate in two steps, each of which transfers a phosphate group from ATP.

[2] A five-carbon isoprene unit, isopentenyl pyrophosphate (IPP), is formed by the decarboxylation of 5-pyrophosphomevalonate. The reaction requires ATP. [Note: IPP is the precursor of a family of molecules with diverse functions, the isoprenoids. Cholesterol is a sterol isoprenoid. Nonsterol isoprenoids include dolichol (see p. 167) and ubiquinone, or coenzyme Q (see p. 75).]

[3] IPP is isomerized to 3,3-dimethylallyl pyrophosphate (DPP).

[4] IPP and DPP condense to form ten-carbon geranyl pyrophosphate (GPP).

[5] A second molecule of IPP then condenses with GPP to form 15-carbon farnesyl pyrophosphate (FPP). [Note: Covalent attachment of farnesyl to proteins, a process known as "prenylation," is one mechanism for anchoring proteins (such as ras) to plasma membranes.]

[6] Two molecules of FPP combine, releasing pyrophosphate, and are reduced, forming the 30-carbon compound squalene. [Note: Squalene is formed from six isoprenoid units. Because three ATP are hydrolyzed per mevalonate residue converted to IPP, a total of 18 ATP are required to make the polyisoprenoid squalene.]

[7] Squalene is converted to the sterol lanosterol by a sequence of reactions catalyzed by ER-associated enzymes that use molecular oxygen and NADPH. The hydroxylation of linear squalene triggers the cyclization of the structure to lanosterol.

[8] The conversion of lanosterol to cholesterol is a multistep, ER-associated process involving shortening of the side-chain, oxidative removal of methyl groups, reduction of double bonds, and migration of a double bond. Smith-Lemli-Opitz syndrome (SLOS), an autosomal-recessive disorder of cholesterol biosynthesis, is caused by a partial deficiency in *7-dehydrocholesterol-7-reductase*, the enzyme that reduces the double bond in 7-dehydrocholesterol (7-DHC), thereby converting it to cholesterol. SLOS is one of several multisystem, embryonic malformation syndromes associated with impaired cholesterol synthesis. [Note: 7-DHC is converted to vitamin D_3 in the skin (see p. 386).]

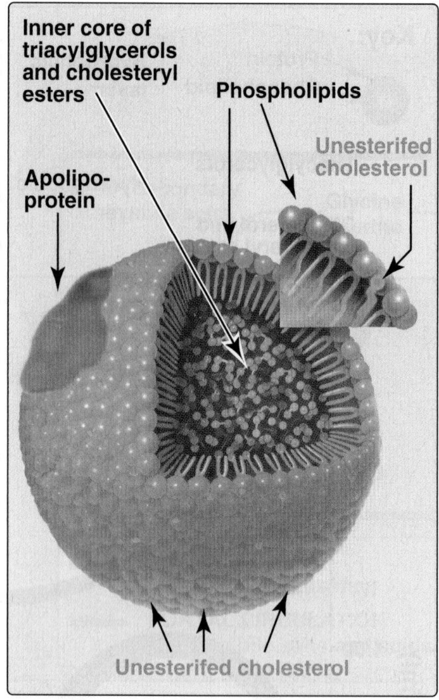

Figure 18.14
Structure of a typical lipoprotein particle.

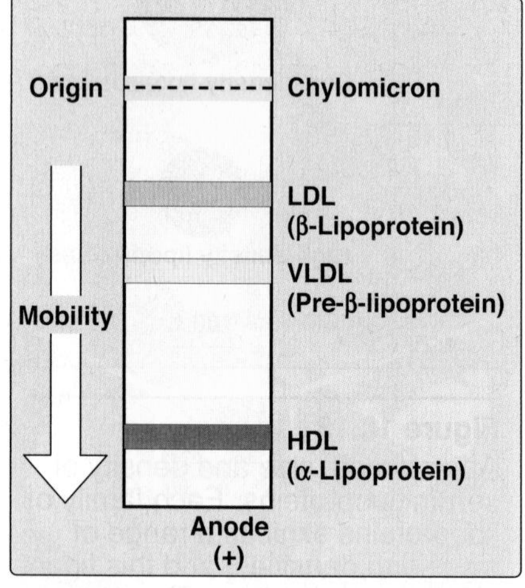

Figure 18.15
Electrophoretic mobility of plasma lipoproteins. The order of low-density lipoprotein (LDL) and very-low-density lipoprotein (VLDL) is reversed if ultracentrifugation is used as the separation technique. HDL = high-density lipoprotein.

cholesteryl esters to the peripheral tissues (Figure 18.16). [Note: TAGs account for close to 90% of the lipids in a chylomicron.]

1. **Synthesis of apolipoproteins:** Apo B-48 is unique to chylomicrons. Its synthesis begins on the rough ER, and it is glycosylated as it moves through the ER and Golgi. [Note: Apo B-48 is so named because it constitutes the N-terminal 48% of the protein encoded by the gene for apo B. Apo B-100, which is synthesized by the liver and found in VLDL and LDL, represents the entire protein encoded by this gene. Posttranscriptional editing (see p. 457) of a cytosine to a uracil in intestinal apo B-100 messenger RNA (mRNA) creates a nonsense (stop) codon (see p. 433), allowing translation of only 48% of the mRNA.]

2. **Assembly of chylomicrons:** The enzymes involved in TAG, cholesterol, and phospholipid synthesis are located in the smooth ER. Assembly of the apolipoproteins and lipid into chylomicrons requires microsomal triglyceride transfer protein ([MTP], see p. 178), which loads apo B-48 with lipid. This occurs before transition from the ER to the Golgi, where the particles are packaged in secretory vesicles. These fuse with the plasma membrane releasing the lipoproteins, which then enter the lymphatic system and, ultimately, the blood. [Note: Chylomicrons leave the lymphatic system via the thoracic duct that empties into the left subclavian vein.]

3. **Modification of nascent chylomicron particles:** The particle released by the intestinal mucosal cell is called a "nascent" chylomicron because it is functionally incomplete. When it reaches the plasma, the particle is rapidly modified, receiving apolipoproteins E (which is recognized by hepatic receptors) and C. The latter includes apo C-II, which is necessary for the activation of *lipoprotein lipase* (*LPL*), the enzyme that degrades the TAG contained in the chylomicron (see below). The source of these apolipoproteins is circulating HDL (see Figure 18.16).

4. **Degradation of triacylglycerol by lipoprotein lipase:** *LPL* is an extracellular enzyme that is anchored by heparan sulfate to the capillary walls of most tissues, but predominantly those of adipose tissue and cardiac and skeletal muscle. Adult liver does not have this enzyme. [Note: A *hepatic lipase* is found on the surface of endothelial cells of the liver. It plays some role in TAG degradation in chylomirons and VLDL and is particularly important in HDL metabolism (see p. 236).] *LPL*, activated by apo C-II on circulating lipoprotein particles, hydrolyzes the TAG contained in these particles to yield fatty acids and glycerol. The fatty acids are stored (by the adipose) or used for energy (by the muscle). If they are not immediately taken up by a cell, the long-chain fatty acids are transported by serum albumin until their uptake does occur. The glycerol is used by the liver, for example, in lipid synthesis or gluconeogenesis. [Note: Patients with a deficiency of *LPL* or apo C-II (type 1 hyperlipoproteinemia, or familial *LPL*-deficiency) show a dramatic accumulation (1,000 mg/dl or greater) of chylomicron-TAG in the plasma (hypertriacylglycerolemia) even in the fasted state. These individuals are at increased risk for acute pancreatitis.]

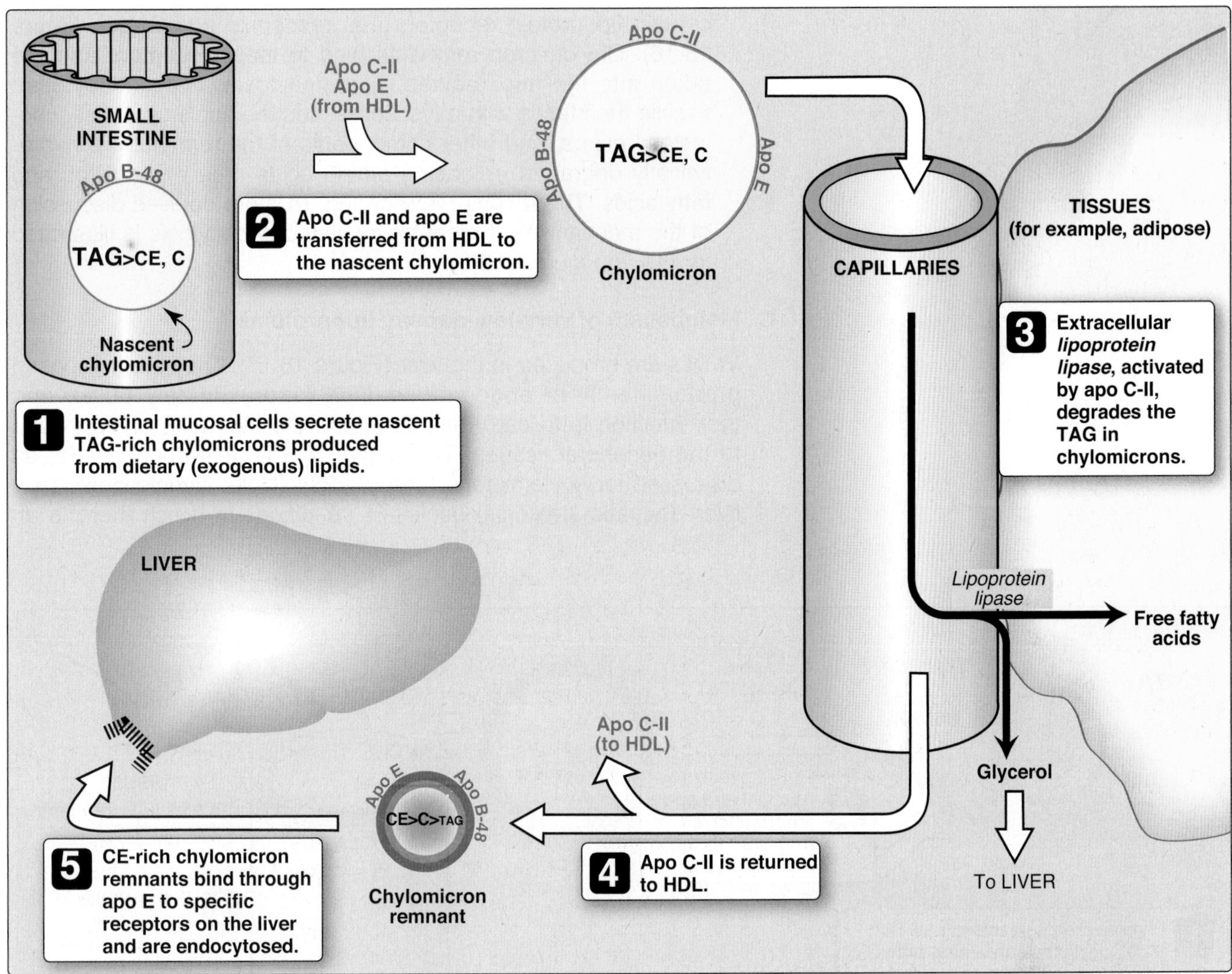

Figure 18.16
Metabolism of chylomicrons. Apo B-48, apo C-II, and apo E are apolipoproteins found as specific components of plasma lipoproteins. The lipoprotein particles are not drawn to scale (see Figure 18.13 for details of their size and density). TAG = triacylglycerol; C = cholesterol; CE = cholesteryl ester; HDL = high-density lipoprotein particle.

5. **Regulation of lipoprotein lipase activity:** *LPL* is synthesized by adipose tissue and by cardiac and skeletal muscle. Expression of the tissue-specific isozymes is regulated by nutritional state and hormonal level. For example, in the fed state (elevated insulin levels), *LPL* synthesis is increased in adipose but decreased in muscle tissue. Fasting (decreased insulin) favors *LPL* synthesis in muscle. [Note: The highest concentration of *LPL* is in cardiac muscle, reflecting the use of fatty acids to provide much of the energy needed for cardiac function.]

6. **Formation of chylomicron remnants:** As the chylomicron circulates, and more than 90% of the TAG in its core is degraded by *LPL*, the particle decreases in size and increases in density. In addition, the C apolipoproteins (but not apo E) are returned to HDL. The remaining particle, called a "remnant," is rapidly removed from the circulation by the liver, whose cell membranes

contain lipoprotein receptors that recognize apo E (see Figure 18.16). Chylomicron remnants bind to these receptors and are taken into the hepatocytes by endocytosis. The endocytosed vesicle then fuses with a lysosome, and the apolipoproteins, cholesteryl esters, and other components of the remnant are hydrolytically degraded, releasing amino acids, free cholesterol, and fatty acids. The receptor is recycled. (A more detailed discussion of the mechanism of receptor-mediated endocytosis is illustrated for LDL in Figure 18.20.)

C. Metabolism of very-low-density lipoproteins

VLDLs are produced in the liver (Figure 18.17). They are composed predominantly of endogenous TAG (approximately 60%), and their function is to carry this lipid from the liver (site of synthesis) to the peripheral tissues. There, the TAG is degraded by *LPL*, as discussed for chylomicrons (see p. 228). [Note: Nonalcoholic "fatty liver" (hepatic steatosis) occurs in conditions in which there is an

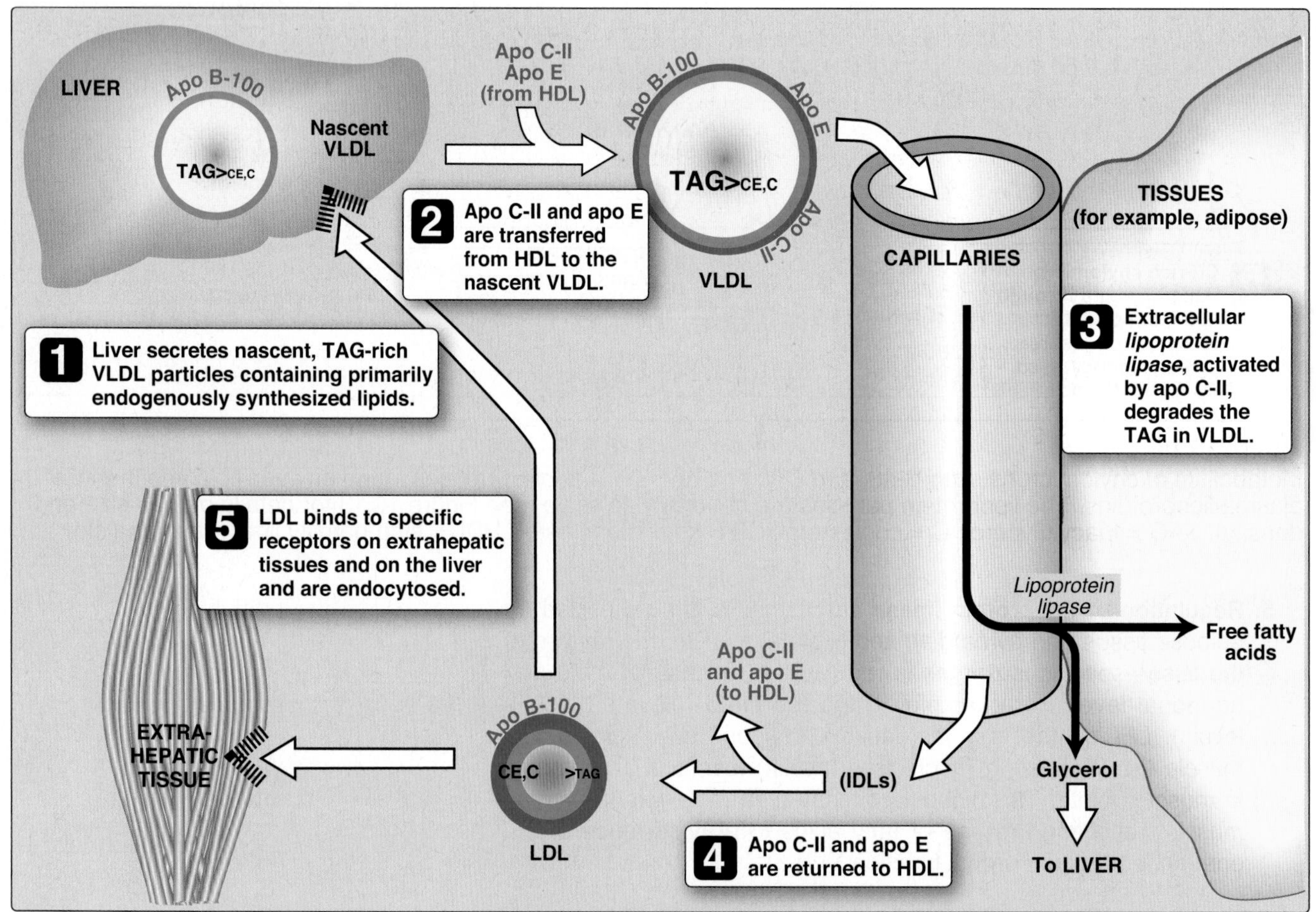

Figure 18.17
Metabolism of very-low-density lipoprotein (VLDL) and low-density lipoprotein (LDL). Apo B-100, apo C-II, and apo E are apolipoproteins found as specific components of plasma lipoprotein particles. The lipoproteins are not drawn to scale (see Figure 18.13 for details of their size and density). TAG = triacylglycerol; HDL = high-density lipoprotein particle; IDLs = intermediate-density lipoprotein particles; C = cholesterol; CE = cholesteryl ester.

imbalance between hepatic TAG synthesis and the secretion of VLDL. Such conditions include obesity and type 2 diabetes mellitus.]

1. **Release from liver:** VLDLs are secreted directly into the blood by the liver as nascent particles containing apo B-100. They must obtain apo C-II and apo E from circulating HDL (see Figure 18.17). As with chylomicrons, apo C-II is required for activation of *LPL*. [Note: Abetalipoproteinemia is a rare hypolipoproteinemia caused by a defect in MTP, leading to an inability to load apo B with lipid. As a consequence, few VLDLs or chylomicrons are formed, and TAGs accumulate in the liver and intestine.]

2. **Modification in the circulation:** As VLDLs pass through the circulation, TAG is degraded by *LPL*, causing the VLDLs to decrease in size and become denser. Surface components, including the C and E apolipoproteins, are returned to HDL, but the particles retain apo B-100. Additionally, some TAGs are transferred from VLDL to HDL in an exchange reaction that concomitantly transfers cholesteryl esters from HDL to VLDL. This exchange is accomplished by *cholesteryl ester transfer protein* (*CETP*) as shown in Figure 18.18.

3. **Conversion to low-density lipoproteins:** With these modifications, the VLDL is converted in the plasma to LDL. Intermediate-sized particles, the intermediate-density lipoproteins (IDLs), or VLDL remnants, are observed during this transition. IDLs can also be taken up by liver cells through receptor-mediated endocytosis that uses apo E as the ligand. [Note: Apo E is normally present in three isoforms, E-2, (the least common), E-3 (the most common), and E-4. Apo E-2 binds poorly to receptors, and patients who are homozygotic for apo E-2 are deficient in the clearance of chylomicron remnants and IDLs. These individuals have familial type III hyperlipoproteinemia (familial dysbetalipoproteinemia, or broad beta disease), with hypercholesterolemia and premature atherosclerosis. Not as yet well understood is the fact that the E-4 isoform confers increased susceptibility to and decreased age of onset of the late-onset form of Alzheimer disease. The effect is dose dependent, with homozygotes being at greatest risk. Estimates of the risk vary.]

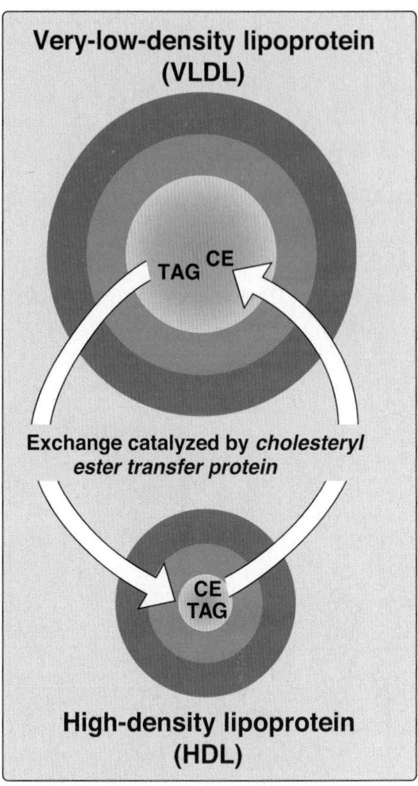

Figure 18.18
Transfer of cholesteryl ester (CE) from HDL to VLDL in exchange for triacylglycerol (TAG).

D. Metabolism of low-density lipoproteins

LDL particles contain much less TAG than their VLDL predecessors and have a high concentration of cholesterol and cholesteryl esters (Figure 18.19).

1. **Receptor-mediated endocytosis:** The primary function of LDL particles is to provide cholesterol to the peripheral tissues (or return it to the liver). They do so by binding to cell surface membrane LDL receptors that recognize apo B-100 (but not apo B-48). Because these LDL receptors can also bind apo E, they are known as apo B-100/apo E receptors. A summary of the uptake and degradation of LDL particles is presented in Figure 18.20. [Note: The numbers in brackets below refer to corresponding numbers on that figure.] A similar mechanism of receptor-mediated endocytosis is used for the cellular uptake and degradation of chylomicron remnants and IDLs by the liver.

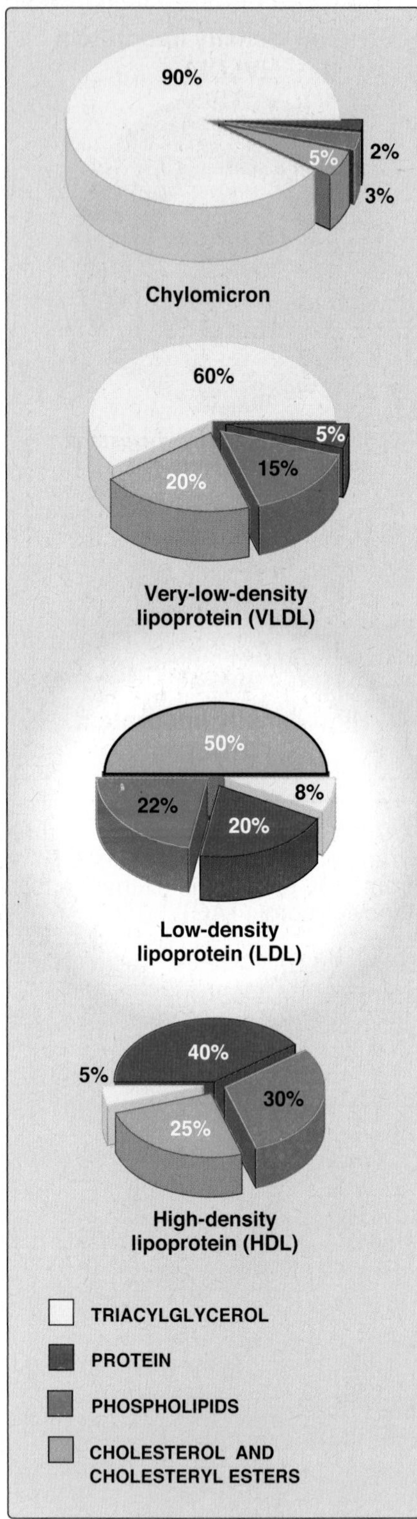

Figure 18.19
Composition of the plasma lipoproteins. Note the high concentration of cholesterol and cholesteryl esters in LDL.

[1] LDL receptors are negatively charged glycoproteins that are clustered in pits on cell membranes. The cytosolic side of the pit is coated with the protein clathrin, which stabilizes the pit.

[2] After binding, the LDL–receptor complex is taken in by endocytosis. [Note: A deficiency of functional LDL receptors causes a significant elevation in plasma LDL-C. Patients with such deficiencies have type II hyperlipidemia (familial hypercholesterolemia, or FH) and premature atherosclerosis. Autosomal-dominant hypercholesterolemia can also be caused by increased activity of a *protease, proprotein convertase subtilisin/kexin type 9* (*PCSK9*), which promotes degradation of the receptor, and by defects in apo B-100 that reduce its binding to the receptor.]

[3] The vesicle containing LDL loses its clathrin coat and fuses with other similar vesicles, forming larger vesicles called endosomes.

[4] The pH of the endosome falls (due to the proton-pumping activity of endosomal *ATPase*), which allows separation of the LDL from its receptor. The receptors then migrate to one side of the endosome, whereas the LDLs stay free within the lumen of the vesicle. [Note: This structure is called CURL, the compartment for uncoupling of receptor and ligand.]

[5] The receptors can be recycled, whereas the lipoprotein remnants in the vesicle are transferred to lysosomes and degraded by lysosomal *acid hydrolases*, releasing free cholesterol, amino acids, fatty acids, and phospholipids. These compounds can be reutilized by the cell. [Note: Storage diseases caused by rare autosomal-recessive deficiencies in the ability to hydrolyze lysosomal cholesteryl esters (late-onset Wolman disease), or to transport free cholesterol out of the lysosome (Niemann-Pick disease, Type C) have been identified.]

2. **Effect of endocytosed cholesterol on cellular cholesterol homeostasis:** The chylomicron remnant-, IDL-, and LDL-derived cholesterol affects cellular cholesterol content in several ways (see Figure 18.20). First, expression of the gene for *HMG CoA reductase* is inhibited by high cholesterol, as a result of which, de novo cholesterol synthesis decreases. Additionally, degradation of the *reductase* is accelerated. Second, synthesis of new LDL receptor protein is reduced by decreasing the expression of the LDL receptor gene, thus limiting further entry of LDL cholesterol into cells. [Note: Regulation of the LDL receptor gene involves a SRE and SREBP-2, as was seen in the regulation of the gene for *HMG CoA reductase* (see p. 222). This allows coordinate regulation of the expression of these proteins.] Third, if the cholesterol is not required immediately for some structural or synthetic purpose, it is esterified by *acyl CoA:cholesterol acyltransferase* (*ACAT*). *ACAT* transfers a fatty acid from a fatty acyl CoA to cholesterol, producing a cholesteryl ester that can be stored in the cell (Figure 18.21). The activity of *ACAT* is enhanced in the presence of increased intracellular cholesterol.

3. **Uptake of chemically modified LDL by macrophage scavenger receptors:** In addition to the highly specific and regulated receptor-mediated pathway for LDL uptake described above,

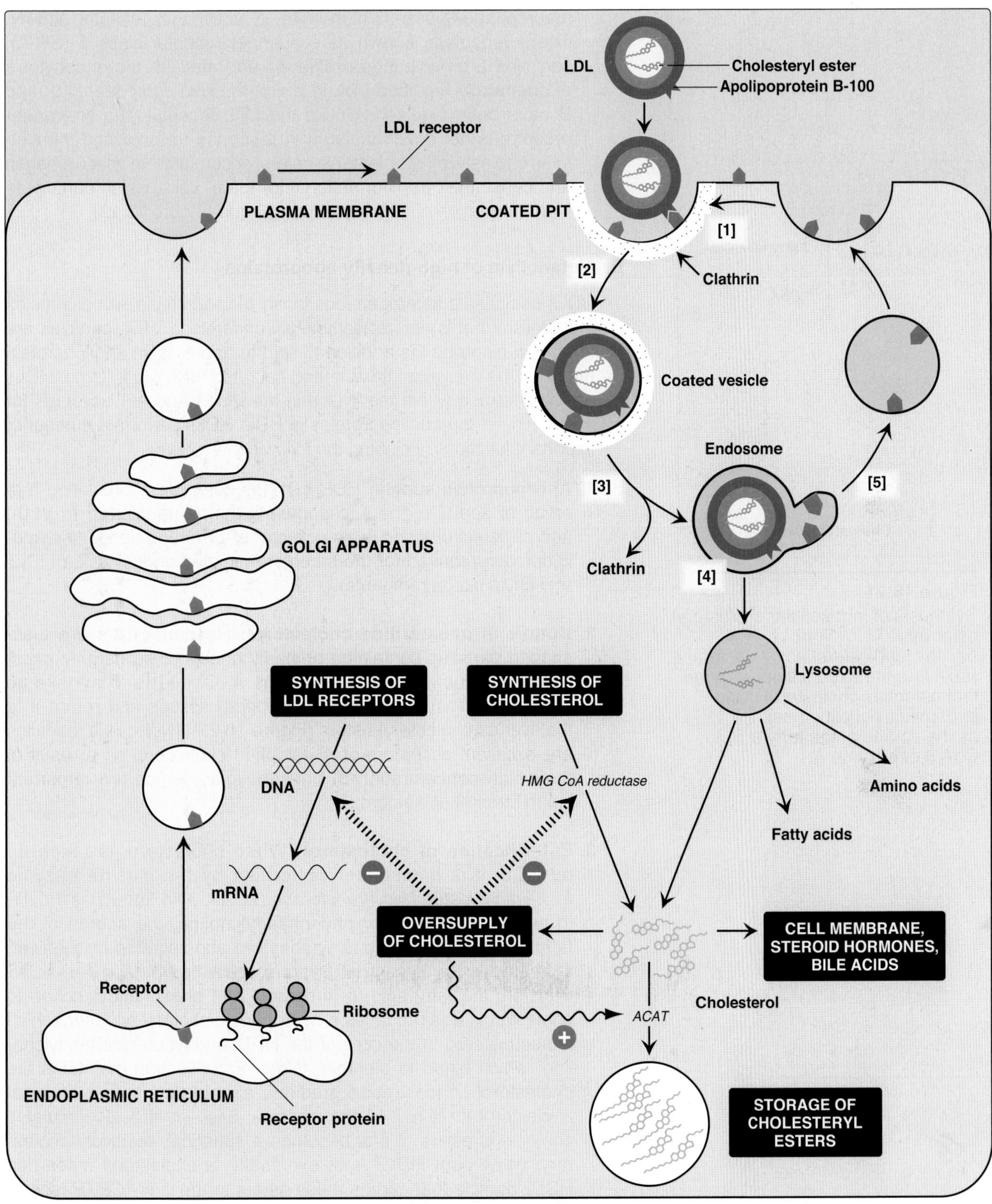

Figure 18.20
Cellular uptake and degradation of low-density lipoprotein (LDL). [Note: Oversupply of cholesterol accelerates the degradation of *HMG CoA reductase*. It also decreases synthesis of the *reductase* by preventing expression of its gene as seen with the LDL receptor.] *ACAT* = *acyl CoA:cholesterol acyltransferase*; HMG CoA = hydroxymethylglutaryl coenzyme A; mRNA = messenger RNA.

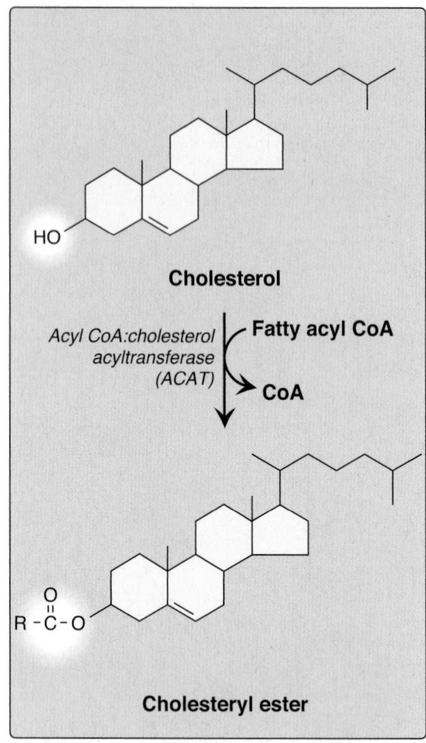

Figure 18.21
Synthesis of intracellular cholesteryl ester by *ACAT*. [Note: *Lecithin:cholesterol acyl transferase* (*LCAT*) is the extracellular enzyme that esterifies cholesterol using phosphatidylcholine (lecithin) as the source of the fatty acid.] CoA = coenzyme A.

macrophages possess high levels of scavenger receptor activity. These receptors, known as scavenger receptor class A (SR-A), can bind a broad range of ligands and mediate the endocytosis of chemically modified LDL in which the lipid components or apo B have been oxidized. Unlike the LDL receptor, the scavenger receptor is not downregulated in response to increased intracellular cholesterol. Cholesteryl esters accumulate in macrophages and cause their transformation into "foam" cells, which participate in the formation of atherosclerotic plaque (Figure 18.22).

E. Metabolism of high-density lipoproteins

HDLs comprise a heterogeneous family of lipoproteins with a complex metabolism that is not yet completely understood. HDL particles are formed in blood by the addition of lipid to apo A-1, an apolipoprotein made by the liver and intestine and secreted into blood. [Note: HDLs are also formed within the liver and intestine.] Apo A-1 accounts for about 70% of the apolipoproteins in HDL. HDLs perform a number of important functions, including the following.

1. **Apolipoprotein supply:** HDL particles serve as a circulating reservoir of apo C-II (the apolipoprotein that is transferred to VLDL and chylomicrons and is an activator of *LPL*) and apo E (the apolipoprotein required for the receptor-mediated endocytosis of IDLs and chylomicron remnants).

2. **Uptake of unesterified cholesterol:** Nascent HDLs are disc-shaped particles containing primarily phospholipid (largely phosphatidylcholine) and apolipoproteins A, C, and E. They take up cholesterol from nonhepatic (peripheral) tissues and return it to the liver as cholesteryl esters (Figure 18.23). [Note: HDL particles are excellent acceptors of unesterified cholesterol as a result of their high concentration of phospholipids, which are important solubilizers of cholesterol.]

3. **Esterification of cholesterol:** When cholesterol is taken up by HDL, it is immediately esterified by the plasma enzyme *lecithin:cholesterol acyltransferase* (*LCAT*, also known as *PCAT*, in which "P" stands for phosphatidylcholine, the source of the fatty acid). This enzyme is synthesized and secreted by the liver. *LCAT* binds to nascent HDL, and is activated by apo A-I. *LCAT* transfers the fatty acid from carbon 2 of phosphatidylcholine to cholesterol. This produces a hydrophobic cholesteryl ester, which is sequestered in the core of the HDL, and lysophosphatidylcholine, which binds to albumin. [Note: Esterification maintains the cholesterol concentration gradient, allowing continued efflux of cholesterol to HDL.] As the discoidal nascent HDL accumulates cholesteryl esters, it first becomes a spherical, relatively cholesteryl ester–poor HDL3 and, eventually, a cholesteryl ester–rich HDL2 particle that carries these esters to the liver. *CETP* (see p. 231) moves some of the cholesteryl esters from HDL to VLDL in exchange for TAG, relieving product inhibition of *LCAT*. Because VLDLs are catabolized to LDL, the cholesteryl esters transferred by *CETP* are ultimately taken up by the liver (see p. 236).

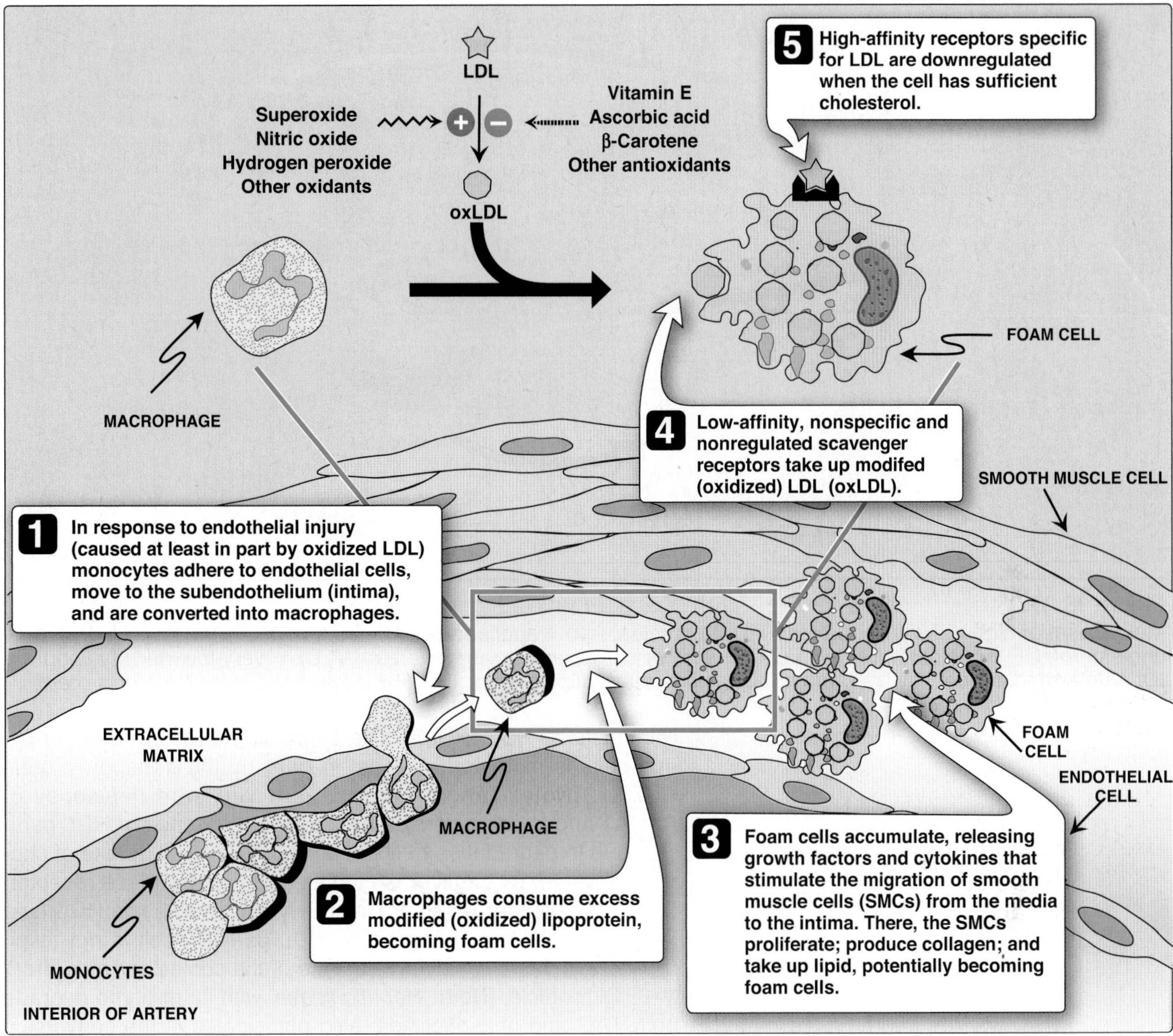

Figure 18.22
Role of oxidized lipoproteins in plaque formation in an arterial wall. LDL = low-density lipoprotein.

4. **Reverse cholesterol transport:** The selective transfer of cholesterol from peripheral cells to HDL, from HDL to the liver for bile acid synthesis or disposal via the bile, and to steroidogenic cells for hormone synthesis, is a key component of cholesterol homeostasis. This process of reverse cholesterol transport is, in part, the basis for the inverse relationship seen between plasma HDL concentration and atherosclerosis and for HDL's designation as the "good" cholesterol carrier. [Note: Exercise and estrogen raise HDL levels.] Reverse cholesterol transport involves efflux of cholesterol from peripheral cells to HDL, esterification of the cholesterol by *LCAT*, binding of the cholesteryl ester–rich HDL (HDL2) to liver (and steroidogenic cells), the selective transfer of the cholesteryl esters into these cells, and the release of

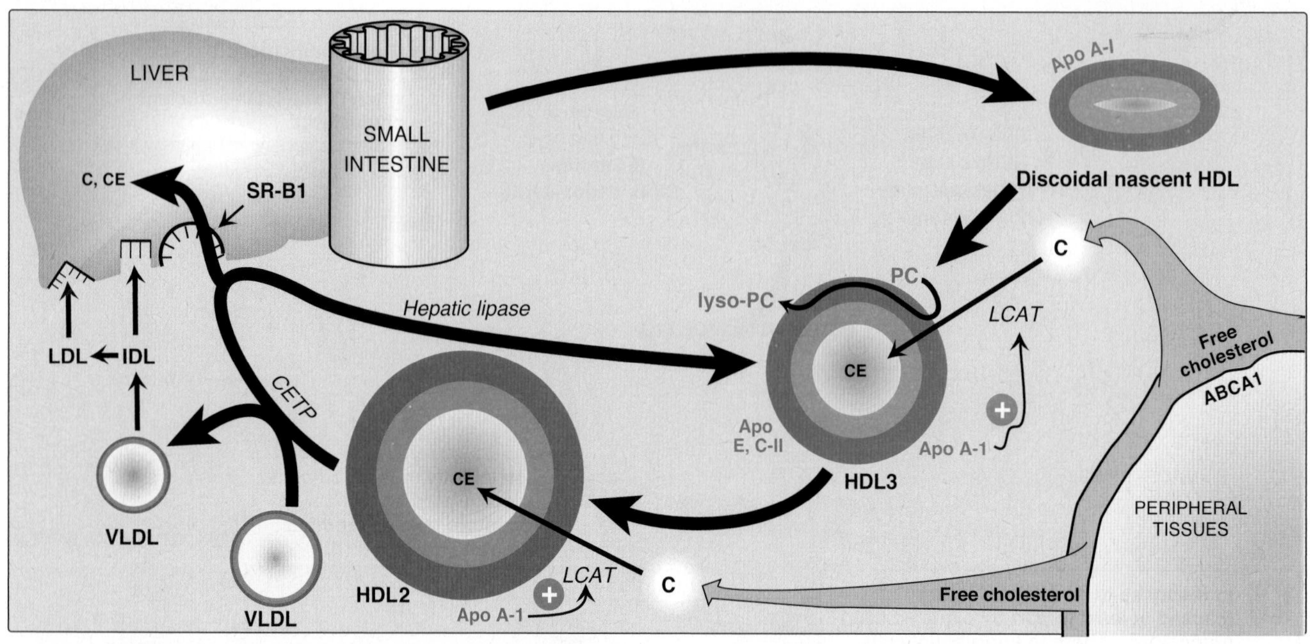

Figure 18.23
Metabolism of high-density lipoprotein (HDL) particles. Apo = apolipoprotein; ABCA1 = transport protein; C = cholesterol; CE = cholesteryl ester; *LCAT = lecithin:cholesterol acyltransferase*; VLDL = very-low-density lipoprotein; IDL = intermediate-density lipoprotein; LDL = low-density lipoprotein; *CETP = cholesteryl ester transfer protein*; SR-B1 = scavenger receptor B1.

lipid-depleted HDL (HDL3). The efflux of cholesterol from peripheral cells is mediated, at least in part, by the transport protein ABCA1. [Note: Tangier disease is a very rare deficiency of ABCA1 and is characterized by the virtual absence of HDL particles due to degradation of lipid-poor apo A-1.] The uptake of cholesteryl esters by the liver is mediated by a cell-surface receptor, SR-B1 (scavenger receptor class B type 1) that binds HDL (see p. 234 for SR-A receptors). The HDL particle itself is not taken up. Instead, there is selective uptake of the cholesteryl ester from the HDL particle. [Note: *Hepatic lipase*, with its ability to degrade both TAG and phospholipids, also participates in the conversion of HDL2 to HDL3.]

> ABCA1 is an ATP-binding cassette (ABC) protein. ABC proteins use energy from ATP hydrolysis to transport materials, including lipids, in and out of cells and across intracellular compartments. In addition to Tangier disease, defects in specific ABC proteins result in sitosterolemia, X-linked adrenoleukodystrophy, respiratory distress syndrome due to decreased surfactant secretion, and cystic fibrosis.

F. Role of lipoprotein (a) in heart disease

Lipoprotein (a), or Lp(a), is a particle that, when present in large quantities in the plasma, is associated with an increased risk of coronary heart disease. Lp(a) is nearly identical in structure to an LDL particle.

Its distinguishing feature is the presence of an additional apolipoprotein molecule, apo(a), that is covalently linked at a single site to apo B-100. Circulating levels of Lp(a) are determined primarily by genetics. However, factors such as diet may play some role, as trans fatty acids have been shown to increase Lp(a), whereas ω-3 fatty acids decrease it. [Note: Apo(a) is structurally homologous to plasminogen, the precursor of a blood *protease* whose target is fibrin, the main protein component of blood clots (See Chapter 34 online). It is hypothesized that elevated Lp(a) slows the breakdown of blood clots that trigger heart attacks because it competes with plasminogen for binding to fibrin. The physiologic function of Lp(a) in unknown. Niacin reduces Lp(a), as well as LDL-cholesterol and TAGs, and raises HDL.]

VII. STEROID HORMONES

Cholesterol is the precursor of all classes of steroid hormones: glucocorticoids (for example, cortisol), mineralocorticoids (for example, aldosterone), and the sex hormones (that is, androgens, estrogens, and progestins) as shown in Figure 18.24). [Note: Glucocorticoids and mineralocorticoids are collectively called corticosteroids.] Synthesis and secretion occur in the adrenal cortex (cortisol, aldosterone, and androgens), ovaries and placenta (estrogens and progestins), and testes (testosterone). Steroid hormones are transported by the blood from their sites of synthesis to their target organs. Because of their hydrophobicity, they must be complexed with a plasma protein. Plasma albumin can act as a nonspecific carrier and does carry aldosterone. However, specific steroid-carrier plasma proteins bind the steroid hormones more tightly than does albumin (for example, corticosteroid-binding globulin, or transcortin, is responsible for transporting cortisol). A number of genetic diseases are caused by deficiencies in specific steps in the biosynthesis of steroid hormones. Some representative diseases are described in Figure 18.25.

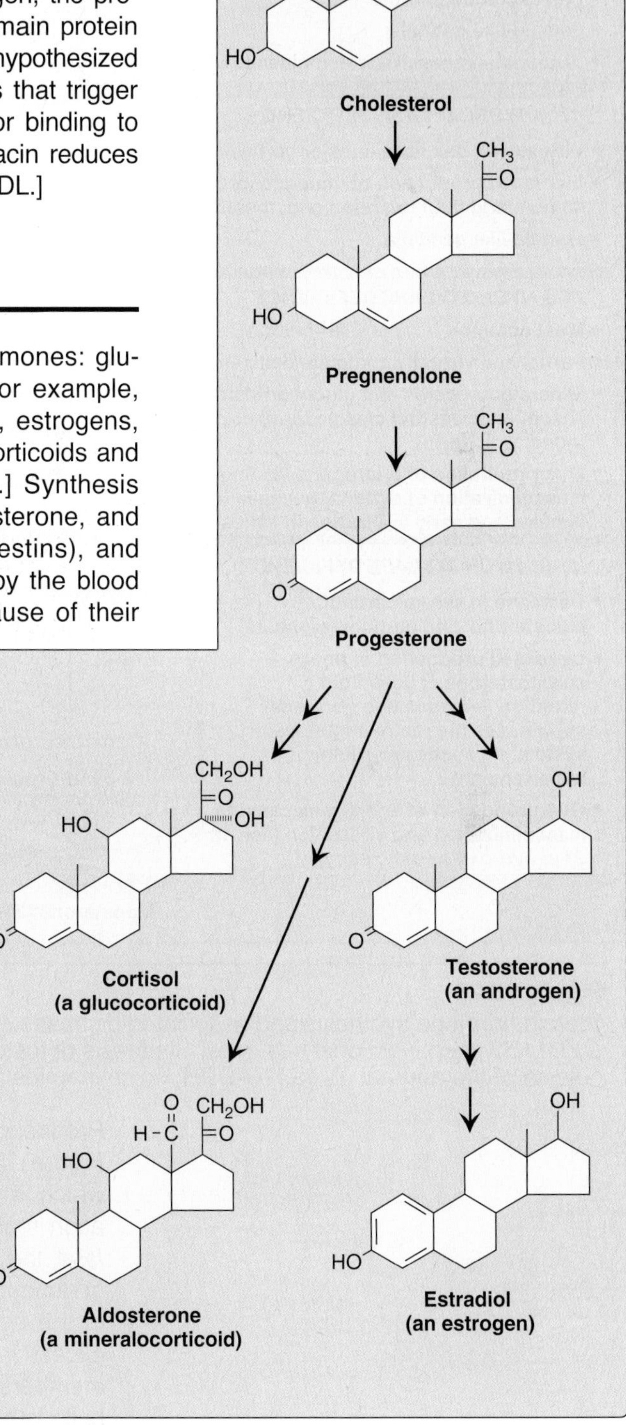

Figure 18.24
Key steroid hormones.

A. Synthesis of steroid hormones

Synthesis involves shortening the hydrocarbon chain of cholesterol and hydroxylation of the steroid nucleus. The initial and rate-limiting reaction converts cholesterol to the 21-carbon pregnenolone. It is catalyzed by the *cholesterol side-chain cleavage enzyme* (*desmolase, $P450_{scc}$*), a cytochrome P450 (CYP) *mixed-function oxidase* of the inner mitochondrial membrane (see p. 149). NADPH and O_2 are required for the reaction. The cholesterol substrate can be newly synthesized, taken up from lipoproteins, or released by an *esterase* from cholesteryl esters stored in the cytosol of steroidogenic tissues. The cholesterol moves to the outer mitochondrial membrane. An important control point is the subsequent movement from the outer to the inner mitochondrial membrane. This process is mediated by StAR (steroidogenic acute regulatory) protein.

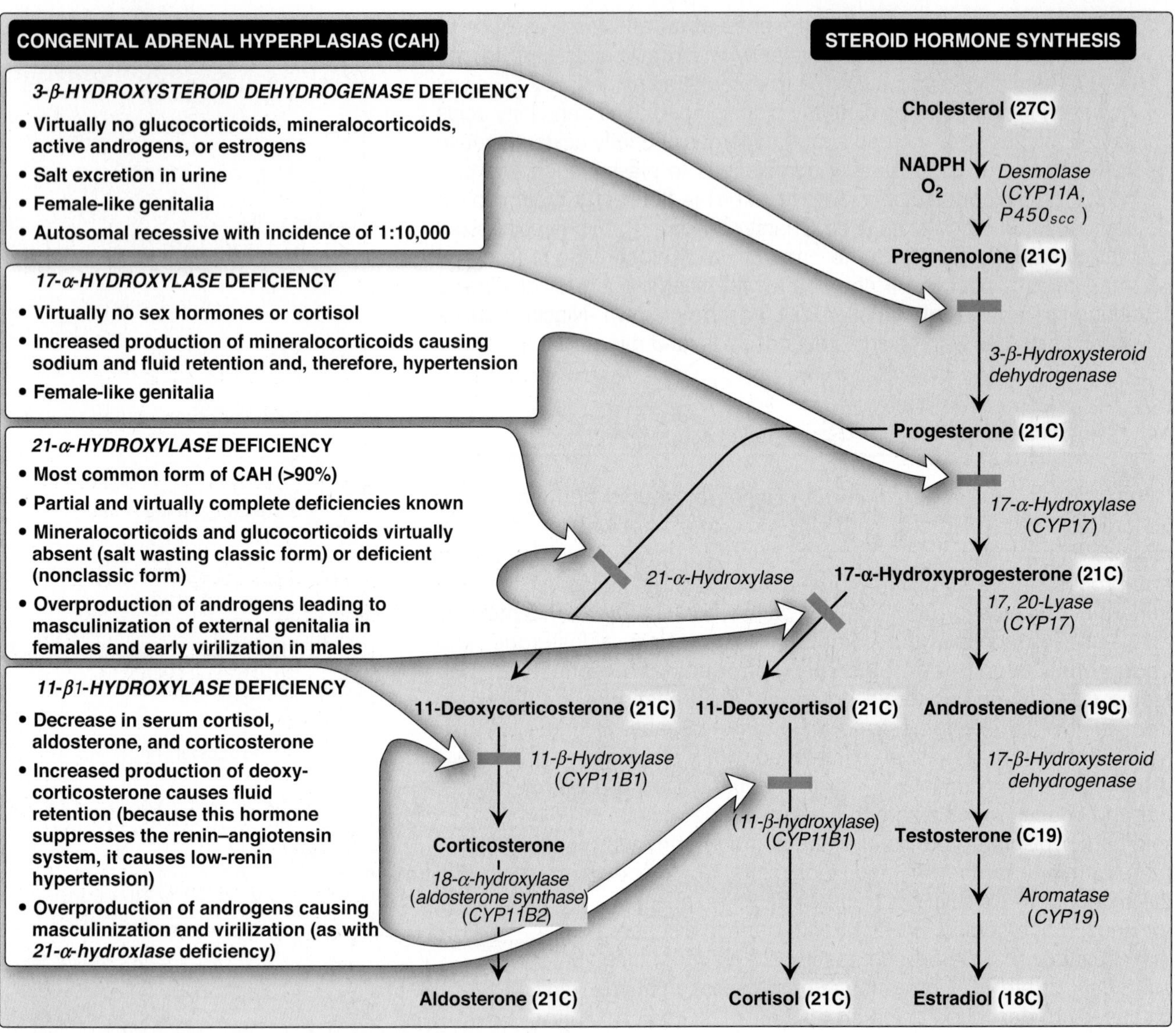

Figure 18.25
Steroid hormone synthesis and associated diseases. [Note: *3-β-Hydroxysteroid dehydrogenase*, *CYP17*, and *CYP11B2* are bifunctional enzymes. Synthesis of testosterone and the estrogens from cholesterol occurs primarily outside of the adrenal gland.] NADPH = nicotinamide adenine dinucleotide phosphate; CYP = cytochrome P450.

Pregnenolone is the parent compound for all steroid hormones (see Figure 18.25). It is oxidized and then isomerized to progesterone, which is further modified to the other steroid hormones by hydroxylation reactions that occur in the ER and mitochondria. Like *desmolase*, the enzymes primarily are CYP proteins. A defect in the activity or amount of an enzyme in this pathway can lead to a deficiency in the synthesis of hormones beyond the affected step and to an excess in the hormones or metabolites before that step. Because all members of the pathway have potent biologic activity, serious metabolic imbalances occur with enzyme deficiencies (see Figure 18.25). Collectively these disorders are known as the congenital adrenal hyperplasias. [Note: Addison disease, due to autoimmune destruction of the adrenal cortex, is characterized by adrenocortical insufficiency.]

B. Secretion of adrenal cortical steroid hormones

Steroid hormones are secreted on demand from their tissues of origin in response to hormonal signals. The corticosteroids and androgens are made in different regions of the adrenal cortex and are secreted into blood in response to different signals.

1. **Cortisol:** Its production in the middle layer (zona fasciculata) of the adrenal cortex is controlled by the hypothalamus, to which the pituitary gland is attached (Figure 18.26). In response to severe stress (for example, infection), corticotropin-releasing hormone (CRH), produced by the hypothalamus, travels through capillaries to the anterior lobe of the pituitary, where it induces the production and secretion of adrenocorticotropic hormone (ACTH). The polypeptide ACTH, the "stress hormone," stimulates the adrenal cortex to synthesize and secrete the glucocorticoid cortisol. Cortisol allows the body to respond to stress through its effects on intermediary metabolism (for example, increased gluconeogenesis) and the inflammatory and immune responses. As cortisol levels rise, the release of CRH and ACTH is inhibited. [Note: ACTH binds to a membrane G protein–coupled receptor, resulting in cyclic AMP (cAMP) production and activation of *protein kinase A* (*PKA*) (see p. 94). *PKA* phosphorylates and activates both the *esterase* that converts cholesteryl ester to free cholesterol and StAR protein.]

2. **Aldosterone:** Its production in the outer layer (zona glomerulosa) of the adrenal cortex is induced by a decrease in the plasma Na^+/K^+ ratio, and by the hormone angiotensin II. Angiotensin II (an octapeptide) is produced from angiotensin I (a decapeptide) by *angiotensin-converting enzyme* (*ACE*), an enzyme found predominantly in the lungs but also distributed widely in the body. [Note: Angiotensin I is produced in the blood by cleavage of an inactive precursor, angiotensinogen, secreted by the liver. Cleavage is accomplished by the enzyme *renin*, made and secreted by the kidney.] Angiotensin II binds to cell-surface receptors. However, in contrast to ACTH, its effects are mediated through the phosphatidylinositol 4,5-bisphosphate pathway (see p. 205) and not by cAMP. Aldosterone's primary effect is on the kidney tubules, where it stimulates sodium and water uptake and potassium excretion (Figure 18.27). [Note: An effect of aldosterone is an increase in blood pressure. Competitive inhibitors of *ACE* are used to treat *renin*-dependent hypertension.]

3. **Androgens:** Both the inner (zona reticularis) and middle layers of the adrenal cortex produce androgens, primarily dehydroepiandrosterone and androstenedione. Although adrenal androgens themselves are weak, they are converted in peripheral tissues to testosterone, a stronger androgen, and to estrogens.

> Estrogens are derived from androstenedione and testosterone by *aromatase* (*CYP19*). *Aromatase* inhibitors are used in the treatment of estrogen-responsive breast cancer in postmenopausal women.

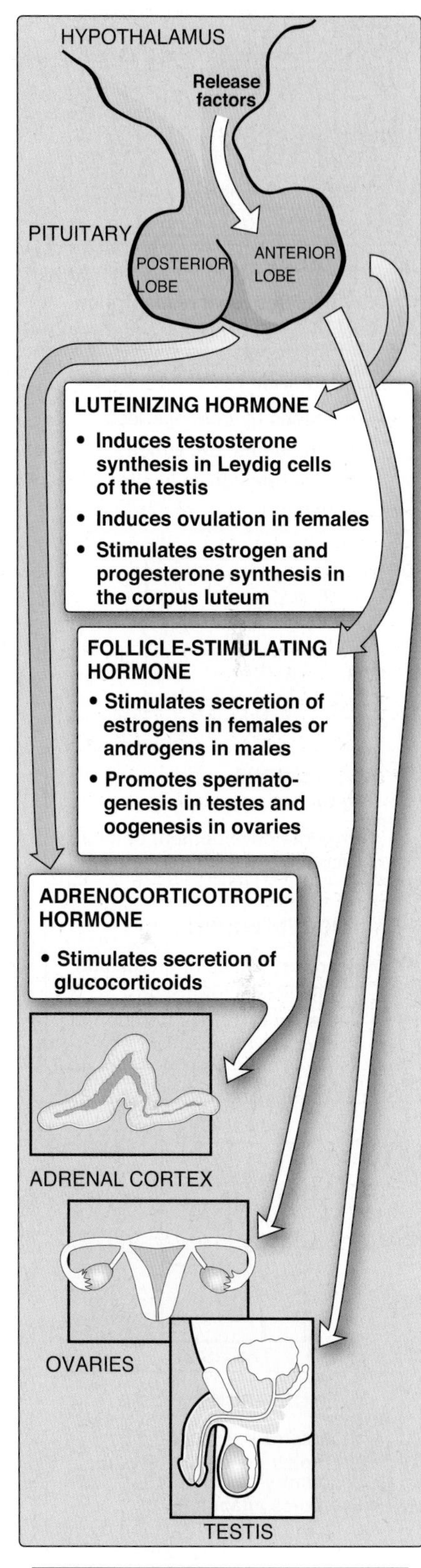

Figure 18.26
Pituitary hormone stimulation of steroid hormone synthesis and secretion.

ADRENAL CORTEX

ALDOSTERONE
- **Stimulates renal reabsorption of Na^+ and excretion of K^+**

CORTISOL
- **Increases gluconeogenesis**
- **Anti-inflammatory action**
- **Protein breakdown in muscle**

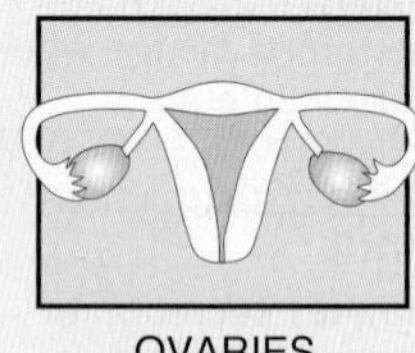

OVARIES

ESTROGENS
- **Control menstrual cycle**
- **Promote development of female secondary sex characteristics**

PROGESTERONE
- **Secretory phase of uterus and mammary glands**
- **Implantation and maturation of fertilized ovum**

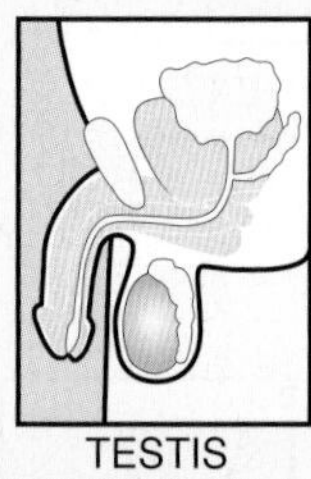

TESTIS

TESTOSTERONE
- **Stimulates spermatogenesis**
- **Promotes development of male secondary sex characteristics**
- **Promotes anabolism**
- **Masculinization of the fetus**

Figure 18.27
Actions of steroid hormones.

C. Secretion of steroid hormones from gonads

The testes and ovaries synthesize hormones necessary for sexual differentiation and reproduction. A single hypothalamic-releasing factor, gonadotropin-releasing hormone, stimulates the anterior pituitary to release the glycoproteins luteinizing hormone (LH) and follicle-stimulating hormone (FSH). Like ACTH, LH and FSH bind to surface receptors and cause an increase in cAMP. LH stimulates the testes to produce testosterone and the ovaries to produce estrogens and progesterone (see Figure 18.27). FSH regulates the growth of ovarian follicles and stimulates testicular spermatogenesis.

D. Mechanism of steroid hormone action

Each steroid hormone diffuses across the plasma membrane of its target cell and binds to a specific cytosolic or nuclear receptor. These receptor–ligand complexes accumulate in the nucleus, dimerize, and bind to specific regulatory DNA sequences (hormone-response elements [HREs]) in association with coactivator proteins, thereby causing promoter activation and increased transcription of targeted genes (Figure 18.28). An HRE is found in the promoter or an enhancer element (see p. 424) for genes that respond to a specific steroid hormone, thus insuring coordinated regulation of these genes. Hormone–receptor complexes can also inhibit transcription in association with corepressors. [Note: The binding of a hormone to its receptor causes a conformational change in the receptor that uncovers its DNA-binding domain, allowing the complex to interact through a zinc-finger motif with the appropriate sequence on the DNA. Receptors for the steroid hormones, plus those for thyroid hormone, retinoic acid (see p. 382), and 1,25-dihydroxycholecalciferol (vitamin D, see p. 386), are members of a "superfamily" of structurally related gene regulators that function in a similar way.]

E. Further metabolism of steroid hormones

Steroid hormones are generally converted into inactive metabolic excretion products in the liver. Reactions include reduction of unsaturated bonds and the introduction of additional hydroxyl groups. The resulting structures are made more soluble by conjugation with glucuronic acid or sulfate (from 3'-phosphoadenosyl-5'-phosphosulfate, see p. 162). Approximately 20%–30% of these metabolites are secreted into the bile and then excreted in the feces, whereas the remainder are released into the blood and filtered from the plasma in the kidney, passing into the urine. These conjugated metabolites are fairly water soluble and do not need protein carriers.

VIII. CHAPTER SUMMARY

Cholesterol is a **hydrophobic** compound, with a single hydroxyl group located at carbon 3 of the A ring, to which a fatty acid can be attached, producing an even more hydrophobic **cholesteryl ester**. Cholesterol is synthesized by virtually all human tissues, although primarily by **liver**, **intestine**, **adrenal cortex**, and **reproductive tissues** (Figure 18.29). All the carbon atoms in cholesterol are provided by **acetyl coenzyme A (CoA)**, and **nicotinamide adenine dinucleotide phosphate** provides the reducing equivalents. The pathway is driven by hydrolysis of the high-energy thioester bond of acetyl CoA and the terminal phosphate bond of adenosine triphosphate. Cholesterol is synthesized in the **cyto-**

plasm.The **rate-limiting and regulated step** in cholesterol synthesis is catalyzed by the smooth endoplasmic reticulum–membrane protein, ***hydroxymethylglutaryl coenzyme A*** (***HMG CoA***) ***reductase***, which produces **mevalonate** from HMG CoA. The enzyme is regulated by a number of mechanisms: 1) **Expression of the gene for the *reductase*** is activated when cholesterol levels are low, via the transcription factor, **sterol regulatory element–binding protein-2** (**SREBP-2**), bound to a sterol regulatory element (**SRE**), resulting in increased enzyme and, therefore, more cholesterol, synthesis; 2) **degradation** of the *reductase* is accelerated when cholesterol levels are high; 3) *reductase* activity is controlled by ***adenosine monophosphate*** (***AMP***)***–activated protein kinase*** ([***AMPK***], which phosphorylates and **inactivates** the *reductase*) and an **insulin-activated protein *phosphatase*** (which dephosphorylates and **activates** it); and 4) expression of the gene for the *reductase* is upregulated by insulin and downregulated by glucagon. **Statins** are **competitive inhibitors** of *HMG CoA reductase*. These drugs are used to decrease plasma cholesterol in patients with **hypercholesterolemia**. The ring structure of cholesterol cannot be degraded in humans.

Cholesterol can be eliminated from the body either by **conversion to bile salts** or by **secretion into the bile**. **Bile salts** and **phosphatidylcholine** are quantitatively the most important organic components of bile. The rate-limiting step in bile acid synthesis is catalyzed by ***cholesterol-7-α-hydroxylase***, which is **inhibited** by **bile acids**. Before the bile acids leave the liver, they are conjugated to a molecule of either **glycine** or **taurine**, producing the **conjugated bile salts glycocholic** or **taurocholic acid** and **glycochenodeoxycholic** or **taurochenodeoxycholic acid**. Bile salts (deprotonated) are more amphipathic than bile acids (protonated) and, therefore, are more effective emulsifiers of dietary fat. In the intestine, bacteria can remove the glycine and taurine and can remove a hydroxyl group from the steroid nucleus, producing the **secondary bile salts**, **deoxycholic** and **lithocholic acids**. More than 95% of the bile salts are efficiently reabsorbed in the intestinal ileum by a sodium–bile salt cotransporter, returned to the blood, and carried by albumin back to the liver where they are taken up by the hepatic form of the cotransporter and reused (**enterohepatic circulation, which bile acid sequestrants reduce**). If more cholesterol enters the bile than can be solubilized by the available bile salts and phosphatidylcholine, **cholesterol gallstone disease** (**cholelithiasis**) can occur.

The plasma lipoproteins include **chylomicrons**, **very-low-density lipoproteins** (**VLDLs**), **low-density lipoproteins** (**LDLs**), and **high-density lipoproteins** (**HDLs**). They function to keep lipids (primarily **triacylglycerol** [**TAG**] and **cholesteryl esters**) soluble as they transport them between tissues. Lipoproteins are composed of a **neutral lipid** (**TAG**, **cholesteryl esters**, or both) core surrounded by a shell of amphipathic **apolipoproteins**, **phospholipid**, and **unesterified cholesterol**. **Chylomicrons** are assembled in **intestinal mucosal cells** from **dietary lipids** (primarily **TAG**). Each nascent chylomicron particle has one molecule of **apolipoprotein** (**apo**) **B-48**. They are released from the cells into the lymphatic system and travel to the blood, where they receive **apo C-II** and **apo E** from **HDLs**. Apo C-II activates endothelial ***lipoprotein lipase*** (***LPL***), which degrades the TAG in chylomicrons to fatty acids and glycerol. The **fatty acids** that are released are **stored** (in the **adipose**) or used for **energy** (by the **muscle**). The **glycerol** is metabolized by the **liver**. Patients with a **deficiency** of ***LPL*** or **apo C-II** show a dra-

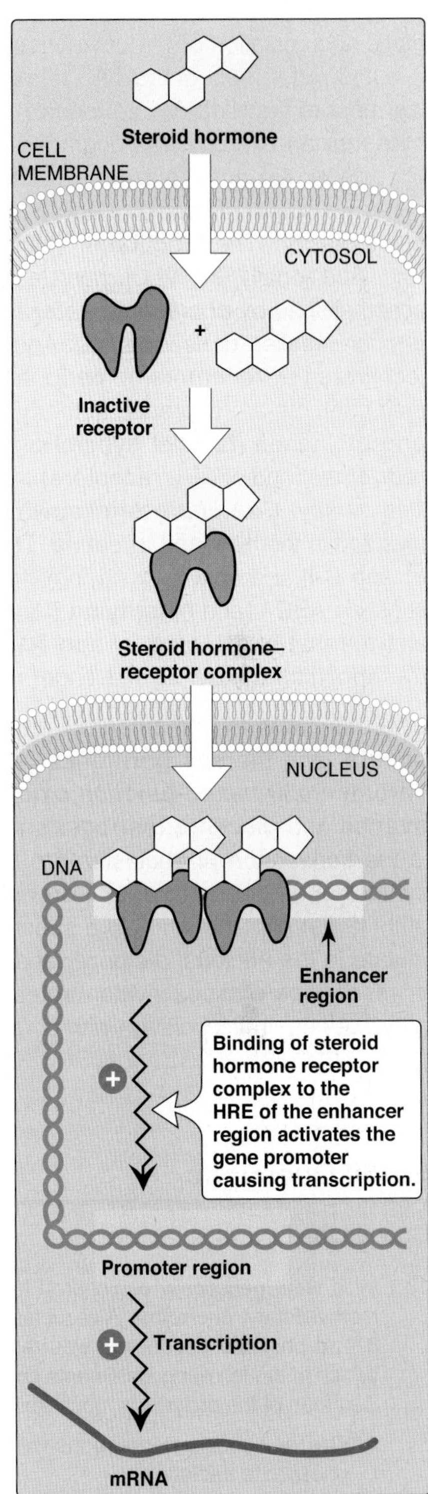

Figure 18.28
Activation of transcription by interaction of steroid hormone–receptor complex with hormone response element (HRE). The receptor contains domains that bind the hormone, DNA, and proteins that relax the DNA. mRNA = messenger RNA.

matic accumulation of chylomicrons in the plasma (**type I hyperlipoproteinemia**, or **familial *LPL* deficiency**) even if fasted. After most of the TAG is removed, apo C-II is returned to the HDL, and the **chylomicron remnant**, carrying most of the **dietary cholesterol**, binds to a **receptor** on the **liver** that recognizes **apo E**. The particle is **endocytosed**, and its contents degraded by **lysosomal enzymes**. Defective uptake of these remnants causes type III hyperlipoproteinemia. **Nascent VLDLs** are produced in the **liver** and are composed predominantly of **TAG**. They contain a single molecule of **apo B-100**. Like nascent chylomicrons, VLDLs receive **apo C-II** and **apo E** from **HDL** in the plasma. The **function** of VLDL is to **carry hepatic TAG** to the **peripheral tissues** where ***LPL*** degrades the lipid. Additionally, the VLDL particle receives **cholesteryl esters** from **HDL in exchange for TAG**. This process is accomplished by ***cholesteryl ester transfer protein* (*CETP*)**. Eventually, VLDL in the **plasma** is **converted to LDL**, a much smaller, denser particle. Apo C-II and apo E are returned to HDL, but the LDL retains **apo B-100**, which is recognized by **receptors** on **peripheral tissues** and the **liver**. LDLs undergo **receptor-mediated endocytosis**, and their contents are degraded in the **lysosomes**. A **deficiency of functional LDL receptors** causes **type II hyperlipoproteinemia (familial hypercholesterolemia)**. The endocytosed cholesterol decreases synthesis of ***HMG CoA reductase*** (and of **LDL receptors**) through prevention of SREBP-2 binding to the SRE. Some of it can also be esterified by ***acyl CoA:cholesterol acyltransferase*** (***ACAT***) and stored. **HDL** are created by **lipidation of apo A-1** synthesized in the **liver** and **intestine**. They have a number of functions, including: 1) serving as a **circulating reservoir of apo C-II** and **apo E** for chylomicrons and VLDL; 2) removing **unesterified cholesterol** from from peripheral tissues via ABCA1and **esterifying it** using ***lecithin:cholesterol acyl transferase* (*LCAT*)**, a liver-synthesized plasma enzyme that is activated by **apo A-1**; and 3) delivering these cholesteryl esters to the liver (**reverse cholesterol transport**) for uptake via scavenger receptor-B1(SR-B1).

Cholesterol is the precursor of all classes of steroid hormones, which include **glucocorticoids**, **mineralocorticoids**, and the **sex hormones** (**androgens**, **estrogens**, and **progestins**). **Synthesis**, using primarily **cytochrome P450 *mixed-function oxidases***, occurs in the **adrenal cortex** (**cortisol**, **aldosterone**, and **androgens**), **ovaries** and **placenta** (**estrogens** and **progestins**), and **testes** (**testosterone**). The initial and rate-limiting step is the conversion of cholesterol to **pregnenolone** by the side-chain cleavage enzyme ***$P450_{scc}$***. Deficiencies in synthesis lead to **congenital adrenal hyperplasia.** Each steroid hormone diffuses across the plasma membrane of its target cell and binds to a specific **cytosolic** or **nuclear receptor**. These **receptor–ligand complexes** accumulate in the nucleus, dimerize, and **bind** to specific regulatory DNA sequences (**hormone-response elements**) in association with coactivator proteins, thereby causing **promoter activation** and **increased transcription** of targeted genes. In association with corepressors, **transcription is decreased**.

Study Questions

Choose the ONE best answer.

18.1 Mice were genetically engineered to contain hydroxymethylglutaryl coenzyme A reductase in which serine 871, a phosphorylation site, was replaced by alanine. Which of the following statements concerning the modified form of the enzyme is most likely to be correct?

A. The enzyme is nonresponsive to adenosine triphosphate depletion.

B. The enzyme is nonresponsive to statin drugs.

C. The enzyme is nonresponsive to the sterol response element–sterol response element–binding protein system.

D. The enzyme is unable to be degraded by the ubiquitin–proteasome system.

Correct answer = A. The reductase is regulated by covalent phosphorylation and dephosphorylation. Depletion of adenosine triphosphate results in a rise in adenosine monophosphate (AMP), which activates AMP kinase (AMPK), thereby phosphorylating and inactivating the enzyme. In the absence of the serine, a common phosphorylation site, the enzyme cannot be phosphorylated by AMPK. The enzyme is also regulated physiologically through changes in transcription and degradation and pharmacologically by statin drugs (competitive inhibitors), but none of these depends on serine phosphorylation.

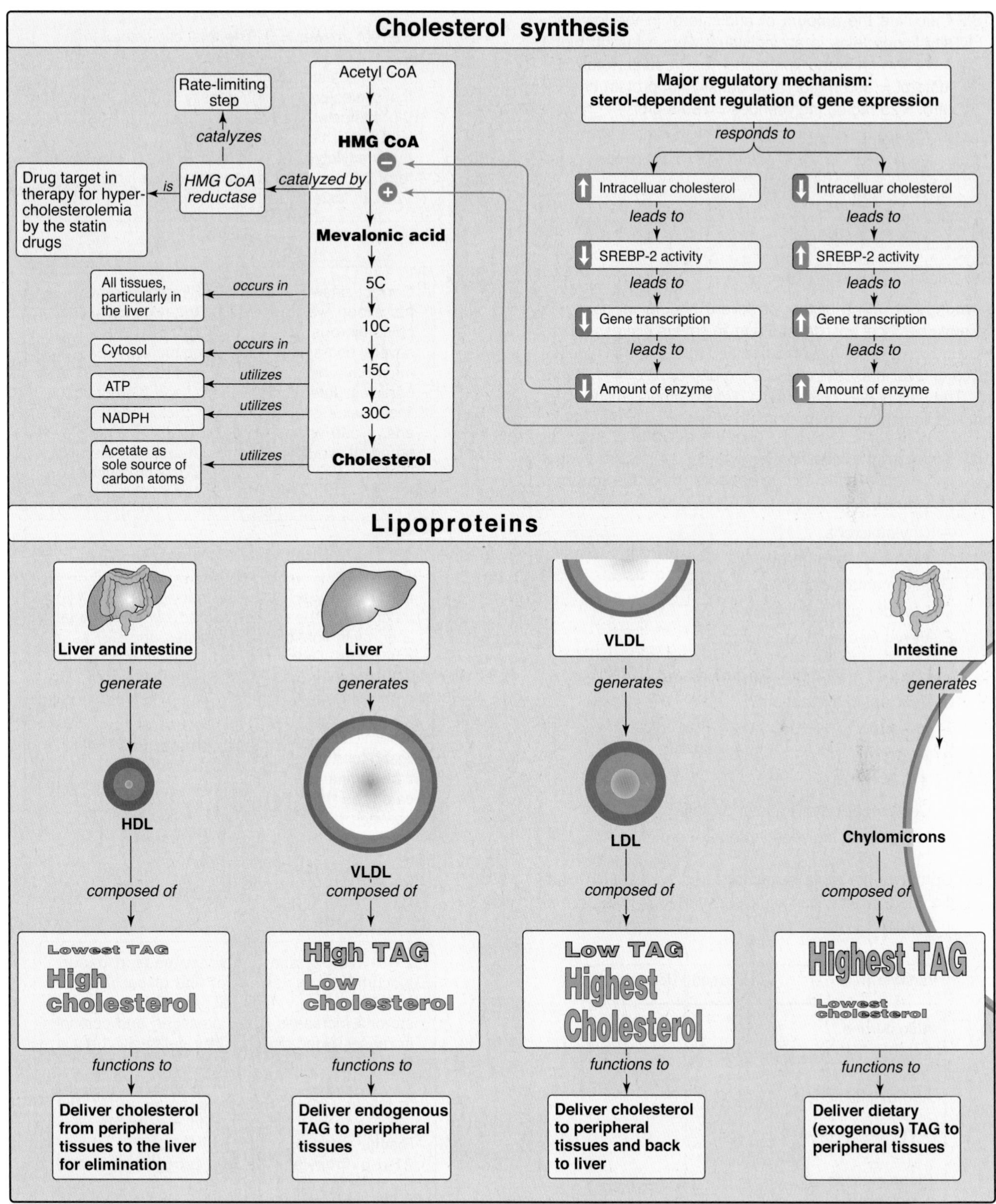

Figure 18.29

Concept map for cholesterol and the lipoproteins. HMG CoA = hydroxymethylglutaryl coenzyme A; SREBP = sterol regulatory element–binding protein; HDL = high-density lipoprotein; VLDL = very-low-density lipoprotein; LDL = low-density lipoprotein; TAG = triacylglycerol; NADP(H) = nicotinamide adenine dinucleotide phosphate.

18.2 Calculate the amount of cholesterol in the low-density lipoproteins in an individual whose fasting blood gave the following lipid-panel test results: total cholesterol = 300 mg/dl, high-density lipoprotein cholesterol = 25 mg/dl, triglycerides = 150 mg/dl.

A. 55 mg/dl
B. 95 mg/dl
C. 125 mg/dl
D. 245 mg/dl

Correct answer = D. The total cholesterol in the blood of a fasted individual is equal to the sum of the cholesterol in low-density lipoproteins plus the cholesterol in high-density lipoproteins plus the cholesterol in very-low-density lipoproteins (VLDLs). This last term is calculated by dividing the triacylglycerol value by 5 because cholesterol accounts for about 1/5 of the volume of VLDL in fasted blood.

For Questions 18.3 and 18.4:

A young girl with a history of severe abdominal pain was taken to her local hospital at 5 a.m. in severe distress. Blood was drawn, and the plasma appeared milky, with the triacylglycerol level in excess of 2,000 mg/dl (normal = 4–150 mg/dl). The patient was placed on a diet extremely limited in fat but supplemented with medium-chain triglycerides.

18.3 Which of the following lipoprotein particles are most likely responsible for the appearance of the patient's plasma?

A. Chylomicrons
B. High-density lipoproteins
C. Intermediate-density lipoproteins
D. Low-density lipoproteins
E. Very-low-density lipoproteins

Correct answer = A. The milky appearance of her blood was a result of triacylglycerol-rich chylomicrons. Because 5 a.m. is presumably several hours after her evening meal, the patient must have difficulty degrading these lipoprotein particles. Intermediate-, low-, and high-density lipoproteins contain primarily cholesteryl esters, and, if one or more of these particles was elevated, it would cause hypercholesterolemia. Very-low-density lipoproteins do not cause the described "milky appearance" in plasma.

18.4 Which one of the following proteins is most likely to be deficient in this patient?

A. Apo A-I
B. Apo B-48
C. Apo C-II
D. Cholesteryl ester transfer protein
E. Microsomal triglyceride transfer protein

Correct answer = C. The triacylglycerol (TAG) in chylomicrons is degraded by endothelial lipoprotein lipase, which requires apo C-II as a coenzyme. Deficiency of the enzyme or coenzyme results in decreased ability to degrade chylomicrons to their remnants, which get cleared by the liver. Apo A-I is the coenzyme for lecithin:cholesterol acyltransferase; apo B-48 is the ligand for the hepatic receptor that binds chylomicron remnants; cholesteryl ester transfer protein catalyzes the cholesteryl ester–TAG exchange between high-density and very-low-density lipoproteins (VLDLs); and microsomal triglyceride transfer protein is involved in the formation, not degradation, of chylomicrons (and VLDLs).

18.5 Complete the table below for an individual with classic 21-α-hydroxylase deficiency relative to a normal individual.

Variable	Increased	Decreased
Aldosterone		
Cortisol		
Androstenedione		
Adrenocorticotropic hormone		
Blood glucose		
Blood pressure		

How might the results be changed if this individual were deficient in 17-α-hydroxylase, rather than 21-α-hydroxylase?

21-α-Hydroxylase deficiency causes mineralocorticoids (aldosterone) and glucocorticoids (cortisol) to be virtually absent. Because aldosterone increases blood pressure, and cortisol increases blood glucose, their deficiencies result in a decrease in blood pressure and blood glucose, respectively. Cortisol normally feeds back to inhibit adrenocorticotropic hormone (ACTH) release by the pituitary, and, so, its absence results in an elevation in ACTH. The loss of 21-α-hydroxylase pushes progesterone and pregnenolone to androgen synthesis, therefore, causes androstenedione levels to rise.

With 17-α-hydroxylase deficiency, sex hormone synthesis would be inhibited. Mineralocorticoid production would be increased, leading to hypertension.

UNIT IV: Nitrogen Metabolism

Amino Acids: Disposal of Nitrogen 19

I. OVERVIEW

Unlike fats and carbohydrates, amino acids are not stored by the body. That is, no protein exists whose sole function is to maintain a supply of amino acids for future use. Therefore, amino acids must be obtained from the diet, synthesized de novo, or produced from normal protein degradation. Any amino acids in excess of the biosynthetic needs of the cell are rapidly degraded. The first phase of catabolism involves the removal of the α-amino groups (usually by transamination and subsequent oxidative deamination), forming ammonia and the corresponding α-keto acids, the "carbon skeletons" of amino acids. A portion of the free ammonia is excreted in the urine, but most is used in the synthesis of urea (Figure 19.1), which is quantitatively the most important route for disposing of nitrogen from the body. In the second phase of amino acid catabolism, described in Chapter 20, the carbon skeletons of the α-keto acids are converted to common intermediates of energy-producing metabolic pathways. These compounds can be metabolized to CO_2 and water, glucose, fatty acids, or ketone bodies by the central pathways of metabolism described in Chapters 8–13 and 16.

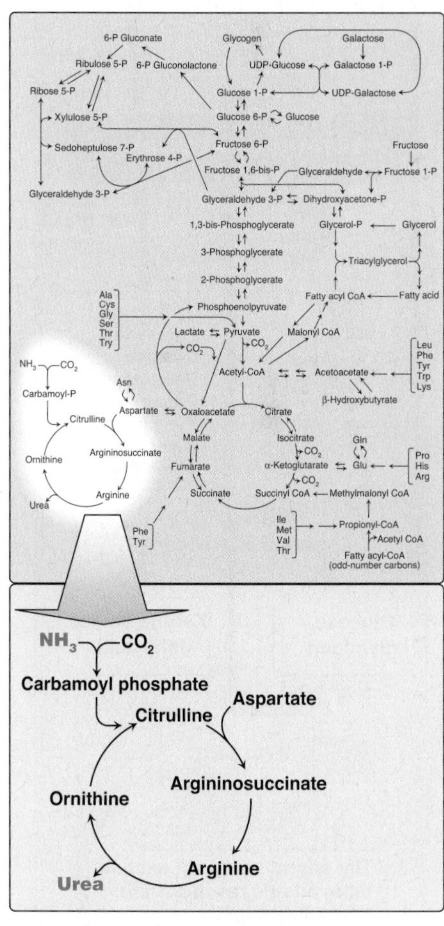

Figure 19.1
Urea cycle shown as part of the essential pathways of energy metabolism. (See Figure 8.2, p. 92, for a more detailed view of intermediary metabolism.)

II. OVERALL NITROGEN METABOLISM

Amino acid catabolism is part of the larger process of the metabolism of nitrogen-containing molecules. Nitrogen enters the body in a variety of compounds present in food, the most important being amino acids contained in dietary protein. Nitrogen leaves the body as urea, ammonia, and other products derived from amino acid metabolism. The role of body proteins in these transformations involves two important concepts: the amino acid pool and protein turnover.

A. Amino acid pool

Free amino acids are present throughout the body, such as in cells, blood, and the extracellular fluids. For the purpose of this discussion, envision all of these amino acids as if they belonged to a single entity, called the amino acid pool. This pool is supplied by three sources: 1) amino acids provided by the degradation of endogenous

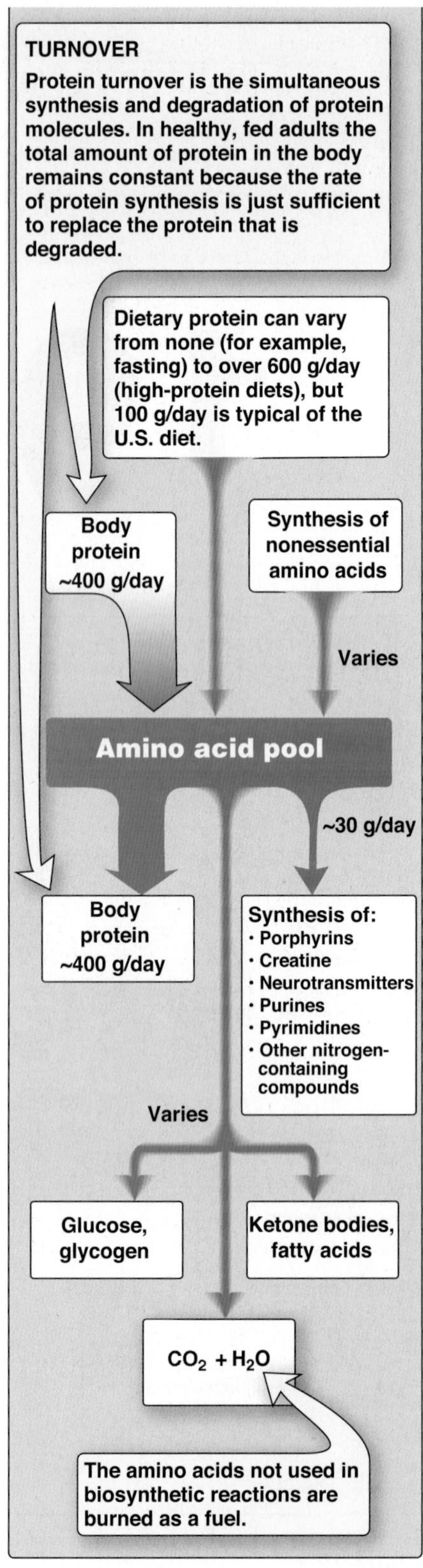

Figure 19.2
Sources and fates of amino acids.

(body) proteins, most of which are reutilized; 2) amino acids derived from exogenous (dietary) protein; and 3) nonessential amino acids synthesized from simple intermediates of metabolism (Figure 19.2). Conversely, the amino pool is depleted by three routes: 1) synthesis of body protein; 2) consumption of amino acids as precursors of essential nitrogen-containing small molecules; and 3) conversion of amino acids to glucose, glycogen, fatty acids, and ketone bodies, or oxidation to $CO_2 + H_2O$ (see Figure 19.2). Although the amino acid pool is small (comprising about 90–100 g of amino acids) in comparison with the amount of protein in the body (about 12 kg in a 70-kg man), it is conceptually at the center of whole-body nitrogen metabolism.

In healthy, well-fed individuals, the input to the amino acid pool is balanced by the output. That is, the amount of amino acids contained in the pool is constant. The amino acid pool is said to be in a steady state, and the individual is said to be in nitrogen balance.

B. Protein turnover

Most proteins in the body are constantly being synthesized and then degraded, permitting the removal of abnormal or unneeded proteins. For many proteins, regulation of synthesis determines the concentration of protein in the cell, with protein degradation assuming a minor role. For other proteins, the rate of synthesis is constitutive (that is, essentially constant), and cellular levels of the protein are controlled by selective degradation.

1. **Rate of turnover:** In healthy adults, the total amount of protein in the body remains constant because the rate of protein synthesis is just sufficient to replace the protein that is degraded. This process, called protein turnover, leads to the hydrolysis and resynthesis of 300–400 g of body protein each day. The rate of protein turnover varies widely for individual proteins. Short-lived proteins (for example, many regulatory proteins and misfolded proteins) are rapidly degraded, having half-lives measured in minutes or hours. Long-lived proteins, with half-lives of days to weeks, constitute the majority of proteins in the cell. Structural proteins, such as collagen, are metabolically stable and have half-lives measured in months or years.

2. **Protein degradation:** There are two major enzyme systems responsible for degrading proteins: the adenosine triphosphate (ATP)-dependent ubiquitin-proteasome system of the cytosol, and the ATP-independent degradative enzyme system of the lysosomes. Proteasomes selectively degrade damaged or short-lived proteins. Lysosomes use *acid hydrolases* (see p. 162) to nonselectively degrade intracellular proteins ("autophagy") and extracellular proteins ("heterophagy"), such as plasma proteins, that are taken into the cell by endocytosis.

a. **Ubiquitin–proteasome proteolytic pathway:** Proteins selected for degradation by the cytosolic ubiquitin-proteasome system are first modified by the covalent attachment of ubiquitin (Ub), a small, globular, nonenzymic protein that is highly conserved across eukaryotic species. Ubiquitination of the target substrate occurs through isopeptide linkage of the α-carboxyl group of the C-terminal glycine of Ub to the ε-amino group of a lysine on the protein substrate by a three-step, enzyme-catalyzed, ATP-dependent process. [Note: Enzyme 1 (E1, or activating enzyme) activates Ub, which is then transferred to E2 (conjugating enzyme). E3 (a *ligase*) identifies the protein to be degraded and interacts with E2-Ub.] The consecutive addition of four or more Ub molecules to the target protein generates a polyubiquitin chain. Proteins tagged with Ub are recognized by a large, barrel-shaped, macromolecular, proteolytic complex called a proteasome (Figure 19.3). The proteasome unfolds, deubiquitinates, and cuts the target protein into fragments that are then further degraded by cytosolic *proteases* to amino acids, which enter the amino acid pool. Ub is recycled. It is noteworthy that the selective degradation of proteins by the ubiquitin-proteosome complex (unlike simple hydrolysis by proteolytic enzymes) requires energy in the form of ATP.

b. **Chemical signals for protein degradation:** Because proteins have different half-lives, it is clear that protein degradation cannot be random but, rather, is influenced by some structural aspect of the protein. For example, some proteins that have been chemically altered by oxidation or tagged with ubiquitin are preferentially degraded. The half-life of a protein is also influenced by the amino (N)-terminal residue. For example, proteins that have serine as the N-terminal amino acid are long-lived, with a half-life of more than 20 hours, whereas those with aspartate at their N-terminus have a half-life of only 3 minutes. Additionally, proteins rich in sequences containing proline, glutamate, serine, and threonine (called PEST sequences after the one-letter designations for these amino acids) are rapidly degraded and, therefore, have short half-lives.

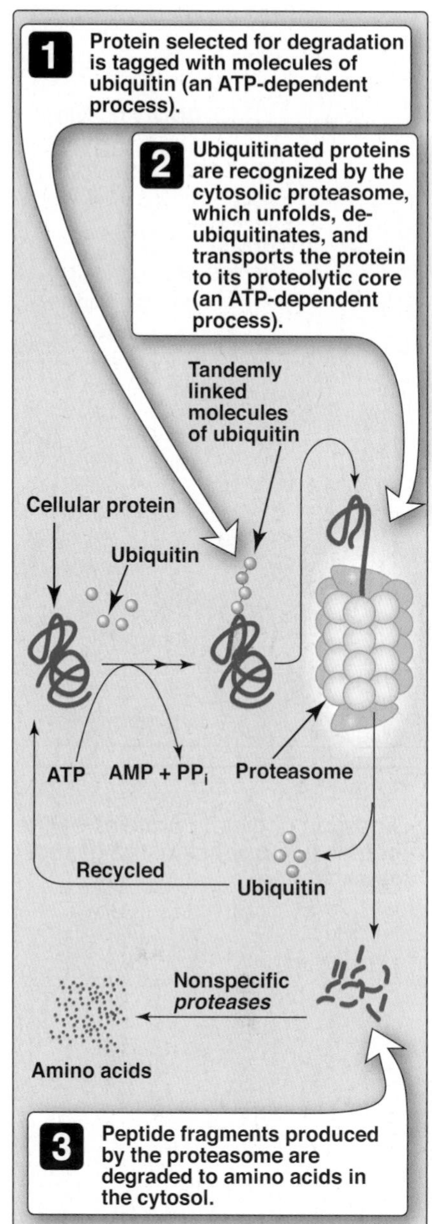

Figure 19.3
The ubiquitin–proteasome degradation pathway of proteins. AMP = adenosine monophosphate; PP_i = pyrophosphate.

III. DIGESTION OF DIETARY PROTEINS

Most of the nitrogen in the diet is consumed in the form of protein, typically amounting to 70–100 g/day in the American diet (see Figure 19.2). Proteins are generally too large to be absorbed by the intestine. [Note: An example of an exception to this rule is that newborns can take up maternal antibodies in breast milk.] They must, therefore, be hydrolyzed to yield di- and tripeptides as well as individual amino acids, which can be absorbed. Proteolytic enzymes responsible for degrading proteins are produced by three different organs: the stomach, the pancreas, and the small intestine (Figure 19.4).

A. Digestion by gastric secretion

The digestion of proteins begins in the stomach, which secretes gastric juice, a unique solution containing hydrochloric acid and the proenzyme pepsinogen.

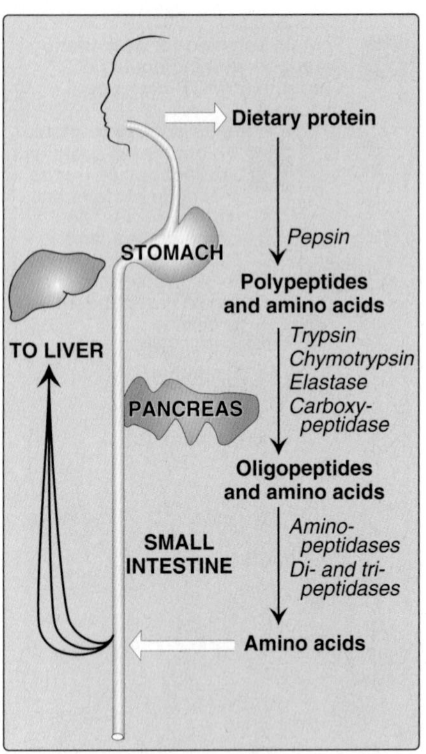

Figure 19.4
Digestion of dietary proteins by the proteolytic enzymes of the gastrointestinal tract.

1. **Hydrochloric acid:** Stomach acid is too dilute (pH 2–3) to hydrolyze proteins. The acid, secreted by the parietal cells of the stomach, functions instead to kill some bacteria and to denature proteins, thereby making them more susceptible to subsequent hydrolysis by *proteases*.

2. **Pepsin:** This acid-stable *endopeptidase* is secreted by the chief cells of the stomach as an inactive zymogen (or proenzyme), pepsinogen. [Note: In general, zymogens contain extra amino acids in their sequences that prevent them from being catalytically active. Removal of these amino acids permits the proper folding required for an active enzyme.] Pepsinogen is activated to *pepsin*, either by hydrochloric acid or autocatalytically by *pepsin* molecules that have already been activated. *Pepsin* releases peptides and a few free amino acids from dietary proteins.

B. Digestion by pancreatic enzymes

On entering the small intestine, large polypeptides produced in the stomach by the action of *pepsin* are further cleaved to oligopeptides and amino acids by a group of pancreatic *proteases* that include both *endopeptidases* (cleave within) and *exopeptidases* (cut at an end). [Note: Bicarbonate (HCO_3^-), also secreted by the pancreas, raises the pH.]

1. **Specificity:** Each of these enzymes has a different specificity for the amino acid R-groups adjacent to the susceptible peptide bond (Figure 19.5). For example, *trypsin* cleaves only when the carbonyl group of the peptide bond is contributed by arginine or lysine. These enzymes, like *pepsin* described above, are synthesized and secreted as inactive zymogens.

2. **Release of zymogens:** The release and activation of the pancreatic zymogens is mediated by the secretion of cholecystokinin and secretin, two polypeptide hormones of the digestive tract (see p. 176).

3. **Activation of zymogens:** *Enteropeptidase* (formerly called *enterokinase*), an enzyme synthesized by and present on the luminal surface of intestinal mucosal cells of the brush border membrane, converts the pancreatic zymogen trypsinogen to *trypsin* by removal of a hexapeptide from the N-terminus of trypsinogen. *Trypsin* subsequently converts other trypsinogen molecules to *trypsin* by cleaving a limited number of specific peptide bonds in the zymogen. *Enteropeptidase*, thus, unleashes a cascade of proteolytic activity because *trypsin* is the common activator of all the pancreatic zymogens (see Figure 19.5).

4. **Abnormalities in protein digestion:** In individuals with a deficiency in pancreatic secretion (for example, due to chronic pancreatitis, cystic fibrosis, or surgical removal of the pancreas), the digestion and absorption of fat and protein are incomplete. This results in the abnormal appearance of lipids in the feces (a condition called steatorrhea; see p. 177) as well as undigested protein.

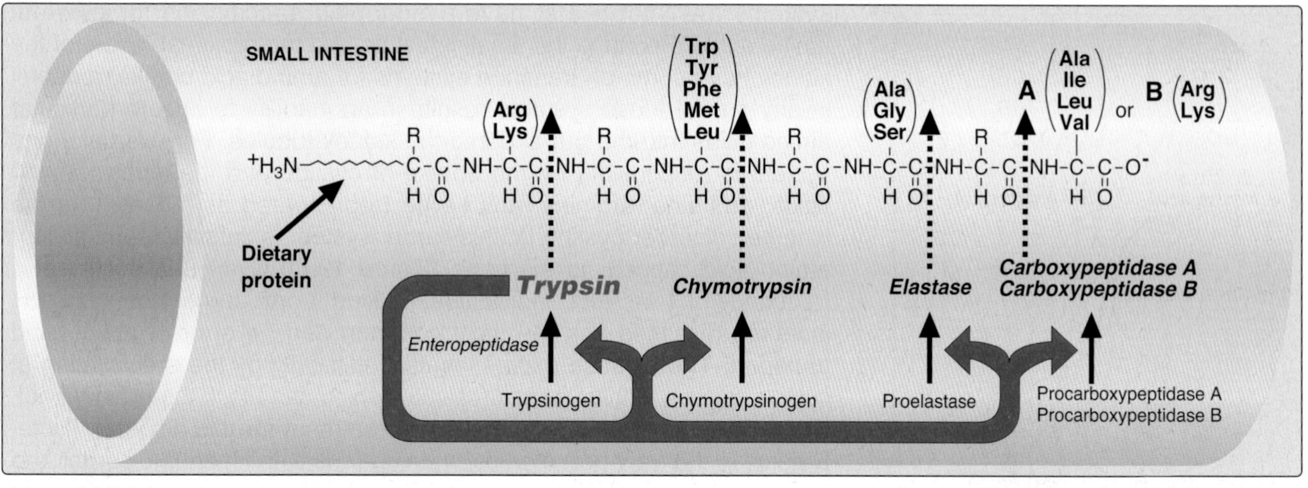

Figure 19.5
Cleavage of dietary protein in the small intestine by pancreatic *proteases*. The peptide bonds susceptible to hydrolysis are shown for each of the five major pancreatic *proteases*. [Note: The first three are serine *endopeptidases*, whereas the last two are *exopeptidases*. Each is produced from an inactive zymogen.]

Celiac disease (celiac sprue) is a disease of malabsorption resulting from immune-mediated damage to the small intestine in response to ingestion of gluten (or gliadin produced from gluten), a protein found in wheat, barley and rye.

C. Digestion of oligopeptides by enzymes of the small intestine

The luminal surface of the intestine contains *aminopeptidase,* an *exopeptidase* that repeatedly cleaves the N-terminal residue from oligopeptides to produce even smaller peptides and free amino acids.

D. Absorption of amino acids and small peptides

Free amino acids are taken into the enterocytes by a sodium-linked secondary transport system of the apical membrane. Di- and tripeptides, however, are taken up by a proton-linked transport system. The peptides are hydrolyzed in the cytosol to amino acids that are released into the portal system by facilitated diffusion. Therefore, only free amino acids are found in the portal vein after a meal containing protein. These amino acids are either metabolized by the liver or released into the general circulation. [Note: Branched-chain amino acids are important examples of amino acids that are not metabolized by the liver but, instead, are sent from the liver primarily to muscle via the blood.]

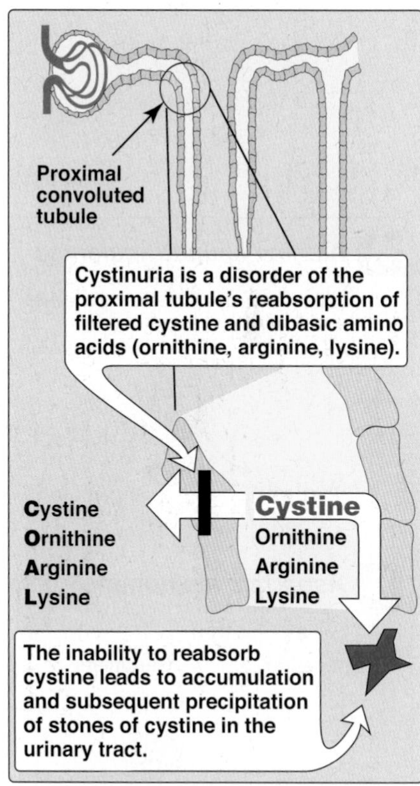

Figure 19.6
Genetic defect seen in cystinuria. [Note: Cystinuria is distinct from cystinosis, a rare defect in the transport of cystine out of lysosomes that results in the formation of cystine crystals within the lysosome and tissue damage.]

IV. TRANSPORT OF AMINO ACIDS INTO CELLS

The concentration of free amino acids in the extracellular fluids is significantly lower than that within the cells of the body. This concentration gradient is maintained because active transport systems, driven by the hydrolysis of ATP, are required for movement of amino acids from the extracellular space into cells. At least seven different transport

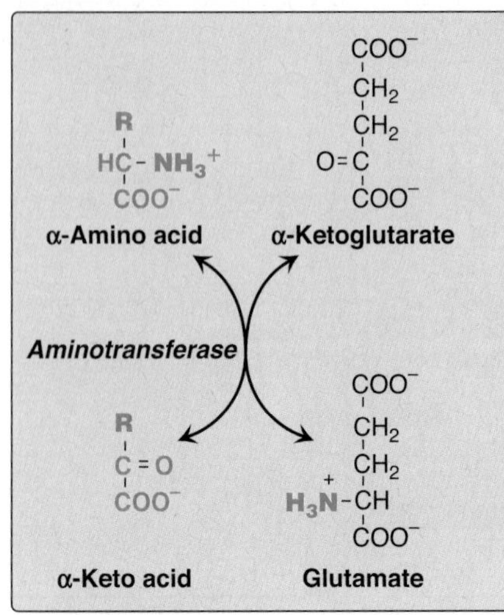

Figure 19.7
Aminotransferase reaction using α-ketoglutarate as the amino group acceptor.

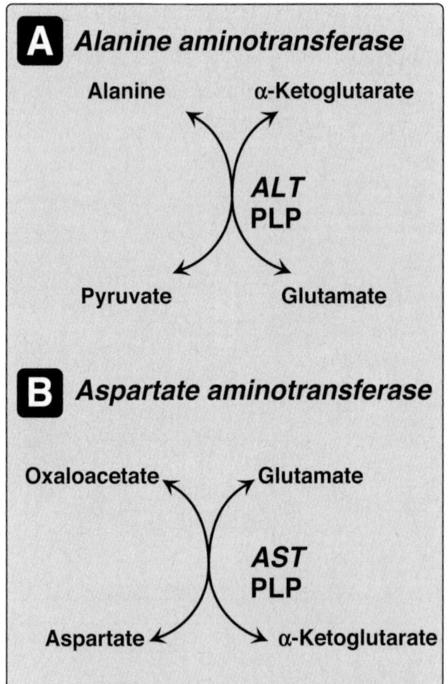

Figure 19.8
Reactions catalyzed during amino acid catabolism. A. *Alanine aminotransferase* (*ALT*). B. *Aspartate aminotransferase* (*AST*). PLP = pyridoxal phosphate (see p. 251).

systems are known that have overlapping specificities for different amino acids. Because the small intestine and the proximal tubule of the kidney have common transport systems for amino acid uptake, a defect in any one of these systems results in an inability to absorb particular amino acids into the gut and into the kidney tubules. For example, one system is responsible for the uptake of cystine and the dibasic amino acids, ornithine, arginine, and lysine (represented as "COAL"). In the inherited disorder cystinuria, this carrier system is defective, and all four amino acids appear in the urine (Figure 19.6). Cystinuria occurs at a frequency of 1 in 7,000 individuals, making it one of the most common inherited diseases and the most common genetic error of amino acid transport. The disease expresses itself clinically by the precipitation of cystine to form kidney stones (calculi), which can block the urinary tract. Oral hydration is an important part of treatment for this disorder. [Note: Defects in the transport of tryptophan can result in Hartnup disorder and pellagra-like (see p. 380) dermatologic and neurologic symptoms.]

V. REMOVAL OF NITROGEN FROM AMINO ACIDS

The presence of the α-amino group keeps amino acids safely locked away from oxidative breakdown. Removing the α-amino group is essential for producing energy from any amino acid and is an obligatory step in the catabolism of all amino acids. Once removed, this nitrogen can be incorporated into other compounds or excreted as urea, with the carbon skeletons being metabolized. This section describes transamination and oxidative deamination, reactions that ultimately provide ammonia and aspartate, the two sources of urea nitrogen (see p. 253).

A. Transamination: the funneling of amino groups to glutamate

The first step in the catabolism of most amino acids is the transfer of their α-amino group to α-ketoglutarate (Figure 19.7), producing an α-keto acid (derived from the original amino acid) and glutamate. α-Ketoglutarate plays a pivotal role in amino acid metabolism by accepting the amino groups from most amino acids, thereby becoming glutamate. Glutamate produced by transamination can be oxidatively deaminated (see below) or used as an amino group donor in the synthesis of nonessential amino acids. This transfer of amino groups from one carbon skeleton to another is catalyzed by a family of enzymes called *aminotransferases* (also called *transaminases*). These enzymes are found in the cytosol and mitochondria of cells throughout the body. All amino acids, with the exception of lysine and threonine, participate in transamination at some point in their catabolism. [Note: These two amino acids lose their α-amino groups by deamination (see pp. 265–266).]

1. **Substrate specificity of aminotransferases:** Each *aminotransferase* is specific for one or, at most, a few amino group donors. *Aminotransferases* are named after the specific amino group donor, because the acceptor of the amino group is almost always α-ketoglutarate. Two important *aminotransferase* reactions are catalyzed by *alanine aminotransferase* (*ALT*) *and aspartate aminotransferase* (*AST*), *as shown in* Figure 19.8).

   a. **Alanine aminotransferase:** *ALT* is present in many tissues. The enzyme catalyzes the transfer of the amino group of alanine to α-ketoglutarate, resulting in the formation of pyruvate and glutamate. The reaction is readily reversible. However, during amino acid catabolism, this enzyme (like most *aminotransferases*) functions in the direction of glutamate synthesis. [Note: Glutamate, in effect, acts as a "collector" of nitrogen from most amino acids.]

b. **Aspartate aminotransferase:** *AST* is an exception to the rule that *aminotransferases* funnel amino groups to form glutamate. During amino acid catabolism, *AST* transfers amino groups from glutamate to oxaloacetate, forming aspartate, which is used as a source of nitrogen in the urea cycle (see p. 253). Like other transaminations, the *AST* reaction is reversible.

2. **Mechanism of action of aminotransferases:** All *aminotransferases* require the coenzyme pyridoxal phosphate (a derivative of vitamin B_6; see p. 378), which is covalently linked to the ε-amino group of a specific lysine residue at the active site of the enzyme. *Aminotransferases* act by transferring the amino group of an amino acid to the pyridoxal part of the coenzyme to generate pyridoxamine phosphate. The pyridoxamine form of the coenzyme then reacts with an α-keto acid to form an amino acid, at the same time regenerating the original aldehyde form of the coenzyme. Figure 19.9 shows these two component reactions for the reaction catalyzed by *AST*.

3. **Equilibrium of transamination reactions:** For most transamination reactions, the equilibrium constant is near 1. This allows the reaction to function in both amino acid degradation through removal of α-amino groups (for example, after consumption of a protein-rich meal) and biosynthesis of nonessential amino acids through addition of amino groups to the carbon skeletons of α-keto acids (for example, when the supply of amino acids from the diet is not adequate to meet the synthetic needs of cells).

4. **Diagnostic value of plasma aminotransferases:** *Aminotransferases* are normally intracellular enzymes, with the low levels found in the plasma representing the release of cellular contents during normal cell turnover. Elevated plasma levels of *aminotransferases* indicate damage to cells rich in these enzymes. For example, physical trauma or a disease process can cause cell lysis, resulting in release of intracellular enzymes into the blood. Two *aminotransferases*, *AST* and *ALT*, are of particular diagnostic value when they are found in the plasma.

a. **Liver disease:** Plasma *AST* and *ALT* are elevated in nearly all liver diseases but are particularly high in conditions that cause extensive cell necrosis, such as severe viral hepatitis, toxic injury, and prolonged circulatory collapse. *ALT* is more specific than *AST* for liver disease, but the latter is more sensitive because the liver contains larger amounts of *AST*. Serial measurements of *AST* and *ALT* (so-called "liver function tests") are often useful in determining the course of liver damage. Figure 19.10 shows the early release of *ALT* into the serum, following ingestion of a liver toxin. [Note: Elevated serum bilirubin results from hepatocellular damage that decreases the hepatic conjugation and excretion of bilirubin (see p. 284).]

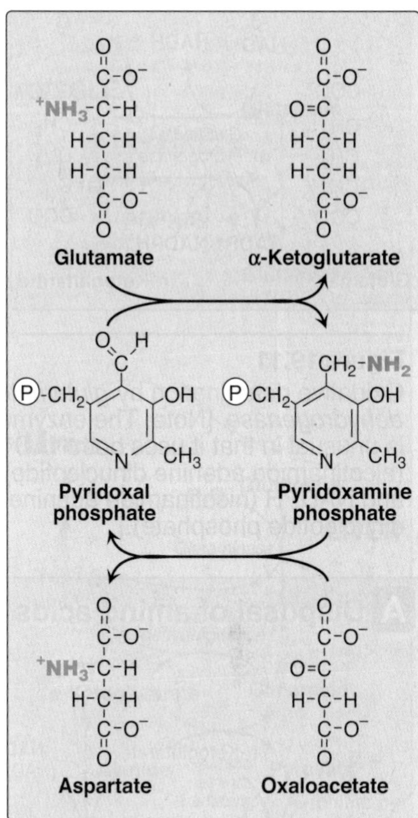

Figure 19.9
Cyclic interconversion of pyridoxal phosphate and pyridoxamine phosphate during the *aspartate aminotransferase* reaction. Ⓟ = phosphate group.

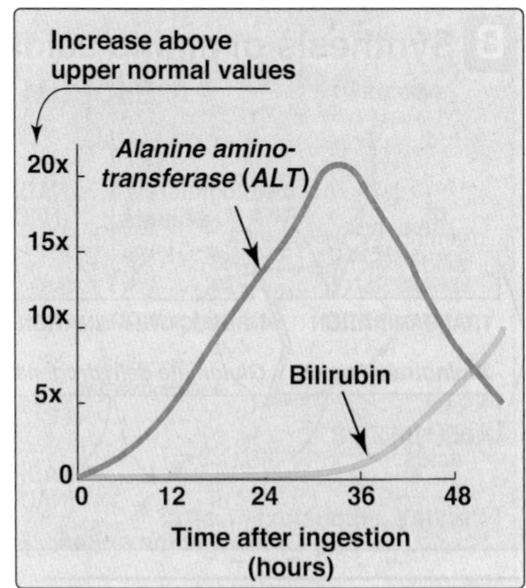

Figure 19.10
Pattern of serum *ALT* and bilirubin in the plasma, following poisoning with the toxic mushroom Amanita phalloides.

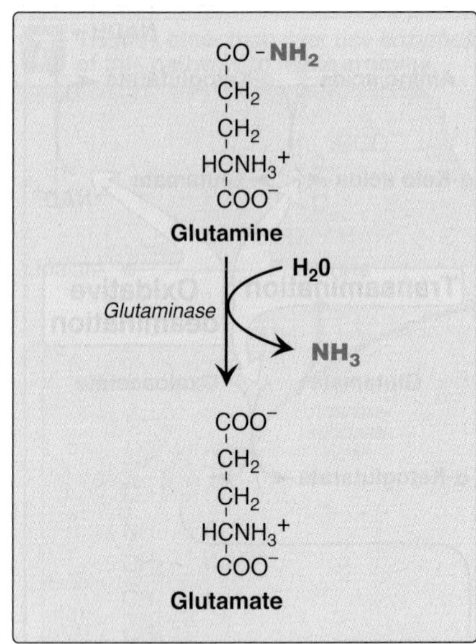

Figure 19.17
Hydrolysis of glutamine to form ammonia (NH_3).

B. Overall stoichiometry of the urea cycle

$$\text{Aspartate} + NH_3 + HCO_3^- + 3\,\text{ATP} + H_2O \longrightarrow$$
$$\text{urea} + \text{fumarate} + 2\,\text{ADP} + \text{AMP} + 2\,P_i + PP_i$$

Because four high-energy phosphate bonds are consumed in the synthesis of each molecule of urea, the synthesis of urea is irreversible, with a large, negative ΔG (see p. 70). One nitrogen of the urea molecule is supplied by free NH_3, and the other nitrogen by aspartate. Glutamate is the immediate precursor of both ammonia (through oxidative deamination by *glutamate dehydrogenase*) and aspartate nitrogen (through transamination of oxaloacetate by *AST*). In effect, both nitrogen atoms of urea arise from glutamate, which, in turn, gathers nitrogen from other amino acids (Figure 19.15).

C. Regulation of the urea cycle

N-Acetylglutamate (NAG) is an essential activator for *CPS I*, the rate-limiting step in the urea cycle. It increases the affinity of *CPS I* for ATP. NAG is synthesized from acetyl CoA and glutamate by *N-acetylglutamate synthase* (Figure 19.16) in a reaction for which arginine is an activator. The cycle is also regulated by substrate availability (short-term regulation) and enzyme induction (long term).

VII. METABOLISM OF AMMONIA

Ammonia is produced by all tissues during the metabolism of a variety of compounds, and it is disposed of primarily by formation of urea in the liver. However, the level of ammonia in the blood must be kept very low, because even slightly elevated concentrations (hyperammonemia) are toxic to the central nervous system (CNS). Therefore, there must be a metabolic mechanism by which nitrogen is moved from peripheral tissues to the liver for ultimate disposal as urea, at the same time maintaining low levels of circulating ammonia.

A. Sources of ammonia

Amino acids are quantitatively the most important source of ammonia because most Western diets are high in protein and provide excess amino acids, which travel to the liver and undergo transdeamination (that is, the linking of *aminotransferase* and *glutamate dehydrogenase* reactions), producing ammonia. [Note: Liver catabolizes straight-chain amino acids, primarily.] However, substantial amounts of ammonia can be obtained from other sources.

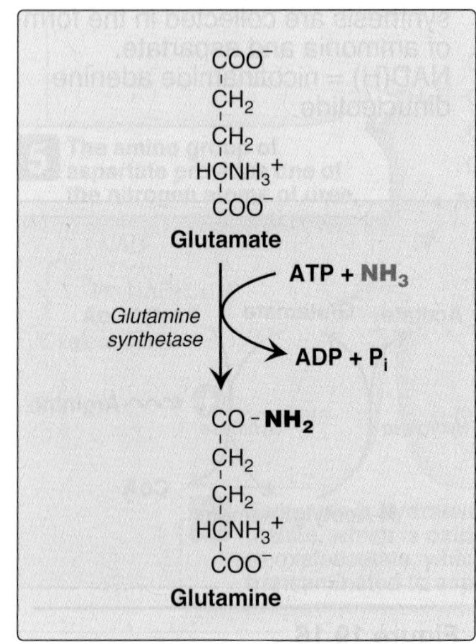

Figure 19.18
Synthesis of glutamine.
ADP = adenosine diphosphate;
P_i = inorganic phosphate.

1. **From glutamine:** An important source of plasma glutamine is from the catabolism of branched-chain amino acids in skeletal muscle. This glutamine is taken up by cells of the intestine, the liver, and the kidney.The liver and kidneys generate ammonia from glutamine by the actions of *glutaminase* (Figure 19.17) and *glutamate dehydrogenase*. In the kidneys, most of this ammonia is excreted into the urine as NH_4^+, which provides an important mechanism for maintaining the body's acid–base balance through the excretion of protons. In the liver, the ammonia is detoxified to urea and excreted. [Note: α-Ketoglutarate, the second product of *glutamate dehydrogenase*, is a glucogenic precursor in liver and kidney.]

Ammonia is also generated by intestinal *glutaminase*. The intestinal mucosal cells obtain glutamine either from the blood or from digestion of dietary protein. [Note: Intestinal glutamine metabolism also produces alanine, which is used by the liver for gluconeogenesis, and citrulline, which is used by the kidneys to synthesize arginine.]

2. **From bacterial action in the intestine:** Ammonia is formed from urea by the action of bacterial *urease* in the lumen of the intestine. This ammonia is absorbed from the intestine by way of the portal vein, and virtually all is removed by the liver via conversion to urea.

3. **From amines:** Amines obtained from the diet and monoamines that serve as hormones or neurotransmitters give rise to ammonia by the action of *monoamine oxidase* (see p. 286).

4. **From purines and pyrimidines:** In the catabolism of purines and pyrimidines, amino groups attached to the ring atoms are released as ammonia (see Figure 22.15 and p. 304).

B. Transport of ammonia in the circulation

Although ammonia is constantly produced in the tissues, it is present at very low levels in blood. This is due both to the rapid removal of blood ammonia by the liver and to the fact that several tissues, particularly muscle, release amino acid nitrogen in the form of glutamine or alanine, rather than as free ammonia (see Figure 19.13).

1. **Urea:** Formation of urea in the liver is quantitatively the most important disposal route for ammonia. Urea travels in the blood from the liver to the kidneys, where it passes into the glomerular filtrate.

2. **Glutamine:** This amide of glutamate provides a nontoxic storage and transport form of ammonia (Figure 19.18). The ATP-requiring formation of glutamine from glutamate and ammonia by *glutamine synthetase* occurs primarily in skeletal muscle and liver but is also important in the CNS, where it is the major mechanism for the removal of ammonia in the brain. Glutamine is found in plasma at concentrations higher than other amino acids, a finding consistent with its transport function. [Note: The liver keeps blood ammonia levels low through *glutaminase* and the urea cycle in periportal (close to inflow of blood) hepatocytes and via *glutamine synthetase* as an ammonia "scavenger" in the perivenous hepatocytes.] The metabolism of ammonia is summarized in Figure 19.19.

C. Hyperammonemia

The capacity of the hepatic urea cycle exceeds the normal rates of ammonia generation, and the levels of serum ammonia are normally low (5–35 µmol/l). However, when liver function is compromised, due either to genetic defects of the urea cycle or liver disease, blood levels can rise above 1,000 µmol/l. Such hyperammonemia is a medical emergency, because ammonia has a direct neurotoxic effect on the CNS. For example, elevated concentrations of ammonia in the blood cause the symptoms of ammonia intoxication, which include tremors, slurring of speech, somnolence (drowsiness), vomiting, cerebral edema, and blurring of vision. At high concentrations, ammonia can cause coma and death. There are two major types of hyperammonemia.

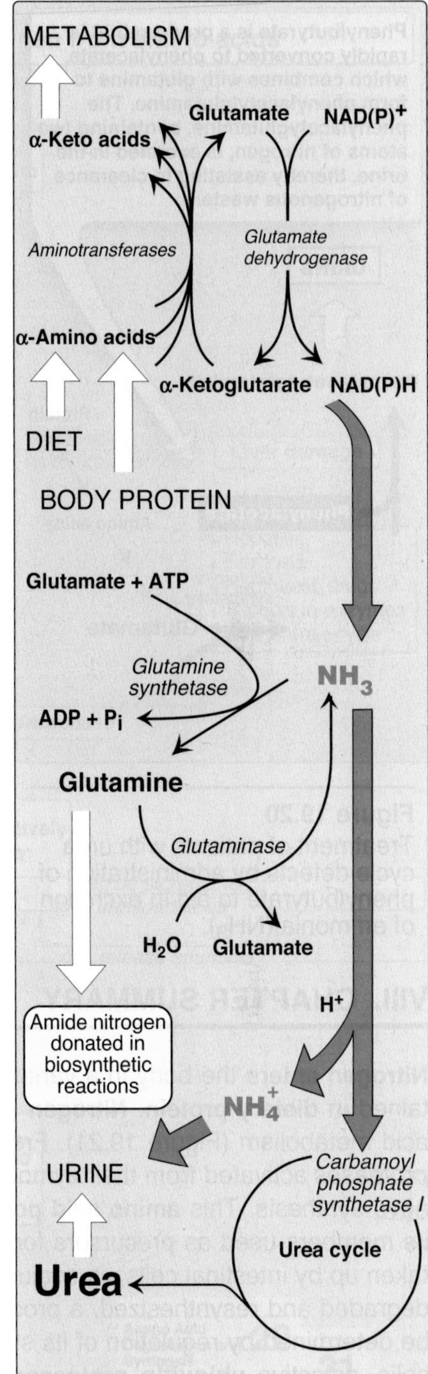

Figure 19.19
Metabolism of ammonia (NH_3). [Note: *Glutamate dehydrogenase* is one of several sources of NH_3.] Urea content in the urine is reported as urinary urea nitrogen, or UUN. Urea in blood is reported as BUN (blood urea nitrogen). The enzymes *glutamate dehydrogenase*, *glutamine synthetase*, and *carbamoyl phosphate synthetase I* fix NH_3 into organic molecules.

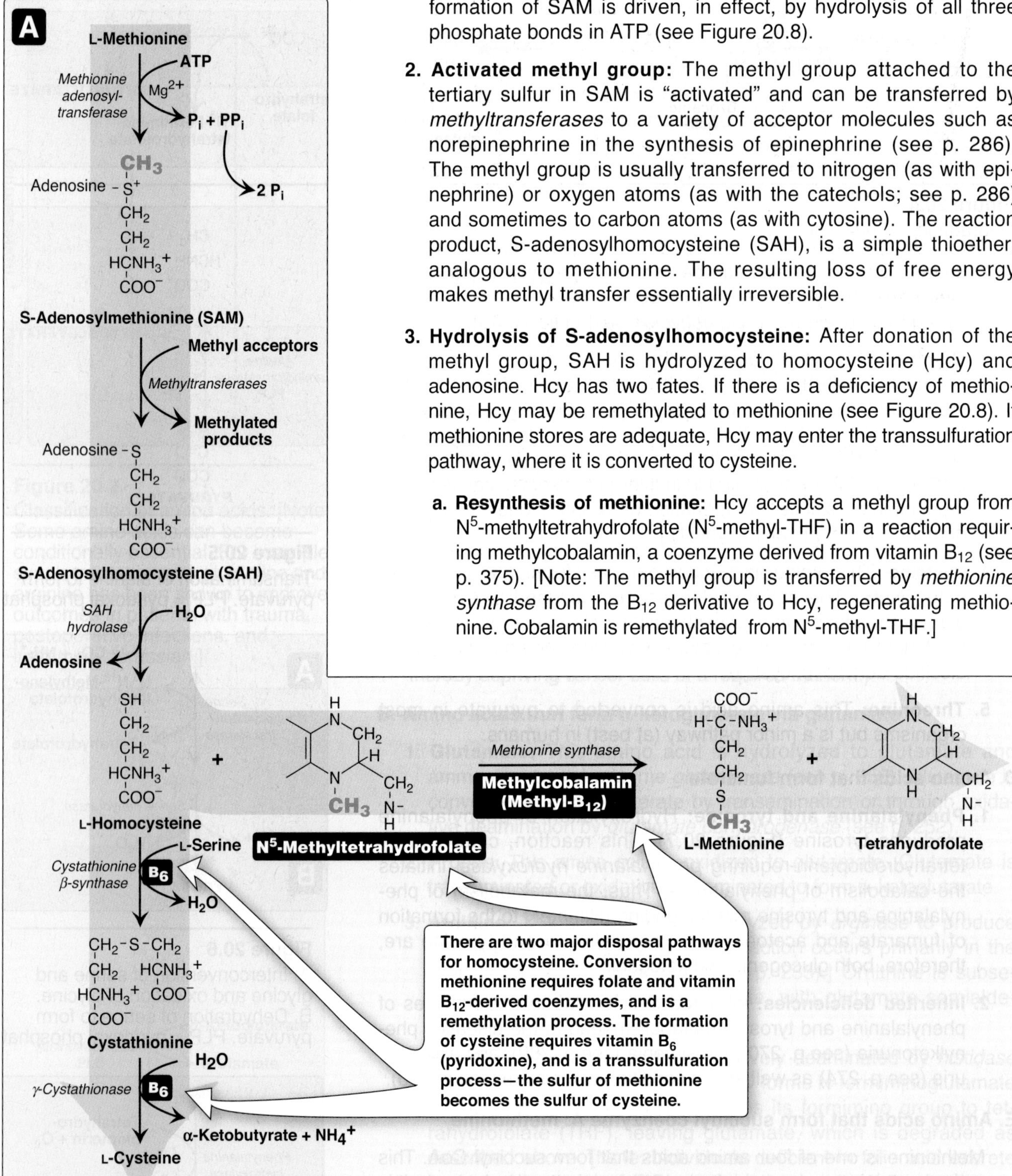

formation of SAM is driven, in effect, by hydrolysis of all three phosphate bonds in ATP (see Figure 20.8).

2. **Activated methyl group:** The methyl group attached to the tertiary sulfur in SAM is "activated" and can be transferred by *methyltransferases* to a variety of acceptor molecules such as norepinephrine in the synthesis of epinephrine (see p. 286). The methyl group is usually transferred to nitrogen (as with epinephrine) or oxygen atoms (as with the catechols; see p. 286) and sometimes to carbon atoms (as with cytosine). The reaction product, S-adenosylhomocysteine (SAH), is a simple thioether, analogous to methionine. The resulting loss of free energy makes methyl transfer essentially irreversible.

3. **Hydrolysis of S-adenosylhomocysteine:** After donation of the methyl group, SAH is hydrolyzed to homocysteine (Hcy) and adenosine. Hcy has two fates. If there is a deficiency of methionine, Hcy may be remethylated to methionine (see Figure 20.8). If methionine stores are adequate, Hcy may enter the transsulfuration pathway, where it is converted to cysteine.

    a. **Resynthesis of methionine:** Hcy accepts a methyl group from N^5-methyltetrahydrofolate (N^5-methyl-THF) in a reaction requiring methylcobalamin, a coenzyme derived from vitamin B_{12} (see p. 375). [Note: The methyl group is transferred by *methionine synthase* from the B_{12} derivative to Hcy, regenerating methionine. Cobalamin is remethylated from N^5-methyl-THF.]

Figure 20.8
Degradation and resynthesis of methionine. [Note: The resynthesis of methionine from homocysteine is the only reaction in which tetrahydrofolate both carries and donates a methyl ($-CH_3$) group. In all other reactions, SAM is the methyl group carrier and donor.] PP_i = pyrophosphate; P_i = inorganic phosphate.

b. **Synthesis of cysteine:** Hcy condenses with serine, forming cystathionine, which is hydrolyzed to α-ketobutyrate and cysteine (see Figure 20.8). This vitamin B_6–requiring sequence has the net effect of converting serine to cysteine and Hcy to α-ketobutyrate, which is oxidatively decarboxylated to form propionyl CoA. Propionyl CoA is converted to succinyl CoA (see p. 194). Because Hcy is synthesized from the essential amino acid methionine, cysteine is not an essential amino acid as long as sufficient methionine is available.

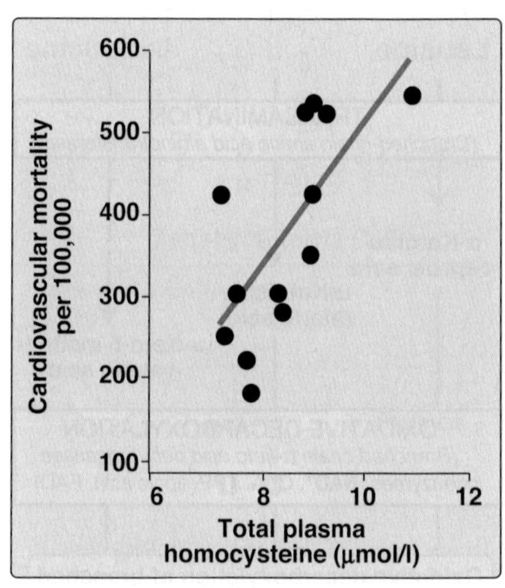

Figure 20.9
Association between cardiovascular disease mortality and total plasma homocysteine.

4. **Relationship of homocysteine to vascular disease:** Elevations in plasma Hcy levels promote oxidative damage, inflammation, and endothelial dysfunction and are an independent risk factor for occlusive vascular disease (Figure 20.9). Mild elevations are seen in about 7% of the population. Epidemiologic studies have shown that plasma Hcy levels are inversely related to plasma levels of folate, B_{12}, and B_6, the three vitamins involved in the conversion of Hcy to methionine or cysteine. Supplementation with these vitamins has been shown to reduce circulating levels of Hcy. However, in patients with established cardiovascular disease, vitamin therapy does not decrease cardiovascular events or death. This raises the question as to whether Hcy is a cause of the vascular damage or merely a marker of such damage. [Note: Large elevations in plasma Hcy as a result of rare deficiencies in *cystathionine β-synthase* of the transsulfuration pathway are seen in patients with classic homocystinuria. These individuals experience premature vascular disease, with about 25% dying from thrombotic complications before age 30 years.] Deficiencies in the remethylation reaction also result in a rise in Hcy.

> Elevated homocysteine and decreased folic acid levels in pregnant women are associated with increased incidence of neural tube defects (improper closure, as in spina bifida) in the fetus. Periconceptual supplementation with folate reduces the risk of such defects.

F. Other amino acids that form succinyl coenzyme A

Degradation of valine, isoleucine, and threonine also results in the production of succinyl CoA, a TCA cycle intermediate and glucogenic compound.

1. **Valine and isoleucine:** These amino acids are branched-chain amino acids (BCAAs) that generate propionyl CoA, which is converted to methylmalonyl CoA and then succinyl CoA by biotin- and vitamin B_{12}–requiring reactions (Figure 20.10).

2. **Threonine:** This amino acid is dehydrated to α-ketobutyrate, which is converted to propionyl CoA and then to succinyl CoA. Propionyl CoA, then, is generated by the catabolism of the amino acids methionine, valine, isoleucine, and threonine. [Note: Propionyl CoA also is generated by the oxidation of odd-numbered fatty acids (see p. 193).]

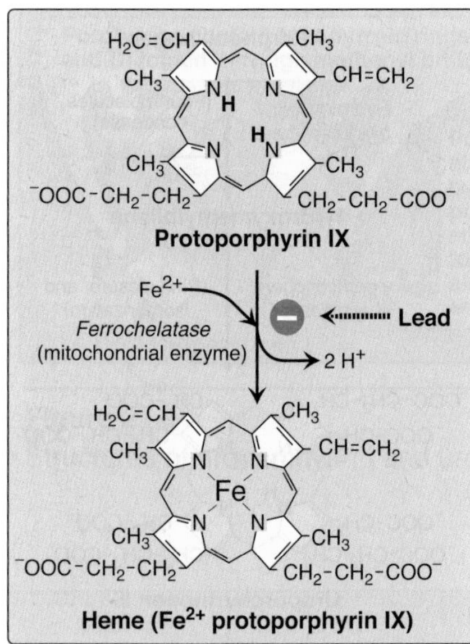

Figure 21.5
Pathway of porphyrin synthesis: formation of heme. (Continued from Figures 21.3 and 21.4.) Fe^{2+} = ferrous iron.

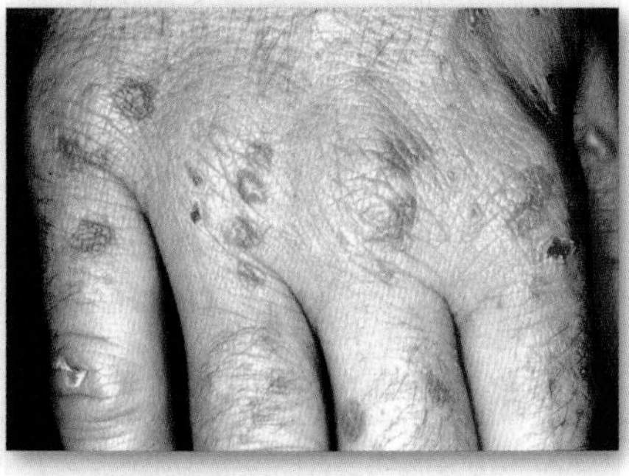

Figure 21.6
Skin eruptions in a patient with porphyria cutanea tarda.

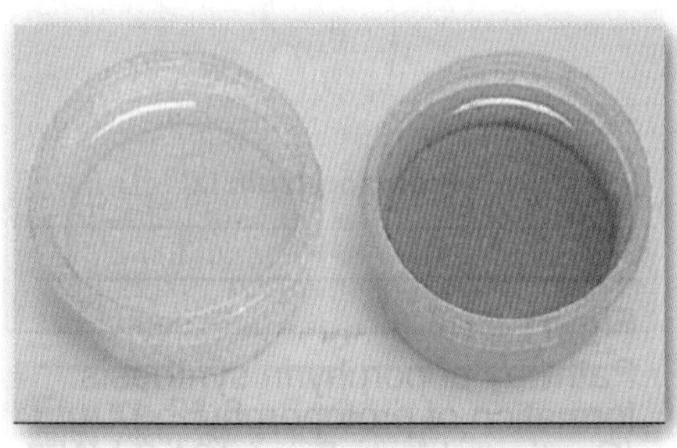

Figure 21.7
Urine from a patient with porphyria cutanea tarda (right) and from a patient with normal porphyrin excretion (left).

general, individuals with an enzyme defect prior to the synthesis of the tetrapyrroles manifest abdominal and neuropsychiatric signs, whereas those with enzyme defects leading to the accumulation of tetrapyrrole intermediates show photosensitivity (that is, their skin itches and burns [pruritus] when exposed to visible light). [Note: Photosenstivity is a result of the oxidation of colorless porphyrinogens to colored porphyrins, which are photosensitizing molecules thought to participate in the formation of superoxide radicals from oxygen. These reactive oxygen species can oxidatively damage membranes and cause the release of destructive enzymes from lysosomes.]

a. **Chronic hepatic porphyria:** Porphyria cutanea tarda, the most common porphyria, is a chronic disease of the liver. The disease is associated with a deficiency in *uroporphyrinogen decarboxylase,* but clinical expression of the enzyme deficiency is influenced by various factors, such as hepatic iron overload, exposure to sunlight, alcohol ingestion, estrogen therapy, and the presence of hepatitis B or C or HIV infections. Clinical onset is typically during the fourth or fifth decade of life. Porphyrin accumulation leads to cutaneous symptoms (Figure 21.6) as well as urine that is red to brown in natural light (Figure 21.7) and pink to red in fluorescent light.

b. **Acute hepatic porphyrias:** Acute hepatic porphyrias (*ALA dehydratase* deficiency porphyria, acute intermittent porphyria, hereditary coproporphyria, and variegate porphyria) are characterized by acute attacks of gastrointestinal (GI), neuropsychiatric, and motor symptoms that may be accompanied by photosensitivity. Porphyrias leading to accumulation of ALA and porphobilinogen, such as acute intermittent porphyria, cause abdominal pain and neuropsychiatric disturbances, ranging from anxiety to delirium. Symptoms of the acute hepatic porphyrias are often precipitated by use of drugs, such as barbiturates and ethanol, which induce the synthesis of the heme-containing *CYP* microsomal drug oxidation system. This further decreases the amount of available heme, which, in turn, promotes increased synthesis of *ALAS1*.

c. **Erythropoietic porphyrias:** The chronic erythropoietic porphyrias (congenital erythropoietic porphyria and erythropoietic protoporphyria) are characterized by skin rashes and blisters that appear in early childhood. [Note: Patients with erythropoietic protoporphyria are also at risk for hepatobiliary disease.]

2. **Increased δ-aminolevulinic acid synthase activity:** One common feature of the porphyrias is a decreased synthesis of heme. In the liver, heme normally functions as a repressor of the gene for *ALAS1*. Therefore, the absence of this end product results in an increase in the synthesis of *ALAS1* (derepression). This causes an increased synthesis of intermediates that occur prior to the genetic block. The accumulation of these toxic intermediates is the major pathophysiology of the porphyrias.

3. **Treatment:** During acute porphyria attacks, patients require medical support, particularly treatment for pain and vomiting. The severity of acute symptoms of the porphyrias can be diminished

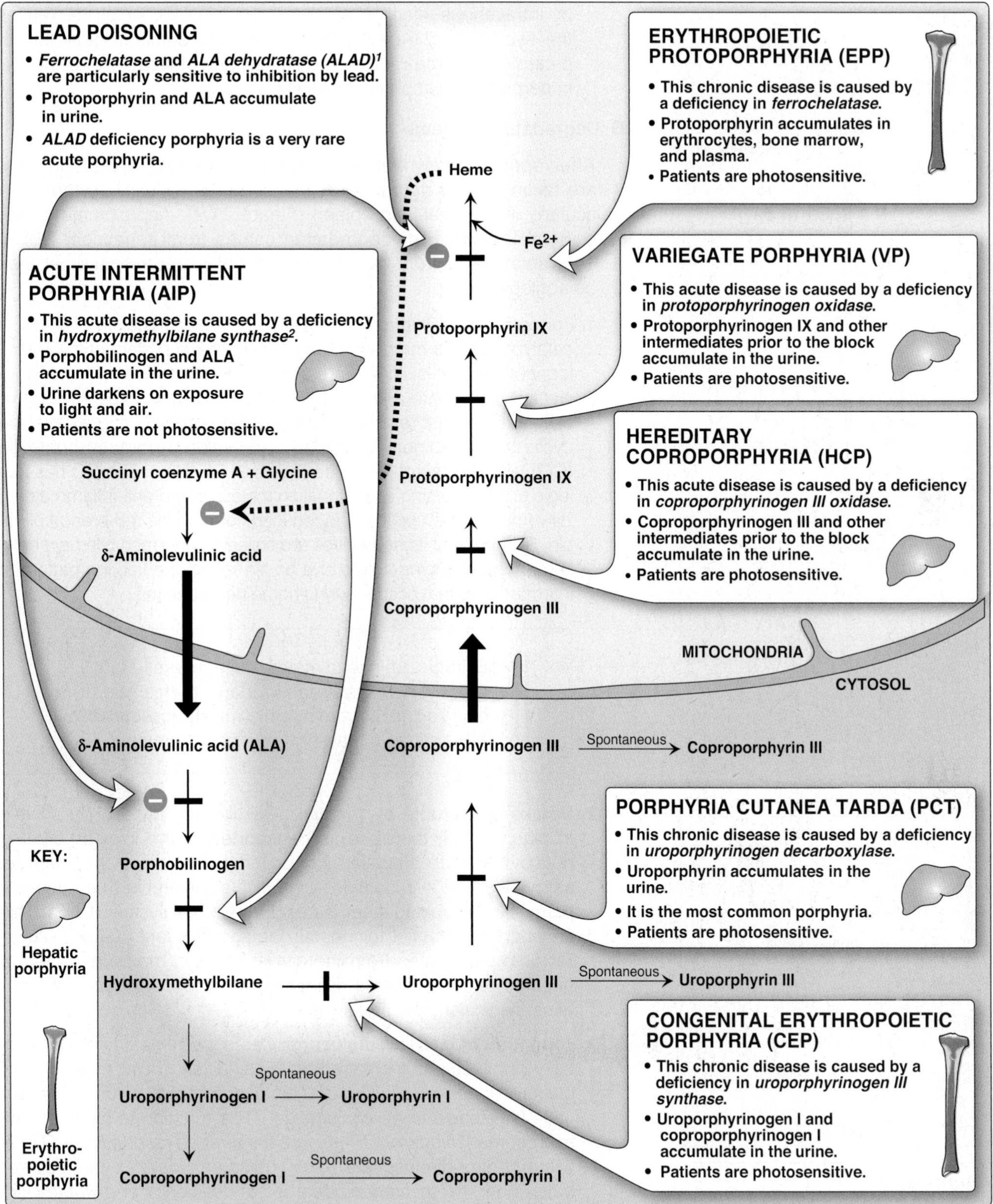

Figure 21.8

Summary of heme synthesis. [1]Also referred to as *porphobilinogen synthase*. [2]Also referred to as *porphobilinogen deaminase*. [Note: Deficiencies in *ALA synthase-1* (*ALAS1*) are unknown. Deficiencies in *ALAS2* result in an anemia, not a porphyria.]

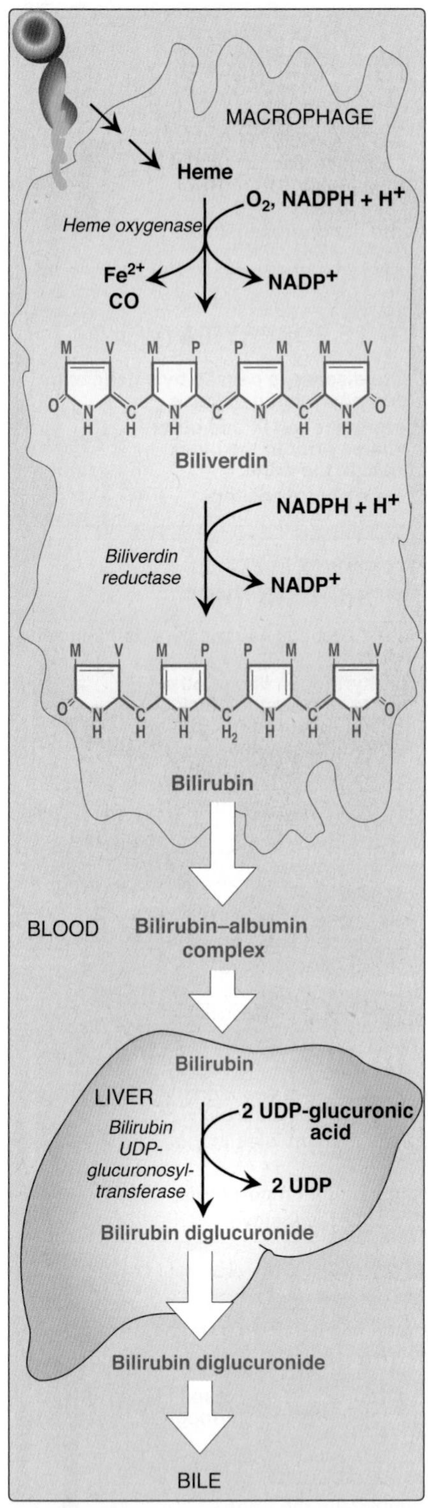

Figure 21.9
Formation of bilirubin from heme and its conversion to bilirubin diglucuronide. UDP = uridine diphosphate; CO = carbon monoxide; NADP(H) = nicotinamide adenine dinucleotide phosphate.

by intravenous injection of hemin and glucose, which decreases the synthesis of *ALAS1*. Protection from sunlight, ingestion of β-carotene (a free-radical scavenger), and phlebotomy are helpful in porphyrias with photosensitivity.

D. Degradation of heme

After approximately 120 days in the circulation, red blood cells are taken up and degraded by the reticuloendothelial system, particularly in the liver and spleen (Figure 21.9). Approximately 85% of heme destined for degradation comes from senescent RBCs. The remainder is from the degradation of heme proteins other than hemoglobin.

1. **Formation of bilirubin:** The first step in the degradation of heme is catalyzed by the microsomal *heme oxygenase* system of the reticuloendothelial cells. In the presence of nicotinamide adenine dinucleotide phosphate and O_2, the enzyme catalyzes three successive oxygenations that result in opening of the porphyrin ring (converting cyclic heme to linear biliverdin), production of carbon monoxide (CO), and release of Fe^{2+} (see Figure 21.9). [Note: The CO has biologic function, acting as a signaling molecule and anti-inflammatory.] Biliverdin, a green pigment, is reduced, forming the red-orange bilirubin. Bilirubin and its derivatives are collectively termed bile pigments. [Note: The changing colors of a bruise reflect the varying pattern of intermediates that occurs during heme degradation.]

> Bilirubin, unique to mammals, appears to function at low levels as an antioxidant. In this role, it is oxidized to biliverdin, which is then reduced by *biliverdin reductase*, regenerating bilirubin.

2. **Uptake of bilirubin by the liver:** Bilirubin is only slightly soluble in plasma and, therefore, is transported to the liver by binding noncovalently to albumin. [Note: Certain anionic drugs, such as salicylates and sulfonamides, can displace bilirubin from albumin, permitting bilirubin to enter the central nervous system (CNS). This causes the potential for neural damage in infants (see p. 285).] Bilirubin dissociates from the carrier albumin molecule; enters a hepatocyte via facilitated diffusion; and binds to intracellular proteins, particularly the protein ligandin.
3. **Formation of bilirubin diglucuronide:** In the hepatocyte, the solubility of bilirubin is increased by the addition of two molecules of glucuronic acid, producing bilirubin diglucuronide. [Note: This process is referred to as conjugation.] The reaction is catalyzed by microsomal *bilirubin UDP-glucuronosyltransferase* (*bilirubin UGT*) using uridine diphosphate (UDP)-glucuronic acid as the glucuronate donor. [Note: Varying degrees of deficiency of *bilirubin UGT* result in Crigler-Najjar I and II and Gilbert syndrome, with Crigler-Najjar I being the most severe deficiency.]
4. **Secretion of bilirubin into bile:** Bilirubin diglucuronide (conjugated bilirubin [CB]) is actively transported against a concentration gradient into the bile canaliculi and then into the bile. This

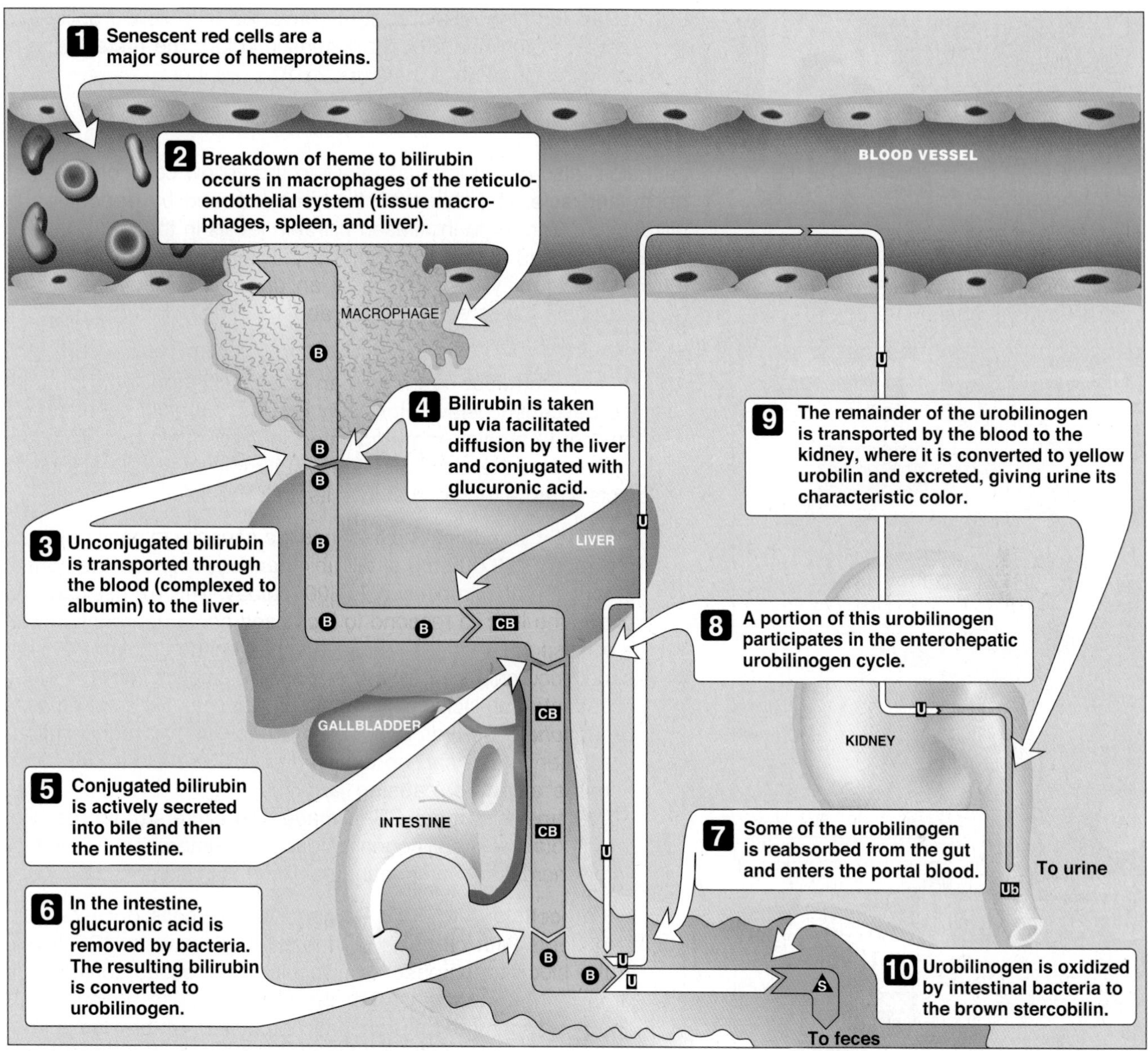

Figure 21.10
Catabolism of heme B = bilirubin; CB = conjugated bilirubin; U = urobilinogen; Ub = urobilin; S = stercobilin.

energy-dependent, rate-limiting step is susceptible to impairment in liver disease. [Note: A rare deficiency in the protein required for transport of CB out of the liver results in Dubin-Johnson syndrome.] Unconjugated bilirubin (UCB) is normally not secreted into bile.

5. **Formation of urobilins in the intestine:** Bilirubin diglucuronide is hydrolyzed and reduced by bacteria in the gut to yield urobilinogen, a colorless compound. Most of the urobilinogen is oxidized by intestinal bacteria to stercobilin, which gives feces the characteristic brown color. However, some of the urobilinogen is reabsorbed from the gut and enters the portal blood. A portion of this urobilinogen participates in the enterohepatic urobilinogen cycle in which it is taken up by the liver and then resecreted into the bile. The remainder of the urobilinogen is transported by the

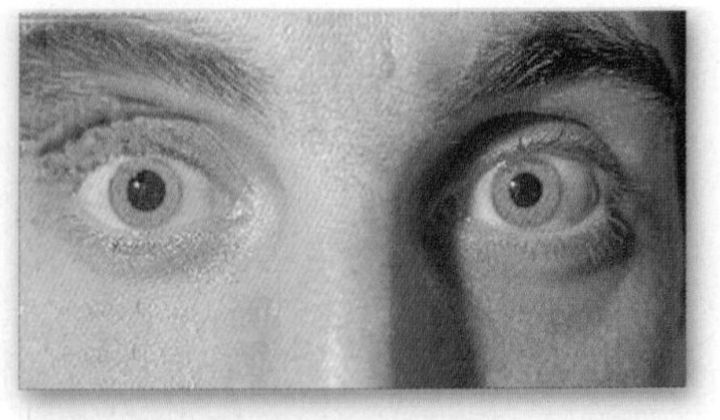

Figure 21.11
Jaundiced patient, with the sclerae of his eyes appearing yellow.

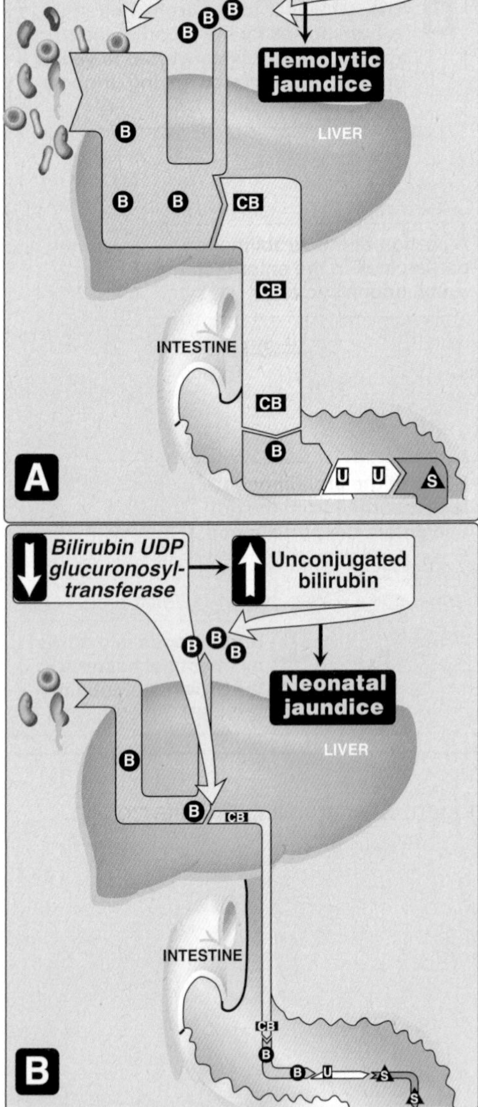

Figure 21.12
Alterations in the metabolism of heme.
A. Hemolytic jaundice. B. Neonatal jaundice.
CB = conjugated bilirubin; B = bilirubin;
U = urobilinogen; S = stercobilin;
UDP = uridine diphosphate.

blood to the kidney, where it is converted to yellow urobilin and excreted, giving urine its characteristic color. The metabolism of bilirubin is summarized in Figure 21.10.

E. Jaundice

Jaundice (also called icterus) refers to the yellow color of skin, nail beds, and sclerae (whites of the eyes) caused by deposition of bilirubin, secondary to increased bilirubin levels in the blood (hyperbilirubinemia) as shown in Figure 21.11. Although not a disease, jaundice is usually a symptom of an underlying disorder. [Note: Blood bilirubin levels are normally about 1 mg/dl. Jaundice is seen at 2–3 mg/dl.]

1. **Types of jaundice:** Jaundice can be classified into three major types described below. However, in clinical practice, jaundice is often more complex than indicated in this simple classification. For example, the accumulation of bilirubin may be a result of defects at more than one step in its metabolism.

   a. **Hemolytic jaundice:** The liver has the capacity to conjugate and excrete over 3,000 mg of bilirubin per day, whereas the normal production of bilirubin is only 300 mg/day. This excess capacity allows the liver to respond to increased heme degradation with a corresponding increase in conjugation and secretion of bilirubin diglucuronide. However, extensive hemolysis (for example, in patients with sickle cell anemia or *pyruvate kinase* or *glucose 6-phosphate dehydrogenase* deficiency) may produce bilirubin faster than it can be conjugated. UCB levels in the blood become elevated, causing jaundice (Figure 21.12A). [Note: With hemolysis, more CB is made and excreted into the bile, the amount of urobilinogen entering the enterohepatic circulation is increased, and urinary urobilinogen is increased.]

   b. **Hepatocellular jaundice:** Damage to liver cells (for example, in patients with cirrhosis or hepatitis) can cause UCB levels in the blood to increase as a result of decreased conjugation. Urobilinogen is increased in the urine because hepatic damage decreases the enterohepatic circulation of this compound, allowing more to enter the blood, from which it is filtered into the urine. The urine consequently darkens, whereas stools may be a pale, clay color. Plasma levels of *alanine* and *aspartate transaminases* (*AST* and *ALT*, respectively; see p. 251) are elevated. [Note: If CB is made but is not efficiently secreted from the liver into bile (intrahepatic cholestasis), it can diffuse ("leak") into the blood, causing a conjugated hyperbilirubinemia.]

   c. **Obstructive jaundice:** In this instance, jaundice is not caused by overproduction of bilirubin or decreased conjugation but, instead, results from obstruction of the common bile duct (extrahepatic cholestasis). For example, the presence of a tumor or bile stones may block the duct, preventing passage of CB into the intestine. Patients with obstructive jaundice experience GI pain and nausea and produce stools that are a pale, clay color. The liver "regurgitates" CB into the blood (hyperbilirubinemia). The CB is eventually excreted in the urine (which darkens upon standing), and is referred to as "urinary bilirubin." Urinary urobilinogen is absent.

2. **Jaundice in newborns:** The majority of newborn infants (60% of full term and 80% of preterm) show a rise in UCB in the first postnatal week (and a transient, "physiologic" jaundice) because the activity of hepatic *bilirubin UGT* is low at birth (it reaches adult levels in about 4 weeks) as shown in Figures 21.12B and 21.13. Elevated UCB, in excess of the binding capacity of albumin (20–25 mg/dl), can diffuse into the basal ganglia, cause toxic encephalopathy (kernicterus) and a pathologic jaundice. Therefore, newborns with significantly elevated bilirubin levels are treated with blue fluorescent light (phototherapy), as shown in Figure 21.14, which converts bilirubin to more polar and, therefore, water-soluble isomers. These photoisomers can be excreted into the bile without conjugation to glucuronic acid. [Note: Because of solubility differences, only UCB crosses the blood brain barrier, and only CB appears in urine.]

3. **Determination of bilirubin concentration:** Bilirubin is commonly measured by the van den Bergh reaction, in which diazotized sulfanilic acid reacts with bilirubin to form red azodipyrroles that are measured colorimetrically. In aqueous solution, the water-soluble CB reacts rapidly with the reagent (within one minute), and is said to be "direct-reacting." The UCB, which is much less soluble in aqueous solution, reacts more slowly. However, when the reaction is carried out in methanol, both CB and UCB are soluble and react with the reagent, providing the total bilirubin value. The "indirect-reacting" bilirubin, which corresponds to the UCB, is obtained by subtracting the direct-reacting bilirubin from the total bilirubin. [Note: In normal plasma, only about 4% of the total bilirubin is conjugated or direct-reacting, because most is secreted into bile.]

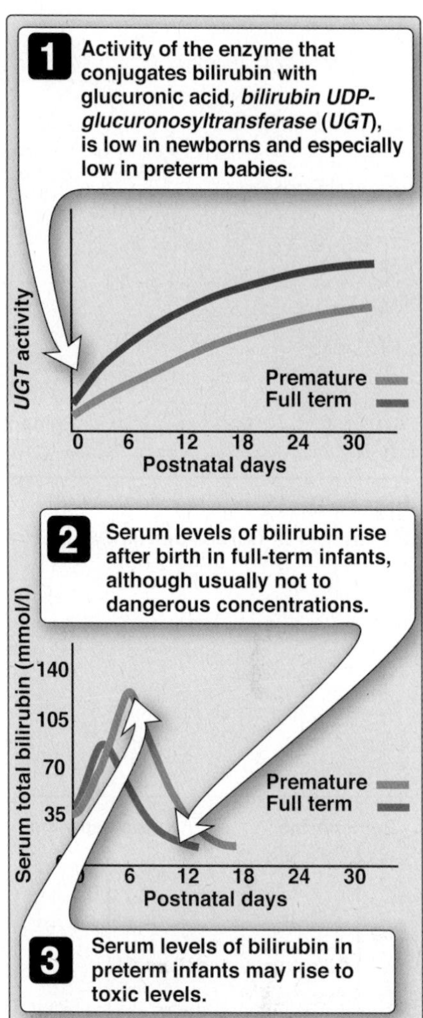

Figure 21.13
Neonatal jaundice. UDP = uridine diphosphate.

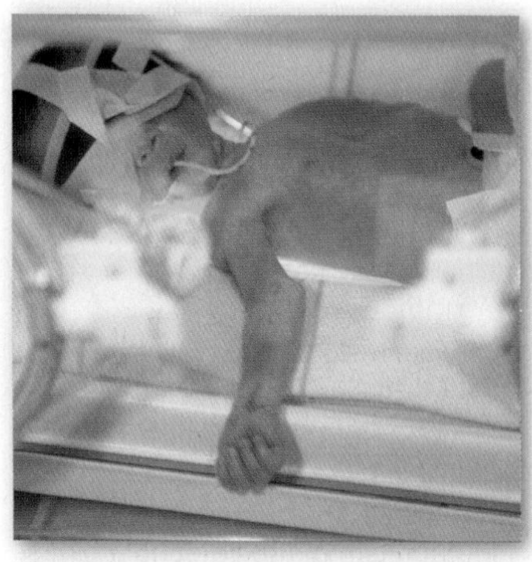

Figure 21.14
Phototherapy in neonatal jaudice.

III. OTHER NITROGEN-CONTAINING COMPOUNDS

A. Catecholamines

Dopamine, norepinephrine, and epinephrine are biologically active (biogenic) amines that are collectively termed catecholamines. Dopamine and norepinephrine are synthesized in the brain and function as neurotransmitters. Norepinephrine is also synthesized in the adrenal medulla, as is epinephrine.

1. **Function:** Outside the CNS, norepinephrine and its methylated derivative, epinephrine, are hormone regulators of carbohydrate and lipid metabolism. Norepinephrine and epinephrine are released from storage vesicles in the adrenal medulla in response to fright, exercise, cold, and low levels of blood glucose. They increase the degradation of glycogen and triacylglycerol as well as increase blood pressure and the output of the heart. These effects are part of a coordinated response to prepare the individual for stress, and are often called the "fight-or-flight" reactions.

2. **Synthesis:** The catecholamines are synthesized from tyrosine, as shown in Figure 21.15. Tyrosine is first hydroxylated by *tyrosine hydroxylase* to form 3,4-dihydroxyphenylalanine (DOPA) in a reaction analogous to that described for the hydroxylation of phenylalanine (see p. 270). The tetrahydrobiopterin (BH_4)-requiring

Tyrosine hydroxylase
Tetrahydro-biopterin + O_2
Dihydro-biopterin + H_2O
Tyrosine
3,4-Dihydroxy-phenylalanine (DOPA)
Aromatic amino acid decarboxylase
PLP
CO_2
Dopamine
Ascorbate + O_2
Cu^{2+}
Dopamine β-hydroxylase
Dehydro-ascorbate + H_2O
Norepinephrine
Phenylethanolamine-N-methyl-transferase
S-Adenosyl-methionine
S-Adenosyl-homocysteine
Epinephrine

Figure 21.15
Synthesis of catecholamines. PLP = pyridoxal phosphate; Cu^{2+} = copper.

enzyme is abundant in the CNS, the sympathetic ganglia, and the adrenal medulla and is the rate-limiting step of the pathway. DOPA is decarboxylated in a reaction requiring PLP (see p. 378) to form dopamine, which is hydroxylated by *dopamine β-hydroxylase* to yield norepinephrine in a reaction that requires ascorbate (vitamin C) and copper. Epinephrine is formed from norepinephrine by an N-methylation reaction using S-adenosylmethionine (SAM) as the methyl donor (see p. 264).

> Parkinson disease, a neurodegenerative movement disorder, is due to insufficient dopamine production as a result of the idiopathic loss of dopamine-producing cells in the brain. Administration of L-DOPA (levodopa) is the most common treatment. Dopamine cannot cross the blood brain barrier.

3. **Degradation:** The catecholamines are inactivated by oxidative deamination catalyzed by *monoamine oxidase* (*MAO*) and by O-methylation carried out by *catechol-O-methyltransferase* (*COMT*) using SAM as the methyl donor (Figure 21.16). The two reactions can occur in either order. The aldehyde products of the *MAO* reaction are oxidized to the corresponding acids. The metabolic products of these reactions are excreted in the urine as vanillylmandelic acid (VMA) from epinephrine and norepinephrine and homovanillic acid from dopamine. [Note: VMA is increased with pheochromocytomas, rare tumors of the adrenal gland characterized by excessive production of catecholamines.]

4. **Monoamine oxidase inhibitors:** *MAO* is found in neural and other tissues, such as the intestine and liver. In the neuron, this enzyme oxidatively deaminates and inactivates any excess neurotransmitter molecules (norepinephrine, dopamine, or serotonin) that may leak out of synaptic vesicles when the neuron is at rest. *MAO* inhibitors may irreversibly or reversibly inactivate the enzyme, permitting neurotransmitter molecules to escape

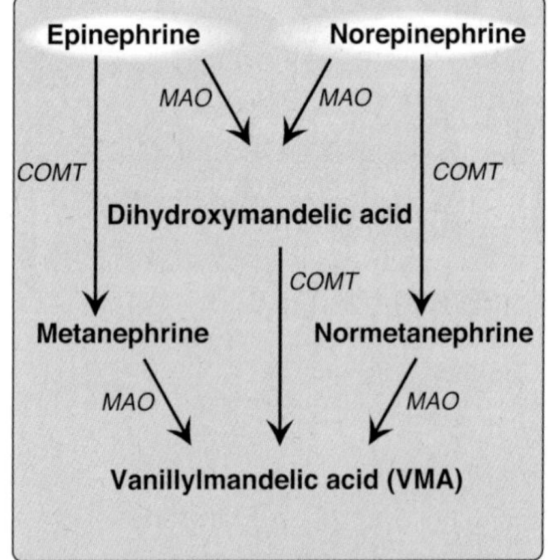

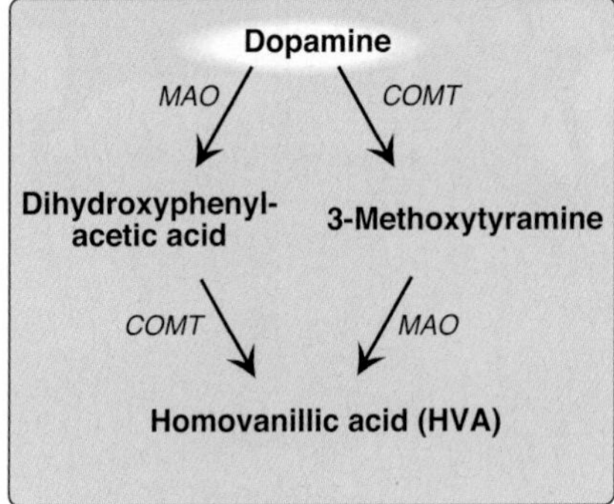

Figure 21.16
Metabolism of the catecholamines by *catechol-O-methyltranferase* (*COMT*) and *monoamine oxidase* (*MAO*).

degradation and, therefore, to both accumulate within the presynaptic neuron and to leak into the synaptic space. This causes activation of norepinephrine and serotonin receptors and may be responsible for the antidepressant action of these drugs.

B. Histamine

Histamine is a chemical messenger that mediates a wide range of cellular responses, including allergic and inflammatory reactions and gastric acid secretion. A powerful vasodilator, histamine is formed by decarboxylation of histidine in a reaction requiring PLP (Figure 21.17). It is secreted by mast cells as a result of allergic reactions or trauma. Histamine has no clinical applications, but agents that interfere with the action of histamine have important therapeutic applications.

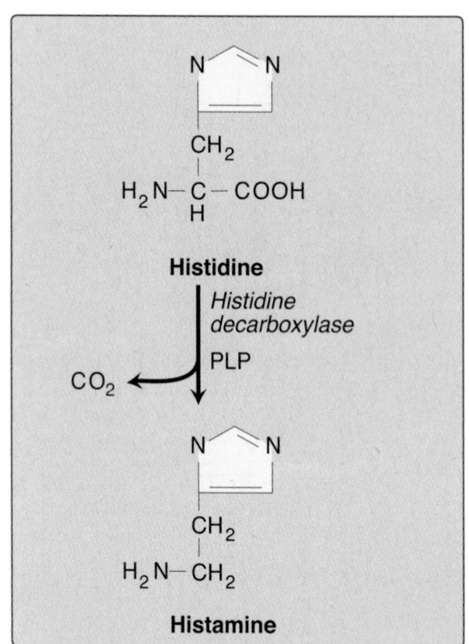

Figure 21.17
Biosynthesis of histamine. PLP = pyridoxal phosphate.

C. Serotonin

Serotonin, also called 5-hydroxytryptamine (5-HT), is synthesized and stored at several sites in the body (Figure 21.18). The largest amount by far is found in the intestinal mucosa. Smaller amounts occur in the CNS, where it functions as a neurotransmitter, and in platelets. Serotonin is synthesized from tryptophan, which is hydroxylated in a BH_4-requiring reaction analogous to that catalyzed by *phenylalanine hydroxylase*. The product, 5-hydroxytryptophan, is decarboxylated to serotonin, which is degraded by *MAO*. Serotonin has multiple physiologic roles including pain perception, regulation of sleep, appetite, temperature, blood pressure, cognitive functions, and mood (causes a feeling of well-being). [Note: Selective serotonin reuptake inhibitors (SSRIs) maintain serotonin levels, thereby functioning as antidepressants.]

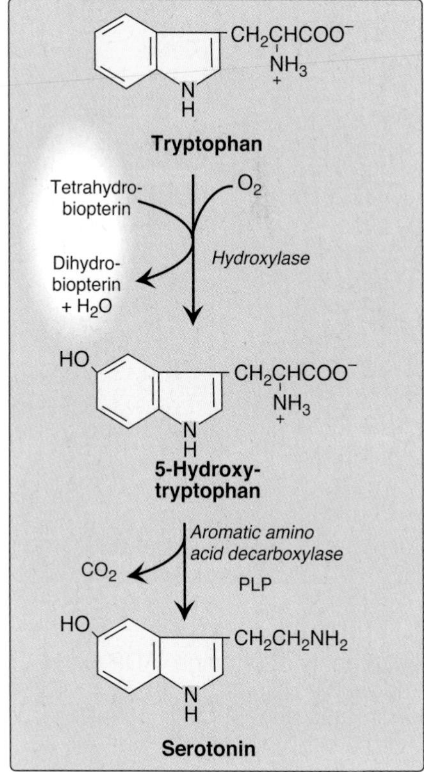

Figure 21.18
Synthesis of serotonin. [Note: Serotonin is converted to melatonin in the pineal gland.] PLP = pyridoxal phosphate.

D. Creatine

Creatine phosphate (also called phosphocreatine), the phosphorylated derivative of creatine found in muscle, is a high-energy compound that provides a small but rapidly mobilized reserve of high-energy phosphates that can be reversibly transferred to adenosine diphosphate (Figure 21.19) to maintain the intracellular level of adenosine triphosphate (ATP) during the first few minutes of intense muscular contraction. [Note: The amount of creatine phosphate in the body is proportional to the muscle mass.]

1. **Synthesis:** Creatine is synthesized in liver and kidney tissue from glycine and the guanidino group of arginine, plus a methyl group from SAM (see Figure 21.19). Animal products are dietary sources. Creatine is reversibly phosphorylated to creatine phosphate by *creatine kinase*, using ATP as the phosphate donor. [Note: The presence of *creatine kinase* (*MB* isozyme) in the plasma is indicative of heart damage and is used in the diagnosis of myocardial infarction (see p. 65).]

2. **Degradation:** Creatine and creatine phosphate spontaneously cyclize at a slow but constant rate to form creatinine, which is excreted in the urine. The amount excreted is proportional to the total creatine phosphate content of the body and, therefore, can be used to estimate muscle mass. When muscle mass decreases for any reason (for example, from paralysis or muscular dystrophy),

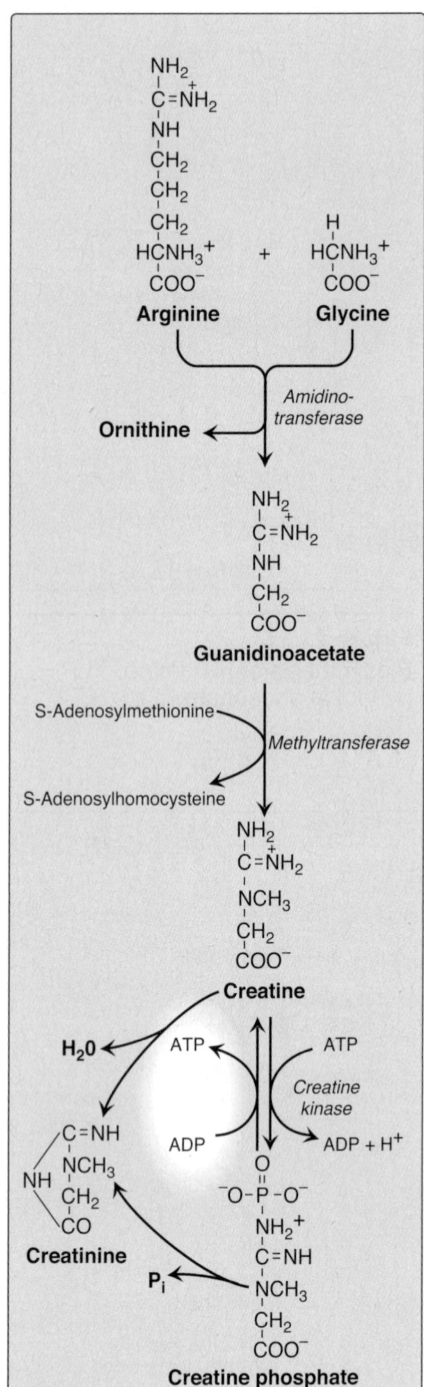

Figure 21.19
Synthesis of creatine. ADP = adenosine diphosphate; P_i = inorganic phosphate.

the creatinine content of the urine falls. In addition, any rise in blood creatinine is a sensitive indicator of kidney malfunction, because creatinine normally is rapidly removed from the blood and excreted. A typical adult male excretes about 1–2 g of creatinine per day.

E. Melanin

Melanin is a pigment that occurs in several tissues, particularly the eye, hair, and skin. It is synthesized from tyrosine in melanocytes (pigment-forming cells) of the epidermis. It functions to protect underlying cells from the harmful effects of sunlight. [Note: A defect in melanin production results in oculocutaneous albinism, the most common type being due to defects in copper-containing *tyrosinase* (see p. 273).]

IV. CHAPTER SUMMARY

Amino acids are precursors of many nitrogen-containing compounds including **porphyrins**, which, in combination with ferrous (Fe^{2+}) iron, form **heme** (Figure 21.20). The major sites of **heme biosynthesis** are the **liver**, which synthesizes a number of heme proteins (particularly *cytochrome P450* enzymes), and the **erythrocyte-producing cells** of the bone marrow, which are active in hemoglobin synthesis. In the liver, the rate of heme synthesis is highly variable, responding to alterations in the cellular heme pool caused by fluctuating demands for hemeproteins. In contrast, heme synthesis in erythroid cells is relatively constant and is matched to the rate of globin synthesis. **Porphyrin synthesis** start with **glycine** and **succinyl coenzyme A**. The **committed step** in heme synthesis is the formation of δ-aminolevulinic acid (ALA). This reaction is catalyzed by ***ALA synthase-1*** (***ALAS1***) in liver (inhibited by **hemin**, the oxidized form of heme that accumulates in the cell when heme is being underutilized) and ***ALAS2*** in erythroid tissues (regulated by **iron**). **Porphyrias** are caused by inherited (primarily **autosomal-dominant**) or acquired defects in heme synthesis, resulting in the accumulation and increased excretion of porphyrins or porphyrin precursors. Enzymic defects early in the pathway cause **abdominal pain** and **neuropsychiatric symptoms**, whereas later defects cause **photosensitivity**. **Degradation** of hemeproteins occurs in the **reticuloendothelial system**, particularly in the **liver** and **spleen**. The first step in the degradation of heme is the production by ***heme oxygenase*** of the green pigment **biliverdin**, which is subsequently reduced to **bilirubin**. Bilirubin is transported to the liver, where its solubility is increased by the addition of two molecules of **glucuronic acid**. Bilirubin diglucuronide is transported into the **bile canaliculi**, where it is first hydrolyzed and reduced by bacteria in the gut to yield **urobilinogen**, then oxidized by intestinal bacteria to **stercobilin**. **Jaundice** refers to the yellow color of the skin and sclerae that is caused by deposition of bilirubin, secondary to increased bilirubin levels in the blood. Three commonly encountered type of jaundice are **hemolytic jaundice**, **obstructive jaundice**, and **hepatocellular jaundice**. Other important N-containing compounds derived from amino acids include the **catecholamines** (dopamine, norepinephrine, and epinephrine), **creatine**, **histamine**, **serotonin**, and **melanin**.

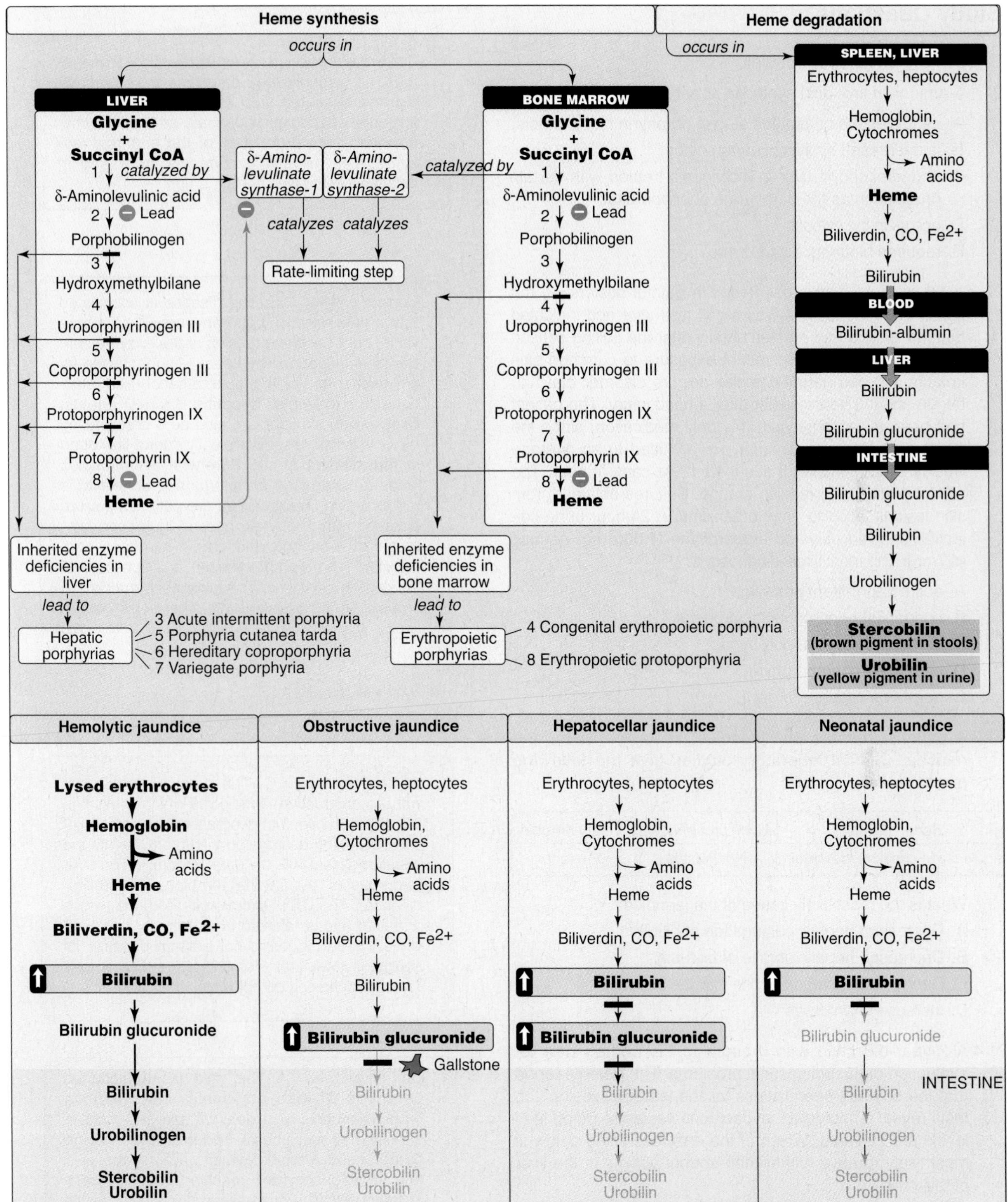

Figure 21.20
Key concept map for heme metabolism. ▬ = Block in the pathway. [Note: Hepatocellular jaundice can be caused by decreased conjugation of bilirubin or decreased secretion of conjugated bilirubin into bile.] CoA = coenzyme A; CO = carbon monoxide.

Study Questions

Choose the ONE best answer.

21.1 δ-Aminolevulinic acid synthase activity:

A. catalyzes the committed step in porphyrin biosynthesis.

B. is decreased by iron in erythrocytes.

C. is decreased in liver in individuals treated with certain drugs such as the barbiturate phenobarbital.

D. occurs in the cytosol.

E. requires biotin as a coenzyme.

Correct answer = A. δ-Aminolevulinic acid synthase is cytosolic and catalyzes the rate-limiting and regulated step of porphyrin synthesis. It requires pyridoxal phosphate as a coenzyme. Iron increases production of the erythroid isozyme. The hepatic isozyme is increased in patients treated with certain drugs.

21.2 A 50-year-old man presented with painful blisters on the backs of his hands. He was a golf instructor and indicated that the blisters had erupted shortly after the golfing season began. He did not have recent exposure to common skin irritants. He had partial complex seizure disorder that had begun about 3 years earlier after a head injury. The patient had been taking phenytoin (his only medication) since the onset of the seizure disorder. He admitted to an average weekly ethanol intake of about 18 12-oz cans of beer. The patient's urine was reddish orange. Cultures obtained from skin lesions failed to grow organisms. A 24-hour urine collection showed elevated uroporphyrin (1,000 mg; normal, <27mg). The most likely diagnosis is:

A. acute intermittent porphyria.

B. congenital erythropoietic porphyria.

C. erythropoietic protoporphyria.

D. hereditary coproporphyria.

E. porphyria cutanea tarda.

Correct answer = E. The disease is associated with a deficiency in uroporphyrinogen decarboxylase, but clinical expression of the enzyme deficiency is influenced by hepatic injury caused by environmental (for example, ethanol) and infectious (for example, hepatitis B virus) agents. Exposure to sunlight can also be a precipitating factor. Clinical onset is typically during the fourth or fifth decade of life. Porphyrin accumulation leads to cutaneous symptoms and urine that is red to brown. Treatment of the patient's seizure disorder with phenytoin caused increased synthesis of δ-aminolevulinic acid synthase and, therefore, of uroporphyrinogen, the substrate of the deficient enzyme. The laboratory and clinical findings are inconsistent with other porphyrias.

21.3 A patient presents with jaundice, abdominal pain, and nausea. Clinical laboratory studies give the following results:

Serum bilirubin	Urine urobilinogen	Urinary bilirubin
Increase in conjugated bilirubin	Not present	Present

What is the most likely cause of the jaundice?

A. Decreased hepatic conjugation of bilirubin

B. Decreased hepatic uptake of bilirubin

C. Decreased secretion of bile into the intestine

D. Increased hemolysis

Correct answer = C. The data are consistent with an obstructive jaundice in which a block in the common bile duct decreases the secretion of bile containing conjugated bilirubin (CB) into the intestine (stool will be pale in color). The liver "regurgitates" the CB into the blood (hyperbilirubinemia). The CB is excreted in the urine (which darkens) and is referred to as "urinary bilirubin." Urinary urobilinogen is not present because its source is intestinal urobilinogen, which is low. The other choices do not match the data.

21.4 A 2-year-old child was brought to his pediatrician for evaluation of gastrointestinal problems. The parents report that the boy has been listless for the last few weeks. Lab tests reveal a microcytic, hypochromic anemia. Blood lead levels are elevated. Which of the enzymes listed below is most likely to have higher-than-normal activity in the liver of this child?

A. δ-Aminolevulinic acid synthase

B. Bilirubiun UDP-glucuronosyltransferase

C. Ferrochelatase

D. Heme oxygenase

E. Porphobilinogen synthase

Correct answer = A. This child has the acquired porphyria of lead poisoning. Lead inhibits δ-aminolevulinic acid dehydratase and, consequently, heme synthesis. The decrease in heme derepresses δ-aminolevulinic acid synthase-1 (the hepatic isozyme), resulting in an increase in its activity. The decrease in heme also results in decreased hemoglobin synthesis, and anemia is seen. Ferrochelatase is directly inhibited by lead. The other choices are enzymes of heme degradation.

Nucleotide Metabolism

22

I. OVERVIEW

Ribonucleoside and deoxyribonucleoside phosphates (nucleotides) are essential for all cells. Without them, neither ribonucleic acid (RNA) nor deoxyribonucleic acid (DNA) can be produced, and, therefore, proteins cannot be synthesized or cells proliferate. Nucleotides also serve as carriers of activated intermediates in the synthesis of some carbohydrates, lipids, and conjugated proteins (for example, uridine diphosphate [UDP]-glucose and cytidine diphosphate [CDP]-choline) and are structural components of several essential coenzymes, such as coenzyme A, flavin adenine dinucleotide (FAD[H_2]), nicotinamide adenine dinucleotide (NAD[H]), and nicotinamide adenine dinucleotide phosphate (NADP[H]). Nucleotides, such as cyclic adenosine monophosphate (cAMP) and cyclic guanosine monophosphate (cGMP), serve as second messengers in signal transduction pathways. In addition, nucleotides play an important role as "energy currency" in the cell. Finally, nucleotides are important regulatory compounds for many of the pathways of intermediary metabolism, inhibiting or activating key enzymes. The purine and pyrimidine bases found in nucleotides can be synthesized de novo or can be obtained through salvage pathways that allow the reuse of the preformed bases resulting from normal cell turnover. [Note: Little of the purines and pyrimidines supplied by diet are utilized and are degraded instead.]

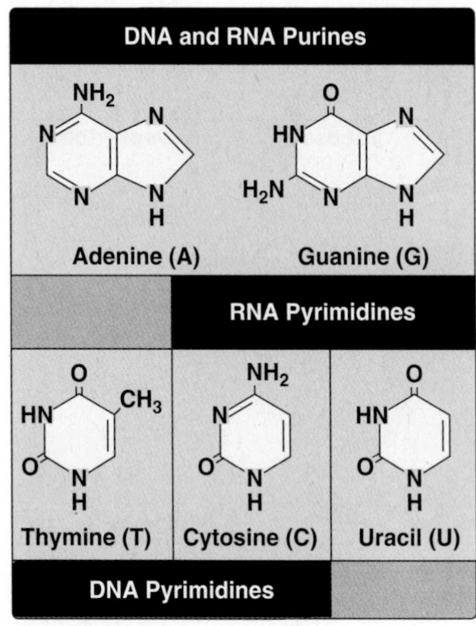

Figure 22.1
Purines and pyrimidines commonly found in DNA and RNA.

II. NUCLEOTIDE STRUCTURE

Nucleotides are composed of a nitrogenous base; a pentose monosaccharide; and one, two, or three phosphate groups. The nitrogen-containing bases belong to two families of compounds: the purines and the pyrimidines.

A. Purine and pyrimidine structures

Both DNA and RNA contain the same purine bases: adenine (A) and guanine (G). Both DNA and RNA contain the pyrimidine

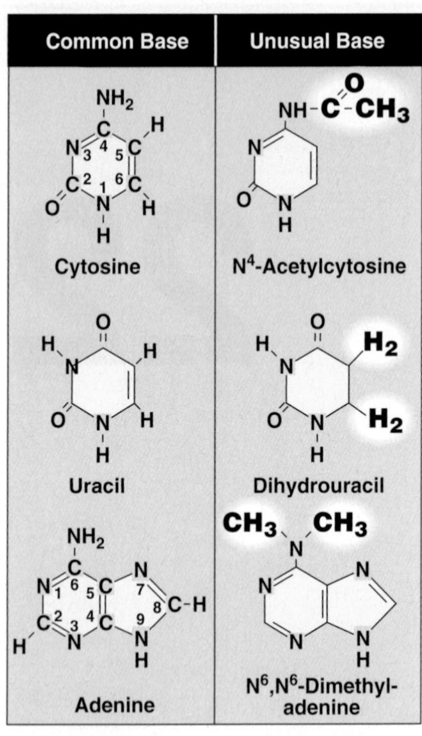

Figure 22.2
Examples of unusual bases.

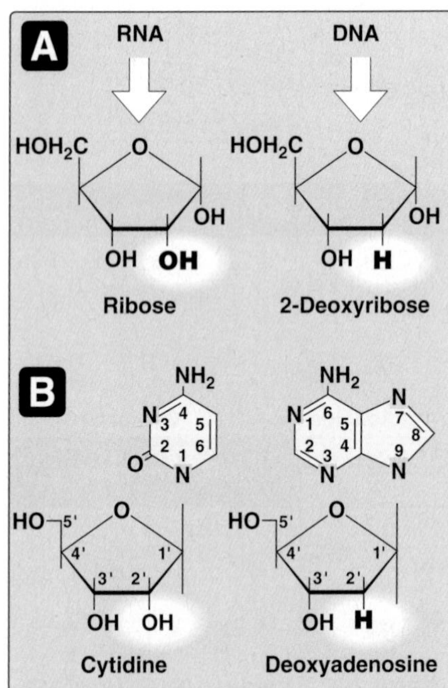

Figure 22.3
A. Pentoses found in nucleic acids.
B. Examples of the numbering systems for purine- and pyrimidine-containing nucleosides.

cytosine (C), but they differ in their second pyrimidine base: DNA contains thymine (T), whereas RNA contains uracil (U). T and U differ in that only T has a methyl group (Figure 22.1). Unusual (modified) bases are occasionally found in some species of DNA and RNA (for example, in some viral DNA) and in transfer RNA (tRNA). Base modifications include methylation, glycosylation, acetylation, and reduction. Some examples of unusual bases are shown in Figure 22.2. [Note: The presence of an unusual base in a nucleotide sequence may aid in its recognition by specific enzymes or protect it from being degraded by *nucleases*.]

B. Nucleosides

The addition of a pentose sugar to a base through a glycosidic bond produces a nucleoside. If the sugar is ribose, a ribonucleoside is produced, and if the sugar is 2-deoxyribose, a deoxyribonucleoside is produced (Figure 22.3A). The ribonucleosides of A, G, C, and U are named adenosine, guanosine, cytidine, and uridine, respectively. The deoxyribonucleosides of A, G, C, and T have the added prefix, "deoxy-" (for example, deoxyadenosine). [Note: The compound deoxythymidine is often simply called thymidine, with the "deoxy-" prefix being understood, because it is incorporated into DNA only.] The carbon and nitrogen atoms in the rings of the base and the sugar are numbered separately (Figure 22.3B). Note that the carbons in the pentose are numbered 1' to 5'. Thus, when the 5'-carbon of a nucleoside (or nucleotide) is referred to, a carbon atom in the pentose, rather than an atom in the base, is being specified.

C. Nucleotides

The addition of one or more phosphate groups to a nucleoside produces a nucleotide. The first phosphate group is attached by an ester linkage to the 5'-OH of the pentose, forming a nucleoside 5'-phosphate or a 5'-nucleotide. The type of pentose is denoted by the prefix in the names "5'-ribonucleotide" and "5'-deoxyribonucleotide." If one phosphate group is attached to the 5'-carbon of the pentose, the structure is a nucleoside monophosphate, like adenosine monophosphate [AMP] also called adenylate). If a second or third phosphate is added to the nucleoside, a nucleoside diphosphate (for example, adenosine diphosphate [ADP] or triphosphate (for example, adenosine triphosphate [ATP]) results (Figure 22.4). The second and third phosphates are each connected to the nucleotide by a "high-energy" bond. [Note: The phosphate groups are responsible for the negative charges associated with nucleotides and cause DNA and RNA to be referred to as "nucleic acids."]

III. SYNTHESIS OF PURINE NUCLEOTIDES

The atoms of the purine ring are contributed by a number of compounds, including amino acids (aspartate, glycine, and glutamine), CO_2, and N^{10}-formyltetrahydrofolate (Figure 22.5). The purine ring is constructed primarily in the liver by a series of reactions that add the donated carbons and nitrogens to a preformed ribose 5-phosphate. (See p. 147 for the synthesis of ribose 5-phosphate by the pentose phosphate pathway.)

A. Synthesis of 5-phosphoribosyl-1-pyrophosphate

5-Phosphoribosyl-1-pyrophosphate (PRPP) is an "activated pentose" that participates in the synthesis and salvage of purines and pyrimidines. Synthesis of PRPP from ATP and ribose 5-phosphate is catalyzed by *PRPP synthetase* (Figure 22.6). This X-linked enzyme is activated by inorganic phosphate and inhibited by purine nucleotides (end-product inhibition). [Note: The sugar moiety of PRPP is ribose, and, therefore, ribonucleotides are the end products of de novo purine synthesis. When deoxyribonucleotides are required for DNA synthesis, the ribose sugar moiety is reduced (see p. 297).]

B. Synthesis of 5-phosphoribosylamine

Synthesis of 5-phosphoribosylamine from PRPP and glutamine is shown in Figure 22.7. The amide group of glutamine replaces the pyrophosphate group attached to carbon 1 of PRPP. This is the committed step in purine nucleotide biosynthesis. The enzyme, *glutamine:phosphoribosylpyrophosphate amidotransferase*, is inhibited by the purine 5'-nucleotides AMP and guanosine monophosphate ([GMP] also called guanylate), the end products of the pathway. The rate of the reaction is also controlled by the intracellular concentration of PRPP. [Note: The concentration of PRPP is normally far below the Michaelis constant (K_m) for the *amidotransferase*. Therefore, any small change in the PRPP concentration causes a proportional change in rate of the reaction (see p. 59).]

C. Synthesis of inosine monophosphate, the "parent" purine nucleotide

The next nine steps in purine nucleotide biosynthesis leading to the synthesis of inosine monophosphate ([IMP] whose base is hypoxanthine) are illustrated in Figure 22.7. Four steps in this pathway require ATP as an energy source, and two steps in the pathway require N^{10}-formyltetrahydrofolate as a one-carbon donor (see p. 267). [Note: Hypoxanthine is found in tRNA (see p. 437).]

D. Synthetic inhibitors of purine synthesis

Some synthetic inhibitors of purine synthesis (for example, the sulfonamides), are designed to inhibit the growth of rapidly dividing microorganisms without interfering with human cell functions (see Figure 22.7). Other purine synthesis inhibitors, such as structural analogs of

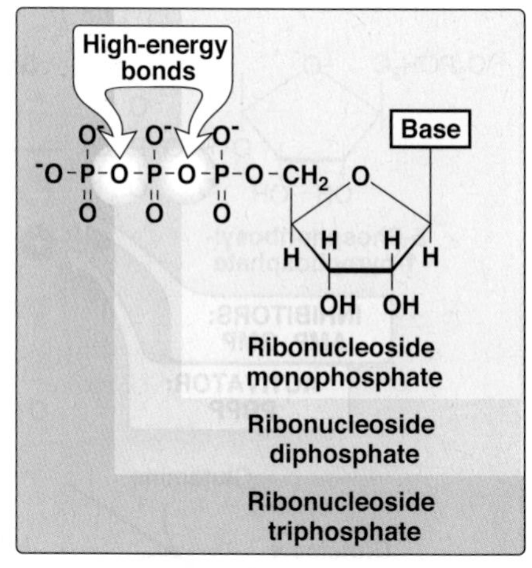

Figure 22.4
Ribonucleoside monophosphate, diphosphate, and triphosphate.

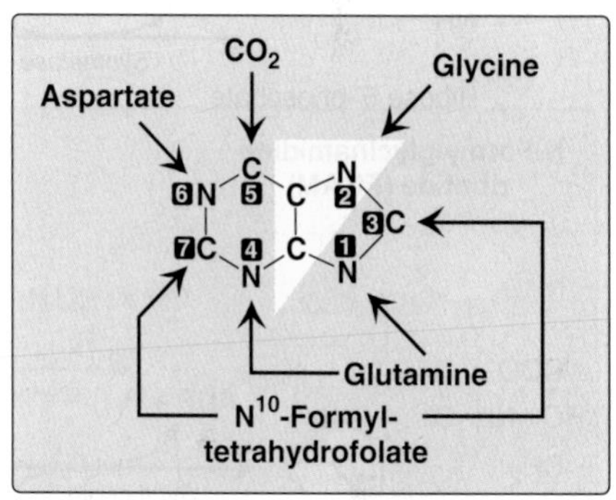

Figure 22.5
Sources of the individual atoms in the purine ring. The order in which the atoms are added is shown by the numbers in the black boxes (see Figure 22.7).

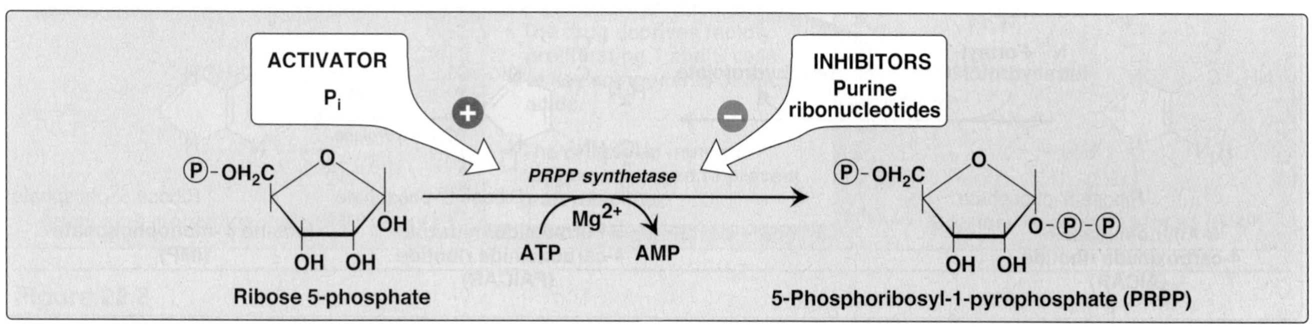

Figure 22.6
Synthesis of PRPP, showing the activator and inhibitors of the reaction. [Note: This is not the committed step of purine synthesis because PRPP is used in other pathways.] Ⓟ= phosphate; P_i = inorganic phosphate; AMP = adenosine monophosphate.

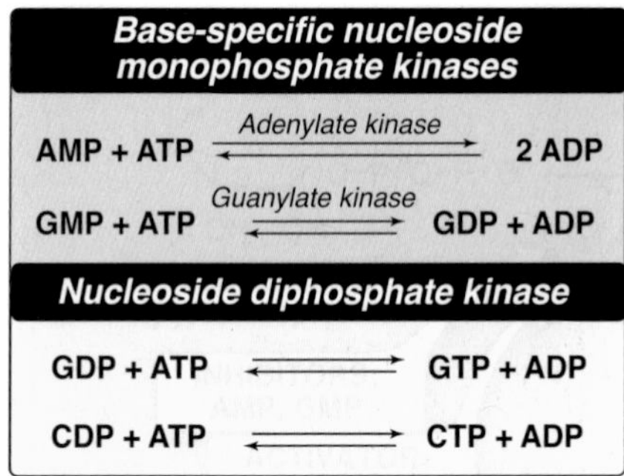

Figure 22.9
Conversion of nucleoside monophosphates to nucleoside diphosphates and triphosphates. AMP = adenosine monophosphate; ADP = adenosine diphosphate; GMP = guanosine monophosphate; GDP = guanosine diphosphate; GTP = guanosine triphosphate; CDP = cytidine diphosphate; CTP = cytidine triphosphate.

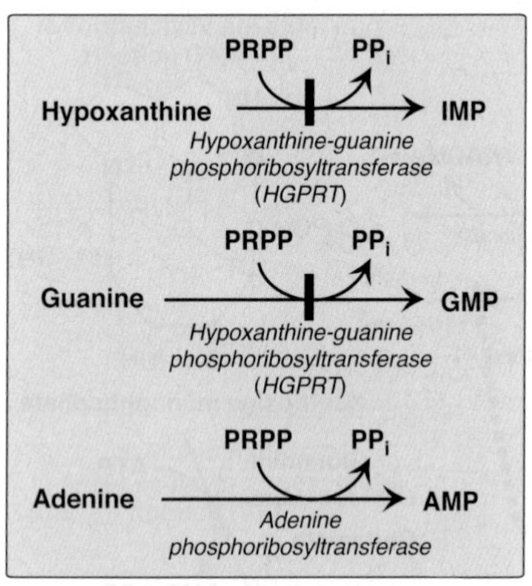

Figure 22.10
Salvage pathways of purine nucleotide synthesis. [Note: Virtually complete deficiency of *HGPRT* results in Lesch-Nyhan syndrome. Partial deficiencies of *HGPRT* are known. As the amount of functional enzyme increases, the severity of the symptoms decreases.] IMP = inosine monophosphate; GMP = guanosine monophosphate; AMP = adenosine monophosphate; PRPP = 5-phosphoribosyl-1- pyrophosphate; PP_i = pyrophosphate.

tion in each pathway is inhibited by the end product of that pathway. This provides a mechanism for diverting IMP to the synthesis of the purine present in lesser amounts. If both AMP and GMP are present in adequate amounts, the de novo pathway of purine synthesis is turned off at the *amidotransferase* step.

F. Conversion of nucleoside monophosphates to nucleoside diphosphates and triphosphates

Nucleoside diphosphates are synthesized from the corresponding nucleoside monophosphates by base-specific *nucleoside monophosphate kinases* (Figure 22.9). [Note: These *kinases* do not discriminate between ribose or deoxyribose in the substrate.] ATP is generally the source of the transferred phosphate because it is present in higher concentrations than the other nucleoside triphosphates. *Adenylate kinase* is particularly active in the liver and in muscle, where the turnover of energy from ATP is high. Its function is to maintain equilibrium among the adenine nucleotides (AMP, ADP, and ATP). Nucleoside diphosphates and triphosphates are interconverted by *nucleoside diphosphate kinase*, an enzyme that, unlike the *monophosphate kinases*, has broad substrate specificity.

G. Salvage pathway for purines

Purines that result from the normal turnover of cellular nucleic acids, or the small amount that is obtained from the diet and not degraded, can be converted to nucleoside triphosphates and used by the body. This is referred to as the "salvage pathway" for purines. [Note: Salvage is particularly important in the brain.]

1. **Salvage of purine bases to nucleotides:** Two enzymes are involved: *adenine phosphoribosyltransferase* (*APRT*) and *hypoxanthine-guanine phosphoribosyltransferase* (*HGPRT*). Both enzymes use PRPP as the source of the ribose 5-phosphate group (Figure 22.10). The release of pyrophosphate and its subsequent hydrolysis by *pyrophosphatase* makes these reactions irreversible. [Note: Adenosine is the only purine nucleoside to be salvaged. It is phosphorylated to AMP by *adenosine kinase*.]

2. **Lesch-Nyhan syndrome:** Lesch-Nyhan is a rare, X-linked recessive disorder associated with a virtually complete deficiency of *HGPRT*. The deficiency results in an inability to salvage hypoxanthine or guanine, from which excessive amounts of uric acid, the end product of purine degradation, are then produced (see p. 298). In addition, the lack of this salvage pathway causes increased PRPP levels and decreased IMP and GMP levels. As a result, *glutamine: phosphoribosylpyrophosphate amidotransferase* (the regulated step in purine synthesis) has excess substrate and decreased inhibitors available, and de novo purine synthesis is increased. The combination of decreased purine reutilization and increased purine synthesis results in increased degradation of purines and the production of large amounts of uric acid, making Lesch-Nyhan a heritable cause of hyperuricemia. In patients with Lesch-Nyhan syndrome, the hyperuricemia frequently results in the formation of uric acid stones in the kidneys (urolithiasis) and the deposition of urate crystals in the joints (gouty arthritis) and soft tissues. In addition, the syndrome is characterized by motor dysfunction, cognitive deficits, and behav-

ioral disturbances that include self-mutilation (for example, biting of lips and fingers) as shown in Figure 22.11).

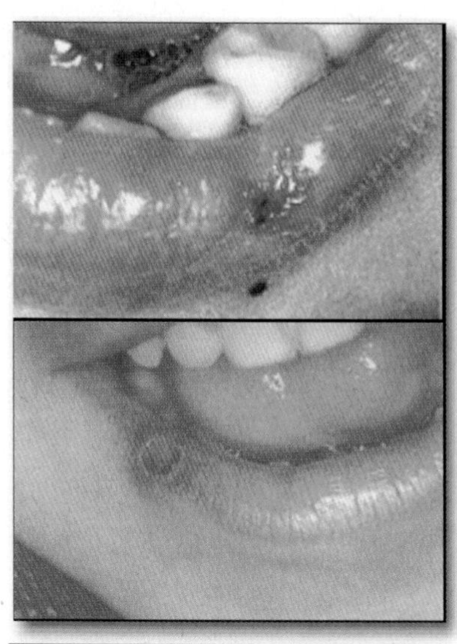

Figure 22.11
Lesions on the lips of Lesch-Nyhan patients caused by self-mutilation.

IV. SYNTHESIS OF DEOXYRIBONUCLEOTIDES

The nucleotides described thus far all contain ribose (ribonucleotides). The nucleotides required for DNA synthesis, however, are 2'-deoxyribonucleotides, which are produced from ribonucleoside diphosphates by the enzyme *ribonucleotide reductase* during the S-phase of the cell cycle (see p. 407). [Note: The same enzyme acts on pyrimidine ribonucleotides.]

A. Ribonucleotide reductase

Ribonucleotide reductase (*ribonucleoside diphosphate reductase*) is composed of two nonidentical dimeric subunits, R1 and R2, and is specific for the reduction of purine nucleoside diphosphates (ADP and GDP) and pyrimidine nucleoside diphosphates (CDP and UDP) to their deoxy forms (dADP, dGDP, dCDP, and dUDP). The immediate donors of the hydrogen atoms needed for the reduction of the 2'-hydroxyl group are two sulfhydryl groups on the enzyme itself, which, during the reaction, form a disulfide bond (Figure 22.12).

1. **Regeneration of reduced enzyme:** In order for *ribonucleotide reductase* to continue to produce deoxyribonucleotides, the disulfide bond created during the production of the 2'-deoxy carbon must be reduced. The source of the reducing equivalents for this purpose is thioredoxin, a peptide coenzyme of *ribonucleotide reductase*. Thioredoxin contains two cysteine residues separated by two amino acids in the peptide chain. The two sulfhydryl groups of thioredoxin donate their hydrogen atoms to *ribonucleotide reductase*, forming a disulfide bond in the process (see p. 19).

2. **Regeneration of reduced thioredoxin:** Thioredoxin must be converted back to its reduced form in order to continue to perform its function. The necessary reducing equivalents are provided by NADPH + H^+, and the reaction is catalyzed by *thioredoxin reductase* (see Figure 22.12).

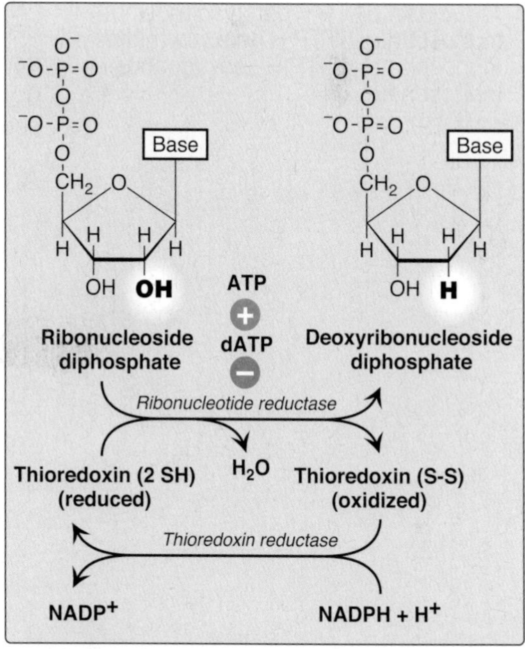

Figure 22.12
Conversion of ribonucleotides to deoxyribonucleotides. NADP(H) = nicotinamide adenine dinucleotide phosphate; dATP = deoxyadenosine triphosphate.

B. Regulation of deoxyribonucleotide synthesis

Ribonucleotide reductase is responsible for maintaining a balanced supply of the deoxyribonucleotides required for DNA synthesis. To achieve this, the regulation of the enzyme is complex. In addition to the catalytic (active) site, there are allosteric sites on the enzyme involved in regulating its activity (Figure 22.13).

1. **Activity sites:** The binding of dATP to allosteric sites (known as the activity sites) on the enzyme inhibits the overall catalytic activity of the enzyme and, therefore, prevents the reduction of any of the four nucleoside diphosphates. This effectively prevents DNA synthesis and explains the toxicity of increased levels of dATP seen in conditions such as

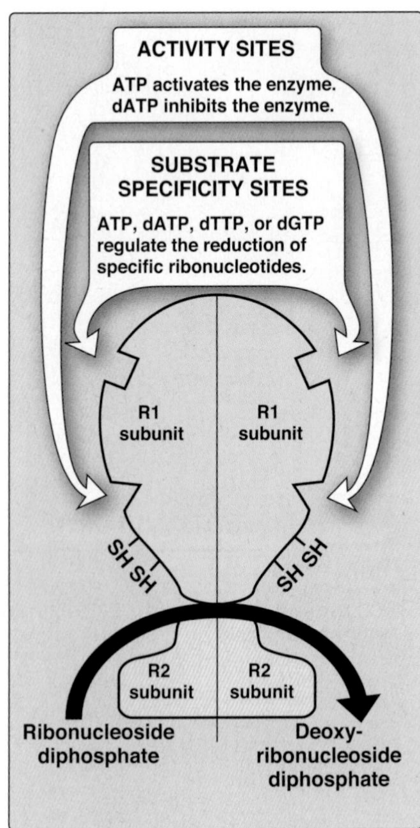

Figure 22.13
Regulation of *ribonucleotide reductase*. dATP = deoxyadenosine triphosphate; dTTP = deoxythymidine triphosphate; dGTP = deoxyguanosine triphosphate.

adenosine deaminase deficiency (see p. 301). In contrast, ATP bound to these sites activates the enzyme.

2. **Substrate specificity sites:** The binding of nucleoside triphosphates to additional allosteric sites (known as the substrate specificity sites) on the enzyme regulates substrate specificity, causing an increase in the conversion of different species of ribonucleotides to deoxyribonucleotides as they are required for DNA synthesis. For example, deoxythymidine triphosphate binding at the specificity sites causes a conformational change that allows reduction of GDP to dGDP at the catalytic site.

> The drug hydroxyurea (hydroxycarbamide) inhibits *ribonucleotide reductase*, thereby inhibiting the generation of substrates for DNA synthesis. Hydroxyurea is an antineoplastic agent and is used in the treatment of cancers such as melanoma. Hydroxyurea is also used in the treatment of sickle cell disease (see p. 36). However, the increase in fetal hemoglobin seen with hydroxyurea is not due to its effect on *ribonucleotide reductase*.

V. DEGRADATION OF PURINE NUCLEOTIDES

Degradation of dietary nucleic acids occurs in the small intestine, where a family of pancreatic enzymes hydrolyzes the nucleic acids to nucleotides. Inside the intestinal mucosal cells, purine nucleotides are sequentially degraded by specific enzymes to nucleosides and free bases, with uric acid as the end product of this pathway. [Note: Purine nucleotides from de novo synthesis are degraded in the liver primarily. The free bases are sent out from liver and salvaged by peripheral tissues.]

A. Degradation of dietary nucleic acids in the small intestine

Ribonucleases and *deoxyribonucleases*, secreted by the pancreas, hydrolyze dietary RNA and DNA to oligonucleotides. Oligonucleotides are further hydrolyzed by pancreatic *phosphodiesterases*, producing a mixture of 3'- and 5'-mononucleotides. In the intestinal mucosal cells, a family of *nucleotidases* removes the phosphate groups hydrolytically, releasing nucleosides that are further degraded by *nucleosidases* (*nucleoside phosphorylases*) to free bases plus (deoxy) ribose 1-phosphate. Dietary purine bases are not used to any appreciable extent for the synthesis of tissue nucleic acids. Instead, they are generally converted to uric acid in intestinal mucosal cells. Most of the uric acid enters the blood and is eventually excreted in the urine. A summary of this pathway is shown in Figure 22.14. [Note: Mammals other than primates express *urate oxidase* (*uricase*) which cleaves the purine ring, generating allantoin. Modified recombinant *urate oxidase* is now used clinically to lower urate levels.]

B Formation of uric acid

A summary of the steps in the production of uric acid and genetic diseases associated with deficiencies of specific degradative enzymes are shown in Figure 22.15. [Note: The bracketed numbers refer to specific reactions in the figure.]

[1] An amino group is removed from AMP to produce IMP by *AMP deaminase* or from adenosine to produce inosine (hypoxanthine-ribose) by *adenosine deaminase.*

[2] IMP and GMP are converted into their nucleoside forms (inosine and guanosine) by the action of *5′-nucleotidase*.

[3] *Purine nucleoside phosphorylase* converts inosine and guanosine into their respective purine bases, hypoxanthine and guanine. [Note: A *mutase* interconverts ribose 1- and ribose 5-phosphate.]

[4] Guanine is deaminated to form xanthine.

[5] Hypoxanthine is oxidized by *xanthine oxidase* to xanthine, which is further oxidized by *xanthine oxidase* to uric acid, the final product of human purine degradation. Uric acid is excreted primarily in the urine.

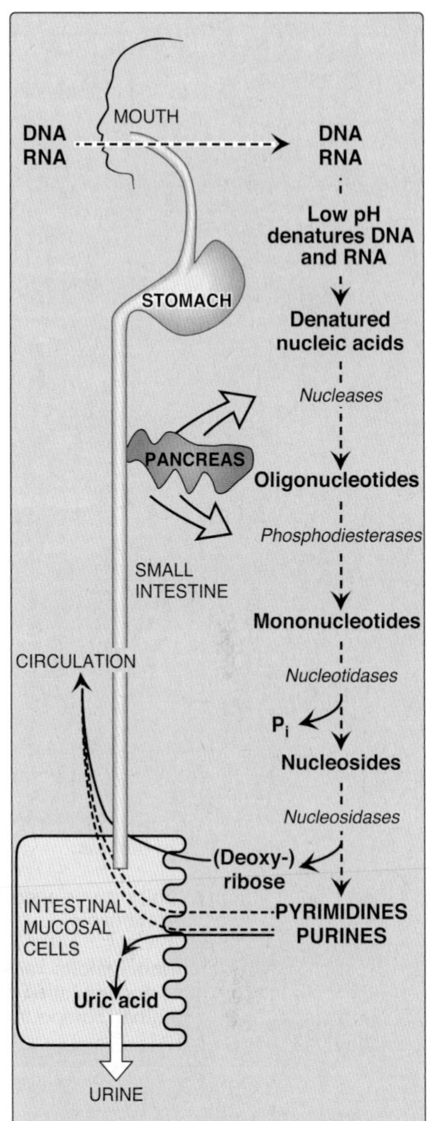

Figure 22.14
Digestion of dietary nucleic acids. [Note: Much of the metabolism of the mononucleotides occurs within the intestinal mucosal cells.] P_i = inorganic phosphate.

C. Diseases associated with purine degradation

1. **Gout:** Gout is a disorder initiated by high levels of uric acid (the end product of purine catabolism) in blood (hyperuricemia), as a result of either the overproduction or underexcretion of uric acid. The hyperuricemia can lead to the deposition of monosodium urate (MSU) crystals in the joints and an inflammatory response to the crystals, causing first acute and then progressing to chronic gouty arthritis. Nodular masses of MSU crystals (tophi) may be deposited in the soft tissues, resulting in chronic tophaceous gout (Figure 22.16). Formation of uric acid stones in the kidney (urolithiasis) may also be seen. [Note: Hyperuricemia, while necessary, is not sufficient to cause gout, but gout is always preceded by hyperuricemia. Hyperuricemia is typically asymptomatic but may be indicative of comorbid conditions such as hypertension.] The definitive diagnosis of gout requires aspiration and examination of synovial fluid (Figure 22.17) from an affected joint (or material from a tophus) using polarized light microscopy to confirm the presence of needle-shaped MSU crystals (Figure 22.18).

   a. **Underexcretion of uric acid:** In over 90% of individuals, hyperuricemia is caused by underexcretion of uric acid. Underexcretion can be primary, due to as-yet-unidentified inherent excretory defects, or secondary to known disease processes that affect how the kidney handles urate (for example, in lactic acidosis, lactate increases renal urate reabsorption, thereby decreasing its excretion) and to environmental factors such as the use of drugs (for example, thiazide diuretics) or exposure to lead (saturnine gout).

   b. **Overproduction of uric acid:** A less common cause of hyperuricemia is from the overproduction of uric acid. Primary hyperuricemia is, for the most part, idiopathic (having no known cause). However, several identified mutations in the gene for X-linked *PRPP synthetase* result in the enzyme having an increased maximal velocity (V_{max}) (see p. 58) for the production of PRPP, a lower K_m (see p. 59) for ribose 5-phosphate, or a decreased sensitivity to purine nucleotides, its allosteric inhibitors (see p. 62). In each case, increased availability of PRPP increases

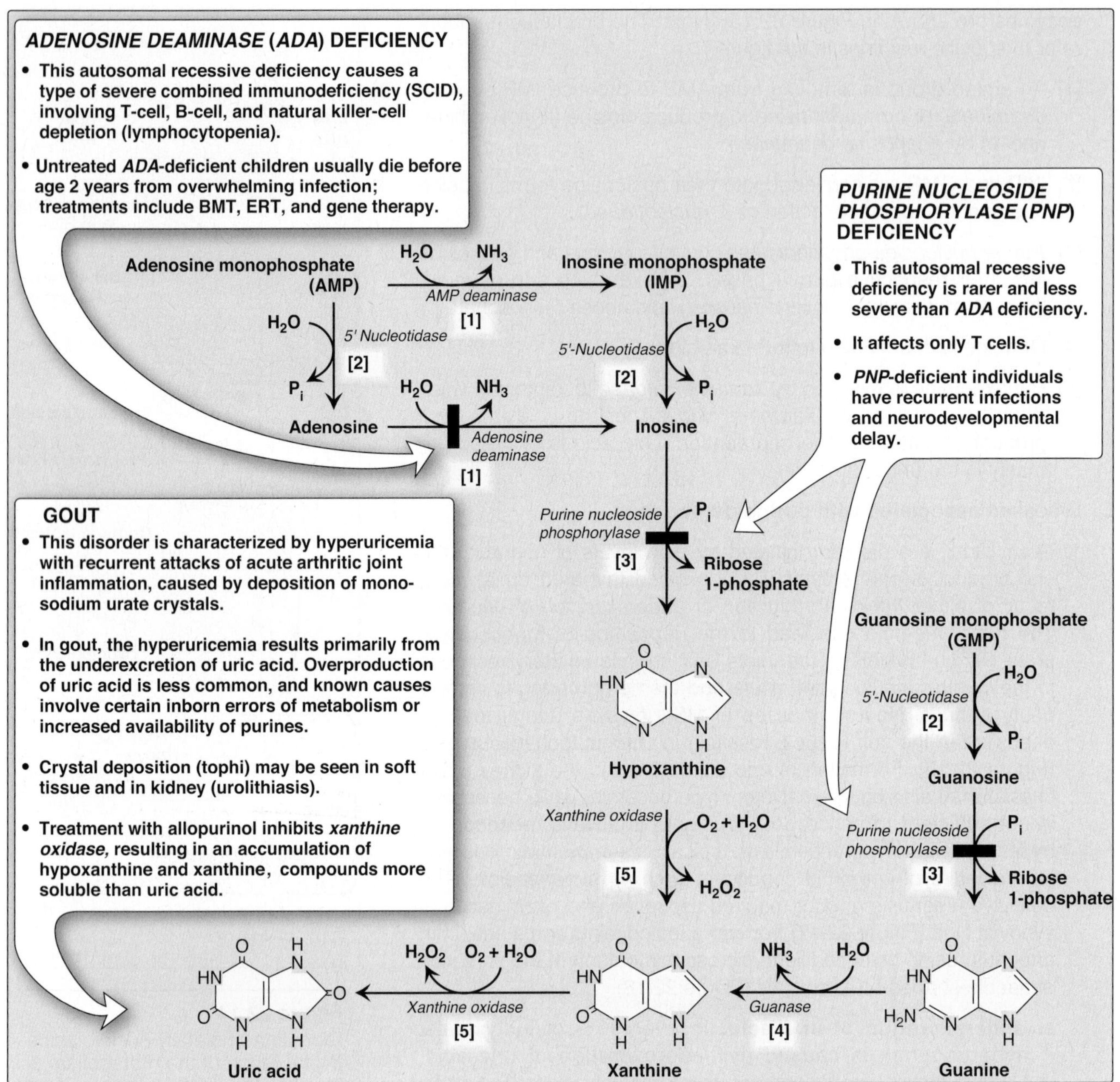

Figure 22.15
The degradation of purine nucleotides to uric acid, illustrating some of the genetic diseases associated with this pathway. [Note: The numbers in brackets refer to the corresponding numbered citations in the text.] BMT = bone marrow transplantation; ERT = enzyme replacement therapy; P_i = inorganic phosphate.

purine production, resulting in elevated levels of plasma uric acid. Lesch-Nyhan syndrome (see p. 296) also causes hyperuricemia as a result of the decreased salvage of hypoxanthine and guanine and the subsequent increased availability of PRPP. Secondary hyperuricemia is typically the consequence of increased availability of purines (for example, in patients with myeloproliferative disorders or who are undergoing chemotherapy and so have a high rate of cell turnover). Hyperuricemia can also be the result of seemingly unrelated metabolic diseases, such as von Gierke disease (see Figure 11.8 on p. 130) or hereditary fructose intolerance (see p. 138).

> A diet rich in meat, seafood (particularly shellfish), and ethanol is associated with increased risk of gout, whereas a diet rich in low-fat dairy products is associated with a decreased risk.

c. **Treatment of gout:** Acute attacks of gout are treated with anti-inflammatory agents. Colchicine; steroidal drugs, such as prednisone; and nonsteroidal drugs, such as indomethacin, are used. [Note: Colchicine prevents formation of microtubules, thereby decreasing the movement of neutrophils into the affected area. Like the other anti-inflammatory drugs, it has no effect on uric acid levels.] Long-term therapeutic strategies for gout involve lowering the uric acid level below its saturation point (6.5 mg/dl), thereby preventing the deposition of urate crystals. Uricosuric agents, such as probenecid or sulfinpyrazone, that increase renal excretion of uric acid, are used in patients who are "underexcretors" of uric acid. Allopurinol, a structural analog of hypoxanthine, inhibits uric acid synthesis and is used in patients who are "overproducers" of uric acid. Allopurinol is converted in the body to oxypurinol, which inhibits *xanthine oxidase* (*XO*), resulting in an accumulation of hypoxanthine and xanthine (see Figure 22.15), compounds more soluble than uric acid and, therefore, less likely to initiate an inflammatory response. In patients with normal levels of *HGPRT*, the hypoxanthine can be salvaged, reducing the levels of PRPP and, therefore, de novo purine synthesis. Febuxostat, a nonpurine inhibitor of *XO*, is also available. [Note: Uric acid levels in the blood normally are close to the saturation point. One reason for this may be the strong antioxidant effects of uric acid.]

2. **Adenosine deaminase deficiency:** *Adenosine deaminase* (*ADA*) is expressed in a variety of tissues, but, in humans, lymphocytes have the highest activity of this cytoplasmic enzyme. A deficiency of *ADA* results in an accumulation of adenosine, which is converted to its ribonucleotide or deoxyribonucleotide forms by cellular *kinases*. As dATP levels rise, *ribonucleotide reductase* is inhibited, thereby preventing the production of all deoxyribose-containing nucleotides (see p. 297). Consequently, cells cannot make DNA and divide. [Note: The dATP and adenosine that accumulate in *ADA* deficiency lead to developmental arrest and apoptosis of lymphocytes.] In its most severe form, this autosomal-recessive disorder causes a type of severe combined immunodeficiency disease (SCID), involving a decrease in T cells, B cells, and natural killer cells. It is estimated that, in the United States, *ADA* deficiency accounts for approximately 14% of all cases of SCID. Treatments include bone marrow transplantation, enzyme replacement therapy, and gene therapy. Without appropriate treatment, children with this disorder usually die from infection by age 2 years. [Note: *Purine nucleoside phosphorylase* deficiency results in a less severe immunodeficiency primarily involving T cells.]

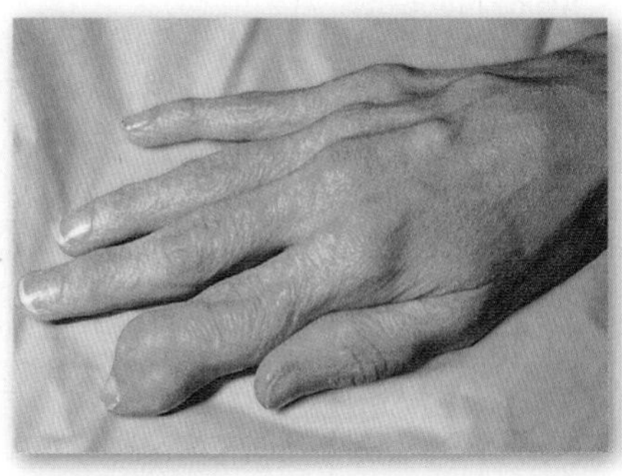

Figure 22.16
Tophaceous gout.

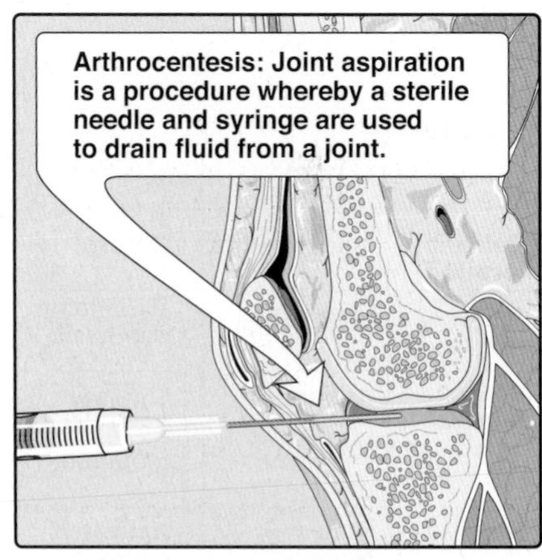

Figure 22.17
Analysis of joint fluid can help to define causes of joint swelling or arthritis, such as infection, gout, and rheumatoid disease.

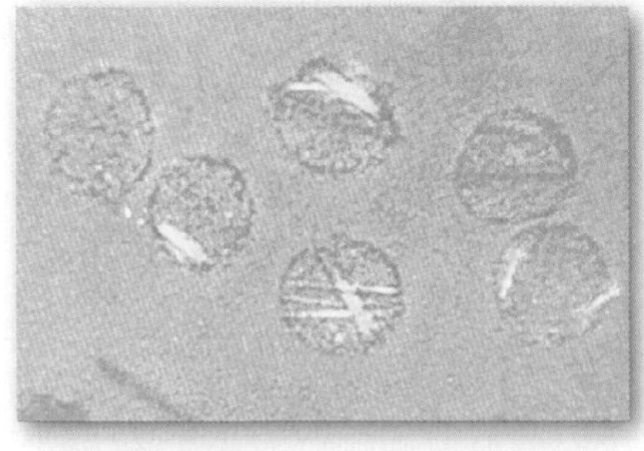

Figure 22.18
Gout can be diagnosed by the presence of negatively birefringent monosodium urate crystals in aspirated synovial fluid examined by polarized-light microscopy. Here, crystals are within polymorphonuclear leukocytes.

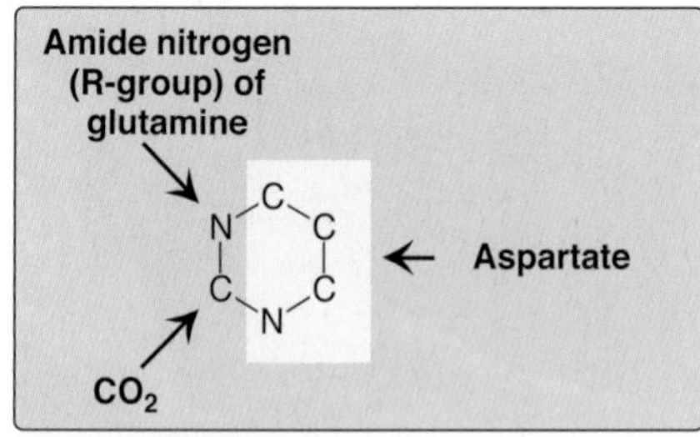

Figure 22.19
Sources of the individual atoms in the pyrimidine ring.

	CPS I	*CPS II*
Cellular location	Mitochondria	Cytosol
Pathway involved	Urea cycle	Pyrimidine synthesis
Source of nitrogen	Ammonia	γ-Amide group of glutamine
Regulators	Activator: N-acetyl-glutamate	Activator: PRPP Inhibitor: UTP

Figure 22.20
Summary of the differences between *carbamoyl phosphate synthetase* (*CPS*) *I* and *II*. PRPP = 5-phosphoribosyl-1-pyrophosphate; UTP = uridine triphosphate.

VI. PYRIMIDINE SYNTHESIS AND DEGRADATION

Unlike the synthesis of the purine ring, which is constructed on a preexisting ribose 5-phosphate, the pyrimidine ring is synthesized before being attached to ribose 5-phosphate, which is donated by PRPP. The sources of the atoms in the pyrimidine ring are glutamine, CO_2, and aspartate (Figure 22.19).

A. Synthesis of carbamoyl phosphate

The regulated step of this pathway in mammalian cells is the synthesis of carbamoyl phosphate from glutamine and CO_2, catalyzed by *carbamoyl phosphate synthetase (CPS) II. CPS II* is inhibited by uridine triphosphate (the end product of this pathway, which can be converted into the other pyrimidine nucleotides), and is activated by PRPP. [Note: Carbamoyl phosphate, synthesized by *CPS I*, is also a precursor of urea (see p. 253). Defects in *ornithine transcarbamylase* of the urea cycle promote pyrimidine synthesis due to increased availability of carbamoyl phosphate. A comparison of the two enzymes is presented in Figure 22.20.]

B. Synthesis of orotic acid

The second step in pyrimidine synthesis is the formation of carbamoylaspartate, catalyzed by *aspartate transcarbamoylase*. The pyrimidine ring is then closed by *dihydroorotase*. The resulting dihydroorotate is oxidized to produce orotic acid (orotate) as shown in Figure 22.21. The enzyme that produces orotate, *dihydroorotate dehydrogenase*, is a flavoprotein associated with the inner mitochondrial membrane. All other enzymes in pyrimidine biosynthesis are cytosolic. [Note: The first three enzymic activities in this pathway (*CPS II, aspartate transcarbamoylase*, and *dihydroorotase*) are actually three different catalytic domains of a single polypeptide known as CAD from the first letter in the name of each domain. (See p. 19 for a discussion of domains.) This is an example of a multfunctional or multicatalytic polypeptide that facilitates the ordered synthesis of an important compound. Synthesis of the purine nucleotide IMP also involves multifunctional proteins.]

C. Formation of a pyrimidine nucleotide

The completed pyrimidine ring is converted to the nucleotide orotidine monophosphate (OMP) in the second stage of pyrimidine nucleotide synthesis (see Figure 22.21). PRPP is again the ribose 5-phosphate donor. The enzyme *orotate phosphoribosyltransferase* produces OMP and releases pyrophosphate, thereby making the reaction biologically irreversible. [Note: Both purine and pyrimidine synthesis require glutamine, aspartic acid, and PRPP as essential precursors.] OMP, the parent pyrimidine mononucleotide, is converted to uridine monophosphate (UMP) by *orotidylate decarboxylase*, which removes the carboxyl group. *Orotate phosphoribosyltransferase* and *orotidylate decarboxylase* are also catalytic domains of a single polypeptide chain called *UMP synthase*. Orotic aciduria (a very rare disorder) may be caused by a deficiency of one or both activities of this bifunctional enzyme, resulting in orotic acid in the urine (see Figure 22.21). UMP is sequentially phosphorylated to UDP and UTP. [Note: The UDP is a substrate for *ribonucleotide reductase*, which generates dUDP. The dUDP is phosphorylated to

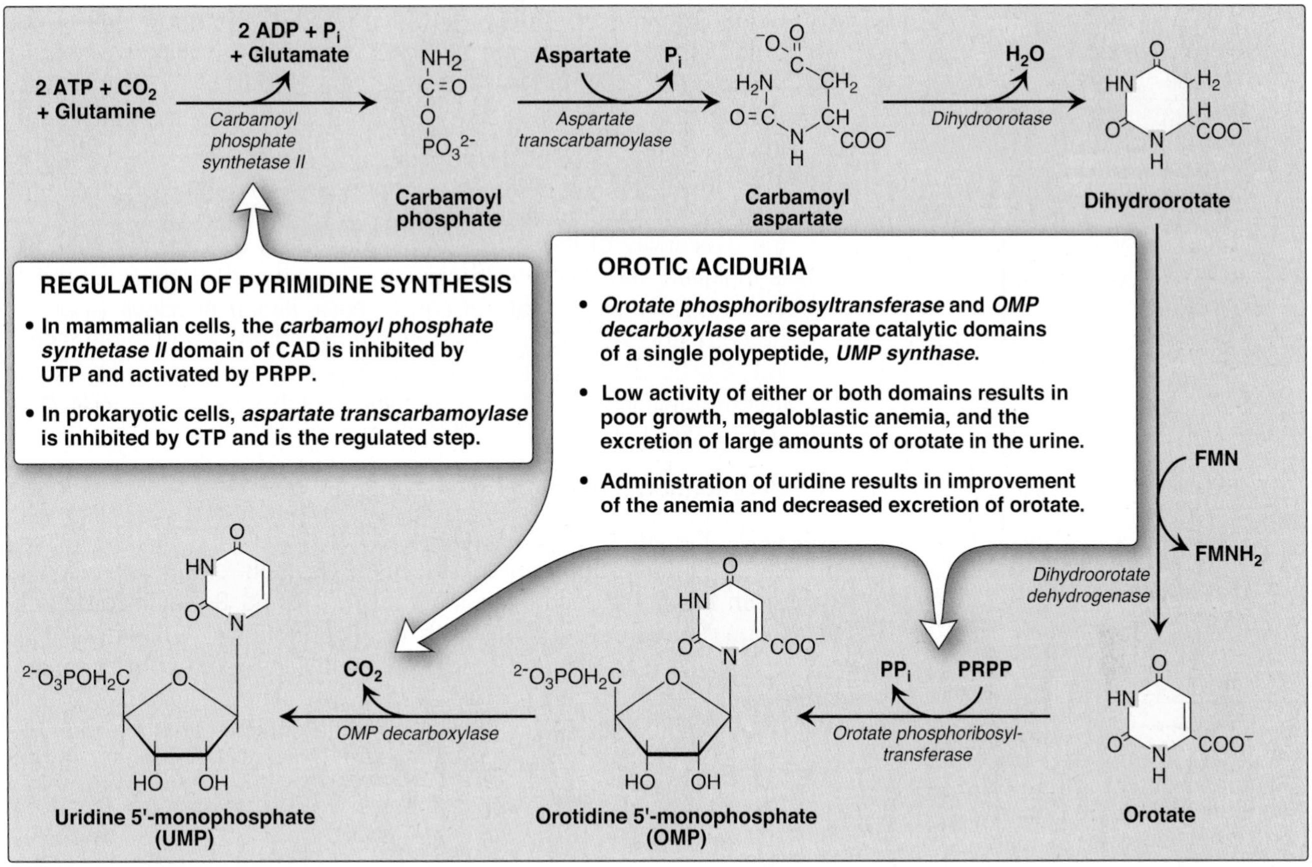

2 ATP + CO_2 + Glutamine → 2 ADP + P_i + Glutamate (*Carbamoyl phosphate synthetase II*) → Carbamoyl phosphate → Aspartate, P_i (*Aspartate transcarbamoylase*) → Carbamoyl aspartate → H_2O (*Dihydroorotase*) → Dihydroorotate → FMN, $FMNH_2$ (*Dihydroorotate dehydrogenase*) → Orotate → PRPP, PP_i (*Orotate phosphoribosyltransferase*) → Orotidine 5'-monophosphate (OMP) → CO_2 (*OMP decarboxylase*) → Uridine 5'-monophosphate (UMP)

REGULATION OF PYRIMIDINE SYNTHESIS

- **In mammalian cells, the *carbamoyl phosphate synthetase II* domain of CAD is inhibited by UTP and activated by PRPP.**
- **In prokaryotic cells, *aspartate transcarbamoylase* is inhibited by CTP and is the regulated step.**

OROTIC ACIDURIA

- ***Orotate phosphoribosyltransferase* and *OMP decarboxylase* are separate catalytic domains of a single polypeptide, *UMP synthase*.**
- **Low activity of either or both domains results in poor growth, megaloblastic anemia, and the excretion of large amounts of orotate in the urine.**
- **Administration of uridine results in improvement of the anemia and decreased excretion of orotate.**

Figure 22.21
De novo pyrimidine synthesis. ADP = adenosine diphosphate; P_i = inorganic phosphate; FMN(H_2) = flavin mononucleotide; CTP = cytidine triphosphate; PRPP = 5-phosphoribosyl-1-pyrophosphate; PP_i = pyrophosphate.

dUTP, which is rapidly hydrolyzed to dUMP by *UTP diphosphatase* (*dUTPase*). *dUTPase*, then, plays an important role in reducing availability of dUTP as a substrate for DNA synthesis, thereby preventing erroneous incorporation of uracil into DNA.]

D. Synthesis of cytidine triphosphate

Cytidine triphosphate (CTP) is produced by amination of UTP by *CTP synthetase* (Figure 22.22), with glutamine providing the nitrogen. [Note: Some CTP is dephosphorylated to cytidine diphosphate (CDP), which is a substrate for *ribonucleotide reductase*. The dCDP product can be phosphorylated to dCTP for DNA synthesis or dephosphoprylated to dCMP that is deaminated to dUMP.]

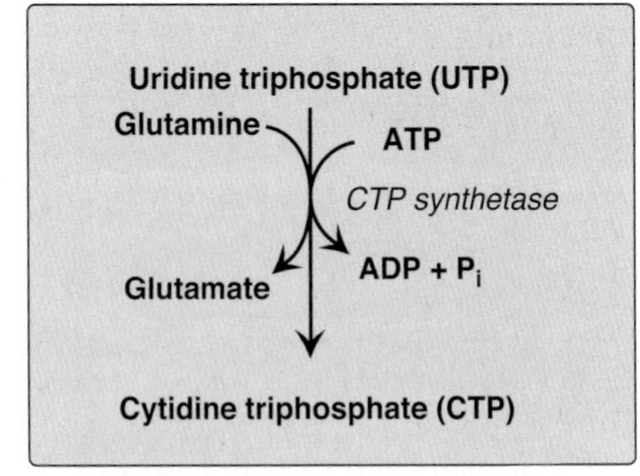

Figure 22.22
Synthesis of CTP from UTP. [Note: CTP, required for RNA synthesis, is converted to dCTP for DNA synthesis.] ADP = adenosine diphosphate; P_i = inorganic phosphate.

E. Synthesis of deoxythymidine monophosphate

dUMP is converted to deoxythymidine monophosphate (dTMP) by *thymidylate synthase*, which uses N^5,N^{10}-methylene tetrahydrofolate as the source of the methyl group (see p. 267 for a discussion of this coenzyme). This is an unusual reaction in that tetrahydrofolate (THF) contributes not only a one-carbon unit but also two hydrogen atoms from the pteridine ring, resulting in the oxidation of THF to dihydrofolate ([DHF] Figure 22.23). Inhibitors of *thymidylate synthase* include thymine analogs such as 5-fluorouracil, which serve as antitumor agents. 5-Fluorouracil is metabolically converted to 5-fluorodeoxyuridine

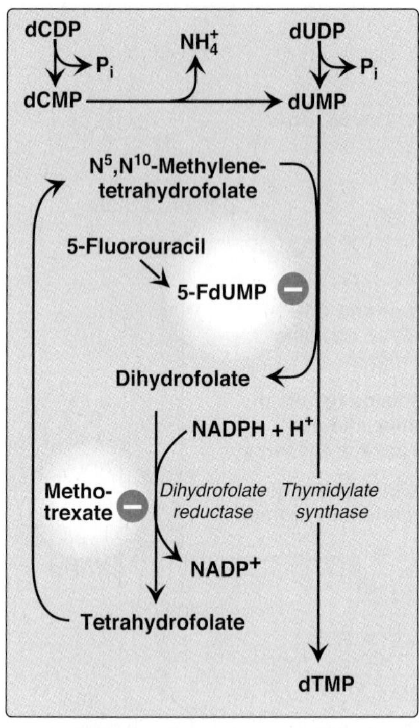

Figure 22.23
Synthesis of dTMP from dUMP, illustrating sites of action of antineoplastic drugs.

monophosphate (5-FdUMP), which becomes permanently bound to the inactivated *thymidylate synthase*, making the drug a "suicide" inhibitor (see p. 60). DHF can be reduced to THF by *dihydrofolate reductase* (see Figure 28.3, p. 374), an enzyme that is inhibited by folate analogs such as methotrexate. By decreasing the supply of THF, these drugs not only inhibit purine synthesis (see Figure 22.7), but, by preventing methylation of dUMP to dTMP, they also decrease the availability of this essential component of DNA. DNA synthesis is inhibited and cell growth slowed. Thus, these drugs are used to decrease the growth rate of cancer cells. [Note: Acyclovir (a purine analog) and AZT (3'-azido-3'-deoxythymidine, a pyrimidine analog) are used to treat infections of herpes simplex virus and human immunodeficiency virus, respectively. Each inhibits the viral *DNA polymerase*.]

F. Degradation and salvage of pyrimidines

Unlike the purine ring, which is not cleaved in humans, the pyrimidine ring is opened and degraded to highly soluble products, β-alanine (from the degradation of CMP and UMP) and β-aminoisobutyrate (from TMP degradation), with the production of NH_3 and CO_2. Pyrimidine bases can be salvaged to nucleosides, which are phosphorylated to nucleotides. However, their high solubility makes pyrimidine salvage less significant clinically than purine salvage. [Note: The salvage of pyrimidine nucleosides is the basis for using uridine in the treatment of hereditary orotic aciduria.]

VII. CHAPTER SUMMARY

Nucleotides are composed of a **nitrogenous base** (**adenine** = **A**, **guanine** = **G**, **cytosine** = **C**, **uracil** = **U**, and **thymine** = **T**); a **pentose**; and one, two, or three **phosphate groups** (Figure 22.24). A and G are **purines**, and C, U, and T are **pyrimidines**. If the sugar is **ribose**, the nucleotide is a **ribonucleoside phosphate** (for example, adenosine monophosphate [AMP]), and it can have several functions in the cell, including being a component of **RNA**. If the sugar is **deoxyribose**, the nucleotide is a **deoxyribonucleoside phosphate** (for example, deoxyAMP), and will be found almost exclusively as a component of **DNA**. The **committed step** in **purine synthesis** uses **5-phosphoribosyl-1-pyrophosphate** ([**PRPP**], an "activated pentose" that provides the ribose-phosphate group for de novo purine and pyrimidine synthesis and salvage) and nitrogen from **glutamine** to produce phosphoribosyl amine. The enzyme is ***glutamine:PRPP amidotransferase*** and is **inhibited** by **AMP** and **guanosine monophosphate** ([**GMP**] the end products of the pathway) and activated by PRPP. Purine nucleotides can also be produced from preformed purine bases by using **salvage reactions** catalyzed by ***adenine phosphoribosyltransferase*** (***APRT***) and ***hypoxanthine-guanine phosphoribosyltransferase*** (***HGPRT***). A near-total deficiency of *HGPRT* causes **Lesch-Nyhan syndrome**, a severe, heritable form of hyperuricemia accompanied by compulsive self-mutilation. All deoxyribonucleotides are synthesized from ribonucleotides by the enzyme ***ribonucleotide reductase***. This enzyme is highly regulated (for example, it is **strongly inhibited by deoxyadenosine triphosphate** [**dATP**], a compound that is overproduced in bone marrow cells in individuals with ***adenosine deaminase*** **deficiency)**. This syndrome causes **severe combined immunodeficiency disease**. The end product of purine degradation is **uric acid**, a compound whose overproduction or undersecretion causes **hyperuricemia** that, if accompanied by the deposition of monosodium urate crystals in joints and soft tissues and an inflammatory response to those crystals, results in **gout**. The first step in **pyrimidine synthesis**, the production of carbamoyl phosphate by ***carbamoyl phosphate synthetase II***, is the **regulated** step in this pathway (it is **inhibited by uridine triphosphate** [**UTP**] and **activated by PRPP**). The UTP produced by this pathway can be converted to cytidine triphosphate. Deoxyuridine monophosphate can be converted to **deoxythymidine monophosphate** using ***thymidylate synthase***, an enzyme targeted by anticancer drugs such as **5-fluorouracil**. The regeneration of tetrahydrofolate from dihydrofolate produced in the *thymidylate synthase* reaction requires ***dihydrofolate reductase***, an enzyme targeted by the drug, **methotrexate**. Pyrimidine degradation results in soluble products.

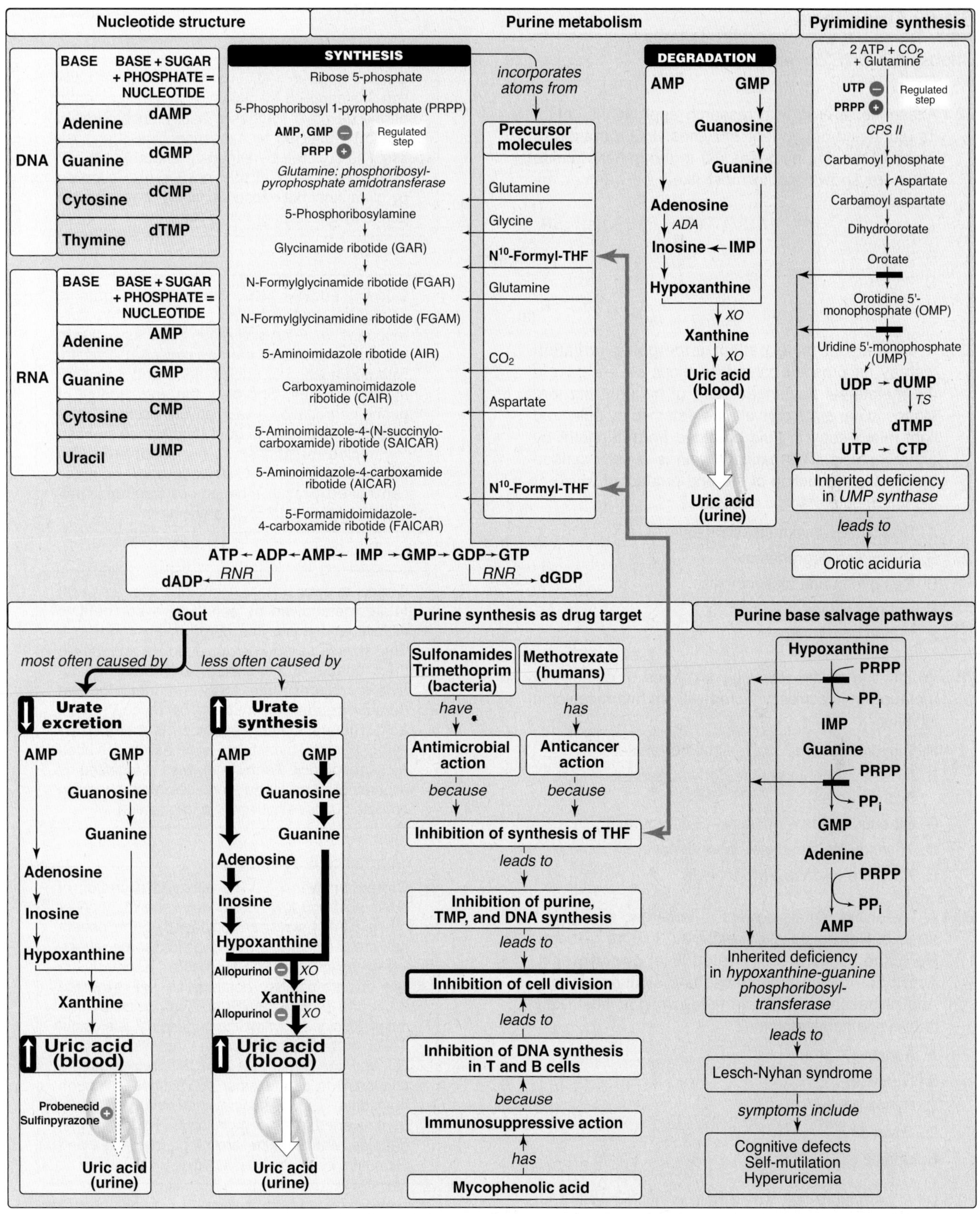

Figure 22.24

Key concept map for nucleotide metabolism. THF = tetrahydrofolate; *ADA= adenosine deaminase; XO = xanthine oxidase; TS = thymidylate synthase; RNR = ribonucleotide reductase; CPS II = carbamyl phosphate synthetase II;* AMP = adenosine monophosphate; GMP = guanosine monophosphate; CMP = cytidine monophosphate; TMP = thymidine monophosphate; IMP = inosine monophosphate; d = deoxy; PP_i = pyrophosphate.

Study Questions

Choose the ONE correct answer.

22.1 Azaserine, a drug with research applications, inhibits glutamine-dependent enzymes. Incorporation of which of the ring nitrogens (N) in the generic purine structure shown would most likely be affected by azaserine?

A. 1

B. 3

C. 7

D. 9

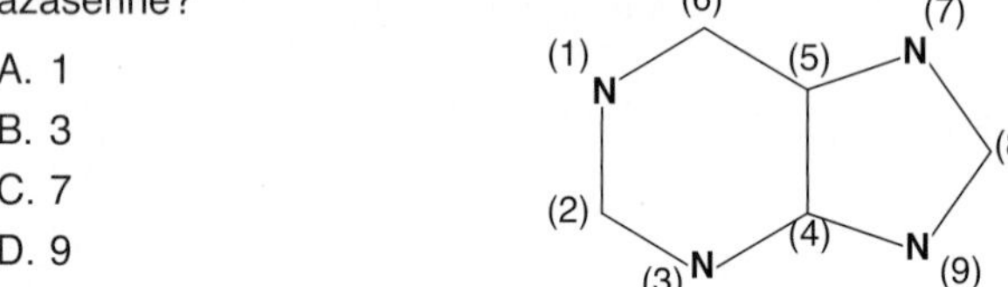

Correct answer = D. The nitrogen (N) at position 9 is supplied by glutamine in the first step of purine de novo synthesis, and its incorporation would be affected by azaserine. The N at position 1 is supplied by aspartate and at position 7 by glycine. The N at position 3 is also supplied by glutamine, but azaserine would have inhibited purine synthesis prior to this step.

22.2 A 42-year-old male patient undergoing radiation therapy for prostate cancer develops severe pain in the metatarsal phalangeal joint of his right big toe. Monosodium urate crystals are detected by polarized light microscopy in fluid obtained from this joint by arthrocentesis. This patient's pain is directly caused by the overproduction of the end product of which of the following metabolic pathways?

A. De novo pyrimidine biosynthesis

B. Pyrimidine degradation

C. De novo purine biosynthesis

D. Purine salvage

E. Purine degradation

Correct answer = E. The patient's pain is caused by gout, resulting from an inflammatory response to the crystallization of excess urate in his joints. Radiation therapy caused cell death, with degradation of nucleic acids and their constituent purines. Uric acid, the end product of purine degradation, is a relatively insoluble compound that can cause gout (and kidney stones). Pyrimidine metabolism is not associated with uric acid production. Overproduction of purines can indirectly result in hyperuricemia. Purine salvage decreases uric acid production.

22.3 Which one of the following enzymes of nucleotide metabolism is correctly paired with its pharmacologic inhibitor?

A. Dihydrofolate reductase—methotrexate

B. Inosine monophosphate dehydrogenase—hydroxyurea

C. Ribonucleotide reductase—5-fluorouracil

D. Thymidylate synthase—allopurinol

E. Xanthine oxidase—probenecid

Correct answer = A. Methotrexate interferes with folate metabolism by acting as a competitive inhibitor of the enzyme dihydrofolate reductase. This starves cells for tetrahydrofolate and makes them unable to synthesize purines and thymidine monophosphate. Inosine monophosphate dehydrogenase is inhibited by mycophenolic acid. Ribonucleotide reductase is inhibited by hydroxyurea. Thymidylate synthase is inhibited by 5-fluorouracil. Xanthine oxidase is inhibited by allopurinol. Probenecid increases renal excretion of urate but does not inhibit its production.

22.4 A 1-year-old female patient is lethargic, weak, and anemic. Her height and weight are low for her age. Her urine contains an elevated level of orotic acid. Activity of uridine monophosphate synthase is low. Administration of which of the following is most likely to alleviate her symptoms?

A. Adenine

B. Guanine

C. Hypoxanthine

D. Thymidine

E. Uridine

Correct answer = E. The elevated excretion of orotic acid and low activity of uridine monophosphate (UMP) synthase indicate that the patient has orotic aciduria, a rare genetic disorder affecting de novo pyrimidine synthesis. Deficiencies in one or both catalytic domains of UMP synthase leave the patient unable to synthesize pyrimidines. Uridine, a pyrimidine nucleoside, is a useful treatment because it bypasses the missing activities and can be salvaged to UMP, which can be converted to all the other pyrimidines. Although thymidine is a pyrimidine nucleoside, it cannot be converted to other pyrimidines. Hypoxanthine, guanine, and adenine are all purine bases and cannot be converted to pyrimidines.

22.5 What laboratory test would help in distinguishing an orotic aciduria caused by ornithine transcarbamylase deficiency from that caused by uridine monophosphate synthase deficiency?

Blood ammonia level would be expected to be elevated in ornithine transcarbamylase deficiency but not in uridine monophosphate synthase deficiency.

UNIT V: Integration of Metabolism

Metabolic Effects of Insulin and Glucagon

23

I. OVERVIEW

Four major tissues play a dominant role in fuel metabolism: liver, adipose, muscle, and brain. These tissues contain unique sets of enzymes, such that each tissue is specialized for the storage, use, or generation of specific fuels. These tissues do not function in isolation, but rather form part of a network in which one tissue may provide substrates to another or process compounds produced by other organs. Communication between tissues is mediated by the nervous system, by the availability of circulating substrates, and by variation in the levels of plasma hormones (Figure 23.1). The integration of energy metabolism is controlled primarily by the actions of two peptide hormones, insulin and glucagon (secreted in response to changing substrate levels in the blood), with the catecholamines epinephrine and norepinephrine (secreted in response to neural signals) playing a supporting role. Changes in the circulating levels of these hormones allow the body to store energy when food is abundant or to make stored energy available such as during "survival crises" (for example, famine, severe injury, and "fight-or-flight" situations). This chapter describes the structure, secretion, and metabolic effects of the two hormones that most profoundly affect energy metabolism.

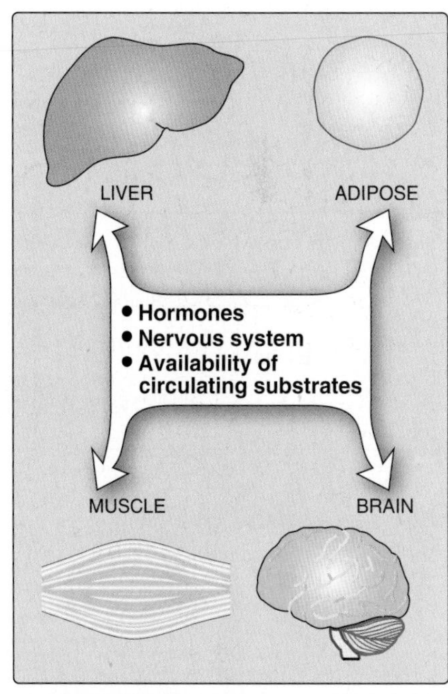

Figure 23.1
Mechanisms of communication between four major tissues.

II. INSULIN

Insulin is a peptide hormone produced by the β cells of the islets of Langerhans, which are clusters of cells that are embedded in the endocrine portion of the pancreas (Figure 23.2). [Note: "Insulin" is from the Latin for island.] The islets make up only about 1%–2% of the total cells of the pancreas. Insulin is the most important hormone coordinating the

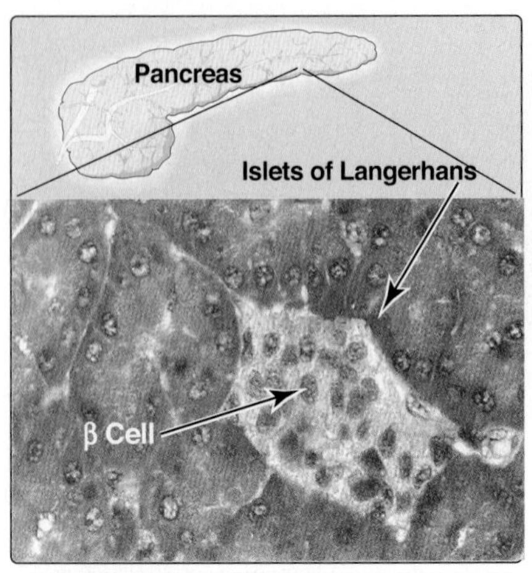

Figure 23.2
Islets of Langerhans.

use of fuels by tissues. Its metabolic effects are anabolic, favoring, for example, synthesis of glycogen, triacylglycerols (TAGs), and protein.

A. Structure of insulin

Insulin is composed of 51 amino acids arranged in two polypeptide chains, designated A (21 amino acids) and B, which are linked together by two disulfide bridges (Figure 23.3A). The insulin molecule also contains an intramolecular disulfide bridge between amino acid residues of the A chain. [Note: Insulin was the first peptide for which the primary structure was determined, and the first therapeutic molecule made by recombinant DNA technology (see p. 470).]

B. Synthesis of insulin

The processing and transport of intermediates that occur during the synthesis of insulin are shown in Figures 23.3B and 23.4. Biosynthesis involves production of two inactive precursors, preproinsulin and proinsulin, that are sequentially cleaved to form the active hormone plus the connecting or C-peptide (see Figure 23.4). [Note: The C-peptide is essential for proper insulin folding. Also, because its half-life in the plasma is longer than that of insulin, the C-peptide is a good indicator of insulin production and secretion.] Insulin is stored in the cytosol in granules that, given the proper stimulus (see below), are released by exocytosis. (See p. 166 for a discussion of the synthesis of secreted proteins.) Insulin is degraded by *insulin-degrading enzyme*, which is present in the liver and, to a lesser extent, in the kidneys. Insulin has a plasma half-life of approximately 6 minutes. This short duration of action permits rapid changes in circulating levels of the hormone.

C. Regulation of insulin secretion

Secretion of insulin is regulated by bloodborne fuels and hormones.

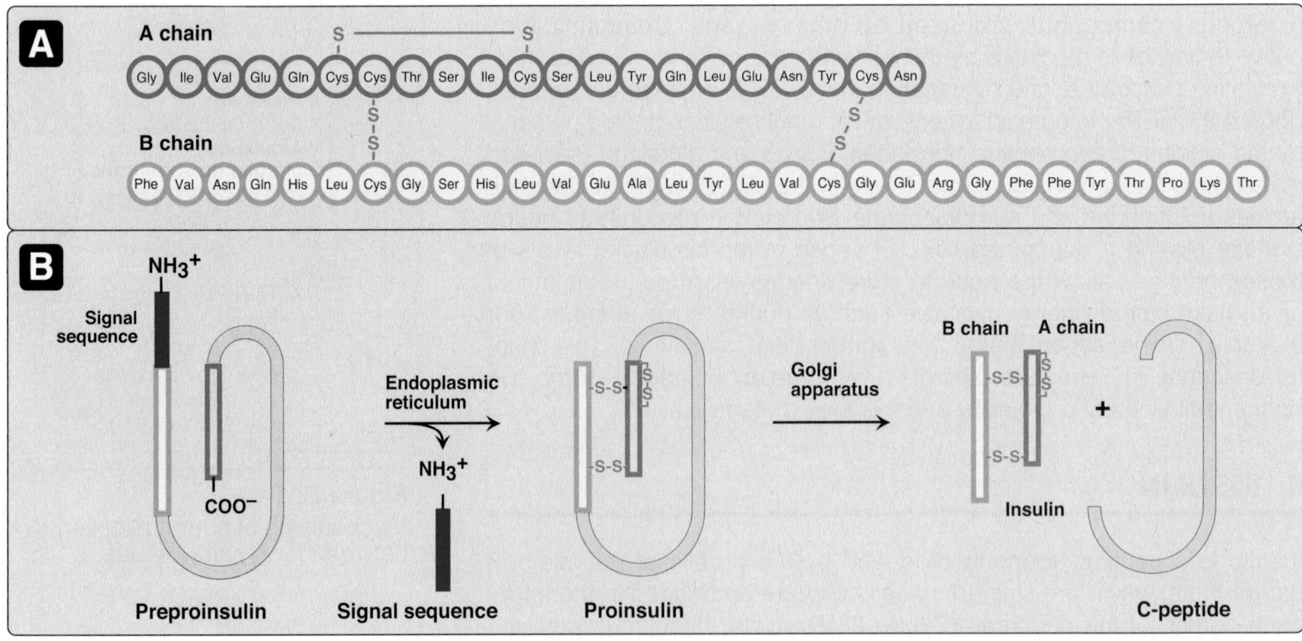

Figure 23.3
A. Structure of insulin. B. Formation of human insulin from preproinsulin.

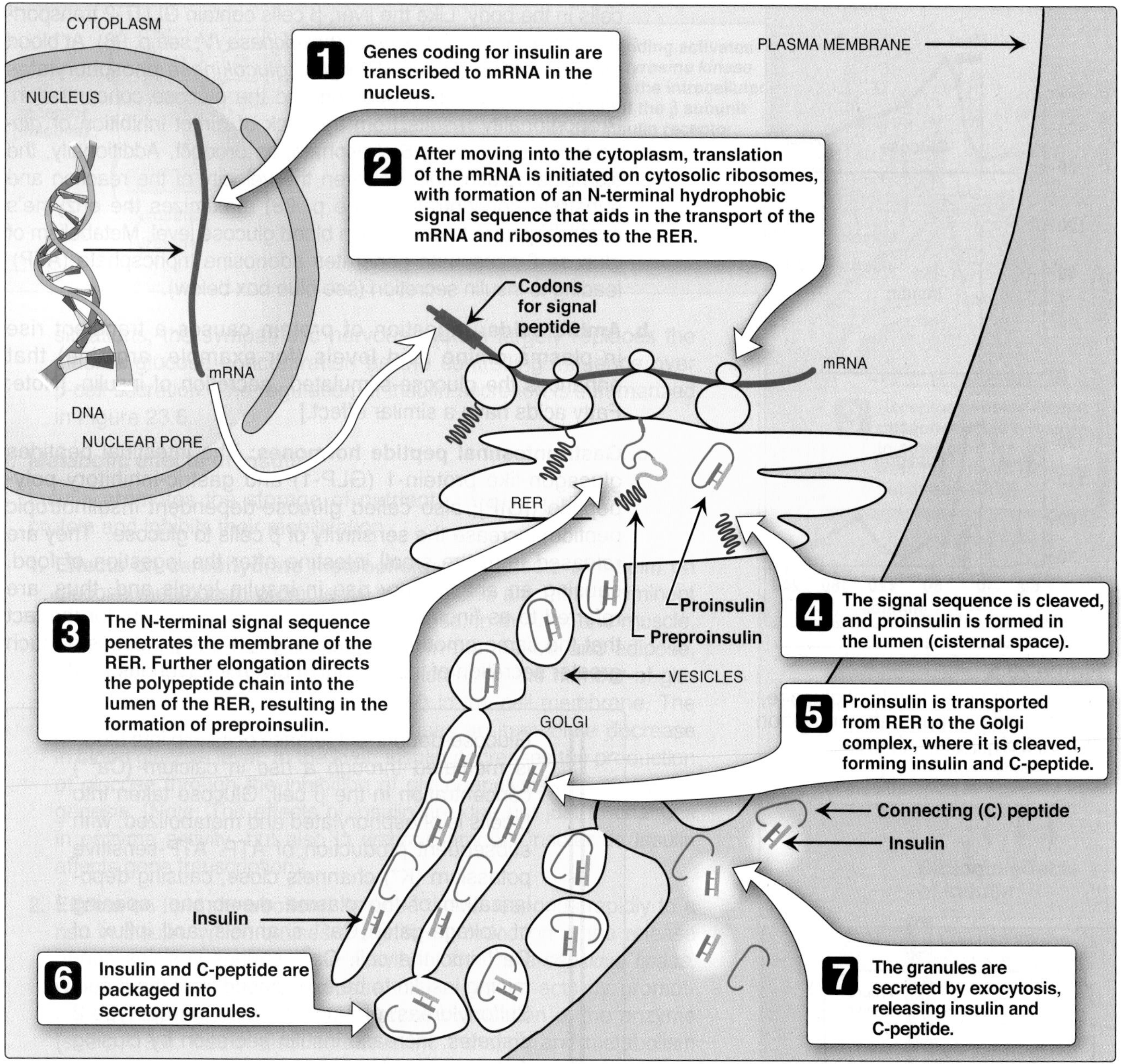

Figure 23.4
Intracellular movements of insulin and its precursors. mRNA = messenger RNA; RER = rough endoplasmic reticulum.

1. **Stimulation of insulin secretion:** Insulin secretion by the pancreatic β cells is closely coordinated with the release of glucagon by pancreatic α cells (Figure 23.5). The relative amounts of insulin and glucagon released by the pancreas are regulated so that the rate of hepatic glucose production is kept equal to the use of glucose by peripheral tissues. In view of its coordinating role, it is not surprising that the β cell responds to a variety of stimuli. In particular, insulin secretion is increased by glucose, amino acids, and gastrointestinal peptide hormones.

   a. **Glucose:** Ingestion of a carbohydrate-rich meal leads to a rise in blood glucose, the primary stimulus for insulin secretion (see Figure 23.5). The β cells are the most important glucose-sensing

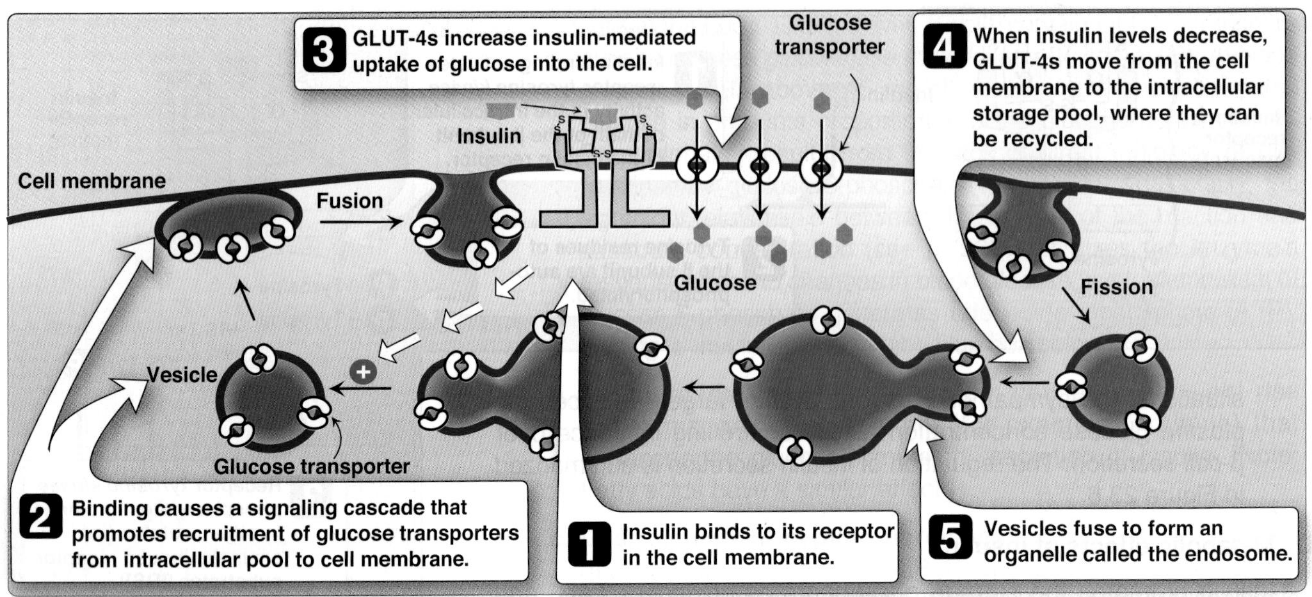

Figure 23.8
Insulin-mediated recruitment of glucose transporters (GLUT-4s) from intracellular stores in skeletal and cardiac muscle and adipose tissue.

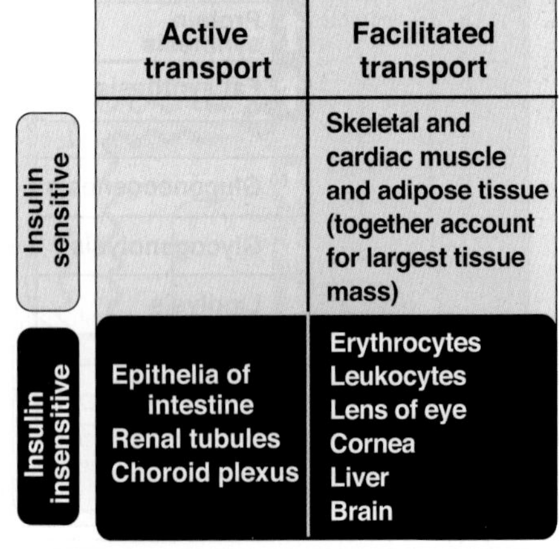

	Active transport	Facilitated transport
Insulin sensitive		Skeletal and cardiac muscle and adipose tissue (together account for largest tissue mass)
Insulin insensitive	Epithelia of intestine Renal tubules Choroid plexus	Erythrocytes Leukocytes Lens of eye Cornea Liver Brain

Figure 23.9
Characteristics of glucose transport in various tissues.

1. **Insulin receptor:** The insulin receptor is synthesized as a single polypeptide that is glycosylated and cleaved into α and β subunits, which are then assembled into a tetramer linked by disulfide bonds (see Figure 23.7). The extracellular α subunit contains the insulin-binding site. A hydrophobic domain in each β subunit spans the plasma membrane. The cytosolic domain of the β subunit is a *tyrosine kinase*, which is activated by insulin. As a result, the insulin receptor is classified as a *tyrosine-kinase* receptor.

2. **Signal transduction:** The binding of insulin to the α subunits of the insulin receptor induces conformational changes that are transmitted to the β subunits. This promotes a rapid autophosphorylation of specific tyrosine residues on each β subunit (see Figure 23.7). Autophosphorylation initiates a cascade of cell-signaling responses, including phosphorylation of a family of proteins called insulin receptor substrates (IRSs). At least four IRSs have been identified that show similar structures but different tissue distributions. Phosphorylated IRS proteins interact with other signaling molecules through specific domains, activating a number of pathways that affect gene expression, cell metabolism, and growth. The actions of insulin are terminated by dephosphorylation of the receptor.

3. **Membrane effects of insulin:** Glucose transport in some tissues, such as muscle and adipose, increases in the presence of insulin (Figure 23.8). Insulin promotes movement of insulin-sensitive glucose transporters (GLUT-4s) from a pool located in intracellular vesicles to the cell membrane. [Note: Movement is the result of a signaling cascade in which an IRS binds to and activates a *kinase* (*phosphoinositide 3-kinase*), leading to phosphorylation of the membrane phospholipid phosphatidylinositol 4,5-bisphosphate to the 3,4,5-trisphosphate form that binds to and activates *phosphoinositide kinase 1*. This *kinase*, in turn, activates *Akt* (*protein kinase B*), resulting in GLUT-4 movement.] In contrast, other

tissues have insulin-insensitive systems for glucose transport (Figure 23.9). For example, hepatocytes; erythrocytes; and cells of the nervous system, intestinal mucosa, renal tubules, and cornea do not require insulin for glucose uptake.

4. **Receptor regulation:** Binding of insulin is followed by internalization of the hormone–receptor complex. Once inside the cell, insulin is degraded in the lysosomes. The receptors may be degraded, but most are recycled to the cell surface. [Note: Elevated levels of insulin promote the degradation of receptors, therby decreasing the number of surface receptors. This is one type of "downregulation."]

5. **Time course of insulin actions:** The binding of insulin provokes a wide range of actions. The most immediate response is an increase in glucose transport into adipocytes and skeletal and cardiac muscle cells that occurs within seconds of insulin binding to its membrane receptor. Insulin-induced changes in enzymic activity in many cell types occur over minutes to hours and reflect changes in the phosphorylation states of existing proteins. Insulin-induced increase in the amount of many enzymes, such as *glucokinase*, liver *pyruvate kinase, acetyl coenzyme A* (*CoA*) *carboxylase* (*ACC*), and *fatty acid synthase*, requires hours to days. These changes reflect an increase in gene expression through increased transcription (mediated by sterol regulatory element–binding protein-1; see p. 184) and translation.

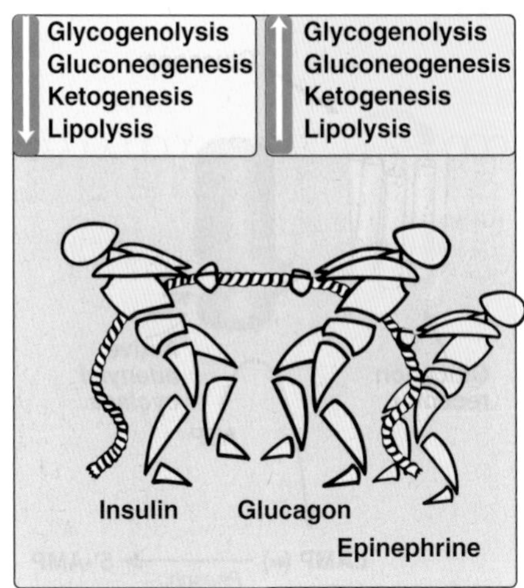

Figure 23.10
Opposing actions of insulin and glucagon plus epinephrine.

III. GLUCAGON

Glucagon is a peptide hormone secreted by the α cells of the pancreatic islets of Langerhans. Glucagon, along with epinephrine, norepinephrine, cortisol, and growth hormone (the "counterregulatory" hormones), opposes many of the actions of insulin (Figure 23.10). Most importantly, glucagon acts to maintain blood glucose levels by activation of hepatic glycogenolysis and gluconeogenesis. Glucagon is composed of 29 amino acids arranged in a single polypeptide chain. [Note: Unlike insulin, the amino acid sequence of glucagon is the same in all mammalian species examined to date.] Glucagon is synthesized as a large precursor molecule (preproglucagon) that is converted to glucagon through a series of selective proteolytic cleavages, similar to those described for insulin biosynthesis (see Figure 23.3). In contrast to insulin, preproglucagon is processed to different products in different tissues, for example, GLP-1 in intestinal L cells. Like insulin, glucagon has a short half-life.

A. Stimulation of glucagon secretion

The α cell is responsive to a variety of stimuli that signal actual or potential hypoglycemia (Figure 23.11). Specifically, glucagon secretion is increased by low blood glucose, amino acids, and catecholamines.

1. **Low blood glucose:** A decrease in plasma glucose concentration is the primary stimulus for glucagon release. During an overnight or prolonged fast, elevated glucagon levels prevent hypoglycemia (see below for a discussion of hypoglycemia).

2. **Amino acids:** Amino acids (for example, arginine) derived from a meal containing protein stimulate the release of glucagon. The glucagon effectively prevents the hypoglycemia that would otherwise occur as a result of the increased insulin secretion that also occurs after a protein meal.

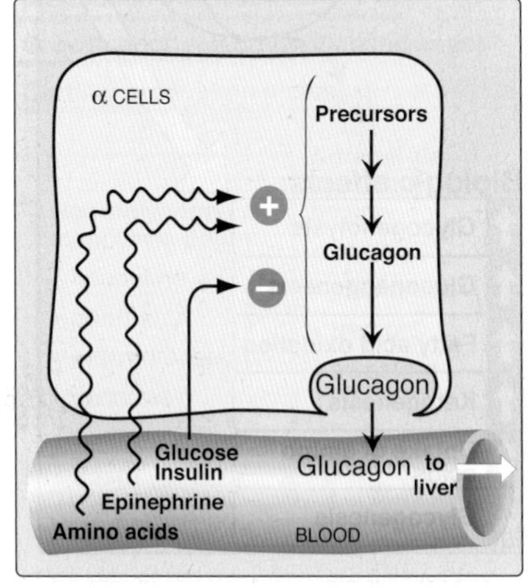

Figure 23.11
Regulation of glucagon release from pancreatic α cells. [Note: Amino acids increase release of insulin and glucagon, whereas glucose increases release of insulin only.]

cogen. [Note: Decreased availability of OAA allows acetyl CoA to be diverted to ketone body synthesis in the liver (see p. 195) and can result in alcoholic ketoacidosis.] Hypoglycemia can produce many of the behaviors associated with alcohol intoxication, such as agitation, impaired judgment, and combativeness. Therefore, alcohol consumption in vulnerable individuals (such as those who are fasted or have engaged in prolonged, strenuous exercise) can produce hypoglycemia that may contribute to the behavioral effects of alcohol. Becuase alcohol consumption can also increase the risk for hypoglycemia in patients using insulin, those in an intensive insulin treatment protocol (see p. 340) are counseled about the increased risk of hypoglycemia that generally occurs many hours after alcohol ingestion. [Note: Chronic alcohol consumption can also result in alcoholic fatty liver due to increased hepatic synthesis of TAGs coupled with impaired formation or release of VLDLs. This occurs as a result of decreased fatty acid oxidation due to a fall in the NAD^+/NADH ratio and increased lipogenesis due to the increased availability of fatty acids (decreased catabolism) and of glyceraldehyde 3-phosphate (the *dehydrogenase* is inhibited by the low NAD^+/NADH ratio). With continued alcohol consumption, alcoholic fatty liver can progress first to alcoholic hepatitis and then to alcoholic cirrhosis (Figure 23.16).]

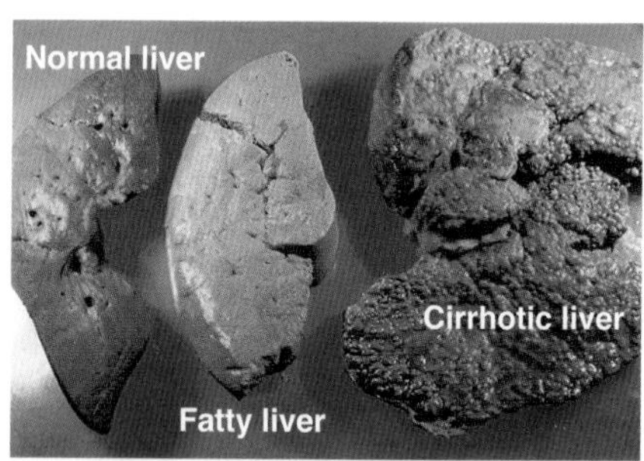

Figure 23.16
Effects of chronic alcohol consumption on liver morphology.

V. CHAPTER SUMMARY

The integration of energy metabolism is controlled primarily by **insulin** and the opposing actions of **glucagon** and the catecholamines, particularly **epinephrine** (Figure 23.17). Changes in the circulating levels of these hormones allow the body to store energy when food is abundant or to make stored energy available in times of physiologic stress (for example, during "survival crises," such as famine). **Insulin** is a peptide hormone produced by the **β cells** of the **islets of Langerhans** of the pancreas. It consists of disulfide-linked A and B chains. A **rise in blood glucose** is the most important signal for insulin **secretion**. The **catecholamines**, secreted in response to stress, trauma, or extreme exercise, **inhibit** insulin **secretion**. Insulin increases glucose uptake (by muscle and adipose) and the synthesis of glycogen, protein, and triacylglycerol: it is an **anabolic** hormone. These actions are mediated by binding to its ***tyrosine kinase*** **receptor**. Binding initiates a cascade of cell-signaling responses, including phosphorylation of a family of proteins called **insulin receptor substrate proteins**. **Glucagon** is a monomeric peptide hormone produced by the **α cells** of the pancreatic islets (both insulin and glucagon synthesis involves formation of inactive precursors that are cleaved to form the active hormones). Glucagon, along with epinephrine, norepinephrine, cortisol, and growth hormone (the **"counterregulatory" hormones**), opposes many of the actions of insulin. Glucagon acts to maintain blood glucose during periods of potential hypoglycemia. Glucagon increases glycogenolysis, gluconeogenesis, fatty acid oxidation, ketogenesis, and uptake of amino acids: it is a **catabolic** hormone. Glucagon **secretion** is **stimulated by low blood glucose, amino acids, and the catecholamines**. Its secretion is **inhibited by elevated blood glucose and by insulin**. Glucagon binds to high-affinity receptors of hepatocytes. Binding results in the activation of ***adenylyl cyclase***, which produces the second messenger **cyclic adenosine monophosphate** (**cAMP**). Subsequent activation of cAMP-dependent ***protein kinase A*** results in the phosphorylation-mediated activation or inhibition of key regulatory enzymes involved in carbohydrate and lipid metabolism. Both insulin and glucagon affect **gene transcription**. **Hypoglycemia** is characterized by low blood glucose accompanied by adrenergic and neuroglycopenic symptoms that are rapidly resolved by the administration of glucose. Insulin-induced, postprandial, and fasting hypoglycemia result in release of glucagon and epinephrine. The rise in **nicotinamide adenine dinucleotide** (**NADH**) that accompanies **ethanol** metabolism inhibits gluconeogenesis, leading to hypoglycemia in individuals with depleted stores. Alcohol consumption also increases the risk for hypoglycemia in patients using insulin. Chronic alcohol consumption can cause fatty liver disease.

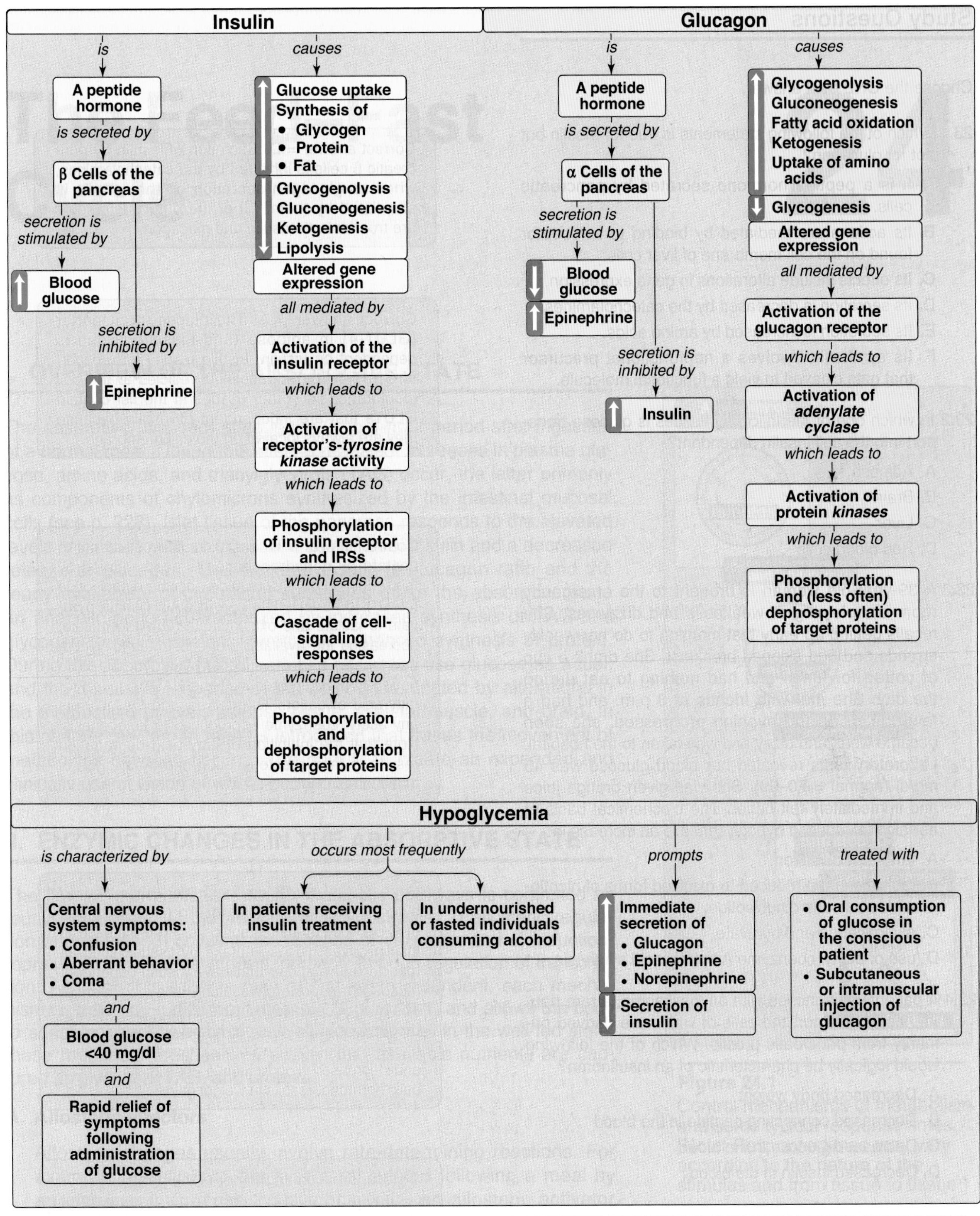

Figure 23.17
Key concept map for the metabolic effects of insulin and glucagon, and hypoglycemia. IRSs = insulin receptor substrates.

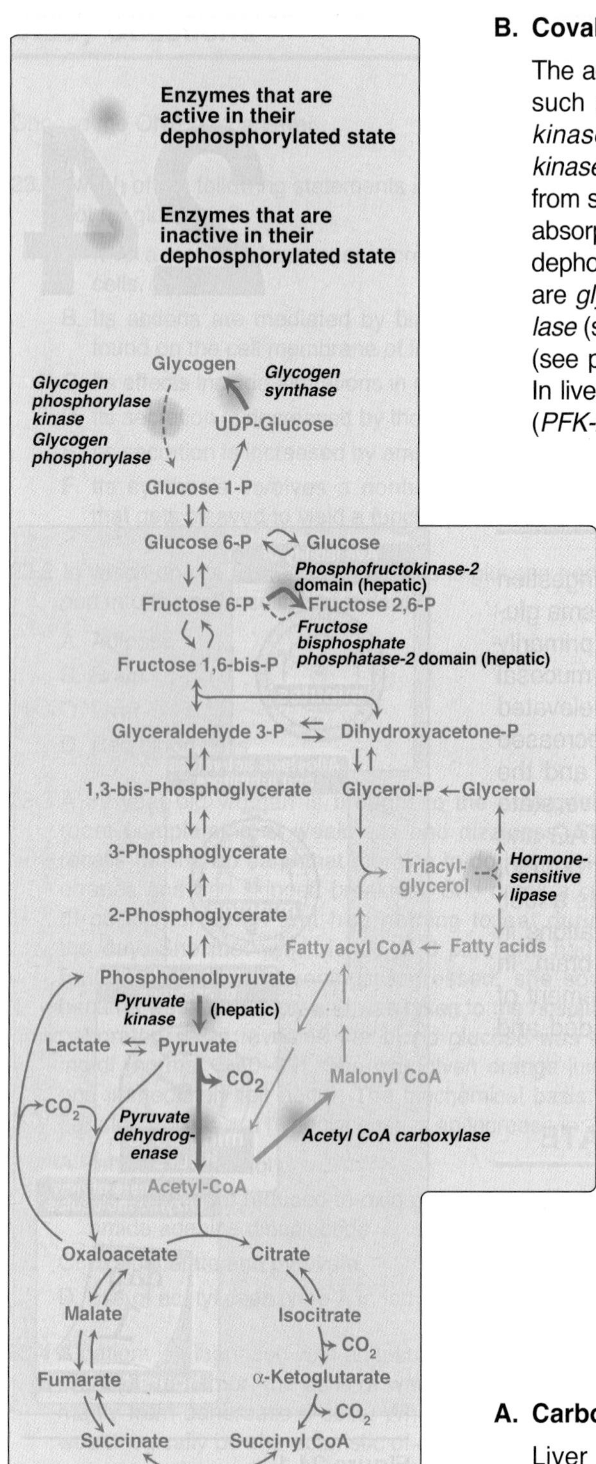

Figure 24.2
Important reactions of intermediary metabolism regulated by enzyme phosphorylation. Blue text = intermediates of carbohydrate metabolism; brown text = intermediates of lipid metabolism. P = phosphate; CoA = coenzyme A.

B. Covalent modification

The activity of many enzymes is regulated by the addition (via *kinases*, such as cyclic adenosine monophosphate [cAMP]-activated *protein kinase A* [*PKA*] and *adenosine monophosphate-activated protein kinase* [*AMPK*]) or removal (via *phosphatases*) of phosphate groups from specific serine, threonine, or tyrosine residues of the protein. In the absorptive state, most of the covalently regulated enzymes are in the dephosphorylated form and are active (Figure 24.2). Three exceptions are *glycogen phosphorylase kinase* (see p. 132), *glycogen phosphorylase* (see p. 132), and *hormone-sensitive lipase* (*HSL*) of adipose tissue (see p. 190), which are inactive in their dephosphorylated form. [Note: In liver, the *phosphatase* domain of bifunctional *phosphofructokinase-2* (*PFK-2*) is inactive when the protein is dephosphorylated (see p. 100).]

C. Induction and repression of enzyme synthesis

Increased (induction of) or decreased (repression of) enzyme synthesis leads to changes in the number of enzyme molecules, rather than influencing the activity of existing enzyme molecules. Enzymes subject to regulation of synthesis are often those that are needed under specific physiologic conditions. For example, in the fed state, elevated insulin levels result in an increase in the synthesis of key enzymes, such as *acetyl coenzyme A (CoA) carboxylase* ([*ACC*] see p. 184) and *fatty acid synthase* (see p.184), involved in anabolic metabolism. In the fasted state, glucagon induces expression of *phosphoenolpyruvate carboxykinase* (*PEPCK*) of gluconeogenesis (see p.120). Both hormones affect transcription factors.

III. LIVER: NUTRIENT DISTRIBUTION CENTER

The liver is uniquely situated to process and distribute dietary nutrients because the venous drainage of the gut and pancreas passes through the hepatic portal vein before entry into the general circulation. Thus, after a meal, the liver is bathed in blood containing absorbed nutrients and elevated levels of insulin secreted by the pancreas. During the absorptive period, the liver takes up carbohydrates, lipids, and most amino acids. These nutrients are then metabolized, stored, or routed to other tissues. In this way, the liver smooths out potentially broad fluctuations in the availability of nutrients for the peripheral tissues.

A. Carbohydrate metabolism

Liver is normally a glucose-producing rather than a glucose-using tissue. However, after a meal containing carbohydrate, the liver becomes a net consumer, retaining roughly 60 of every 100 g of glucose presented by the portal system. This increased use reflects increased glucose uptake by the hepatocytes. Their insulin-independent glucose transporter (GLUT-2) has a low affinity (high K_m) for glucose and, therefore, takes up glucose only when blood glucose is high (see p. 97). Additional mechanisms by which hepatic glucose metabolism is increased include the following. [Note: The numbers in colored circles in the text refer to Figure 24.3.]

1. **Increased phosphorylation of glucose:** The elevated levels of glucose within the hepatocyte (as a result of elevated extracellular levels) allow *glucokinase* to phosphorylate glucose to glucose 6-phosphate (Figure 24.3, ❶). (Recall that *glucokinase* has a high K_m for glucose, is not subject to direct product inhibition, and has a sigmoidal reaction curve; see p.98.).

2. **Increased glycogenesis:** The conversion of glucose 6-phosphate to glycogen is favored by the activation of *glycogen synthase*, both by dephosphorylation and by increased availability of glucose 6-phosphate, its allosteric effector (see Figure 24.3, ❷).

3. **Increased activity of the pentose phosphate pathway:** The increased availability of glucose 6-phosphate, combined with the active use of nicotinamide adenine dinucleotide phosphate (NADPH) in hepatic lipogenesis, stimulates the pentose phosphate pathway ([PPP] see p. 145). This pathway typically accounts for 5%–10% of the glucose metabolized by the liver (see Figure 24.3, ❸).

4. **Increased glycolysis:** In liver, glycolysis is significant only during the absorptive period following a carbohydrate-rich meal. The conversion of glucose to pyruvate is stimulated by the elevated insulin-to-glucagon ratio that results in increased amounts of the regulated enzymes of glycolysis: *glucokinase*, *PFK-1*, and *pyruvate kinase* ([*PK*] see p. 102). Additionally, *PFK-1* is allosterically activated by fructose 2,6-bisphosphate generated by the active (dephosphorylated) *kinase* domain of bifunctional *PFK-2*. *PK* is dephosphorylated and active. *Pyruvate dehydrogenase* (*PDH*), which converts pyruvate to acetyl CoA, is active (dephosphorylated) because pyruvate inhibits *PDH kinase* (see Figure 24.3, ❹). The acetyl CoA either is

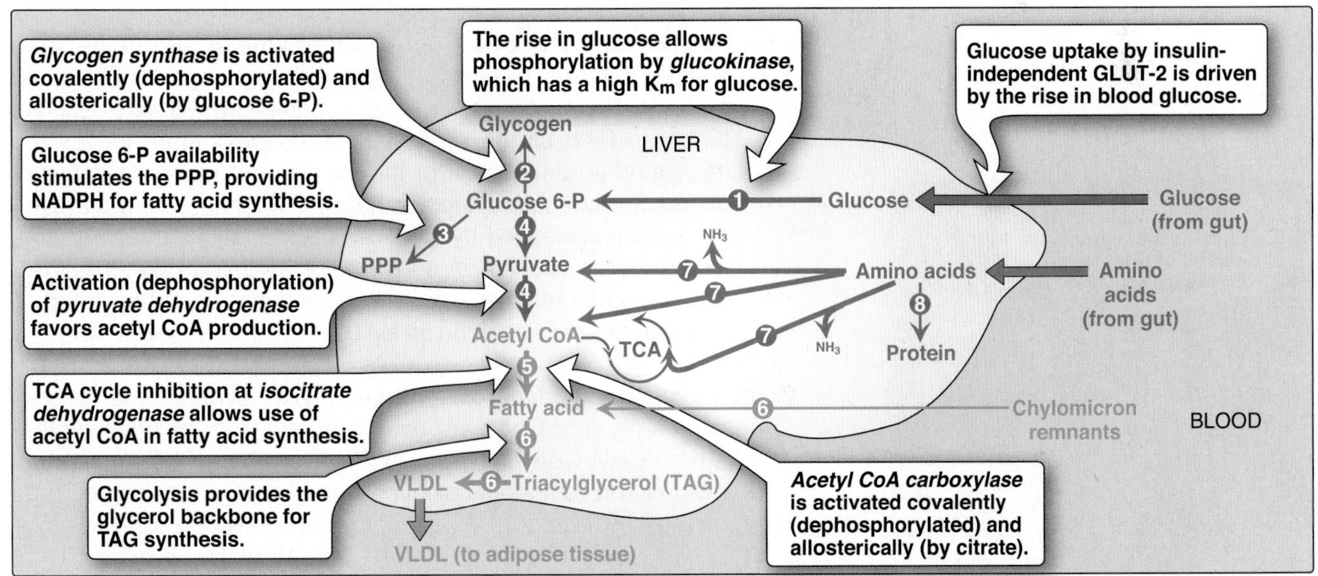

Figure 24.3
Major metabolic pathways in liver in the absorptive state. [Note: The acetyl CoA is also used for cholesterol synthesis.] The numbers in circles, which appear both in the figure and in the text, indicate important pathways for carbohydrate, fat, or protein metabolism. Blue text = intermediates of carbohydrate metabolism; brown text = intermediates of lipid metabolism; green text = intermediates of protein metabolism. P = phosphate; PPP = pentose phosphate pathway; TCA = tricarboxylic acid (cycle); CoA = coenzyme A; VLDL = very-low-density lipoprotein; GLUT = glucose transporter; NADPH = nicotinamide adenine dinucleotide phosphate.

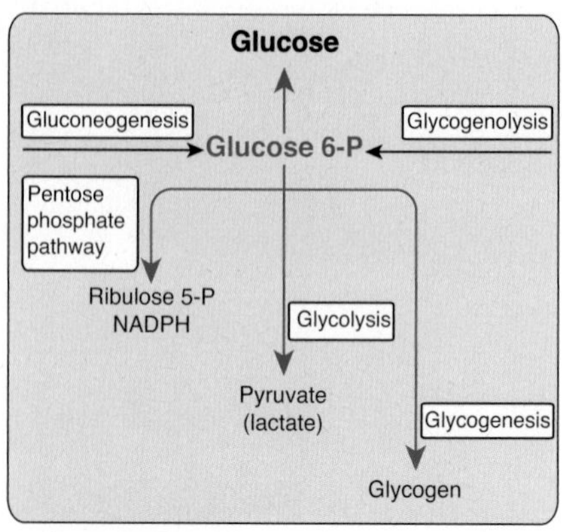

Figure 24.4
Central role of glucose 6-phosphate in metabolism. [Note: The presence of *glucose 6-phosphatase* in liver allows the production of free glucose from glycogenolysis and gluconeogenesis.] NADPH = nicotinamide adenine dinucleotide phosphate; P = phosphate.

used as a substrate for fatty acid (FA) synthesis or is oxidized for energy in the tricarboxylic acid (TCA) cycle. (See Figure 24.4 for the central role of glucose 6-phosphate.)

5. **Decreased production of glucose:** Although glycolysis and glycogenesis (pathways that promote glucose storage) are stimulated in liver in the absorptive state, gluconeogenesis and glycogenolysis (pathways that generate glucose) are decreased. *Pyruvate carboxylase* (*PC*), which catalyzes the first step in gluconeogenesis, is largely inactive due to low levels of acetyl CoA, its allosteric activator (see p. 119). [Note: The acetyl CoA is being used for fatty acid synthesis.] The high insulin-to-glucagon ratio also favors inactivation of other gluconeogenic enzymes such as *fructose 1,6-bisphosphatase* (see Figure 8.17, p. 100). Glycogenolysis is inhibited by dephosphorylation of *glycogen phosphorylase* and *phosphorylase kinase*.

B. Fat metabolism

1. **Increased fatty acid synthesis:** Liver is the primary tissue for de novo synthesis of FAs (see Figure 24.3, ⑤). FA synthesis, a cytosolic process, is favored in the absorptive period by availability of the substrates acetyl CoA (from glucose and amino acid metabolism) and NADPH (from glucose metabolism) and by the activation of *ACC*, both by dephosphorylation and by the presence of its allosteric activator, citrate. [Note: Inactivity of *AMPK* favors dephosphorylation.] *ACC* catalyzes the formation of malonyl CoA from acetyl CoA, the rate-limiting reaction for FA synthesis (see p. 183). [Note: Malonyl CoA inhibits *carnitine palmitoyltransferase-I* (*CPT-I*) of FA oxidation (see p.191). Citrate, thereby, directly activates FA synthesis and indirectly inhibits FA degradation.]

   a. **Source of cytosolic acetyl coenzyme A:** Pyruvate from aerobic glycolysis enters mitochondria and is decarboxylated by *PDH*. The acetyl CoA product is combined with oxaloacetate (OAA) to form citrate via *citrate synthase*. Citrate leaves the mitochondria (as a result of the inhibition of *isocitrate dehydrogenase* by adenosine triphosphate [ATP]) and enters the cytosol. Citrate is cleaved by *ATP-citrate lyase* (induced by insulin), producing the acetyl CoA substrate of *ACC* and OAA. The OAA is reduced to malate, which is oxidatively decarboxylated to pyruvate by *malic enzyme* as NADPH is formed (see p. 187).

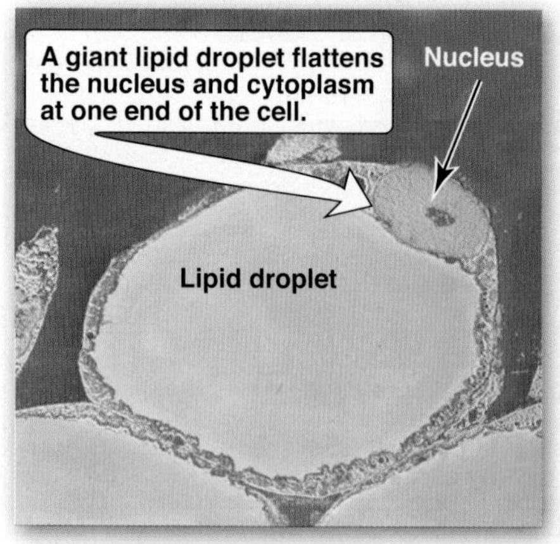

Figure 24.5
Colorized transmission electron micrograph of adipocytes.

2. **Increased triacylglycerol synthesis:** TAG synthesis is favored because fatty acyl CoAs are available both from de novo synthesis from acetyl CoA and from hydrolysis of the TAG component of chylomicron remnants removed from the blood by hepatocytes (see p. 178). Glycerol 3-phosphate, the backbone for TAG synthesis, is provided by glycolysis (see p. 189). The liver packages TAG into very-low-density lipoprotein (VLDL) particles that are secreted into the blood for use by extrahepatic tissues, particularly adipose and muscle tissues (see Figure 24.3, ⑥).

C. Amino acid metabolism

1. **Increased amino acid degradation:** In the absorptive period, more amino acids are present than the liver can use in the synthesis

of proteins and other nitrogen-containing molecules. The surplus amino acids are not stored but are either released into the blood for other tissues to use in protein synthesis or deaminated, with the resulting carbon skeletons being degraded by the liver to pyruvate, acetyl CoA, or TCA cycle intermediates. These metabolites can be oxidized for energy or used in FA synthesis (see Figure 24.3, ❼). The liver has limited capacity to degrade the branched-chain amino acids (BCAAs) leucine, isoleucine, and valine. They pass through the liver essentially unchanged and are preferentially metabolized in muscle (see p. 266).

2. **Increased protein synthesis:** The body does not store protein in the same way that it maintains glycogen or TAG reserves (see p. 327). However, a transient increase in the synthesis of hepatic proteins does occur in the absorptive state, resulting in replacement of any proteins that may have been degraded during the previous postabsorptive period (see Figure 24.3, ❽).

IV. ADIPOSE TISSUE: ENERGY STORAGE DEPOT

Adipose tissue is second only to the liver in its ability to distribute fuel molecules. In a 70-kg man, white adipose tissue (WAT) weighs approximately 14 kg, or about half as much as the total muscle mass. Nearly the entire volume of each adipocyte in WAT can be occupied by a droplet of TAG (Figure 24.5).

A. Carbohydrate metabolism

1. **Increased glucose transport:** Circulating insulin levels are elevated in the absorptive state, resulting in an influx of glucose into adipocytes via insulin-sensitive GLUT-4 recruited to the cell surface from intracellular vesicles (Figure 24.6, ❶). The glucose is phosphorylated by *hexokinase*.

2. **Increased glycolysis:** The increased intracellular availability of glucose results in an enhanced rate of glycolysis (see Figure 24.6, ❷). In adipose tissue, glycolysis serves a synthetic function by supplying glycerol 3-phosphate for TAG synthesis (see p. 189). Recall that adipose tissue lacks *glycerol kinase*.

3. **Increased activity of the pentose phosphate pathway:** Adipose tissue can metabolize glucose by means of the PPP, thereby producing NADPH, which is essential for fat synthesis (see p. 186 and Figure 24.6, ❸). However, in humans, de novo synthesis is not a major source of FA in adipose tissue, except when refeeding a previously fasted individual (see Figure 24.6, ❹).

B. Fat metabolism

Most of the FAs added to the TAG stores of adipocytes after consumption of a lipid-containing meal are provided by the degradation of exogenous (dietary) TAG in chylomicrons sent out by the intestine and endogenous TAG in VLDL sent out by the liver (see Figure 24.6, ❺). The FAs are released from the lipoproteins by the action of *lipoprotein lipase* (*LPL*), an extracellular enzyme attached to the capillary walls in many tissues, particularly adipose and muscle. In adipose

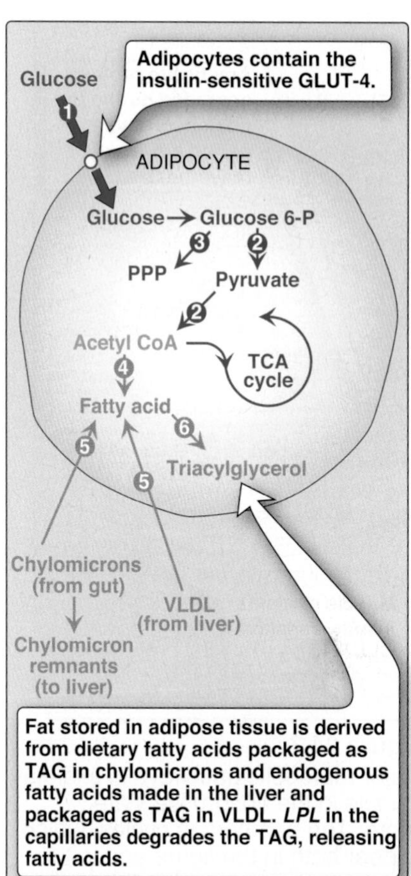

Figure 24.6
Major metabolic pathways in adipose tissue in the absorptive state. [Note: The numbers in the circles, which appear both in the figure and in the corresponding text, indicate important pathways for adipose tissue metabolism.] GLUT = glucose transporter; P = phosphate; PPP = pentose phosphate pathway; CoA = coenzyme A; TCA = tricarboxylic acid; TAG = triacylglycerol; VLDL = very-low-density lipoprotein; *LPL* = *lipoprotein lipase*.

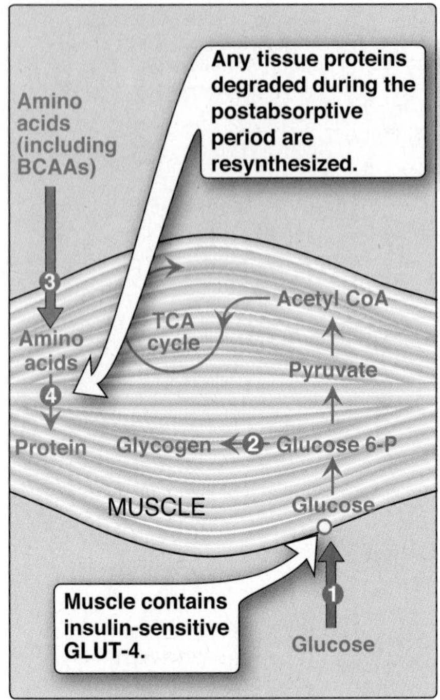

Figure 24.7
Major metabolic pathways in skeletal muscle in the absorptive state. [Note: The numbers in circles, which appear both in the figure and in the text, indicate important pathways for carbohydrate or protein metabolism.] CoA = coenzyme A; P = phosphate; GLUT = glucose transporter; BCAAs = branched-chain amino acids; TCA = tricarboxylic acid.

tissue, *LPL* is upregulated by insulin. Thus, in the fed state, elevated levels of glucose and insulin favor storage of TAG (see Figure 24.6, ➏), all the carbons of which are supplied by glucose. [Note: Elevated insulin favors the dephosphorylated (inactive) form of *HSL* (see p. 190), thereby inhibiting lipolysis in the fed state.]

V. RESTING SKELETAL MUSCLE

In the fed state, muscle takes up glucose via GLUT-4 (for energy and glycogen synthesis) and amino acids (for energy and protein synthesis). [Note: The energy metabolism of skeletal muscle is unique in being able to respond to substantial changes in the demand for ATP that accompanies muscle contraction. At rest, muscle accounts for approximately 30% of the O_2 consumption of the body, whereas during vigorous exercise, it is responsible for up to 90% of the total O_2 consumption. This graphically illustrates the fact that skeletal muscle, despite its potential for transient periods of anaerobic glycolysis, is an oxidative tissue. In contrast to liver, there is no covalent regulation of *PFK-2* in skeletal muscle. In the cardiac isozyme, however, the *kinase* domain is activated by epinephrine-mediated phosphorylation.]

A. Carbohydrate metabolism

1. **Increased glucose transport:** The transient increase in plasma glucose and insulin after a carbohydrate-rich meal leads to an increase in glucose transport into muscle cells by GLUT-4 (see p. 97 and Figure 24.7, ➊), thereby reducing blood glucose. Glucose is phosphorylated to glucose 6-phosphate by *hexokinase* and metabolized to provide the energy needs of the cells.

2. **Increased glycogen synthesis:** The increased insulin-to-glucagon ratio and the availability of glucose 6-phosphate favor glycogen synthesis, particularly if glycogen stores have been depleted as a result of exercise (see p. 126, and Figure 24.7, ➋).

B. Fat metabolism

FAs are released from chylomicrons and VLDL by the action of *LPL* (see pp. 228 and 231). However, fatty acids are of secondary importance as a fuel for resting muscle during the fed state, in which glucose is the primary source of energy.

C. Amino acid metabolism

1. **Increased protein synthesis:** An increase in amino acid uptake and protein synthesis occurs in the absorptive period after ingestion of a meal containing protein (see Figure 24.7, ➌ and ➍). This synthesis replaces protein degraded since the previous meal.

2. **Increased uptake of branched-chain amino acids:** Muscle is the principal site for degradation of the BCAAs (leucine, isoleucine, and valine) because it contains the required *transaminase* (see p. 266). The BCAAs escape metabolism by the liver and are taken up by muscle, where they are used for protein synthesis (see Figure 24.7, ➌) and as sources of energy.

VI. BRAIN

Although contributing only 2% of the adult weight, the brain accounts for a consistent 20% of the basal O_2 consumption of the body at rest. Because the brain is vital to the proper functioning of all organs of the body, special priority is given to its fuel needs. To provide energy, substrates must be able to cross the endothelial cells that line the blood vessels in the brain (the blood–brain barrier [BBB]). In the fed state, the brain exclusively uses glucose as a fuel (GLUT-1 of the BBB is insulin independent), completely oxidizing approximately 140 g/day to CO_2 and H_2O. The brain contains no significant stores of glycogen and is, therefore, completely dependent on the availability of blood glucose (Figure 24.8, ❶). [Note: If blood glucose levels fall below 40 mg/100 ml (normal fasted blood glucose is 70–99 mg/100 ml), cerebral function is impaired (see p. 315).] The brain also lacks significant stores of TAG, and the FAs circulating in the blood make little contribution to energy production because FAs bound to albumin do not efficiently cross the BBB. The intertissue exchanges characteristic of the absorptive period are summarized in Figure 24.9.

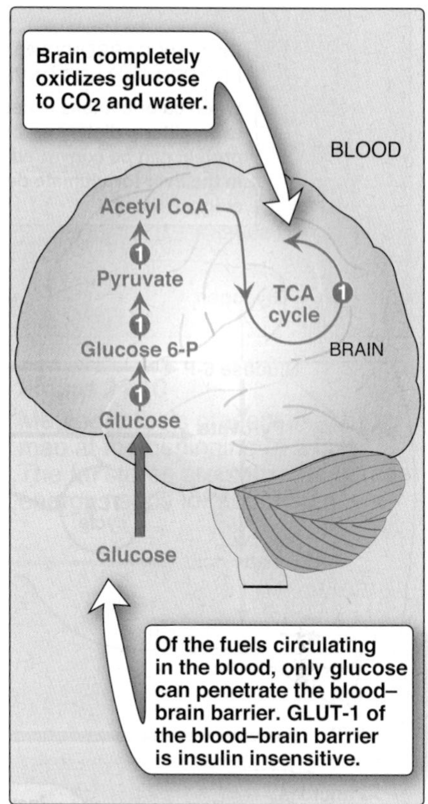

Figure 24 .8
Major metabolic pathways in brain in the absorptive state. [Note: The numbers in circles, which appear both in the figure and in the text, indicate important pathways for carbohydrate metabolism.] CoA = coenzyme A; TCA = tricarboxylic acid; P = phosphate; GLUT = glucose transporter.

VII. OVERVIEW OF FASTING

Fasting begins if no food is ingested after the absorptive period. It may result from an inability to obtain food, the desire to lose weight rapidly, or clinical situations in which an individual cannot eat (for example, because of trauma, surgery, cancer, or burns). In the absence of food, plasma levels of glucose, amino acids, and TAG fall, triggering a decline in insulin secretion and an increase in glucagon and epinephrine release. The decreased insulin/counterregulatory hormone ratio and the decreased availability of circulating substrates make the period of nutrient deprivation a catabolic period characterized by degradation of TAG, glycogen, and protein. This sets into motion an exchange of substrates among liver, adipose tissue, skeletal muscle, and brain that is guided by two priorities: 1) the need to maintain adequate plasma levels of glucose to sustain energy metabolism in the brain, red blood cells, and other glucose-requiring tissues and 2) the need to mobilize fatty acids from adipose tissue and the synthesis and release of ketone bodies from the liver to supply energy to other tissues. [Note: Maintaining glucose requires that the substrates for gluconeogenesis (such as pyruvate, alanine, and glycerol) be available.]

A. Fuel stores

The metabolic fuels available in a normal 70-kg man at the beginning of a fast are shown in Figure 24.10. Note the enormous caloric stores available in the form of TAG compared with those contained in glycogen. [Note: Although protein is listed as an energy source, each protein also has a function (for example, as a structural component of the body, an enzyme, and so forth). Therefore, only about one third of the body's protein can be used for energy production without fatally compromising vital functions.]

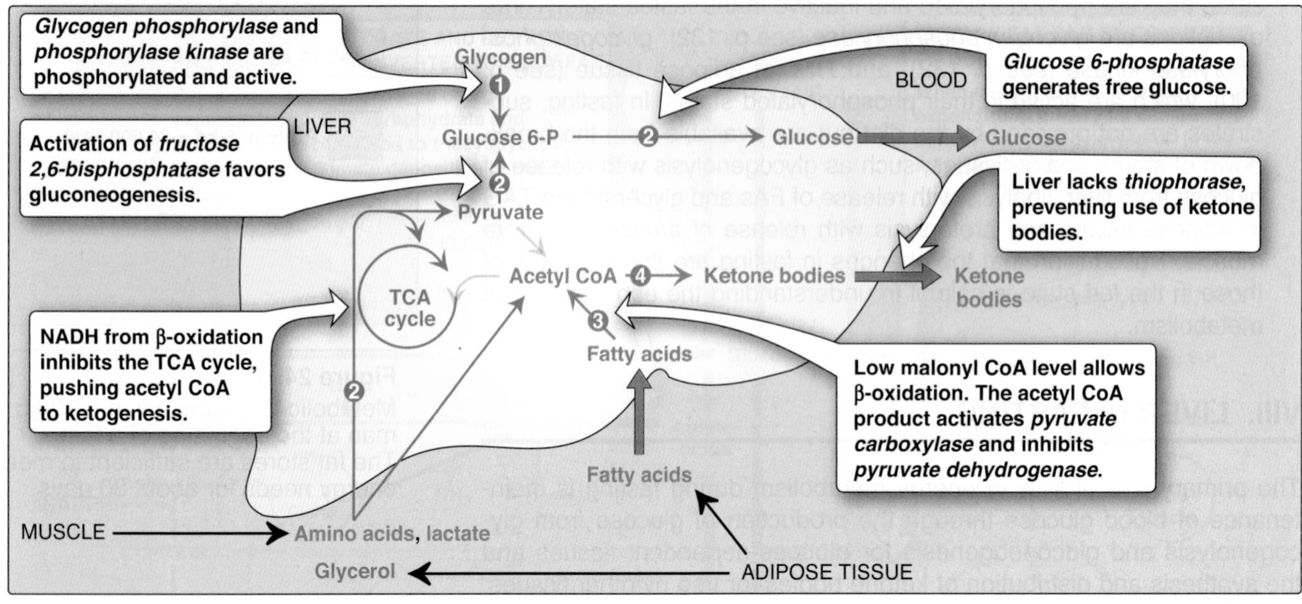

Figure 24.12
Major metabolic pathways in liver during fasting. [Note: The numbers in circles, which appear both in the figure and in the corresponding citation in the text, indicate important metabolic pathways for carbohydrate or fat.] P = phosphate; CoA = coenzyme A; TCA = tricarboxylic acid; NADH = nicotinamide adenine dinucleotide.

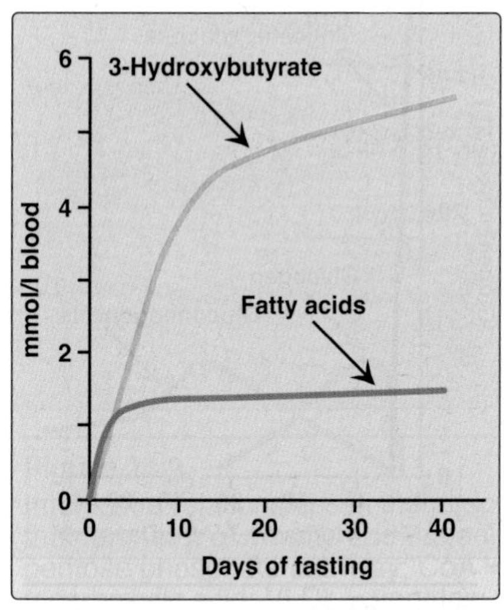

Figure 24.13
Concentrations of fatty acids and 3-hydroxybutyrate in the blood during fasting. [Note: 3-Hydroxybutyrate is made from the reduction of acetoacetate.]

by glucagon (see p. 122), begins 4–6 hours after the last meal and becomes fully active as stores of liver glycogen are depleted (see Figure 24.11). [Note: The decrease in fructose 2,6-bisphosphate simultaneously inhibits glycolysis at *PFK-1* (see p. 99).]

B. Fat metabolism

1. **Increased fatty acid oxidation:** The oxidation of FAs obtained from TAG hydrolysis in adipose tissue is the major source of energy in hepatic tissue in the postabsorptive state (see Figure 24.12, ❸). The fall in malonyl CoA due to phosphorylation (inactivation) of *ACC* by *AMPK* removes the brake on *CPT-1*, allowing β-oxidation to occur (see p. 191). FA oxidation generates NADH, $FADH_2$, and acetyl CoA. The NADH inhibits the TCA cycle. The acetyl CoA is an allosteric activator of *PC* and an allosteric inhibitor of *PDH*, thereby favoring use of pyruvate in gluconeogenesis (see Figure 8.24). [Note: The acetyl CoA cannot be used as a substrate for gluconeogenesis, in part because the *PDH* reaction is irreversible.] Oxidation of NADH and $FADH_2$ coupled with oxidative phosphorylation supplies the energy required by the *PC* and *PEPCK* reactions of gluconeogenesis.

2. **Increased ketone body synthesis:** The liver is unique in being able to synthesize and release ketone bodies, primarily 3-hydroxybutyrate but also acetoacetate, for use as fuel by peripheral tissues (see p. 195) but not by the liver itself because liver lacks *thiophorase*. Ketogenesis, which starts during the first days of fasting (Figure 24.13), is favored when the concentration of acetyl CoA from FA oxidation exceeds the oxidative capacity of the TCA cycle. [Note:

Ketogenesis releases CoA, ensuring its availability for continued FA oxidation.] The availability of circulating water-soluble ketone bodies is important in fasting because they can be used for fuel by most tissues, including brain, once their level in the blood is sufficiently high. This reduces the need for gluconeogenesis from amino acid carbon skeletons, thus preserving essential protein (see Figure 24.11). Ketogenesis as part of the overall hepatic response to fasting is shown in Figure 24.12, ❹. [Note: Ketone bodies are organic acids and, when present at high concentrations, can cause ketoacidosis.]

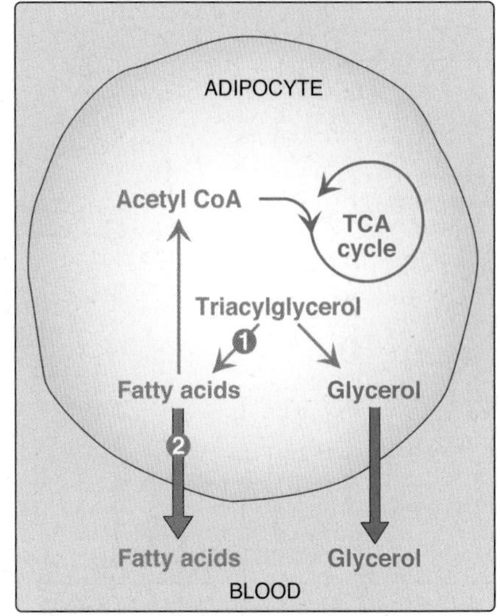

Figure 24.14
Major metabolic pathways in adipose tissue during fasting. [Note: The numbers in the circles, which appear both in the figure and in the corresponding citation in the text, indicate important pathways for fat metabolism.] CoA = coenzyme A; TCA = tricarboxylic acid.

IX. ADIPOSE TISSUE IN FASTING

A. Carbohydrate metabolism

Glucose transport by insulin-sensitive GLUT-4 into the adipocyte and its subsequent metabolism are depressed due to low levels of circulating insulin. This results in decreased TAG synthesis.

B. Fat metabolism

1. **Increased degradation of fat:** The *PKA*-mediated phosphorylation and activation of *HSL* (see p. 190) and subsequent hydrolysis of stored fat are enhanced by the elevated catecholamines norepinephrine and epinephrine. These hormones, which are released from the sympathetic nerve endings in adipose tissue and/or from the adrenal medulla, are physiologically important activators of *HSL* (Figure 24.14, ❶).

2. **Increased release of fatty acids:** FAs obtained from hydrolysis of stored TAG are primarily released into the blood (see Figure 24.14, ❷). Bound to albumin, they are transported to a variety of tissues for use as fuel. The glycerol produced from TAG degradation is used as a gluconeogenic precursor by the liver, which contains *glycerol kinase*. [Note: FA can also be oxidized to acetyl CoA, which can enter the TCA cycle, thereby producing energy for the adipocyte. They also can be re-esterified to glycerol 3-phosphate (from glyceroneogenesis, see p. 190), generating TAG and reducing plasma FA concentration.]

3. **Decreased uptake of fatty acids:** In fasting, *LPL* activity of adipose tissue is low. Consequently, circulating TAG of lipoproteins is not available to adipose tissue.

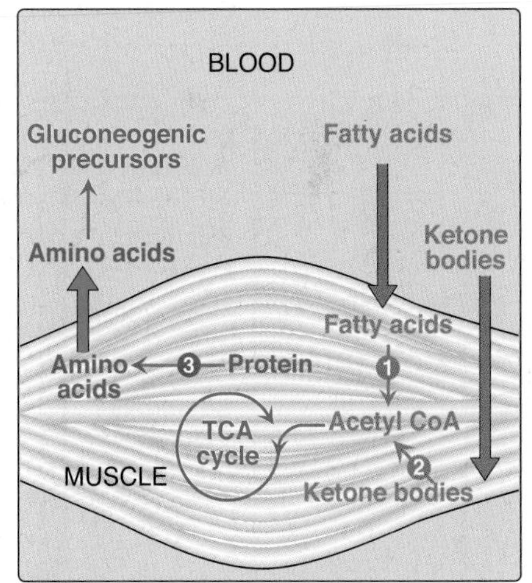

Figure 24.15
Major metabolic pathways in skeletal muscle during fasting. [Note: The numbers in the circles, which appear both in the figure and in the corresponding citation in the text, indicate important pathways for fat or protein metabolism.] CoA = coenzyme A; TCA = tricarboxylic acid.

X. RESTING SKELETAL MUSCLE IN FASTING

Resting muscle switches from glucose to FAs as its major fuel source in fasting. [Note: By contrast, exercising muscle initially uses its glycogen stores as a source of energy. During intense exercise, glucose 6-phosphate derived from glycogen is converted to lactate by anaerobic glycolysis (see p. 103). The lactate is used by liver for gluconeogenesis (Cori cycle; see p.118). As these glycogen reserves are depleted, free FAs provided by the mobilization of TAG from adipose tissue become the

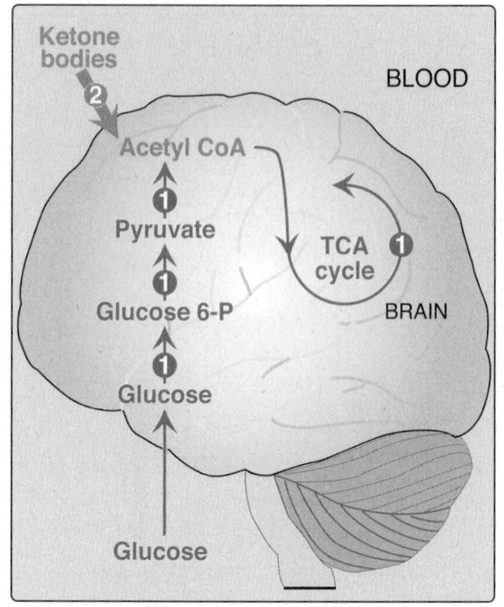

Figure 24.16
Major metabolic pathways in the brain during fasting. [Note: The numbers in the circles, which appear both in the figure and in the corresponding citation in the text, indicate important pathways for metabolism of fat or carbohydrates.] CoA = coenzyme A; TCA = tricarboxylic acid; P = phosphate.

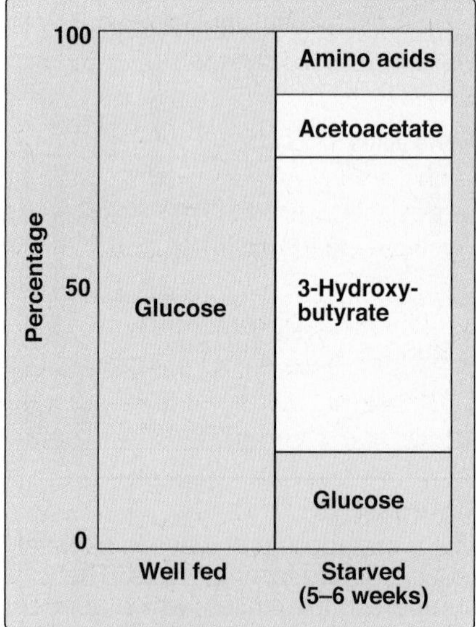

Figure 24.17
Fuel sources used by the brain to meet energy needs in the well fed and starved states.

dominant energy source. The contraction-based rise in AMP activates *AMPK* that phosphorylates and inactivates the muscle isozyme of *ACC*, decreasing malonyl CoA and allowing FA oxidation (see p. 183).

A. Carbohydrate metabolism

Glucose transport into skeletal muscle cells via insulin-sensitive GLUT-4 (see p. 97) and subsequent glucose metabolism are depressed because of low levels of circulating insulin. Therefore, the glucose from hepatic gluconeogenesis is unavailable to muscle (and adipose tissue).

B. Lipid metabolism

During the first 2 weeks of fasting, muscle uses FA from adipose tissue and ketone bodies from the liver as fuels (Figure 24.15, ❶ and ❷). After about 3 weeks of fasting, muscle decreases its use of ketone bodies (thus sparing them for brain) and oxidizes FA almost exclusively. [Note: The acetyl CoA from FA oxidation indirectly inhibits *PDH* (by activation of *PDH kinase*) and spares pyruvate, which is transaminated to alanine and used by liver for gluconeogenesis (glucose–alanine cycle; see p. 253).]

C. Protein metabolism

During the first few days of fasting, there is a rapid breakdown of muscle protein, providing amino acids that are used by the liver for gluconeogenesis (see Figure 24.15, ❸). Because muscle does not have glucagon receptors, muscle proteolysis is initiated by a fall in insulin and sustained by a rise in glucocorticoids. [Note: Alanine and glutamine are quantitatively the most important gluconeogenic amino acids released from muscle. They are produced by the catabolism of BCAAs (see p. 267).] The glutamine is used as a fuel by enterocytes, for example, which send out alanine that is used in hepatic gluconeogenesis. In the second week of fasting, the rate of muscle proteolysis decreases, paralleling a decline in the need for glucose as a fuel for the brain, which has begun using ketone bodies as a source of energy.

XI. BRAIN IN FASTING

During the early days of fasting, the brain continues to use only glucose as a fuel (Figure 24.16, ❶). Blood glucose is maintained by hepatic gluconeogenesis from glucogenic precursors, such as amino acids from proteolysis and glycerol from lipolysis. In prolonged fasting (beyond 2–3 weeks), plasma ketone bodies (see Figure 24.12) reach significantly elevated levels and replace glucose as the primary fuel for the brain (see Figure 24.16, ❷, and Figure 24.17). This reduces the need for protein catabolism for gluconeogenesis: ketone bodies spare glucose and, thus, muscle protein. [Note: As the duration of a fast extends from overnight to days to weeks, blood glucose levels initially drop and then are maintained at the lower level (65–70 mg/dl).] The metabolic changes that occur during fasting ensure that all tissues have an adequate supply of fuel molecules. The response of the major tissues involved in energy metabolism during fasting is summarized in Figure 24.19 (see below).

XII. KIDNEY IN LONG-TERM FASTING

As fasting continues into early starvation and beyond, the kidney plays important roles. The kidney expresses the enzymes of gluconeogenesis, including *glucose 6-phosphatase*, and in late fasting about 50% of gluconeogenesis occurs here. [Note: A portion of this glucose is used by the kidney itself.] The kidney also provides compensation for the acidosis that accompanies the increased production of ketone bodies (organic acids). The glutamine released from the muscle's metabolism of BCAAs is taken up by the kidney and acted upon by renal *glutaminase* and *glutamate dehydrogenase* (see p. 256), producing α-ketoglutarate that can be used as a substrate for gluconeogenesis, plus ammonia (NH_3). The NH_3 picks up protons from ketone body dissociation and is excreted in the urine as ammonium (NH_4^+), thereby decreasing the acid load in the body (Figure 24.18). In long-term fasting, then, there is a switch from nitrogen disposal in the form of urea to disposal in the form of ammonia. [Note: As ketone body concentration rises, enterocytes, typically consumers of glutamine, become consumers of ketone bodies. This allows more glutamine to be available to the kidney.]

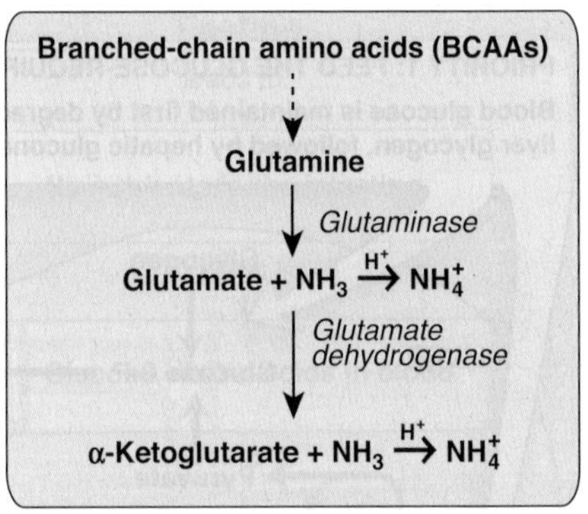

Figure 24.18
Use of glutamine from BCAA catabolism in muscle to generate ammonia (NH_3) used for the excretion of protons (H^+) as ammonium (NH_4^+) in kidney.

XIII. CHAPTER SUMMARY

The flow of intermediates through metabolic pathways is controlled by four mechanisms: 1) the availability of substrates, 2) allosteric activation and inhibition of enzymes, 3) covalent modification of enzymes, and 4) induction-repression of enzyme synthesis. In the absorptive state, the 2–4-hour period after ingestion of a meal, these regulatory mechanisms ensure that available nutrients are captured as **glycogen**, **triacylglycerol** (**TAG**), and **protein** (Figure 24.20). During this interval, transient increases in plasma glucose, amino acids, and TAG occur, the last primarily as components of chylomicrons synthesized by the intestinal mucosal cells. The **pancreas** responds to the elevated levels of glucose with an **increased secretion of insulin** and a **decreased secretion of glucagon** by the **pancreas**. The elevated insulin-to-glucagon ratio and the ready availability of circulating substrates make the absorptive state an **anabolic period** during which virtually all tissues use **glucose** as a fuel. In addition, the **liver** replenishes its **glycogen** stores, replaces any needed **hepatic proteins**, and increases **TAG** synthesis. The latter are packaged in **very-low-density lipoproteins**, which are exported to the peripheral tissues. **Adipose tissue** increases **TAG** synthesis and storage, whereas **muscle** increases **protein** synthesis to replace protein degraded since the previous meal. In the fed state, the **brain** uses glucose exclusively as a fuel. In the **absence of food**, plasma levels of glucose, amino acids, and TAG fall, triggering a **decline** in **insulin secretion** and an **increase in glucagon** and **epinephrine release**. The decreased insulin/counterregulatory hormone ratio and the decreased availability of circulating substrates make the fasting state a **catabolic period**. This sets into motion an **exchange of substrates** among liver, adipose tissue, skeletal muscle, and brain that is guided by two priorities: 1) the need to maintain adequate plasma levels of glucose to sustain energy metabolism of the brain and other glucose-requiring tissues and 2) the need to mobilize fatty acids (FAs) from adipose tissue and release ketone bodies from liver to supply energy to other tissues. To accomplish these goals, the **liver** degrades **glycogen** and initiates **gluconeogenesis**, using **increased fatty acid oxidation** as a source of the energy and reducing equivalents needed for gluconeogenesis and to supply the acetyl coenzyme A building blocks for **ketogenesis**. The **adipose tissue** degrades stored **TAG**, thus providing **FAs** and **glycerol** to the liver. The **muscle** can also use **FAs** as fuel as well as **ketone bodies** supplied by the liver. Muscle **protein** is **degraded** to supply **amino acids** for the liver to use in gluconeogenesis, but deceases as ketone bodies increase. The **brain** can use both **glucose** and **ketone bodies** as fuels. From late fasting into starvation, the **kidneys** play important roles by **synthesizing glucose** and **excreting the protons** from ketone body dissociation as ammonium (**NH_4^+**).

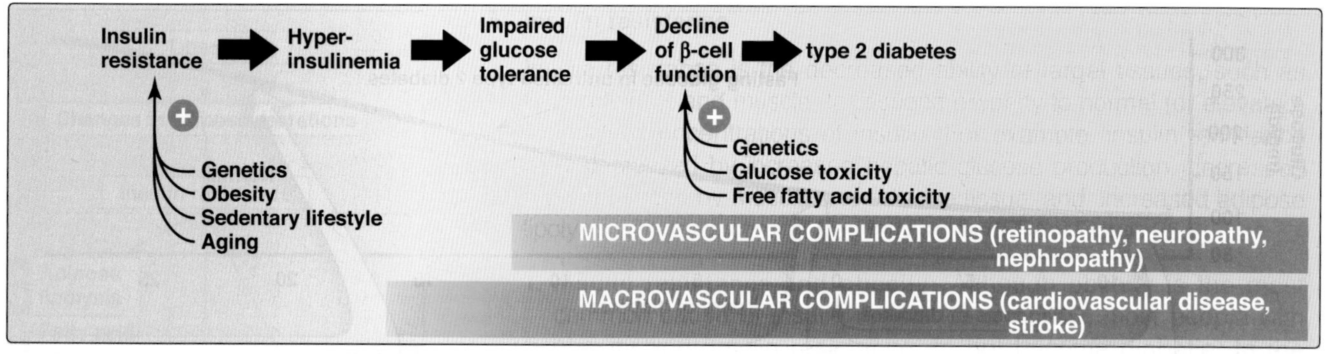

Figure 25.10
Typical progression of type 2 diabetes.

C. Metabolic changes in type 2 diabetes

The metabolic abnormalities of T2D are the result of insulin resistance expressed primarily in liver, muscle, and adipose tissue (Figure 25.11).

1. **Hyperglycemia:** Hyperglycemia is caused by increased hepatic production of glucose, combined with diminished peripheral use. Ketosis is usually minimal or absent in patients with T2D because the presence of insulin, even in the presence of insulin resistance, restrains hepatic ketogenesis.

2. **Dyslipidemia:** In the liver, FAs are converted to TAGs, which are packaged and secreted in VLDL. Chylomicrons are synthesized from dietary lipids by the intestinal mucosal cells following a meal (see p. 177). Because lipoprotein degradation catalyzed by *lipoprotein lipase* in adipose tissue is low in diabetics, the plasma chylomicron and VLDL levels are elevated, resulting in hypertriacylglycerolemia (see Figure 25.10). Low levels of high-density lipoproteins are also associated with T2D, likely as a result of increased degradation.

D. Treatment of type 2 diabetes

The goal in treating T2D is to maintain blood glucose concentrations within normal limits and to prevent the development of long-term complications. Weight reduction, exercise, and medical nutrition therapy (dietary modifications) often correct the hyperglycemia of newly diagnosed T2D. Hypoglycemic agents (for example, metformin, which decreases hepatic output of glucose), sulfonylureas (increase insulin secretion; see p. 310), thiazolidinediones (increase peripheral insulin sensitivity), *α-glucosidase* inhibitors (decrease absorption of dietary carbohydrate) or insulin therapy may be required to achieve satisfactory plasma glucose levels. [Note: Bariatric surgery in morbidly obese individuals with T2D has been shown to result in disease remission in most patients. Remission may not be permanent.]

IV. CHRONIC EFFECTS AND PREVENTION OF DIABETES

As noted previously, available therapies moderate the hyperglycemia of diabetes but fail to completely normalize metabolism. The long-standing elevation of blood glucose is associated with the chronic complications

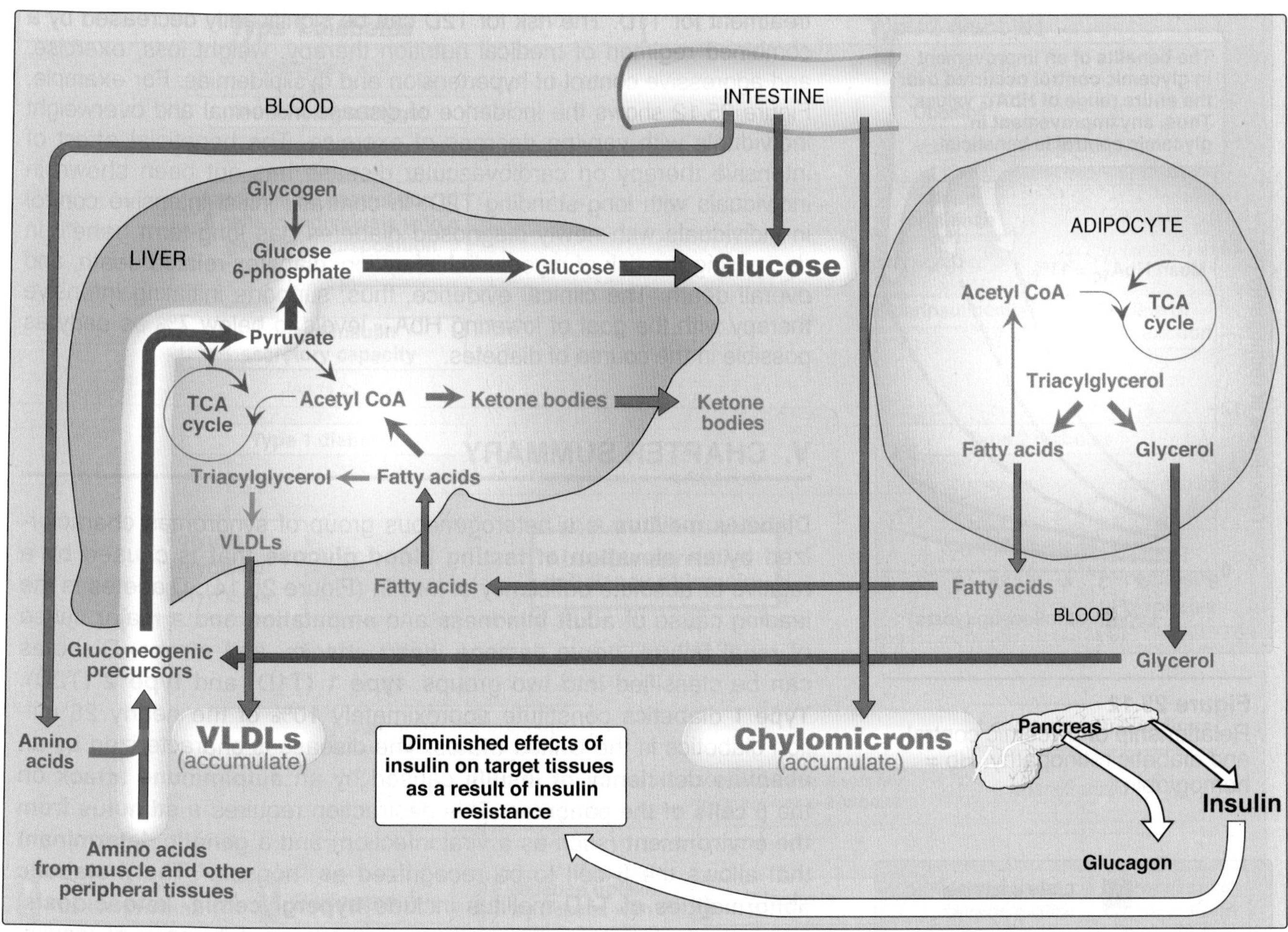

Figure 25.11
Intertissue relationships in type 2 diabetes. [Note: Ketogenesis is restrained as long as insulin action is adequate.] TCA = tricarboxylic acid; CoA = coenzyme A; VLDL = very-low-density lipoprotein.

of diabetes including premature atherosclerosis as well as cardiovascular disease and stroke, retinopathy, nephropathy, and neuropathy. Intensive treatment with insulin (see p. 340) delays the onset and slows the progression of these long-term complications. For example, the incidence of retinopathy decreases as control of blood glucose improves and HbA_{1c} levels decrease (Figure 25.12). The benefits of tight control of blood glucose outweigh the increased risk of severe hypoglycemia in most patients. How hyperglycemia causes the chronic complications of diabetes is unclear. In cells in which entry of glucose is not dependent on insulin, elevated blood glucose leads to increased intracellular glucose and its metabolites. For example, increased intracellular sorbitol contributes to the formation of cataracts (see p. 140) in diabetics. Additionally, hyperglycemia promotes the nonenzymic condensation of glucose with cellular proteins in a reaction analogous to the formation of HbA_{1c} (see p. 34). These glycated proteins undergo additional reactions and become advanced glycation end products (AGEs) that mediate some of the early microvascular changes of diabetes and can reduce wound healing. AGEs bind to their receptors (RAGEs), causing the release of proinflammatory molecules. There is currently no preventative

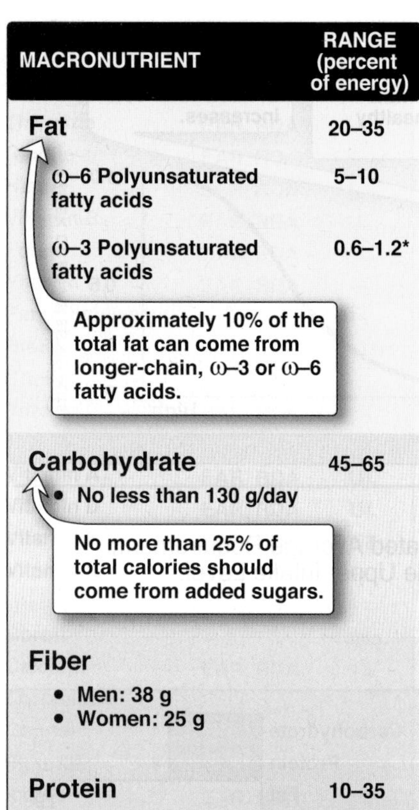

Figure 27.7
Acceptable macronutrient distribution ranges in adults. *A growing body of evidence suggests that higher levels of ω–3 polyunsaturated fatty acids provide protection against coronary heart disease.

In general, a sedentary person requires about 30%–50% more calories than the RMR (see Figure 27.6), whereas a highly active individual may require 100% or more calories above the RMR.

3. **Thermic effect of food:** The production of heat by the body increases as much as 30% above the resting level during the digestion and absorption of food. This is called the thermic effect of food, or diet-induced thermogenesis. The thermic response to food intake may amount to 5%–10% of the TEE.

IV. ACCEPTABLE MACRONUTRIENT DISTRIBUTION RANGES

Acceptable Macronutrient Distribution Ranges (AMDRs) are defined as a range of intakes for a particular macronutrient that is associated with reduced risk of chronic disease while providing adequate amounts of essential nutrients. The AMDR for adults is 45%–65% of their total calories from carbohydrates, 20%–35% from fat, and 10%–35% from protein (Figure 27.7). The biologic properties of dietary fat, carbohydrate, and protein are described below.

V. DIETARY FATS

The incidence of a number of chronic diseases is significantly influenced by the kinds and amounts of nutrients consumed (Figure 27.8). Dietary fats most strongly influence the incidence of coronary heart disease (CHD), but evidence linking dietary fat and the risk for cancer or obesity is much weaker.

> Although earlier recommendations emphasized decreasing the total amount of fat and cholesterol in the diet, data now show that the type of fat is a more important risk factor than the total amount of fat consumed.

A. Plasma lipids and coronary heart disease

Plasma cholesterol may arise from the diet or from endogenous biosynthesis. In either case, cholesterol is transported between the tissues in combination with protein and phospholipids as lipoproteins.

1. **Low-density lipoprotein and high-density lipoprotein:** The level of plasma cholesterol is not precisely regulated but, rather, varies in response to the diet. Elevated levels of total cholesterol (hypercholesterolemia) result in an increased risk for CHD (Figure 27.9). A much stronger correlation exists between CHD and the level of cholesterol in low-density lipoproteins ([LDL-C] see p. 232). As LDL-C increases, CHD increases. In contrast, high levels of high-density lipoprotein cholesterol (HDL-C) have been associated with a decreased risk for heart disease (see p. 235). [Note: Elevated plasma triacylglycerol (TAG) is associated with CHD, but a causative relationship has yet to be demonstrated.] Abnormal levels of plasma lipids (dyslipidemias) act in combination with smoking, obesity, sedentary lifestyle, insulin resistance, and other risk factors to increase the risk of CHD.

2. **Benefits of lowering plasma cholesterol:** Dietary or drug treatment of hypercholesterolemia has been shown to be effective in decreasing LDL-C, increasing HDL-C, and reducing the risk for cardiovascular events. The diet-induced changes of plasma lipoprotein concentrations are modest, typically 10%–20%, whereas treatment with "statin" drugs decreases plasma cholesterol by 30%–60% (see p. 224). [Note: Dietary and drug treatment can lower TAGs.]

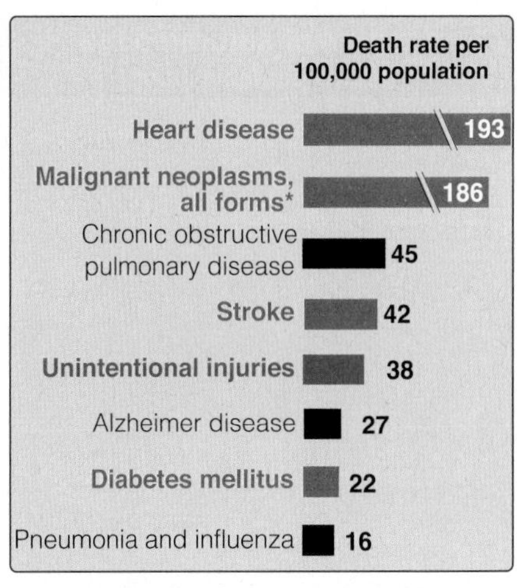

Figure 27.8
Influence of nutrition on some common causes of death in the United States in the year 2010. Red indicates causes of death in which the diet plays a significant role. Blue indicates causes of death in which excessive alcohol consumption plays a part. (*Diet plays a role in only some forms of cancer.)

B. Dietary fats and plasma lipids

TAGs are quantitatively the most important class of dietary fats. The influence of TAGs on blood lipids is determined by the chemical nature of their constituent fatty acids. The absence or presence and number of double bonds (saturated versus mono- and polyunsaturated), the location of the double bonds (ω-6 versus ω-3), and the cis versus trans configuration of the unsaturated fatty acids are the most important structural features that influence blood lipids.

1. **Saturated fat:** TAGs composed primarily of fatty acids whose hydrocarbon chains do not contain any double bonds are referred to as saturated fats. Consumption of saturated fats is positively associated with high levels of total plasma cholesterol and LDL-C and an increased risk of CHD. The main sources of saturated fatty acids are dairy and meat products and some vegetable oils, such as coconut and palm oils (a major source of fat in Latin America and Asia, although not in the United States; Figure 27.10). Most experts strongly advise limiting intake of saturated fats to less than 10% of total caloric intake.

> Saturated fatty acids with carbon chain lengths of 14 (myristic) and 16 (palmitic) are most potent in increasing the serum cholesterol. Stearic acid (18 carbons, found in many foods including chocolate) has little effect on blood cholesterol.

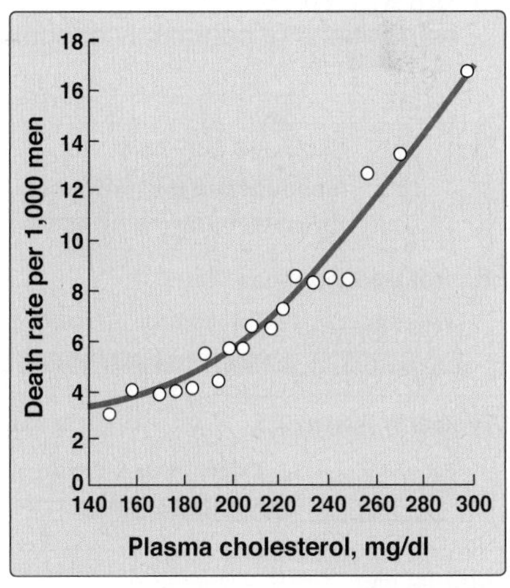

Figure 27.9
Correlation of the death rate from coronary heart disease with the concentration of plasma cholesterol. [Note: The data were obtained from a 6-year study of men with the death rate adjusted for age.]

2. **Monounsaturated fats:** TAGs containing primarily fatty acids with one double bond are referred to as monounsaturated fat. Unsaturated fatty acids are generally derived from vegetables and fish. When substituted for saturated fatty acids in the diet, monounsaturated fats lower both total plasma cholesterol and LDL-C but maintain or increase HDL-C. This ability of monounsaturated fats to favorably modify lipoprotein levels may explain, in part, the observation that Mediterranean cultures, with diets rich in olive oil (high in monounsaturated oleic acid), show a low incidence of CHD. It is recommended that monounsaturated fats account for about 50% of the total fat intake.

   a. **The Mediterranean diet:** The Mediterranean diet is an example of a diet rich in monounsaturated fatty acids, or MUFAs (from olive oil), and polyunsaturated fatty acids, or PUFAs (from fish oils and some nuts), but low in saturated fat. For example, Figure 27.11 shows the composition of the Mediterranean diet in comparison with both a Western diet similar to that consumed in the United States and a typical low-fat diet. The Mediterranean diet contains seasonally fresh food, with an abundance of plant

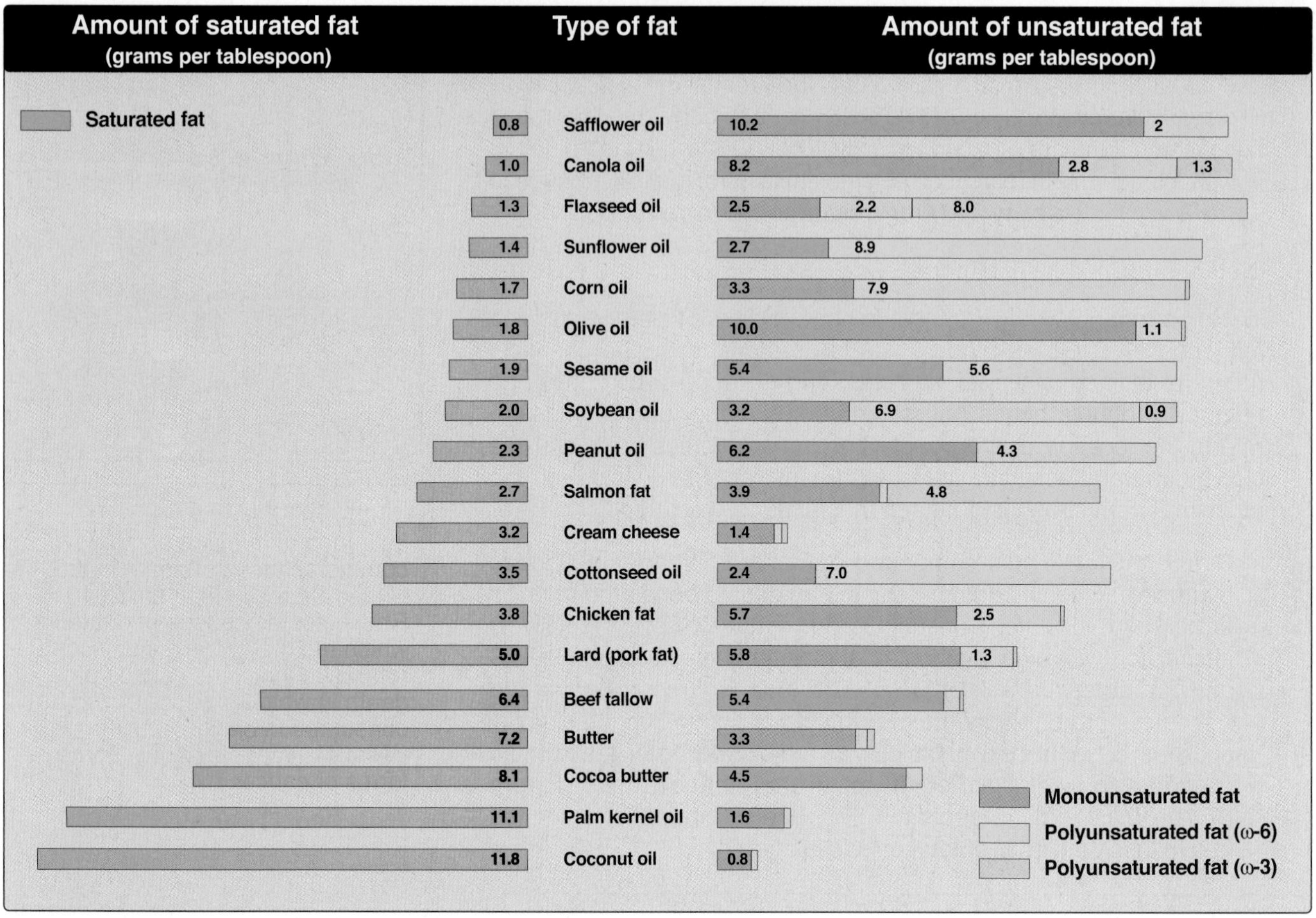

Amount of saturated fat (grams per tablespoon)	Type of fat	Amount of unsaturated fat (grams per tablespoon)
0.8	Safflower oil	10.2, 2
1.0	Canola oil	8.2, 2.8, 1.3
1.3	Flaxseed oil	2.5, 2.2, 8.0
1.4	Sunflower oil	2.7, 8.9
1.7	Corn oil	3.3, 7.9
1.8	Olive oil	10.0, 1.1
1.9	Sesame oil	5.4, 5.6
2.0	Soybean oil	3.2, 6.9, 0.9
2.3	Peanut oil	6.2, 4.3
2.7	Salmon fat	3.9, 4.8
3.2	Cream cheese	1.4
3.5	Cottonseed oil	2.4, 7.0
3.8	Chicken fat	5.7, 2.5
5.0	Lard (pork fat)	5.8, 1.3
6.4	Beef tallow	5.4
7.2	Butter	3.3
8.1	Cocoa butter	4.5
11.1	Palm kernel oil	1.6
11.8	Coconut oil	0.8

Key: Saturated fat; Monounsaturated fat; Polyunsaturated fat (ω-6); Polyunsaturated fat (ω-3)

Figure 27.10
Compositions of commonly encountered dietary fats.

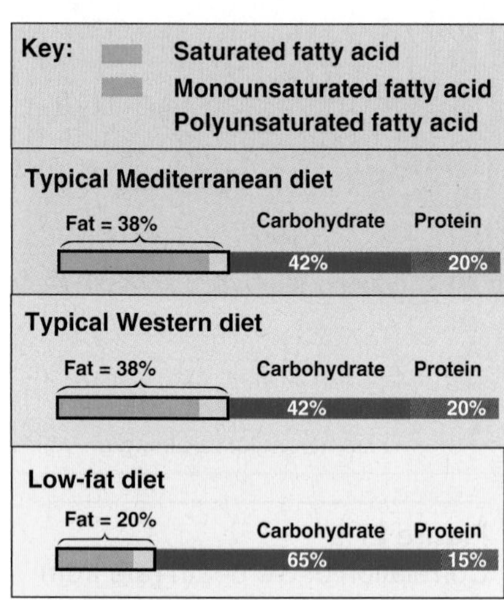

Figure 27.11
Composition of typical Mediterranean, Western, and low-fat diets.

material, low amounts of red meat, and olive oil as the principal source of fat. The Mediterranean diet is associated with decreased serum total cholesterol and LDL-C, decreased TAGs, and increased HDL-C when compared with a typical Western diet higher in saturated fats.

3. **Polyunsaturated fats:** TAGs containing primarily fatty acids with more than one double bond are referred to as polyunsaturated fats. The effects of PUFAs on cardiovascular disease is influenced by the location of the double bonds within the molecule.

   a. **ω-6 Fatty acids:** These are long-chain PUFAs, with the first double bond beginning at the sixth bond position when starting from the methyl (ω) end of the fatty acid molecule. [Note: They are also called n-6 fatty acids (see p. 183).]

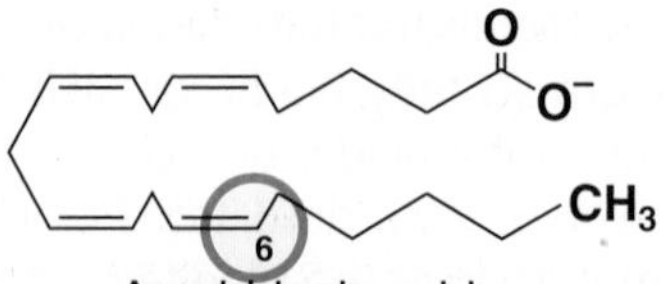

O, O^-, 6, CH_3

Arachidonic acid
(20:4, ω-6)
found in seed oils

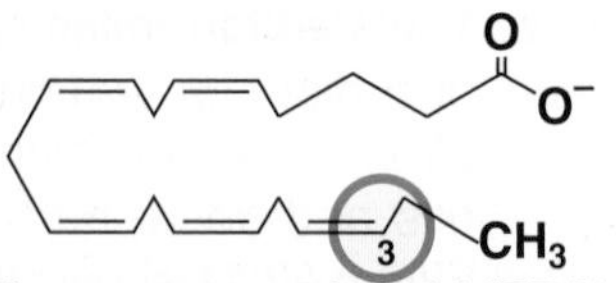

O, O^-, 3, CH_3

Eicosapentaenoic acid (EPA)
(20:5, ω-3)
found in fish oils

Consumption of fats containing ω-6 PUFAs, principally linoleic acid (18:2 [9,12]), obtained from vegetable oils, lowers plasma cholesterol when substituted for saturated fats. Plasma LDL-C is lowered, but HDL-C, which protects against CHD, is also lowered. The powerful benefits of lowering LDLs are only partially offset because of the decreased HDL. Nuts, avocados, olives, soybeans, and various oils, including sunflower, cottonseed, and corn oil, are common sources of these fatty acids (see Figure 27.10). The AMDR for linoleic acid is 5%–10%. [Note: The lower recommendation for PUFAs relative to MUFAs is because of concern that free radical–mediated oxidation (peroxidation) of PUFAs may lead to deleterious products.]

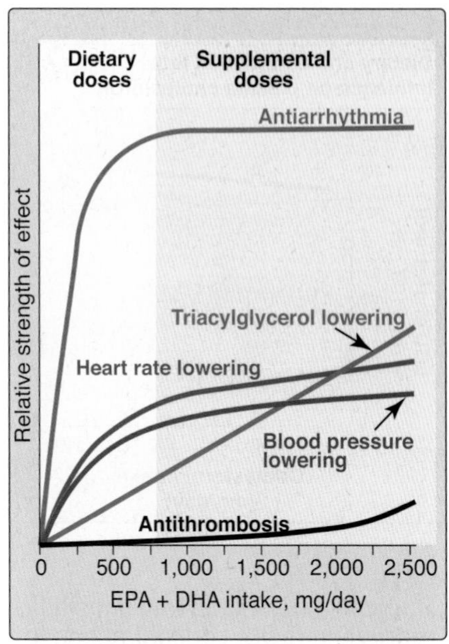

Figure 27.12
Dose responses of physiologic effects of fish oil intake. EPA = eicosapentaenoic acid; DHA = docosahexaenoic acid.

b. ω-3 Fatty acids: These are long-chain PUFAs, with the first double bond beginning at the third bond position from the methyl (ω) end. Dietary ω-3 PUFAs suppress cardiac arrhythmias, reduce serum TAGs, decrease the tendency for thrombosis, lower blood pressure, and substantially reduce risk of cardiovascular mortality (Figure 27.12), but they have little effect on LDL-C or HDL-C levels. Evidence suggests that they have anti-inflammatory effects. The ω-3 PUFAs, principally α-linolenic acid, 18:3(9,12,15), are found in plant oils, such as flaxseed and canola, and some nuts. The AMDR for α-linolenic acid is 0.6%–1.2%. Fish oil contains the long-chain ω-3 docosahexaenoic acid (DHA) and eicosapentaenoic acid (EPA). Two fatty fish (for example, salmon) meals per week are recommended. For patients with documented CHD, 1 g/day of fish oils is recommended, while 2–4 g/day is prescribed to lower TAGs. [Note: The ω-3 long-chain PUFAs are included in infant formulas to promote brain development.] Linoleic and α-linolenic acids are essential fatty acids (EFAs) required for membrane fluidity and synthesis of eicosanoids (see p. 213). EFA deficiency is characterized by scaly dermatitis as a result of the depletion of skin ceramides with long-chain fatty acids (see p. 206).]

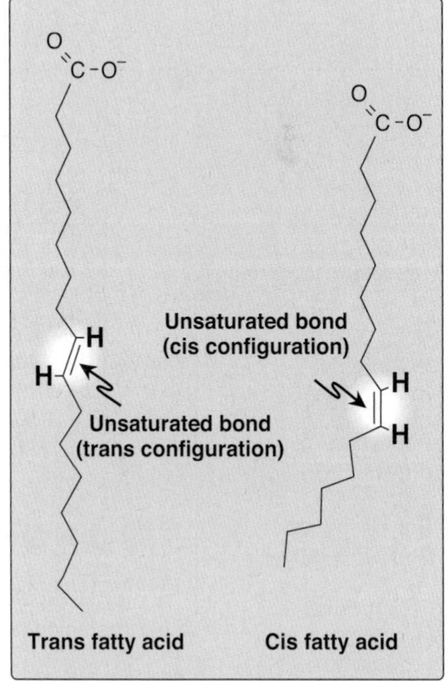

Figure 27.13
Structure of cis and trans fatty acids.

4. **Trans fatty acids:** Trans fatty acids (Figure 27.13) are chemically classified as unsaturated fatty acids but behave more like saturated fatty acids in the body because they elevate serum LDL-C (but not HDL-C), and they increase the risk of CHD. Trans fatty acids do not occur naturally in plants but occur in small amounts in animals. However, trans fatty acids are formed during the hydrogenation of liquid vegetable oils (for example, in the manufacture of margarine and partially hydrogenated vegetable oil). Trans fatty acids are a major component of many commercial baked goods, such as cookies and cakes, and most deep-fried foods. Many manufacturers have reformulated their products to be free of trans fats. Starting in 2006, the U.S. Food and Drug Administration requires that Nutrition Facts labels portray the trans fat content of packaged food. Some municipalities, such as New York City, have banned the use of trans fats in restaurants.

5. **Dietary cholesterol:** Cholesterol is found only in animal products. The effect of dietary cholesterol on plasma cholesterol (Figure 27.14) is less important than the amount and types of fatty acids consumed. Cholesterol consumption should be no more than 300 mg/day.

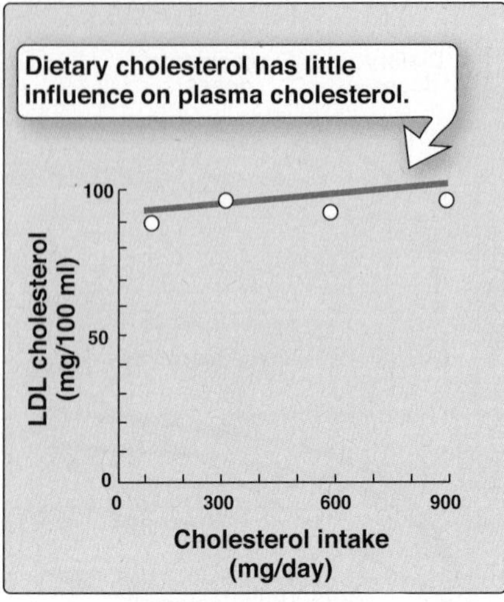

Figure 27.14
Response of plasma low-density lipoprotein (LDL) concentrations to an increase in dietary cholesterol intake.

C. Other dietary factors affecting coronary heart disease

Moderate consumption of alcohol (up to 1 drink a day for women and up to 2 drinks a day for men) decreases the risk of CHD, because there is a positive correlation between moderate alcohol consumption and the plasma concentration of HDL-C. However, because of the potential dangers of alcohol abuse, health professionals are reluctant to recommend increased alcohol consumption to their patients. Red wine may provide cardioprotective benefits in addition to those resulting from its alcohol content (for example, red wine contains phenolic compounds that inhibit lipoprotein oxidation; see p. 235). [Note: These antioxidants are also present in raisins and grape juice.] Figure 27.15 summarizes the effects of dietary fats.

VI. DIETARY CARBOHYDRATES

The primary role of dietary carbohydrate is to provide energy. Although caloric intake in the United States has shown a modest increase since 1971, the incidence of obesity has dramatically increased (see p. 349). During this same period, carbohydrate consumption has significantly increased (as fat consumption decreased), leading some observers to link obesity with carbohydrate consumption. However, obesity has also been related to increasingly inactive lifestyles and to calorie-dense foods served in expanded portion size. Carbohydrates are not inherently fattening.

A. Classification of carbohydrates

Dietary carbohydrates are classified as simple sugars (monosaccharides and disaccharides), complex sugars (polysaccharides), and fiber.

1. **Monosaccharides:** Glucose and fructose are the principal monosaccharides found in food. Glucose is abundant in fruits, sweet corn, corn syrup, and honey. Free fructose is found together with free glucose and sucrose in honey and fruits (for example, apples).

TYPE OF FAT	METABOLIC EFFECTS	EFFECTS ON DISEASE PREVENTION
Trans fatty acid	↑ LDL ↓ HDL	↑ Incidence of coronary heart disease
Saturated fatty acid	↑ LDL Little effect on HDL	↑ Incidence of coronary heart disease; may increase risk of prostate, colon cancer
Monounsaturated fatty acid	↓ LDL Maintain or increase HDL	↓ Incidence of coronary heart disease
Polyunsaturated fatty acids ω–6	↓ LDL ↓ HDL Provide arachidonic acid, which is an important precursor of prostaglandins and leukotrienes	↓ Incidence of coronary heart disease
Polyunsaturated fatty acids ω–3	Little effect on LDL Little effect on HDL Suppress cardiac arrhythmias, reduce serum triacylglycerols, decrease the tendency for thrombosis, lower blood pressure	↓ Incidence of coronary heart disease ↓ Risk of sudden cardiac death

Figure 27.15
Effects of dietary fats. LDL = low-density lipoprotein; HDL = high-density lipoprotein.

a. **High-fructose corn syrup:** High-fructose corn syrups (HFCSs) are corn syrups that have undergone enzymatic processing to convert their glucose into fructose and have then been mixed with pure corn syrup (100% glucose) to produce a desired sweetness. In the United States, HFCS 55 (containing 55% fructose and 42% glucose) is commonly used as a substitute for sucrose in beverages, including soft drinks, with HFCS 42 used in processed foods. The composition and metabolism of HFCS and sucrose are similar, the major difference being that HFCS is ingested as a mixture of monosaccharides (Figure 27.16). Most studies have shown no significant difference between sucrose and HFCS syrup meals in either postprandial glucose or insulin responses. [Note: The rise in the use of HFCS parallels the rise in obesity, but a causal relationship has not been demonstrated.]

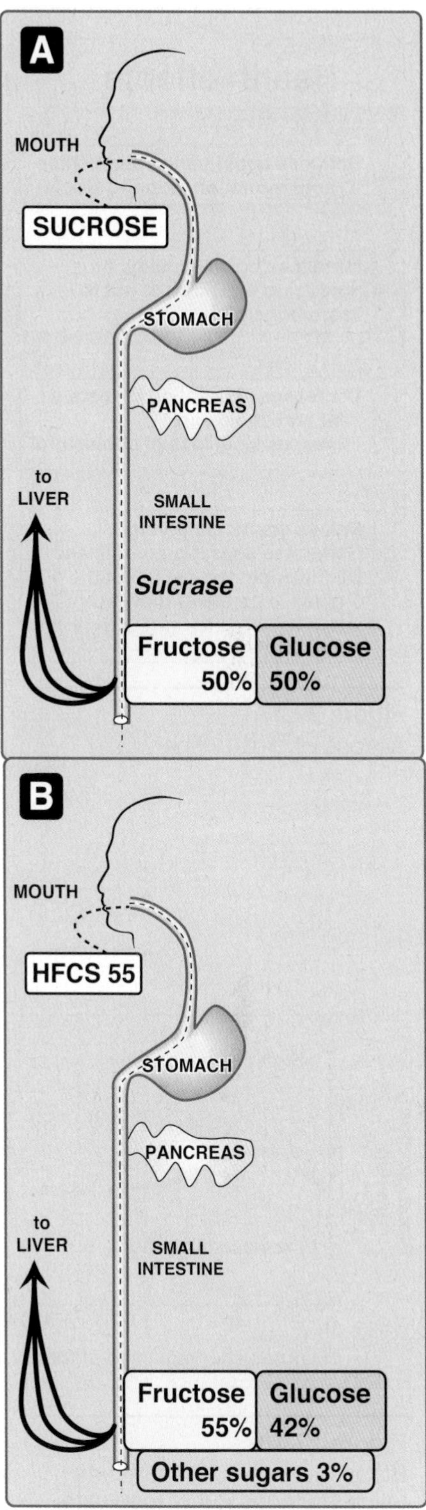

Figure 27.16
Digestion of high-fructose corn syrup (HFCS) 55 or sucrose leads to absorption of glucose plus fructose.

2. **Disaccharides:** The most abundant disaccharides are sucrose (glucose + fructose), lactose (glucose + galactose), and maltose (glucose + glucose). Sucrose is ordinary "table sugar" and is abundant in molasses and maple syrup. Lactose is the principal sugar found in milk. Maltose is a product of enzymic digestion of polysaccharides. It is also found in significant quantities in beer and malt liquors. The term "sugar" refers to monosaccharides and disaccharides. "Added sugars" are those sugars and syrups (such as HFCSs) added to foods during processing or preparation. [Note: Fructose is 1.7 times sweeter than sucrose.]

3. **Polysaccharides:** Complex carbohydrates are polysaccharides (most often polymers of glucose) that do not have a sweet taste. Starch is an example of a complex carbohydrate that is found in abundance in plants. Common sources include wheat and other grains, potatoes, dried peas and beans, and vegetables.

4. **Fiber:** Dietary fiber is defined as the nondigestible, nonstarch carbohydrates and lignin (a noncarbohydrate polymer of aromatic alcohols) present intact in plants. Soluble fiber is the edible parts of plants that is resistant to digestion and absorption in the human small intestine but is completely or partially fermented by bacteria to short-chain fatty acids in the large intestine. Insoluble fiber passes through the digestive track largely intact. Dietary fiber provides little energy but has several beneficial effects. First, it adds bulk to the diet (Figure 27.17). Fiber can absorb 10–15 times its own weight in water, drawing fluid into the lumen of the intestine and increasing bowel motility and promoting normal laxation. Soluble fiber delays gastric emptying and can result in a sensation of fullness. This delayed emptying also results in reduced peaks of blood glucose following a meal. Second, consumption of soluble fiber has now been shown to lower LDL-C levels by increasing fecal bile acid excretion and interfering with bile acid absorption (see p. 225). For example, diets rich (25–50 g/day) in the soluble fiber oat bran are associated with a modest, but significant, reduction in risk for CHD by lowering total cholesterol and LDL-C levels. Also, fiber-rich diets decrease the risk for constipation, hemorrhoids, and diverticulosis. The AI for dietary fiber is 25 g/day for women and 38 g/day for men. However, most American diets are far lower in fiber at approximately 15 g/day. [Note: "Functional fiber" is the term used for isolated fiber that has proven health benefits

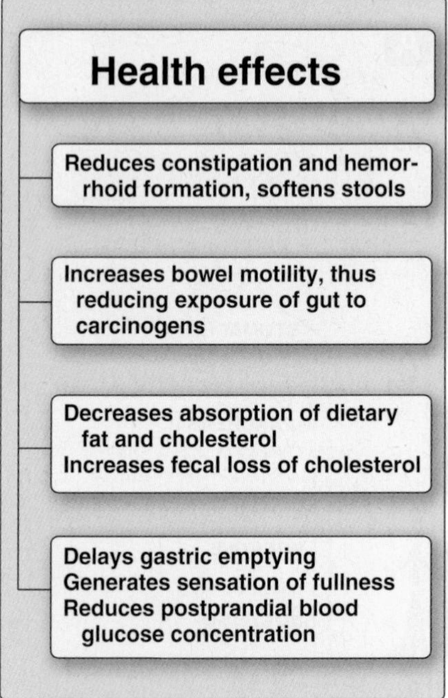

Figure 27.17
Actions of dietary fiber.

such as commercially available fiber supplements. Total fiber is the sum of dietary fiber and functional fiber.]

B. Dietary carbohydrate and blood glucose

Some carbohydrate-containing foods produce a rapid rise followed by a steep fall in blood glucose concentration, whereas others result in a gradual rise followed by a slow decline. Thus, they differ in their glycemic response (GR). [Note: Fiber blunts the GR.] The glycemic index (GI) quantitates these differences in the time course of postprandial glucose concentrations (Figure 27.18). GI is defined as the area under the blood glucose curves seen after ingestion of a meal with carbohydrate-rich food, compared with the area under the blood glucose curve observed after a meal consisting of the same amount (50 g) of carbohydrate either as glucose or white bread. The clinical importance of the GI is unresolved, but evidence suggests that a low-GI diet improves glycemic control in diabetic individuals. Food with a low GI tends to create a sense of satiety over a longer period of time and may be helpful in limiting caloric intake. [Note: How much a typical serving size of a food raises blood glucose is referred to as the glycemic load (GL). A food (for example, carrots) can have a high GI and a low GL.]

C. Requirements for carbohydrate

Carbohydrates are not essential nutrients, because the carbon skeletons of most amino acids can be converted into glucose (see p. 261). However, the absence of dietary carbohydrate leads to ketone body production (see p. 262) and degradation of body protein whose constituent amino acids provide carbon skeletons for gluconeogenesis (see p. 118). The RDA for carbohydrate is set at 130 g/day for adults and children, based on the amount of glucose used by carbohydrate-dependent tissues, such as the brain and erythrocytes. However, this level of intake is usually exceeded to meet energy needs. Adults should consume 45%–65% of their total calories from carbohydrates. It is recommended that added sugar represent no more than 25% of total energy because of concerns that sugar may displace nutrient-rich foods from the diet, potentially leading to deficiencies of certain micronutrients.

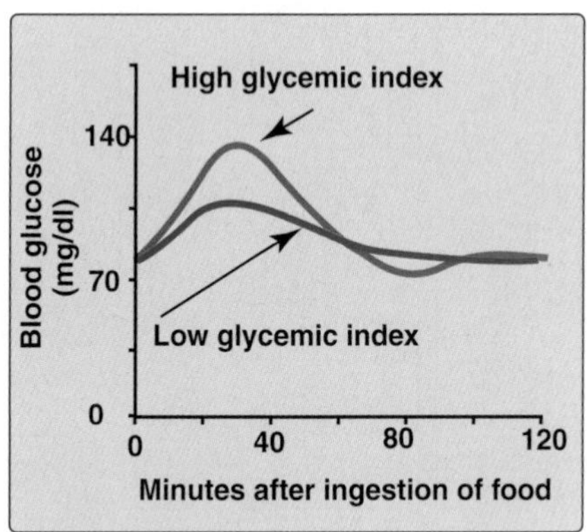

Figure 27.18
Blood glucose concentrations following ingestion of food with low or high glycemic index.

D. Simple sugars and disease

There is no direct evidence that the consumption of simple sugars is harmful. Contrary to folklore, diets high in sucrose do not lead to diabetes or hypoglycemia. Also contrary to popular belief, carbohydrates are not inherently fattening. They yield 4 kcal/g (the same as protein and less than one half that of fat; see Figure 27.5) and result in fat synthesis only when consumed in excess of the body's energy needs. However, there is an association between sucrose consumption and dental caries, particularly in the absence of fluoride treatment.

VII. DIETARY PROTEIN

Humans have no dietary requirement for protein per se, but the protein in food does provide essential amino acids (see Figure 20.2, p. 262). Nine of the 20 amino acids needed for the synthesis of body proteins are essential (that is, they cannot be synthesized in humans).

A. Quality of proteins

The quality of a dietary protein is a measure of its ability to provide the essential amino acids required for tissue maintenance. Most government agencies have adopted the Protein Digestibility–Corrected Amino Acid Score (PDCAAS) as the standard by which to evaluate protein quality. PDCAAS is based on the profile of essential amino acids after correcting for the digestibility of the protein. The highest possible score under these guidelines is 1.00. This amino acid score provides a method to balance intakes of poorer-quality proteins with high-quality dietary proteins.

Source	PDCAAS value
Animal proteins	
Egg	1.00
Milk protein	1.00
Beef/poultry/fish	0.82–0.92
Gelatin	0.08
Plant proteins	
Soybean protein	1.00
Kidney beans	0.68
Whole wheat bread	0.40

Figure 27.19
Relative quality of some common dietary proteins. PDCAAS = protein digestibility–corrected amino acid score.

1. **Proteins from animal sources:** Proteins from animal sources (meat, poultry, milk, and fish) have a high quality because they contain all the essential amino acids in proportions similar to those required for synthesis of human tissue proteins (Figure 27.19), and they are more readily digested. [Note: Gelatin prepared from animal collagen is an exception. It has a low biologic value as a result of deficiencies in several essential amino acids.]

2. **Proteins from plant sources:** Proteins from plant sources have a lower quality than do animal proteins. However, proteins from different plant sources may be combined in such a way that the result is equivalent in nutritional value to animal protein. For example, wheat (lysine deficient but methionine rich) may be combined with kidney beans (methionine poor but lysine rich) to produce an improved biologic value. Therefore, eating foods with different amino acids during the day can result in a dietary combination with a higher biologic value than either of the component proteins (Figure 27.20). [Note: Animal proteins can also complement the biologic value of plant proteins.]

B. Nitrogen balance

Nitrogen balance occurs when the amount of nitrogen consumed equals that of the nitrogen excreted in the urine (primarily as urinary urea nitrogen, or UUN), sweat, and feces. Most healthy adults are normally in nitrogen balance.

1. **Positive nitrogen balance:** This occurs when nitrogen intake exceeds nitrogen excretion. It is observed during situations in which tissue growth occurs, for example, in childhood, pregnancy, or during recovery from an emaciating illness.

2. **Negative nitrogen balance:** This occurs when nitrogen loss is greater than nitrogen intake. It is associated with inadequate dietary protein; lack of an essential amino acid; or during physiologic stresses, such as trauma, burns, illness, or surgery.

> Nitrogen (N) balance can be determined by the formula, N balance = protein N intake (g/24 hrs) – (UUN + 4 g), where 4 g accounts for urinary loss in forms other than UUN plus loss in skin and feces. Alternatively, protein balance = protein intake (g/24 hrs) – [(UUN + 4 g) x 6.25] can be used because there are, on average, 6.25 g N in 1 g protein.

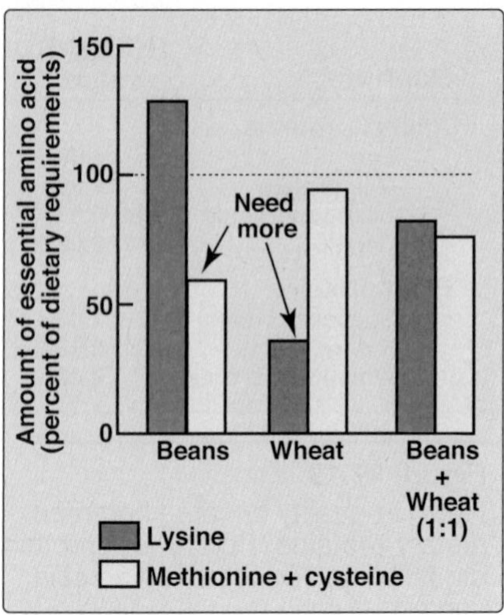

Figure 27.20
Combining two incomplete proteins that have complementary amino acid deficiencies results in a mixture with a higher biologic value.

C. Requirement for protein in humans

The amount of dietary protein required in the diet varies with its biologic value. The greater the proportion of animal protein included in the diet, the less protein is required. The RDA for protein is computed for proteins of mixed biologic value at 0.8 g/kg of body weight for adults, or about 56 g of protein for a 70-kg individual. People who exercise strenuously on a regular basis may benefit from extra protein to maintain muscle mass, and a daily intake of about 1 g/kg has been recommended for athletes. Women who are pregnant or lactating require up to 30 g/day in addition to their basal requirements. To support growth, infants should consume 2 g/kg/day.

1. **Consumption of excess protein:** There is no physiologic advantage to the consumption of more protein than the RDA. Protein consumed in excess of the body's needs is deaminated, and the resulting carbon skeletons are metabolized to provide energy or acetyl coenzyme A for fatty acid synthesis. When excess protein is eliminated from the body as urinary nitrogen, it is often accompanied by increased urinary calcium, thereby increasing the risk of nephrolithiasis and osteoporosis.

2. **The protein-sparing effect of carbohydrate:** The dietary protein requirement is influenced by the carbohydrate content of the diet. When the intake of carbohydrates is low, amino acids are deaminated to provide carbon skeletons for the synthesis of glucose that is needed as a fuel by the central nervous system. If carbohydrate intake is less than 130 g/day, substantial amounts of protein are metabolized to provide precursors for gluconeogenesis. Therefore, carbohydrate is considered to be "protein-sparing," because it allows amino acids to be used for repair and maintenance of tissue protein rather than for gluconeogenesis.

D. Protein-energy (calorie) malnutrition

In developed countries, protein-energy malnutrition (PEM) is most commonly seen in patients with medical conditions that decrease appetite or alter how nutrients are digested or absorbed or in hospitalized patients with major trauma or infections. [Note: Such highly catabolic patients frequently require intravenous (parenteral) or

CHARACTERISTIC	KWASHIORKOR	MARASMUS
Weight for age (% expected)	60–80	<60
Weight for height	Normal or decreased	Markedly decreased
Edema	Present	Absent
Mood	Irritable when picked up; apathetic when left alone	Alert, irritable
Appetite	Poor	Good

Figure 27.21
Features of protein-energy malnutrition in children.

tube-based (enteral) administration of nutrients.] PEM may also be seen in children or the elderly who are malnourished. In developing countries, an inadequate intake of protein and/or energy is the primary cause of PEM. Affected individuals show a variety of symptoms, including a depressed immune system with a reduced ability to resist infection. Death from secondary infection is common. PEM is a spectrum of degrees of malnutrition, and two extreme forms are kwashiorkor and marasmus (Figure 27.21). [Note: PEM is also referred to as protein-energy undernutrition (PEU).]

1. **Kwashiorkor:** Kwashiorkor occurs when protein deprivation is relatively greater than the reduction in total calories. Protein deprivation is associated with severely decreased synthesis of visceral protein. Kwashiorkor is commonly seen in developing countries in children after weaning at about age 1 year, when their diet consists predominantly of carbohydrates. Typical symptoms include stunted growth, skin lesions, depigmented hair, anorexia, enlarged fatty liver, edema, and decreased serum albumin concentration. Edema results from the lack of adequate blood proteins, primarily albumin, to maintain the distribution of water between blood and tissues. It may mask muscle loss. Therefore, chronic malnutrition is reflected in the level of serum albumin. [Note: Because caloric intake from carbohydrates may be adequate, insulin levels suppress lipolysis and proteolysis. Kwashiorkor is nonadapted malnutrition.]

Cachexia, a wasting disorder characterized by loss of appetite and muscle atrophy (with or without increased lipolysis) that cannot be reversed by conventional nutritional support, is seen with a number of chronic diseases, such as cancer and chronic pulmonary and renal disease. It is associated with decreased treatment tolerance and response and decreased survival time.

2. **Marasmus:** Marasmus occurs when calorie deprivation is relatively greater than the reduction in protein. It usually occurs in developing countries in children younger than age 1 year when breast milk is supplemented with watery gruels of native cereals that are usually deficient in both protein and calories. Typical symptoms include arrested growth, extreme muscle wasting and loss of subcutaneous fat (emaciation), weakness, and anemia (Figure 27.22). Individuals with marasmus do not show the edema observed in kwashiorkor.

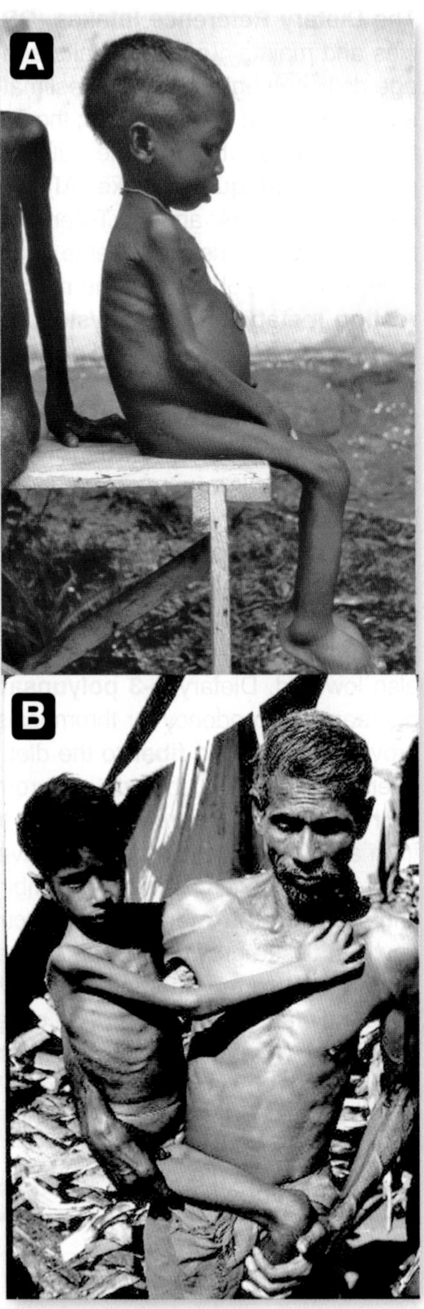

Figure 27.22
A. Listless child with kwashiorkor. Note the swollen belly.
B. Child suffering with marasmus.

27.2 Which one of the following statements concerning dietary fat is correct?

A. Coconut oil is rich in monounsaturated fats, and olive oil is rich in saturated fats.

B. Fatty acids containing trans double bonds, unlike the naturally occurring cis isomers, raise high-density lipoprotein cholesterol levels.

C. The polyunsaturated fatty acids linoleic and linolenic acids are required components.

D. Triacylglycerols obtained from plants generally contain less unsaturated fatty acids than those from animals.

Correct answer = C. We are unable to make linoleic and linolenic fatty acids. Consequently, these fatty acids are essential in the diet. Coconut oil is rich in saturated fats, and olive oil is rich in monounsaturated fats. Trans fatty acids raise plasma levels of low-density lipoprotein cholesterol, not high-density lipoprotein cholesterol. Triacylglycerols obtained from plants generally contain more unsaturated fatty acids than those from animals.

27.3 Given the information that a 70-kg man is consuming a daily average of 275 g of carbohydrate, 75 g of protein, and 65 g of fat, which one of the following conclusions can reasonably be drawn?

A. About 20% of calories are derived from fats.

B. The diet contains a sufficient amount of fiber.

C. The individual is in nitrogen balance.

D. The proportions of carbohydrate, protein, and fat in the diet conform to current recommendations.

E. The total energy intake per day is about 3,000 kcal.

Correct answer = D. The total energy intake is (275 g carbohydrate × 4 kcal/g) + (75 g protein × 4 kcal/g) + (65 g fat × 9 kcal/g) = 1,100 + 300 + 585 = 1,985 total kcal/day. The percentage calories from carbohydrate is 1,100/1,985 = 55, percentage calories from protein is 300/1,985 = 15, and percentage calories derived from fat is 585/1,985 = 30. These are very close to current recommendations. The amount of fiber or nitrogen balance cannot be deduced from the data presented. If the protein is of low biologic value, a negative nitrogen balance is possible.

For Questions 27.4 and 27.5:

A sedentary 50-year-old man weighing 80 kg (176 pounds) requests a physical. He denies any health problems. Routine blood analysis is unremarkable except for plasma total cholesterol of 295 mg/dl. (Reference value is less than 200 mg.) The man refuses drug therapy for his hypercholesterolemia. Analysis of a 1-day dietary recall showed the following:

Kilocalories	3,475 kcal	Cholesterol	822 mg
Protein	102 g	Saturated fat	69 g
Carbohydrate	383 g	Total Fat	165 g
Fiber	6 g		

27.4 Decreasing which one of the following dietary components would have the greatest effect in lowering the patient's plasma cholesterol?

A. Carbohydrate

B. Cholesterol

C. Fiber

D. Monounsaturated fat

E. Polyunsaturated fat

F. Saturated fat

Correct answer = F. The intake of saturated fat most strongly influences plasma cholesterol in this diet. The patient is consuming a high-calorie, high-fat diet with 40% of the fat as saturated fat. The most important dietary recommendations are lower total caloric intake, substitute monounsaturated and polyunsaturated fats for saturated fats, and increase dietary fiber. A decrease in dietary cholesterol would be helpful but is not a primary objective.

27.5 What would you need to know to estimate the total energy expenditure of the patient?

The daily basal energy expenditure (estimated resting metabolic rate/hour x 24 hours) and an activity factor (AF) based on the type and duration of physical activities are needed variables. An additional 10% would be added to account for the thermic effect of food. Note that if the patient were hospitalized, an injury factor (IF) would be included in the calculation, and the AF would be modified. Tables of AFs and IFs are available.

Vitamins

28

I. OVERVIEW

Vitamins are chemically unrelated organic compounds that cannot be synthesized in adequate quantities by humans and, therefore, must be supplied by the diet. Nine vitamins (folic acid, cobalamin, ascorbic acid, pyridoxine, thiamine, niacin, riboflavin, biotin, and pantothenic acid) are classified as water soluble. Because they are readily excreted in the urine, toxicity is rare. However, deficiencies can occur quickly. Four vitamins (A, D, K, and E) are termed fat soluble (Figure 28.1). They are released, absorbed, and transported (in chylomicrons) with dietary fat. They are not readily excreted, and significant quantities are stored in the liver and adipose tissue. In fact, consumption of vitamins A and D in excess of the Dietary Reference Intakes can lead to accumulation of toxic quantities of these compounds. Vitamins are required to perform specific cellular functions. For example, many of the water-soluble vitamins are precursors of coenzymes for the enzymes of intermediary metabolism. In contrast to the water-soluble vitamins, only one fat-soluble vitamin (vitamin K) has a coenzyme function.

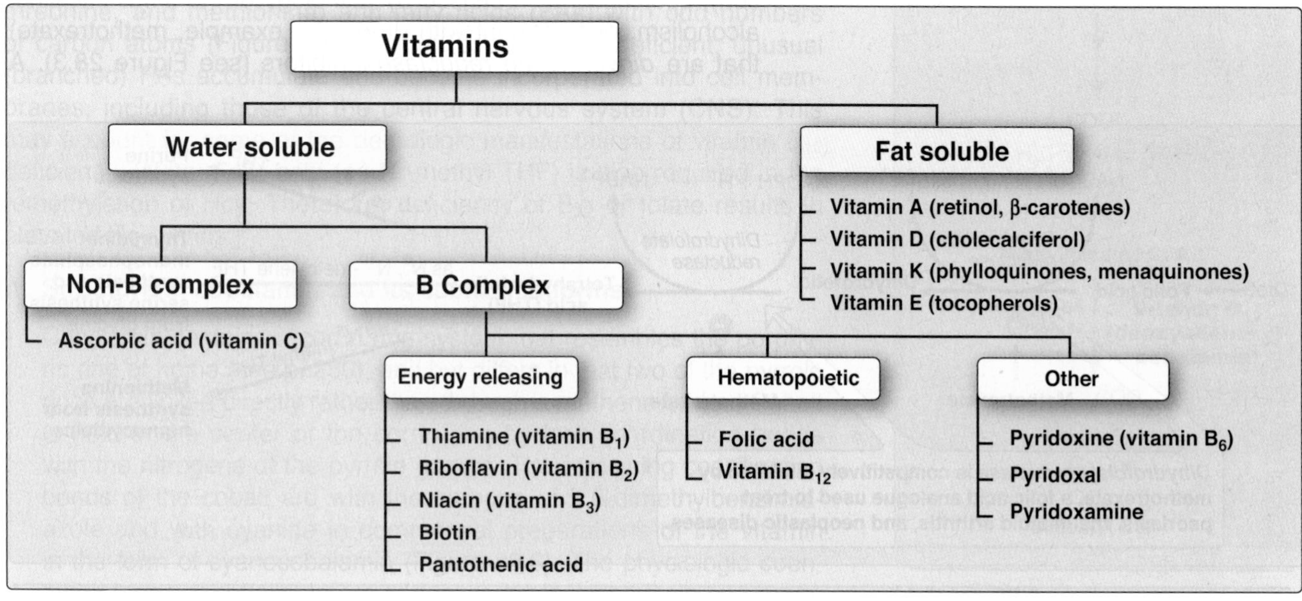

Figure 28.1
Classification of the vitamins.

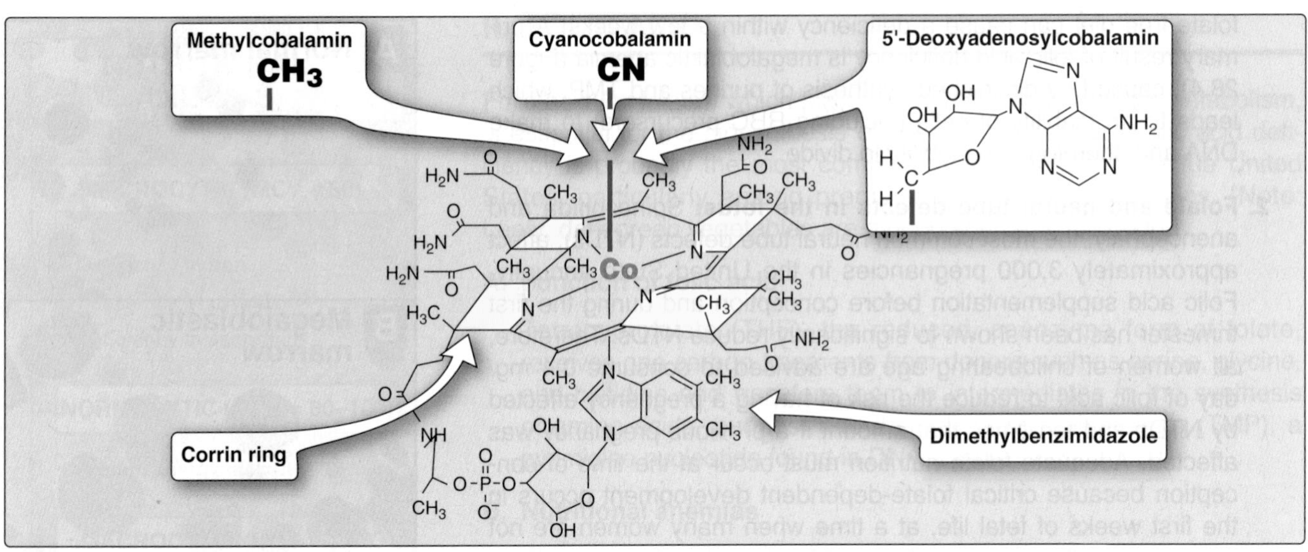

Figure 28.6
Structure of vitamin B_{12} (cyanocobalamin) and its coenzyme forms (methylcobalamin and 5'-deoxyadenosylcobalamin).

B. Distribution of cobalamin

Vitamin B_{12} is synthesized only by microorganisms, and it is not present in plants. Animals obtain the vitamin preformed from their natural bacterial flora or by eating foods derived from other animals. Cobalamin is present in appreciable amounts in liver, red meat, fish, eggs, dairy products, and fortified cereals.

C. Folate trap hypothesis

The effects of cobalamin deficiency are most pronounced in rapidly dividing cells, such as the erythropoietic tissue of bone marrow and the mucosal cells of the intestine. Such tissues need both the N^5,N^{10}-methylene and N^{10}-formyl forms of THF for the synthesis of nucleotides required for DNA replication (see pp. 293 and 303). However, in vitamin B_{12} deficiency, the utilization of the N^5-methyl form of THF in the B_{12}-dependent methylation of homocysteine to methionine is impaired. Because the methylated form cannot be converted directly to other forms of THF, folate is trapped in the N^5-methyl form, which accumulates. The levels of the other forms decrease. Thus, cobalamin deficiency leads to a deficiency of the THF forms needed in purine and TMP synthesis, resulting in the symptoms of megaloblastic anemia.

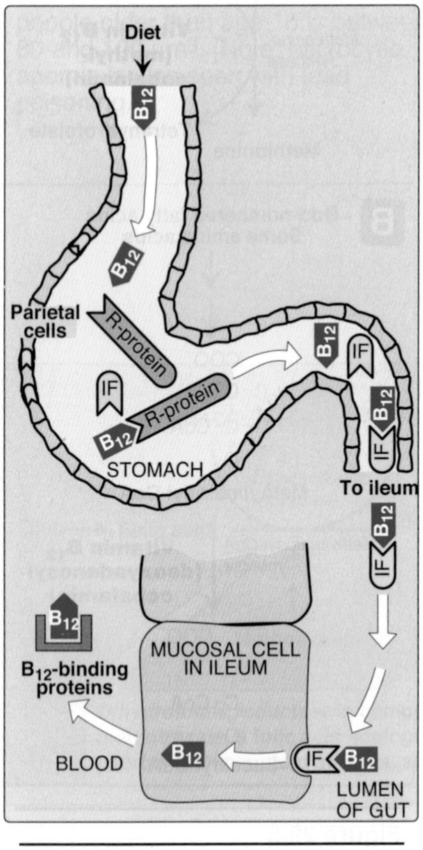

D. Clinical indications for vitamin B_{12}

In contrast to other water-soluble vitamins, significant amounts (2–5 mg) of vitamin B_{12} are stored in the body. As a result, it may take several years for the clinical symptoms of B_{12} deficiency to develop as a result of decreased intake of the vitamin. [Note: Deficiency happens much more quickly if absorption is impaired (see below).] B_{12} deficiency can be determined by the level of methylmalonic acid in blood, which is elevated in individuals with low intake or decreased absorption of the vitamin.

1. **Pernicious anemia:** Vitamin B_{12} deficiency is most commonly seen in patients who fail to absorb the vitamin from the intestine. B_{12}

Figure 28.7
Absorption of vitamin B_{12}. IF = intrinsic factor.

is released from food in the acidic environment of the stomach. [Note: Malabsorption of cobalamin in the elderly is most often due to reduced secretion of gastric acid (achlorhydria).] Free B_{12} then binds a glycoprotein (R-protein), and the complex moves into the intestine. B_{12} is released from the R-protein by pancreatic enzymes and binds another glycoprotein, intrinsic factor (IF). The cobalamin–IF complex travels through the intestine and binds to specific receptors on the surface of mucosal cells in the ileum. The cobalamin is transported into the mucosal cell and, subsequently, into the general circulation, where it is carried by its binding protein (transcobalamin). B_{12} is taken up and stored in the liver, primarily. It is released into bile and efficiently reabsorbed in the ileum. Severe malabsorption of vitamin B_{12} leads to pernicious anemia. This disease is most commonly a result of an autoimmune destruction of the gastric parietal cells that are responsible for the synthesis of IF (lack of IF prevents B_{12} absorption). [Note: Patients who have had a partial or total gastrectomy become IF deficient and, therefore, B_{12} deficient.] Individuals with cobalamin deficiency are usually anemic, and they show neuropsychiatric symptoms later, as the disease develops. The CNS effects are irreversible and occur by mechanisms that appear to be different from those described for megaloblastic anemia. Pernicious anemia requires life-long treatment with either high-dose oral B_{12} or intramuscular injection of cyanocobalamin. [Note: Supplementation works even in the absence of IF because approximately 1% of B_{12} uptake is by IF-independent diffusion.]

> Folic acid supplementation can partially reverse the hematologic abnormalities of B_{12} deficiency and, therefore, can mask a cobalamin deficiency. Thus, to prevent the CNS effects of B_{12} deficiency, therapy for megaloblastic anemia is initiated with both vitamin B_{12} and folic acid until the cause of the anemia can be determined.

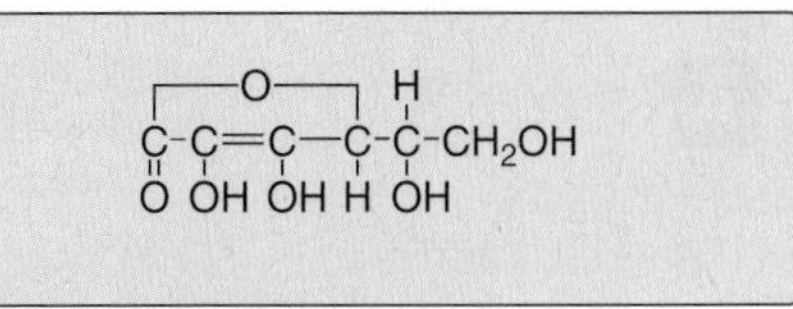

Figure 28.8
Structure of ascorbic acid.

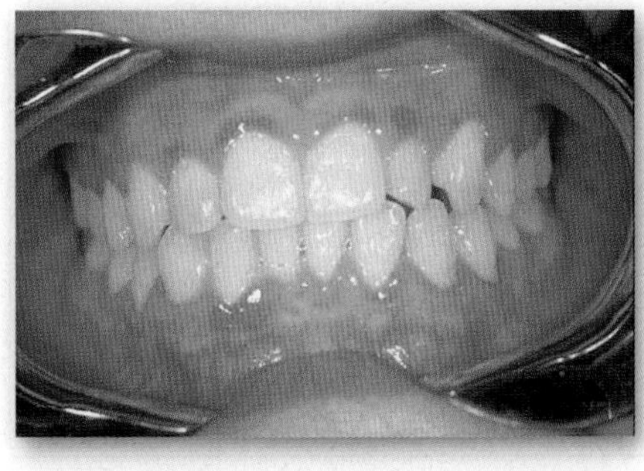

Figure 28.9
Hemorrhage and swollen gums of a patient with scurvy.

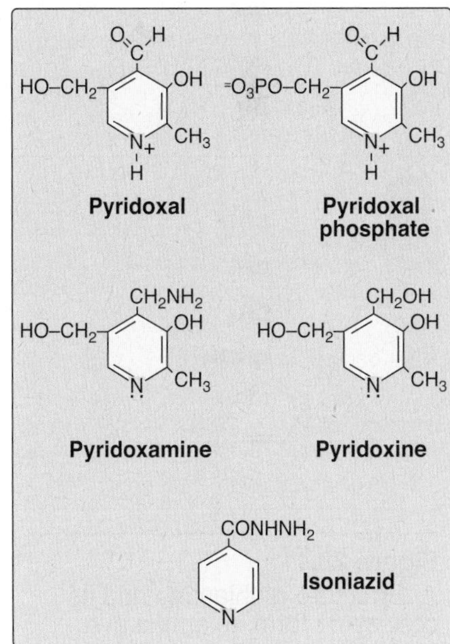

Figure 28.10
Structures of vitamin B_6 and the antituberculosis drug isoniazid.

IV. ASCORBIC ACID (VITAMIN C)

The active form of vitamin C is ascorbic acid (Figure 28.8). The main function of ascorbate is as a reducing agent in several different reactions. Vitamin C has a well-documented role as a coenzyme in hydroxylation reactions (for example, hydroxylation of prolyl and lysyl residues of collagen; see p. 47). Vitamin C is, therefore, required for the maintenance of normal connective tissue as well as for wound healing. Vitamin C also reduces ferric iron to the ferrous form, thereby facilitating the absorption of dietary iron from the intestine.

A. Deficiency of ascorbic acid

A deficiency of ascorbic acid results in scurvy, a disease characterized by sore and spongy gums, loose teeth, fragile blood vessels, swollen joints, fatigue, and a microcytic anemia caused by decreased absorption of iron (Figure 28.9). Many of the deficiency symptoms can be explained by a deficiency in the hydroxylation of collagen, resulting in defective connective tissue.

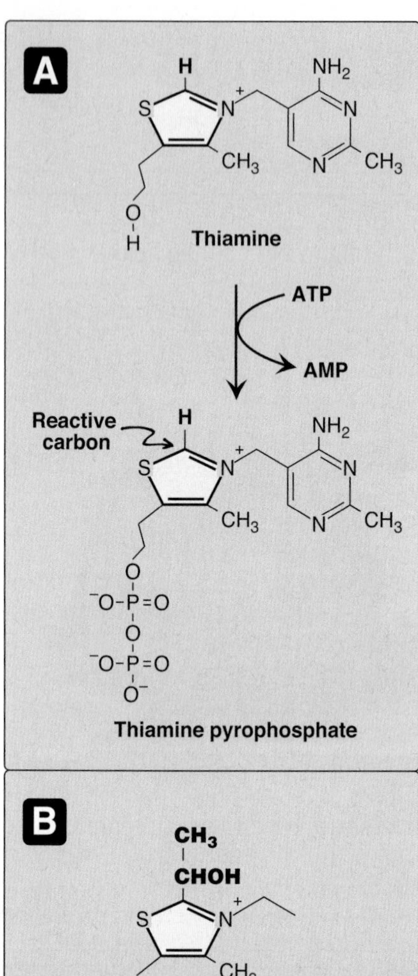

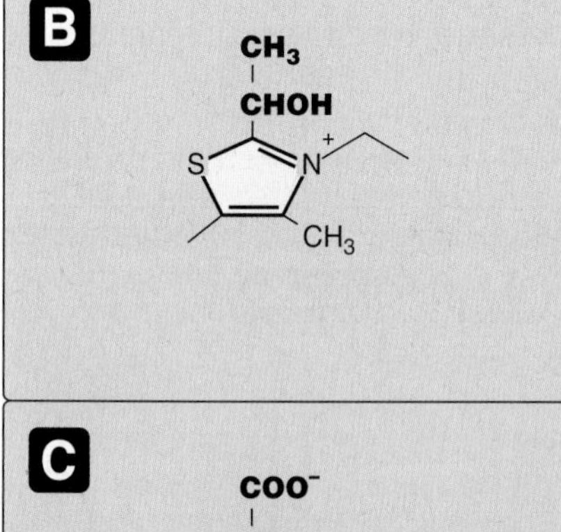

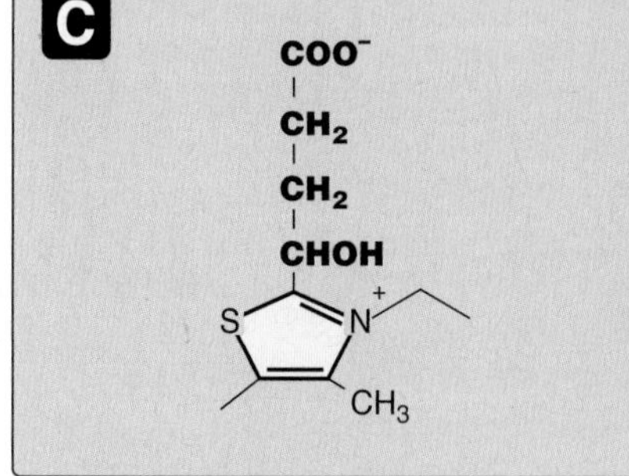

Figure 28.11
A. Structure of thiamine and its coenzyme form, thiamine pyrophosphate. B. Structure of intermediate formed in the reaction catalyzed by *pyruvate dehydrogenase.* C. Structure of intermediate formed in the reaction catalyzed by α-*ketoglutarate dehydrogenase.* AMP = adenosine monophosphate.

B. Prevention of chronic disease

Vitamin C is one of a group of nutrients that includes vitamin E (see p. 391) and β-carotene (see p. 382), which are known as antioxidants. [Note: Ascorbate regenerates the functional, reduced form of vitamin E.] Consumption of diets rich in these compounds is associated with a decreased incidence of some chronic diseases, such as coronary heart disease and certain cancers. However, clinical trials involving supplementation with the isolated antioxidants have failed to demonstrate any convincing beneficial effects.

V. PYRIDOXINE (VITAMIN B_6)

Vitamin B_6 is a collective term for pyridoxine, pyridoxal, and pyridoxamine, all derivatives of pyridine. They differ only in the nature of the functional group attached to the ring (Figure 28.10). Pyridoxine occurs primarily in plants, whereas pyridoxal and pyridoxamine are found in foods obtained from animals. All three compounds can serve as precursors of the biologically active coenzyme, pyridoxal phosphate (PLP). PLP functions as a coenzyme for a large number of enzymes, particularly those that catalyze reactions involving amino acids, for example, in the synthesis of cysteine from Hcy (see p. 264). [Note: PLP is also required by *glycogen phosphorylase* (see p. 128).]

Reaction type	Example
Transamination	Oxaloacetate + glutamate $\rightleftarrows$ aspartate + α-ketoglutarate
Deamination	Serine $\rightarrow$ pyruvate + NH_3
Decarboxylation	Histidine $\rightarrow$ histamine + CO_2
Condensation	Glycine + succinyl CoA $\rightarrow$ δ-aminolevulinic acid

A. Clinical indications for pyridoxine

Isoniazid, a drug commonly used to treat tuberculosis, can induce a vitamin B_6 deficiency by forming an inactive derivative with PLP. Dietary supplementation with B_6 is, thus, an adjunct to isoniazid treatment. Otherwise, dietary deficiencies in pyridoxine are rare but have been observed in newborn infants fed formulas low in B_6, in women taking oral contraceptives, and in alcoholics.

B. Toxicity of pyridoxine

Pyridoxine is the only water-soluble vitamin with significant toxicity. Neurologic symptoms (sensory neuropathy) occur at intakes above 500 mg/day, an amount nearly 400 times the Recommended Dietary Allowance (RDA) and over 5 times the Tolerable Upper Limit (UL). Substantial improvement, but not complete recovery, occurs when the vitamin is discontinued.

VI. THIAMINE (VITAMIN B_1)

Thiamine pyrophosphate (TPP) is the biologically active form of the vitamin, formed by the transfer of a pyrophosphate group from adenosine triphosphate (ATP) to thiamine (Figure 28.11). TPP serves as a coenzyme in the formation or degradation of α-ketols by *transketolase* (Figure 28.12A), and in the oxidative decarboxylation of α-keto acids (Figure 28.12B).

A. Clinical indications for thiamine

The oxidative decarboxylation of pyruvate and α-ketoglutarate, which plays a key role in energy metabolism of most cells, is particularly important in tissues of the CNS. In thiamine deficiency, the activity of these two *dehydrogenase*-catalyzed reactions is decreased, resulting in decreased production of ATP and, therefore, impaired cellular function. TPP is also required by *branched-chain α-keto acid dehydrogenase* of muscle. [Note: It is the *decarboxylase* of each of these *α-keto acid dehydrogenase* multienzyme complexes that requires TPP.] Thiamine deficiency is diagnosed by an increase in erythrocyte *transketolase* activity observed on addition of TPP.]

1. **Beriberi:** This is a severe thiamine-deficiency syndrome found in areas where polished rice is the major component of the diet. Adult beriberi is classified as dry (characterized by peripheral neurologic deficits) or wet (characterized by edema due to cardiac dysfunction). Infantile beriberi is seen in nursing infants whose mothers are deficient in thiamine.

2. **Wernicke-Korsakoff syndrome:** In the United States, thiamine deficiency, which is seen primarily in association with chronic alcoholism, is due to dietary insufficiency or impaired intestinal absorption of the vitamin. Some alcoholics develop Wernicke-Korsakoff syndrome, a thiamine deficiency state characterized by confusion, ataxia, and a rhythmic to-and-fro motion of the eyeballs (nystagmus) with Wernicke encephalopathy as well as memory problems and hallucinations with Korsakoff dementia. The syndrome is treatable with thiamine supplementation, but recovery of memory is typically incomplete.

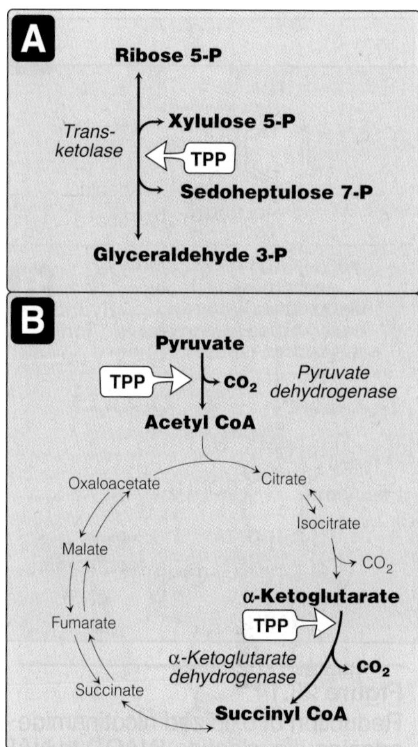

Figure 28.12
Reactions that use thiamine pyrophosphate (TPP) as coenzyme. A. *Transketolase*. B. *Pyruvate dehydrogenase* and *α-ketoglutarate dehydrogenase*. Note that TPP is also used by *branched-chain α-keto acid dehydrogenase*. P = phosphate; CoA = coenzyme A.

VII. NIACIN

Niacin, or nicotinic acid, is a substituted pyridine derivative. The biologically active coenzyme forms are nicotinamide adenine dinucleotide

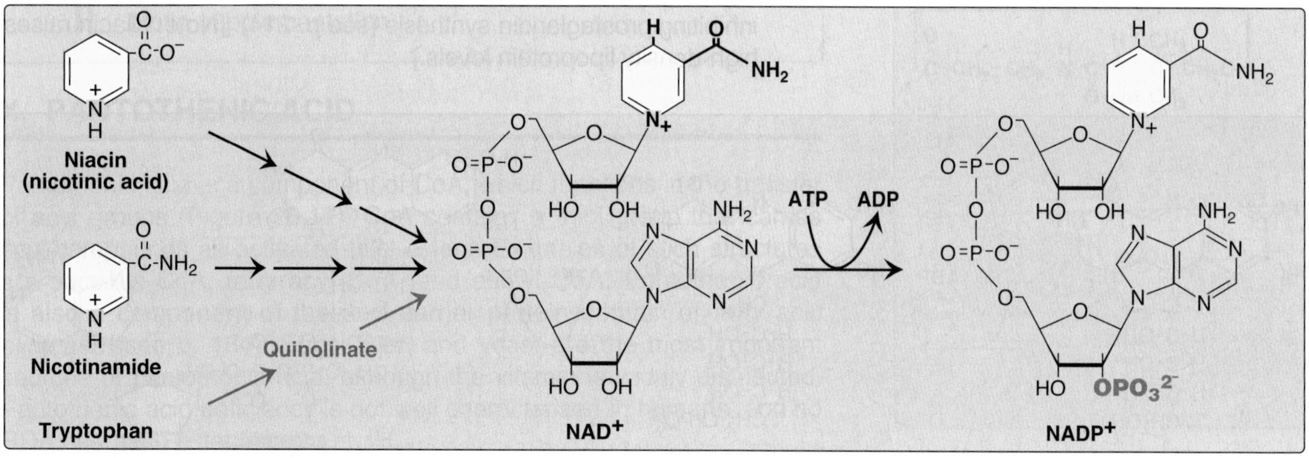

Figure 28.13
Structure and biosynthesis of oxidized nicotinamide adenine dinucleotide (NAD^+) and nicotinamide adenine dinucleotide phosphate ($NADP^+$). ADP = adenosine diphosphate.

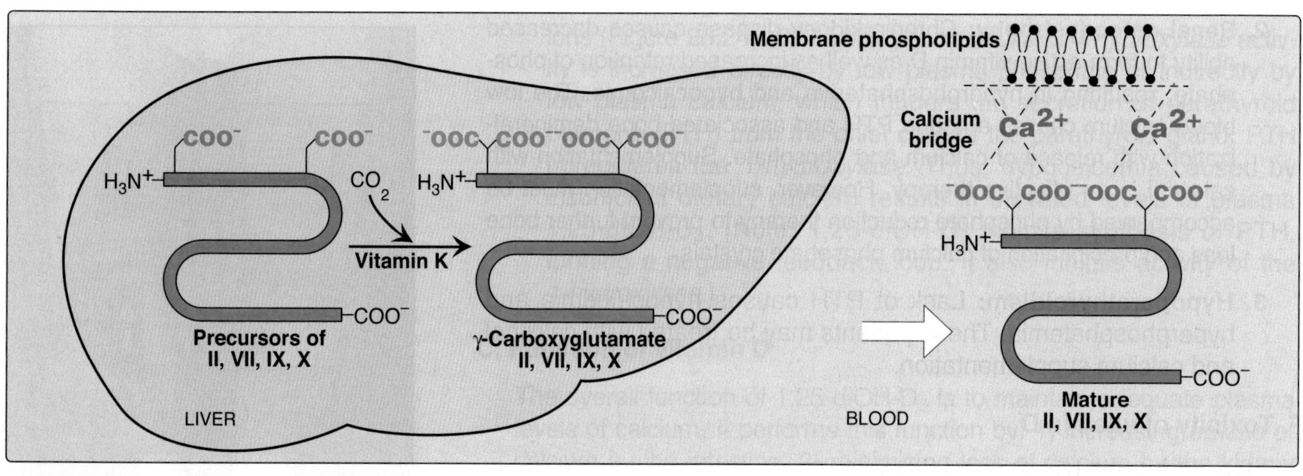

Figure 28.27
Role of vitamin K in blood coagulation.

membrane increases the rate at which the proteolytic conversion of prothrombin to thrombin can occur (Figure 28.27).

3. **γ-Carboxyglutamate residues in other proteins:** Gla residues are also present in proteins other than those involved in forming a blood clot. For example, osteocalcin of bone and proteins C and S (involved in limiting the formation of blood clots) also undergo γ-carboxylation.

B. Distribution and requirement of vitamin K

Vitamin K is found in cabbage, kale, spinach, egg yolk, and liver. There is also extensive synthesis of the vitamin by the bacteria in the gut. The adequate intake for vitamin K is 120 µg/day for adult males and 90 µg for adult females.

C. Clinical indications

1. **Deficiency of vitamin K:** A true vitamin K deficiency is unusual because adequate amounts are generally produced by intestinal bacteria or obtained from the diet. If the bacterial population in the gut is decreased (for example, by antibiotics), the amount of endogenously formed vitamin is depressed, and this can lead to hypoprothrombinemia in the marginally malnourished individual (for example, a debilitated geriatric patient). This condition may require supplementation with vitamin K to correct the bleeding tendency. In addition, certain second-generation cephalosporin antibiotics (for example, cefamandole) cause hypoprothrombinemia, apparently by a warfarin-like mechanism that inhibits *VKOR*. Consequently, their use in treatment is usually supplemented with vitamin K.

2. **Deficiency of vitamin K in the newborn:** Newborns have sterile intestines and, so, initially lack the bacteria that synthesize vitamin K. Because human milk provides only about one fifth of the daily requirement for vitamin K, it is recommended that all newborns receive a single intramuscular dose of vitamin K as prophylaxis against hemorrhagic disease.

D. Toxicity of vitamin K

Prolonged administration of large doses of synthetic vitamin K (menadione) can produce hemolytic anemia and jaundice in the infant, due to toxic effects on the membrane of RBCs. Therefore, it is no longer used to treat vitamin K deficiency. No UL has been set for vitamin K.

XIV. VITAMIN E

The E vitamins consist of eight naturally occurring tocopherols, of which α-tocopherol is the most active (Figure 28.28). The primary function of vitamin E is as an antioxidant in prevention of the nonenzymic oxidation of cell components (for example, peroxidation of polyunsaturated FAs by molecular oxygen and free radicals).

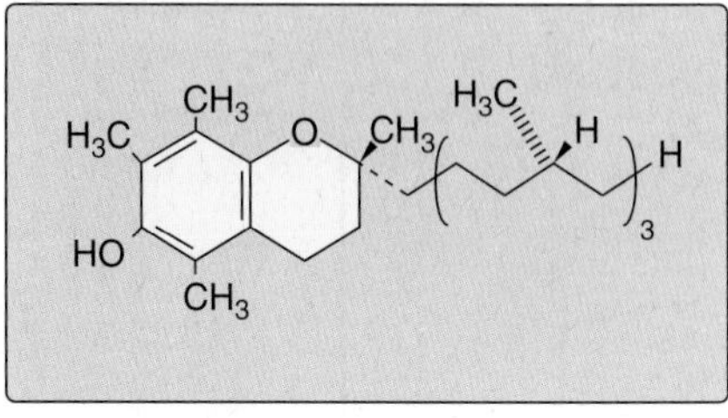

Figure 28.28
Structure of vitamin E.

A. Distribution and requirements of vitamin E

Vegetable oils are rich sources of vitamin E, whereas liver and eggs contain moderate amounts. The RDA for α-tocopherol is 15 mg/day for adults. The vitamin E requirement increases as the intake of polyunsaturated FA increases to limit FA peroxidation.

B. Deficiency of vitamin E

Newborns have low reserves of vitamin E, but breast milk (and formulas) contain the vitamin. Very-low-birth-weight infants may be given supplements to prevent the hemolysis and retinopathy associated with deficiency of vitamin E. When observed in adults, deficiency is usually associated with defective lipid absorption or transport. [Note: Abetalipoproteinemia, caused by a defect in the formation of chylomicrons (and VLDL), results in vitamin E deficiency (see p. 231).]

C. Clinical indications

Vitamin E is not recommended for the prevention of chronic disease, such as coronary heart disease or cancer. Clinical trials using vitamin E supplementation have been uniformly disappointing. For example, subjects in the Alpha-Tocopherol, Beta-Carotene Cancer Prevention Study trial who received high doses of vitamin E not only lacked cardiovascular benefit but also had an increased incidence of stroke.

D. Toxicity of vitamin E

Vitamin E is the least toxic of the fat-soluble vitamins, and no toxicity has been observed at doses of 300 mg/day (UL = 1,000 mg/day).

> Populations consuming diets high in fruits and vegetables show decreased incidence of some chronic diseases. However, clinical trials have failed to show a definitive benefit from supplements of vitamins A, C, or E; multivitamins with folic acid; or antioxidant combinations for the prevention of cancer or cardiovascular disease.

The vitamins are summarized in Figure 28.29.

VITAMIN	OTHER NAMES	ACTIVE FORM	FUNCTION
Folic acid	–	Tetrahydro-folic acid	Transfer one-carbon units; synthesis of methionine, purines, and thymidine monophosphate
Vitamin B_{12}	Cobalamin	Methylcobalamin Deoxyadenosyl cobalamin	Coenzyme for reactions: Homocysteine → methionine Methylmalonyl CoA → succinyl CoA
Vitamin C	Ascorbic acid	Ascorbic acid	Antioxidant Coenzyme for hydroxylation reactions, for example: In procollagen: Proline → hydroxyproline Lysine → hydroxylysine
Vitamin B_6	Pridoxine Pyridoxamine Pyridoxal	Pyridoxal phosphate	Coenzyme for enzymes, particularly in amino acid metabolism
Vitamin B_1	Thiamine	Thiamine pyrophosphate	Coenzyme of enzymes catalyzing: Pyruvate → acetyl CoA α-Ketoglutarate → Succinyl CoA Ribose 5-P + xylulose 5-P → Sedoheptulose 7-P + Glyceraldehyde 3-P Branched-chain α-keto acid oxidation
Niacin	Nicotinic acid Nicotinamide	NAD^+, $NADP^+$	Electron transfer
Vitamin B_2	Riboflavin	FMN, FAD	Electron transfer
Biotin	–	Enzyme-bound biotin	Carboxylation reactions
Pantothenic acid	–	Coenzyme A	Acyl carrier
			WATER SOLUBLE
			FAT SOLUBLE
Vitamin A	Retinol Retinal Retinoic acid β-Carotene	Retinol Retinal Retinoic acid	Maintenance of reproduction Vision Promotion of growth Differentiation and maintenance of epithelial tissues Gene expression
Vitamin D	Cholecalciferol Ergocalciferol	1,25-Dihydroxy-cholecalciferol	Calcium uptake Gene expression
Vitamin K	Menadione Menaquinone Phylloquinone	Menadione Menaquinone Phylloquinon	γ-Carboxylation of glutamate residues in clotting and other proteins
Vitamin E	α-Tocopherol	Any of several tocopherol derivatives	Antioxidant

Figure 28.29 (continued on next page)
Summary of vitamins. P = phosphate; NAD(P) = nicotinamide adenine dinucleotide (phosphate); FMN = flavin mononucleotide; FAD = flavin adenine dinucleotide; CoA = coenzyme A.

DEFICIENCY	SIGNS AND SYMPTOMS	TOXICITY	NOTES
Megaloblastic anemia Neural tube defects	Anemia Birth defects	None	Administration of high levels of folate can mask vitamin B_{12} deficiency
Pernicious anemia Dementia Spinal degeneration	Megaloblastic anemia Neuropsychiatric symptoms	None	Pernicious anemia is treated with intramuscular or high-dose oral vitamin B_{12}
Scurvy	Sore, spongy gums Loose teeth Poor wound healing	None	Benefits of supplementation not established in controlled trials
Rare	Glossitis Neuropathy	Yes	Deficiency can be induced by isoniazid Sensory neuropathy occurs at high doses
Beriberi Wernicke-Korsakoff syndrome (most common in alcoholics)	Tachycardia, vomiting, convulsions Apathy, loss of memory, dysregulated eye movements	None	–
Pellagra	Dermatitis Diarrhea Dementia	None	High doses of niacin used to treat hyperlipidemia
Rare	Dermatitis Angular stomatitis	None	–
Rare	–	None	Consumption of large amounts of raw egg whites (which contains a protein, avidin, that binds biotin) can induce a biotin deficiency
Rare	–	None	–
			WATER SOLUBLE
			FAT SOLUBLE
infertility Night blindness Retardation of growth Xerophthalmia	Increased visual threshold Dryness of cornea	Yes	β-Carotene not acutely toxic, but supplementation is not recommended Excess vitamin A can increase incidence of fractures
Rickets (in children) Osteomalacia (in adults)	Soft, pliable bones	Yes	Vitamin D is not a true vitamin because it can be synthesized in skin; application of sunscreen lotions or presence of dark skin color decreases this synthesis.
Newborn Rare in adults	Bleeding	Rare	Vitamin K produced by intestinal bacteria. Vitamin K deficiency common in newborns Intramuscular treatment with vitamin K is recommended at birth
Rare	Red blood cell fragility leads to hemolytic anemia	None	Benefits of supplementation not established in controlled trials

Figure 28.29 (continued from previous page)
Summary of vitamins.

Study Questions

Choose the ONE best answer.

For Questions 28.1–28.5, match the vitamin deficiency to the clinical consequence.

A. Folic acid
B. Niacin
C. Vitamin A
D. Vitamin B_{12}
E. Vitamin C
F. Vitamin D
G. Vitamin E
H. Vitamin K

28.1 Bleeding

28.2 Diarrhea and dermatitis

28.3 Neural tube defects

28.4 Night blindness

28.5 Sore, spongy gums and loose teeth

Correct answers = H, B, A, C, E. Vitamin K is required for formation of the γ-carboxyglutamate residues in several proteins required for blood clotting. Consequently, a deficiency of vitamin K results in a tendency to bleed. Niacin deficiency is characterized by the three Ds: diarrhea, dermatitis, and dementia (and death if untreated). Folic acid deficiency can result in neural tube defects in the developing fetus. Night blindness is one of the first signs of vitamin A deficiency. Rod cells in the retina detect white and black images and work best in low light, for example, at night. Rhodopsin, the visual pigment of the rod cells, consists of 11-cis retinal bound to the protein opsin. Vitamin C is required for the hydroxylation of proline and lysine during collagen synthesis. Severe vitamin C deficiency (scurvy) results in defective connective tissue, characterized by sore and spongy gums, loose teeth, capillary fragility, anemia, and fatigue.

28.6 A 52-year-old woman presents with fatigue of several months' duration. Blood studies reveal a macrocytic anemia, reduced levels of hemoglobin, elevated levels of homocysteine, and normal levels of methylmalonic acid. Which of the following is most likely deficient in this woman?

A. Folic acid
B. Folic acid and vitamin B_{12}
C. Iron
D. Vitamin C

Correct answer = A. Macrocytic anemia is seen with deficiencies of folic acid, vitamin B_{12}, or both. Vitamin B_{12} is utilized in only two reactions in the body: the remethylation of homocysteine to methionine, which also requires folic acid (as tetrahydrofolate [THF]), and the conversion of methymalonyl coenzyme A to succinyl coenzyme A, which does not require THF. The elevated homocysteine and normal methylmalonic acid levels in the patient's blood reflect a deficiency of folic acid as the cause of the macrocytic anemia. Iron deficiency causes microcytic anemia, as can vitamin C deficiency.

28.7 A 10-month-old African-American girl, whose family recently located from Maine to Virginia, is being evaluated for the bowed appearance of her legs. The parents report that the baby is still being breastfed and takes no supplements. Radiologic studies confirm the suspicion of vitamin D–deficient rickets. Which one of the following statements concerning vitamin D is correct?

A. A deficiency results in an increased secretion of calbindin.
B. Chronic kidney disease results in overproduction of 1,25-dihydroxycholecalciferol (calcitriol).
C. 25-Hydroxycholecalciferol (calcidiol) is the active form of the vitamin.
D. It is required in the diet of individuals with limited exposure to sunlight.
E. Its actions are mediated through binding to G protein–coupled receptors.
F. It opposes the effect of parathyroid hormone.

Correct answer = D. Vitamin D is required in the diet of individuals with limited exposure to sunlight, such as those living at northern latitudes like Maine and those with dark skin. Note that breast milk is low in vitamin D, and the lack of supplementation increases the risk of a deficiency. Vitamin D deficiency results in decreased synthesis of calbindin. Chronic kidney disease decreases production of calcitriol (1,25-dihydroxycholecalciferol), the active form of the vitamin. Vitamin D binds to nuclear receptors and alters gene transcription. Its effects are synergistic with parathyroid hormone.

28.8 Why might a deficiency of vitamin B_6 result in a fasting hypoglycemia? Deficiency of what other vitamin could also result in hypoglycemia?

Vitamin B_6 is required for glycogen degradation by glycogen phosphorylase. A deficiency would result in fasting hypoglycemia. Additionally, a deficiency of biotin (required by pyruvate carboxylase of gluconeogenesis) would also result in fasting hypoglycemia.

UNIT VI: Storage and Expression of Genetic Information

DNA Structure, Replication, and Repair

29

I. OVERVIEW

Nucleic acids are required for the storage and expression of genetic information. There are two chemically distinct types of nucleic acids: deoxyribonucleic acid (DNA) and ribonucleic acid ([RNA], see Chapter 30). DNA, the repository of genetic information, is present not only in chromosomes in the nucleus of eukaryotic organisms, but also in mitochondria and the chloroplasts of plants. Prokaryotic cells, which lack nuclei, have a single chromosome but may also contain nonchromosomal DNA in the form of plasmids. The genetic information found in DNA is copied and transmitted to daughter cells through DNA replication. The DNA contained in a fertilized egg encodes the information that directs the development of an organism. This development may involve the production of billions of cells. Each cell is specialized, expressing only those functions that are required for it to perform its role in maintaining the organism. Therefore, DNA must be able to not only replicate precisely each time a cell divides, but also to have the information that it contains be selectively expressed. Transcription (RNA synthesis) is the first stage in the expression of genetic information (see Chapter 30). Next, the code contained in the nucleotide sequence of messenger RNA molecules is translated (protein synthesis; see Chapter 31), thus completing gene expression. The regulation of gene expression is discussed in Chapter 32.

> The flow of information from DNA to RNA to protein is termed the "central dogma" of molecular biology (Figure 29.1) and is descriptive of all organisms, with the exception of some viruses that have RNA as the repository of their genetic information.

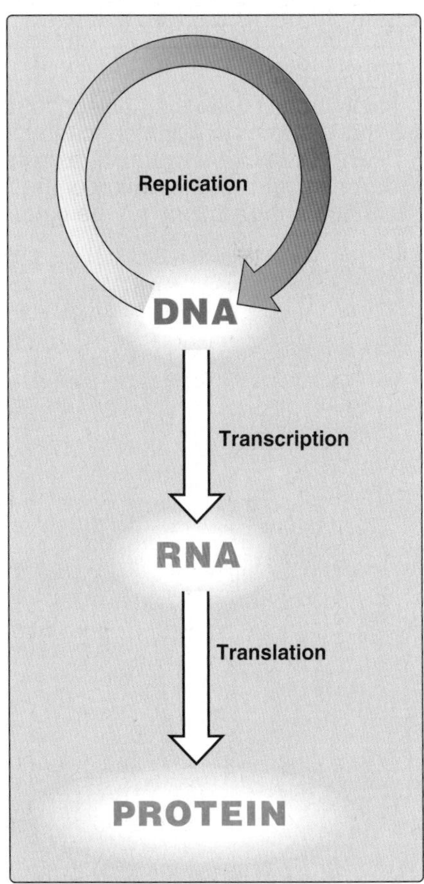

Figure 29.1
The "central dogma" of molecular biology.

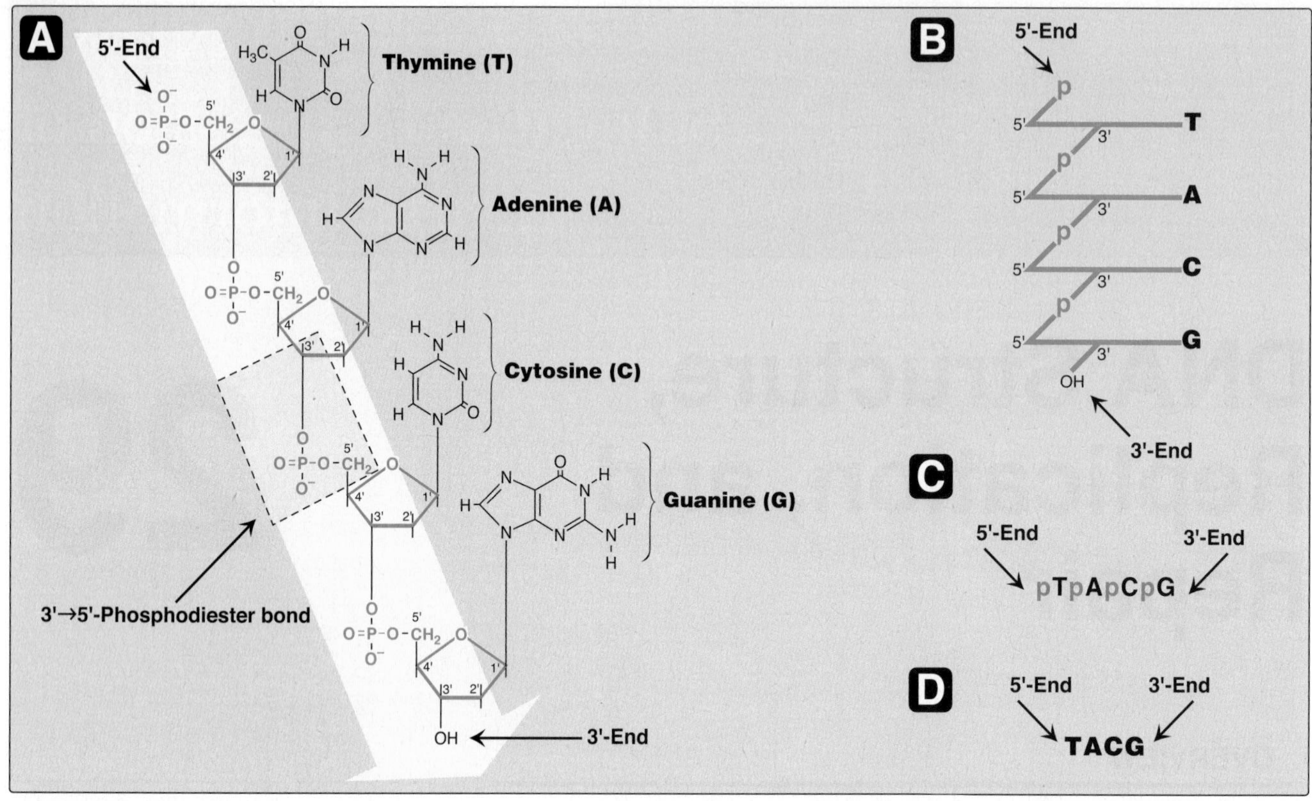

Figure 29.2
A. DNA chain with the nucleotide sequence shown written in the 5'→3' direction. A 3'→5'-phosphodiester bond is shown highlighted in the blue box, and the deoxyribose-phosphate backbone is shaded in yellow. B. The DNA chain written in a more stylized form, emphasizing the deoxyribose–phosphate backbone. C. A simpler representation of the nucleotide sequence. D. The simplest (and most common) representation, with the abbreviations for the bases written in the conventional 5'→3' direction.

II. STRUCTURE OF DNA

DNA is a polymer of deoxyribonucleoside monophosphates (dNMPs) covalently linked by 3'→5'–phosphodiester bonds. With the exception of a few viruses that contain single-stranded (ss) DNA, DNA exists as a double-stranded (ds) molecule, in which the two strands wind around each other, forming a double helix. [Note: The sequence of the linked dNMPs is primary structure, whereas the double helix is secondary structure.] In eukaryotic cells, DNA is found associated with various types of proteins (known collectively as nucleoprotein) present in the nucleus, whereas in prokaryotes, the protein–DNA complex is present in a nonmembrane-bound region known as the nucleoid.

A. 3'→5'-Phosphodiester bonds

Phosphodiester bonds join the 3'-hydroxyl group of the deoxypentose of one nucleotide to the 5'-hydroxyl group of the deoxypentose of an adjacent nucleotide through a phosphoryl group (Figure 29.2). The resulting long, unbranched chain has polarity, with both a 5'-end (the end with the free phosphate) and a 3'-end (the end with the free hydroxyl) that are not attached to other nucleotides. The bases located along the resulting deoxyribose–phosphate backbone are, by convention, always written in sequence from the 5'-end of the chain to the 3'-end. For example, the sequence of bases in the DNA shown in Figure 29.2D (5'-TACG-3') is read "thymine, adenine, cytosine, guanine." Phosphodiester linkages between nucleotides can be hydrolyzed enzymatically by a family of *nucleases*: *deoxyribonucleases* for DNA and *ribonucleases* for RNA, or cleaved hydrolytically by chemicals. [Note: Only RNA is cleaved by alkali.]

B. Double helix

In the double helix, the two chains are coiled around a common axis called the helical axis. The chains are paired in an antiparallel manner (that is, the 5'-end of one strand is paired with the 3'-end of the other strand) as shown in Figure 29.3. In the DNA helix, the hydrophilic deoxyribose–phosphate backbone of each chain is on the outside of the molecule, whereas the hydrophobic bases are stacked inside. The overall structure resembles a twisted ladder. The spatial relationship between the two strands in the helix creates a major (wide) groove and a minor (narrow) groove. These grooves provide access for the binding of regulatory proteins to their specific recognition sequences along the DNA chain. [Note: Certain anticancer drugs, such as dactinomycin (actinomycin D), exert their cytotoxic effect by intercalating into the narrow groove of the DNA double helix, thereby interfering with DNA (and RNA) synthesis.]

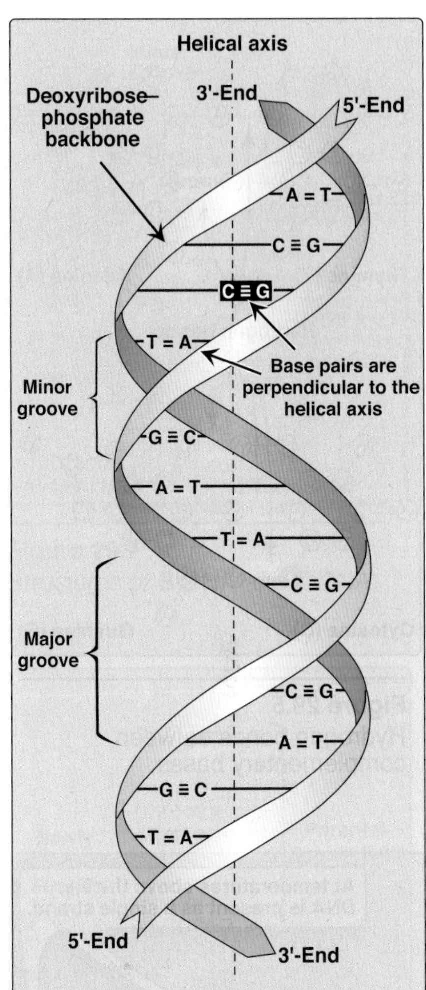

Figure 29.3
DNA double helix, illustrating some of its major structural features.

1. **Base-pairing:** The bases of one strand of DNA are paired with the bases of the second strand, so that an adenine (A) is always paired with a thymine (T) and a cytosine (C) is always paired with a guanine (G). [Note: The base pairs are perpendicular to the helical axis (see Figure 29.3).] Therefore, one polynucleotide chain of the DNA double helix is always the complement of the other. Given the sequence of bases on one chain, the sequence of bases on the complementary chain can be determined (Figure 29.4). [Note: The specific base-pairing in DNA leads to the Chargaff rule, which states that in any sample of dsDNA, the amount of A equals the amount of T, the amount of G equals the amount of C, and the total amount of purines equals the total amount of pyrimidines.] The base pairs are held together by hydrogen bonds: two between A and T and three between G and C (Figure 29.5). These hydrogen bonds, plus the hydrophobic interactions between the stacked bases, stabilize the structure of the double helix.

2. **Separation of the two DNA strands in the double helix:** The two strands of the double helix separate when hydrogen bonds between the paired bases are disrupted. Disruption can occur in the laboratory if the pH of the DNA solution is altered so that the nucleotide bases ionize, or if the solution is heated. [Note: Phosphodiester bonds are not broken by such treatment.] When DNA is heated, the temperature at which one half of the helical structure is lost is defined as the melting temperature (T_m). The loss of helical structure in DNA, called denaturation, can be monitored by measuring its absorbance at 260 nm. [Note: ssDNA has a higher relative absorbance at this wavelength than does dsDNA.] Because there are three hydrogen bonds between G and C but only two between A and T, DNA that contains high concentrations of A and T denatures at a lower temperature than G- and C-rich

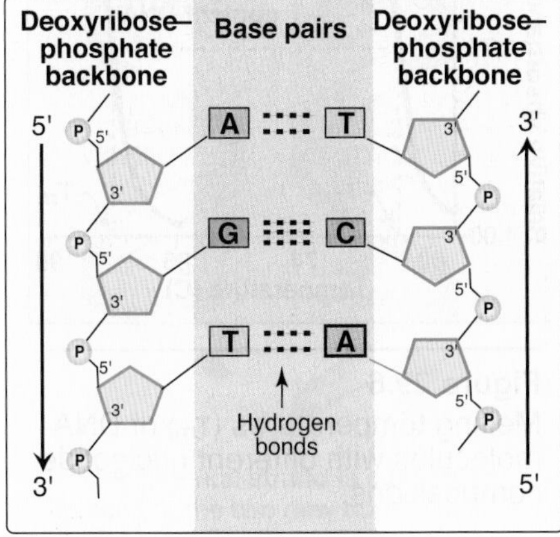

Figure 29.4
Two complementary DNA sequences. T= thymine; A = adenine; C = cytosine; G = guanine.

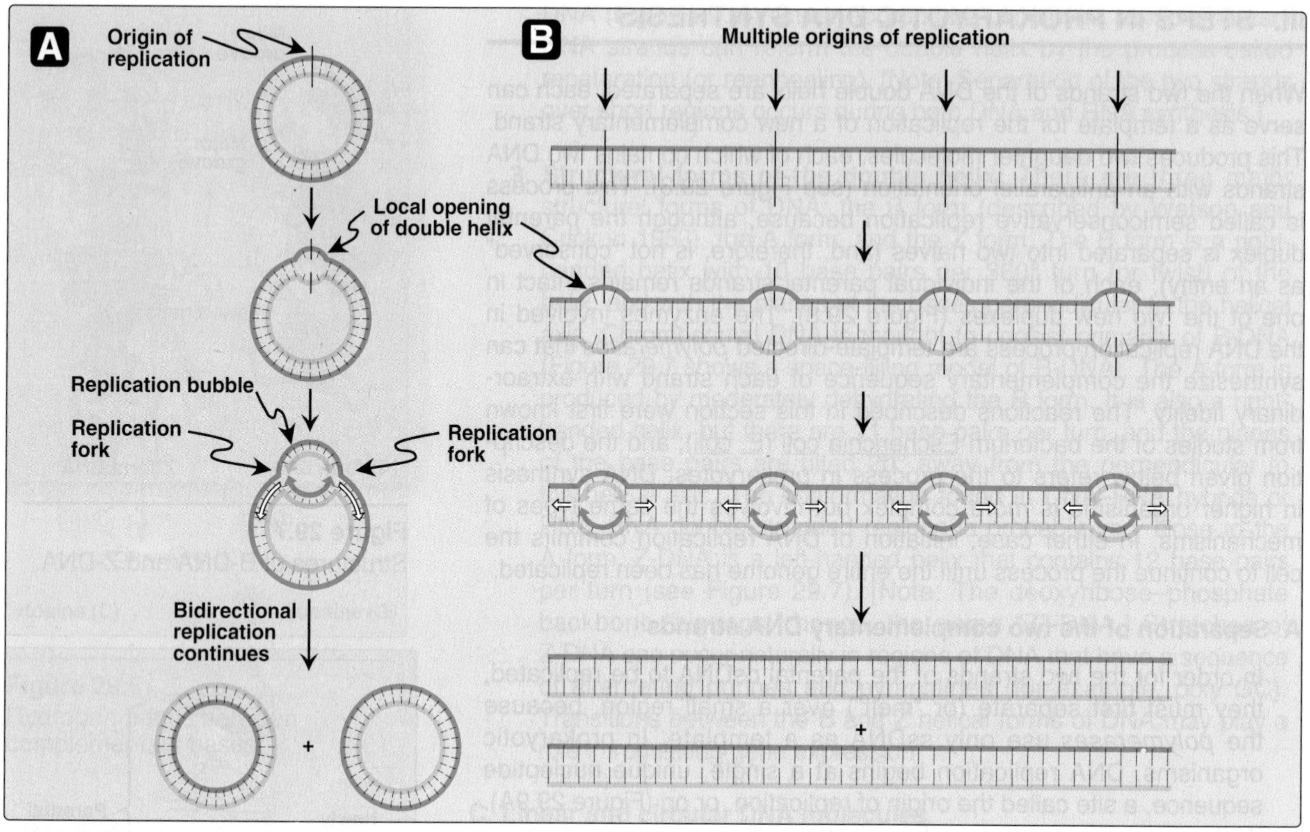

Figure 29.9
Replication of DNA: origins and replication forks. A. Small prokaryotic circular DNA. B. Very long eukaryotic DNA.

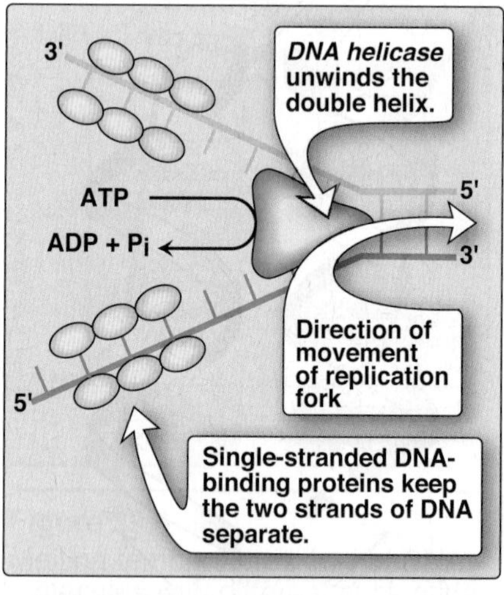

Figure 29.10
Proteins responsible for maintaining the separation of the parental strands and unwinding the double helix ahead of the advancing replication fork (>-). ADP = adenosine diphosphate; P_i = inorganic phosphate.

b. **DNA helicases:** These enzymes bind to ssDNA near the replication fork and then move into the neighboring double-stranded region, forcing the strands apart (in effect, unwinding the double helix). *Helicases* require energy provided by ATP (see Figure 29.10). Unwinding at the replication fork causes supercoiling in other regions of the DNA molecule. [Note: *DnaB* is the principal *helicase* of replication in E. coli. Its binding to DNA requires *DnaC*.]

c. **Single-stranded DNA-binding protein:** This protein binds to the ssDNA generated by *helicases* (see Figure 29.10). Binding is cooperative (that is, the binding of one molecule of single-stranded binding [SSB] protein makes it easier for additional molecules of SSB protein to bind tightly to the DNA strand). The SSB proteins are not enzymes, but rather serve to shift the equilibrium between dsDNA and ssDNA in the direction of the single-stranded forms. These proteins not only keep the two strands of DNA separated in the area of the replication origin, thus providing the single-stranded template required by *polymerases*, but also protect the DNA from *nucleases* that degrade ssDNA.

2. **Solving the problem of supercoils:** As the two strands of the double helix are separated, a problem is encountered, namely, the appearance of positive supercoils in the region of DNA ahead

of the replication fork as a result of overwinding (Figure 29.11), and negative supercoils in the region behind the fork. The accumulating positive supercoils interfere with further unwinding of the double helix. [Note: Supercoiling can be demonstrated by tightly grasping one end of a helical telephone cord while twisting the other end. If the cord is twisted in the direction of tightening the coils, the cord will wrap around itself in space to form positive supercoils. If the cord is twisted in the direction of loosening the coils, the cord will wrap around itself in the opposite direction to form negative supercoils.] To solve this problem, there is a group of enzymes called *DNA topoisomerases*, which are responsible for removing supercoils in the helix by transiently cleaving one or both of the DNA strands.

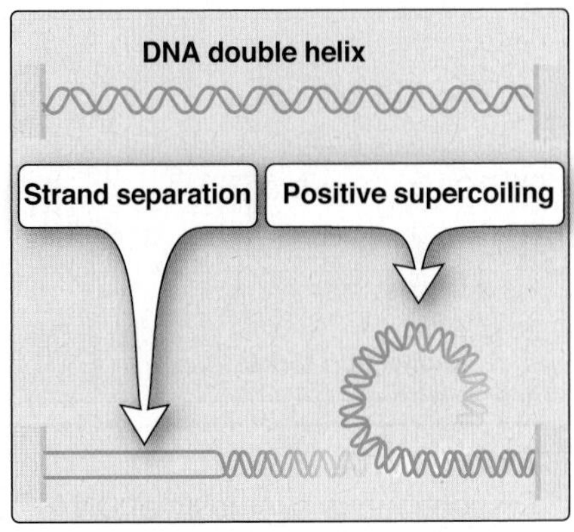

Figure 29.11
Positive supercoiling resulting from DNA strand separation.

a. Type I DNA topoisomerases: These enzymes reversibly cleave one strand of the double helix. They have both strand-cutting and strand-resealing activities. They do not require ATP, but rather appear to store the energy from the phosphodiester bond they cleave, reusing the energy to reseal the strand (Figure 29.12). Each time a transient "nick" is created in one DNA strand, the intact DNA strand is passed through the break before it is resealed, thus relieving ("relaxing") accumulated supercoils. *Type I topoisomerases* relax negative supercoils (that is, those that contain fewer turns of the helix than relaxed DNA) in E. coli, and both negative and positive supercoils (that is, those that contain fewer or more turns of the helix than relaxed DNA) in many prokaryotic cells (but not E. coli) and in eukaryotic cells.

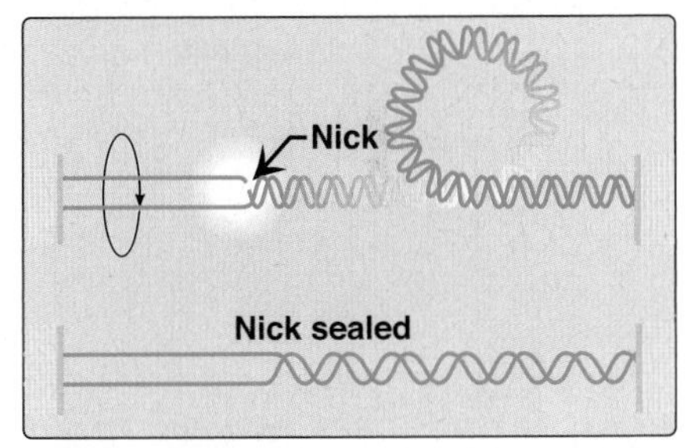

Figure 29.12
Action of *type I DNA topoisomerases.*

b. Type II DNA topoisomerases: These enzymes bind tightly to the DNA double helix and make transient breaks in both strands. The enzyme then causes a second stretch of the DNA double helix to pass through the break and, finally, reseals the break (Figure 29.13). As a result, both negative and positive supercoils can be relieved by this ATP-requiring process. *DNA gyrase*, a *type II topoisomerase* found in bacteria and plants, has the unusual property of being able to introduce negative supercoils into circular DNA using energy from the hydrolysis of ATP. This facilitates the replication of DNA because the negative supercoils neutralize the positive supercoils introduced during opening of the double helix. It also aids in the transient strand separation required during transcription (see p. 420).

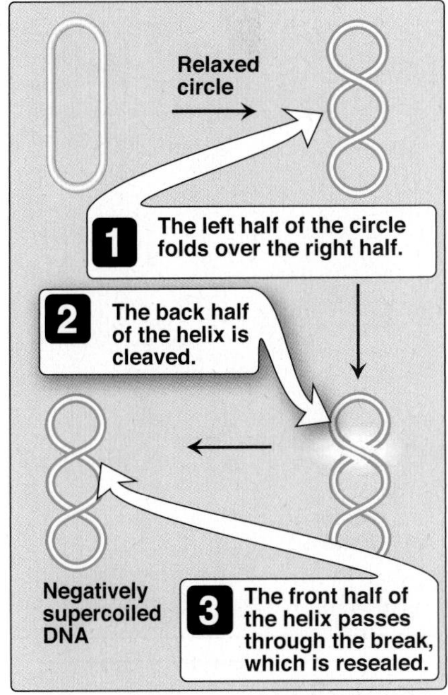

Figure 29.13
Action of *type II DNA topoisomerase.*

> Anticancer agents, such as the camptothecins, target human *type I topoisomerases*, whereas etoposide targets human *type II topoisomerases*. Bacterial *DNA gyrase* is a unique target of a group of antimicrobial agents called fluoroquinolones (for example, ciprofloxacin).

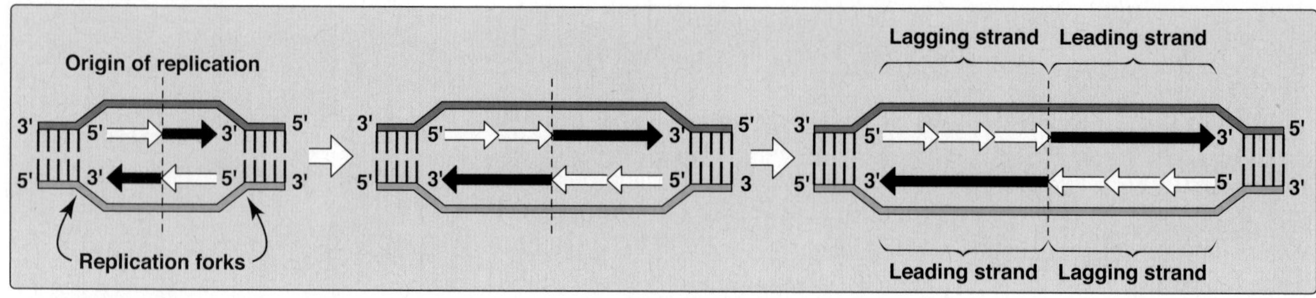

Figure 29.14
Discontinuous synthesis of DNA.

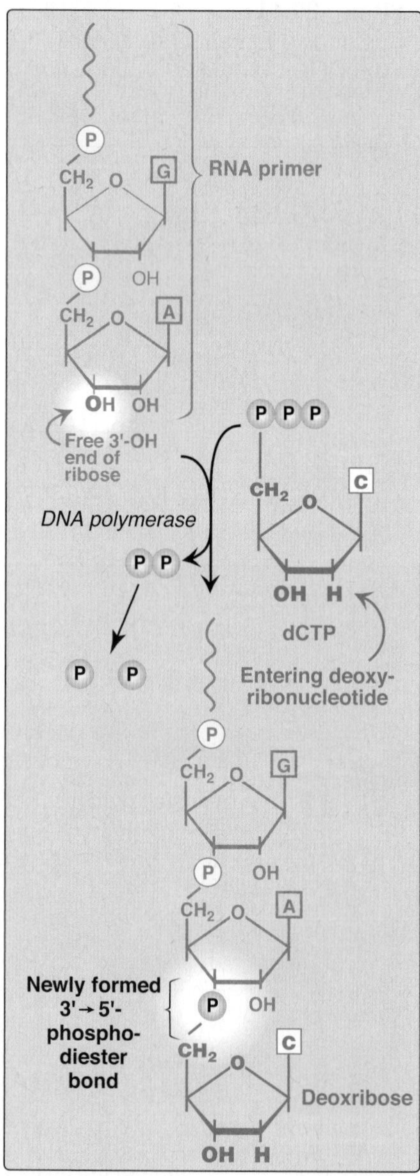

Figure 29.15
Use of an RNA primer to initiate DNA synthesis. P = phosphate.

C. Direction of DNA replication

The *DNA polymerases* responsible for copying the DNA templates are only able to "read" the parental nucleotide sequences in the 3'→5' direction, and they synthesize the new DNA strands only in the 5'→3' (antiparallel) direction. Therefore, beginning with one parental double helix, the two newly synthesized stretches of nucleotide chains must grow in opposite directions, one in the 5'→3' direction toward the replication fork and one in the 5'→3' direction away from the replication fork (Figure 29.14). This feat is accomplished by a slightly different mechanism on each strand.

1. **Leading strand:** The strand that is being copied in the direction of the advancing replication fork is called the leading strand and is synthesized continuously.

2. **Lagging strand:** The strand that is being copied in the direction away from the replication fork is synthesized discontinuously, with small fragments of DNA being copied near the replication fork. These short stretches of discontinuous DNA, termed Okazaki fragments, are eventually joined (ligated) to become a single, continuous strand. The new strand of DNA produced by this mechanism is termed the lagging strand.

D. RNA primer

DNA polymerases cannot initiate synthesis of a complementary strand of DNA on a totally single-stranded template. Rather, they require an RNA primer, which is a short, double-stranded region consisting of RNA base-paired to the DNA template, with a free hydroxyl group on the 3'-end of the RNA strand (Figure 29.15). This hydroxyl group serves as the first acceptor of a deoxynucleotide by action of a *DNA polymerase*. [Note: Recall that *glycogen synthase* also requires a primer (see p. 126).]

1. **Primase:** A specific *RNA polymerase*, called *primase* (*DnaG*), synthesizes the short stretches of RNA (approximately ten nucleotides long) that are complementary and antiparallel to the DNA template. In the resulting hybrid duplex, the U (uracil) in RNA pairs with A in DNA. As shown in Figure 29.16, these short RNA sequences are constantly being synthesized at the replication fork on the lagging strand, but only one RNA sequence at the origin of replication is required on the leading strand. The substrates

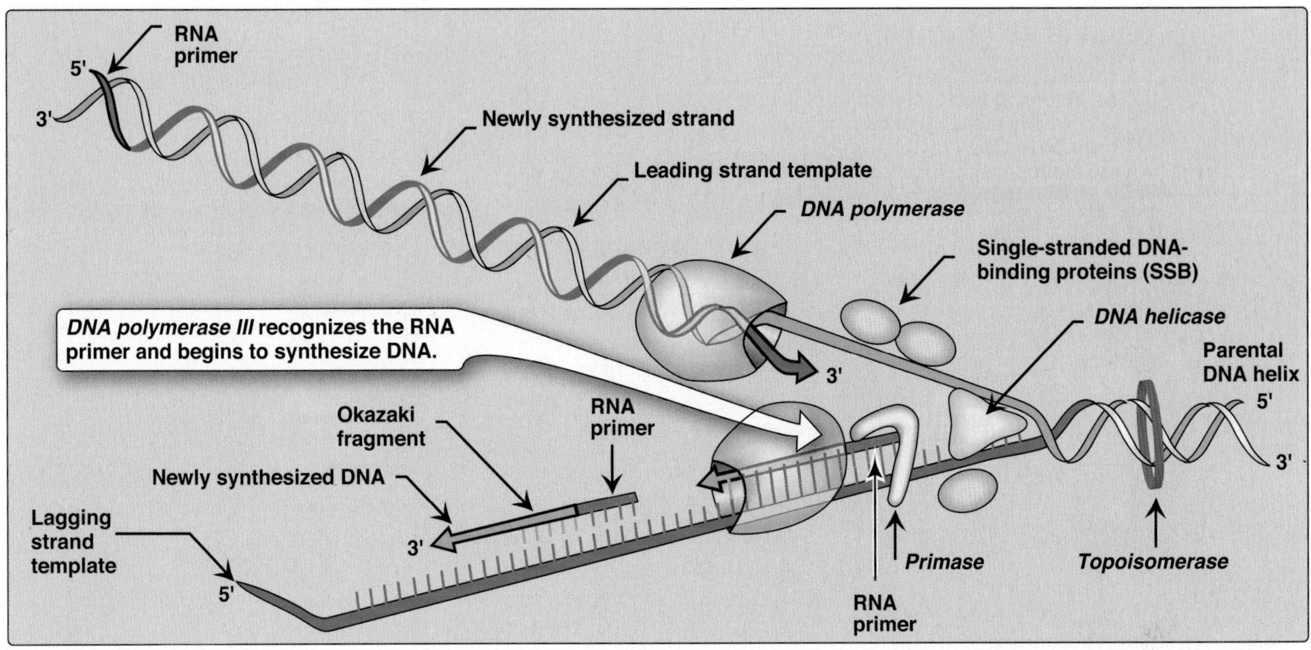

Figure 29.16
Elongation of the leading and lagging strands. [Note: The DNA sliding clamp is not shown.]

for this process are 5'-ribonucleoside triphosphates, and pyrophosphate is released as each ribonucleoside monophosphate is added through formation of a 3'→5' phosphodiester bond. [Note: The RNA primer is later removed as described on p. 405.]

2. **Primosome:** The addition of *primase* converts the prepriming complex of proteins required for DNA strand separation (see p. 399) to a primosome. The primosome makes the RNA primer required for leading strand synthesis and initiates Okazaki fragment formation in lagging strand synthesis. As with DNA synthesis, the direction of synthesis of the primer is 5'→3'.

E. Chain elongation

Prokaryotic (and eukaryotic) *DNA polymerases* (*DNA pols*) elongate a new DNA strand by adding deoxyribonucleotides, one at a time, to the 3'-end of the growing chain (see Figure 29.16). The sequence of nucleotides that are added is dictated by the base sequence of the template strand with which the incoming nucleotides are paired.

1. **DNA polymerase III:** DNA chain elongation is catalyzed by the multisubunit enzyme, *DNA polymerase III* (*DNA pol III*). Using the 3'-hydroxyl group of the RNA primer as the acceptor of the first deoxyribonucleotide, *DNA pol III* begins to add nucleotides along the single-stranded template that specifies the sequence of bases in the newly synthesized chain. *DNA pol III* is a highly "processive" enzyme (that is, it remains bound to the template strand as it moves along and does not diffuse away and then rebind before adding each new nucleotide). The processivity of *DNA pol III* is the result of its β subunit forming a ring that encircles and moves along the template strand of the DNA, thus serving as a sliding

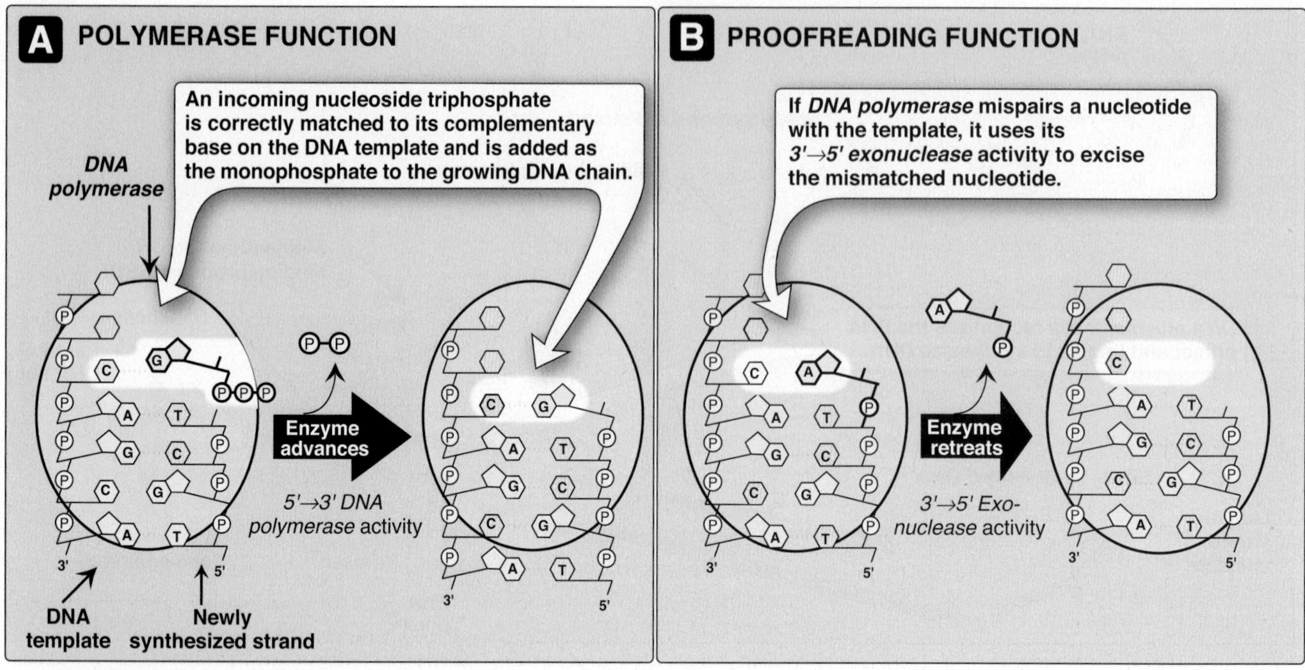

Figure 29.17
3'→5' Exonuclease activity enables *DNA polymerase III* to "proofread" the newly synthesized DNA strand.

DNA clamp. [Note: Clamp formation is facilitated by a protein complex, the clamp loader, and ATP hydrolysis.] The new strand grows in the 5'→3' direction, antiparallel to the parental strand (see Figure 29.16). The nucleotide substrates are 5'-deoxyribonucleoside triphosphates. Pyrophosphate (PP_i) is released when each new deoxynucleoside monophosphate is added to the growing chain (see Figure 29.15). Hydrolysis of PP_i to $2P_i$ means that a total of two high-energy bonds are used to drive the addition of each deoxynucleotide.

The production of PP_i with subsequent hydrolysis to $2P_i$, as seen in DNA replication, is a common theme in biochemistry. Removal of the PP_i product drives a reaction in the forward direction, making it essentially irreversible.

All four substrates (deoxyadenosine triphosphate [dATP], deoxythymidine triphosphate [dTTP], deoxycytidine triphosphate [dCTP], and deoxyguanosine triphosphate [dGTP]) must be present for DNA elongation to occur. If one of the four is in short supply, DNA synthesis stops when that nucleotide is depleted.

2. **Proofreading of newly synthesized DNA:** It is highly important for the survival of an organism that the nucleotide sequence of DNA be replicated with as few errors as possible. Misreading of the template sequence could result in deleterious, perhaps lethal,

mutations. To ensure replication fidelity, *DNA pol III* has a "proofreading" activity (*3'→5' exonuclease*, Figure 29.17) in addition to its *5'→3' polymerase* activity. As each nucleotide is added to the chain, *DNA pol III* checks to make certain the added nucleotide is, in fact, correctly matched to its complementary base on the template. If it is not, the *3'→5' exonuclease* activity removes the error. [Note: The enzyme requires an improperly base-paired 3'-hydroxy terminus and, therefore, does not degrade correctly paired nucleotide sequences.] For example, if the template base is C and the enzyme mistakenly inserts an A instead of a G into the new chain, the *3'→5' exonuclease* activity hydrolytically removes the misplaced nucleotide. The *5'→3' polymerase* activity then replaces it with the correct nucleotide containing G (see Figure 29.17). [Note: The proofreading *exonuclease* activity requires movement in the 3'→5' direction, not 5'→3' like the *polymerase* activity. This is because the excision must be done in the reverse direction from that of synthesis.]

F. Excision of RNA primers and their replacement by DNA

DNA pol III continues to synthesize DNA on the lagging strand until it is blocked by proximity to an RNA primer. When this occurs, the RNA is excised and the gap filled by *DNA pol I*.

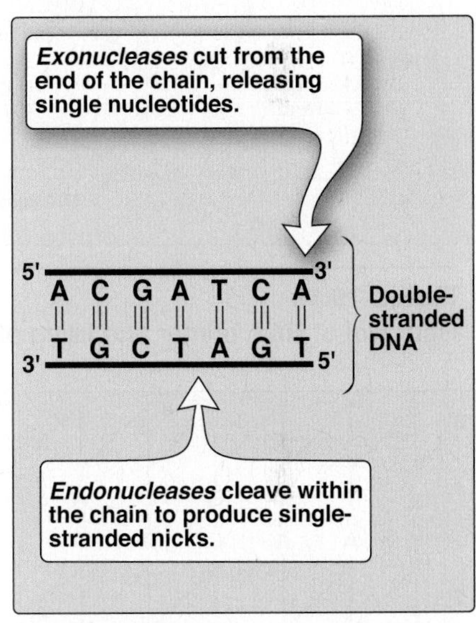

Figure 29.18
Endonuclease versus *exonuclease* activity. [Note: *Restriction endonucleases* (see p. 465) cleave both strands.] T= thymine; A = adenine; C = cytosine; G = guanine.

1. **5'→3' Exonuclease activity:** In addition to having the *5'→3' polymerase* activity that synthesizes DNA and the *3'→5' exonuclease* activity that proofreads the newly synthesized DNA chain like *DNA pol III*, *DNA pol I* also has a *5'→3' exonuclease* activity that is able to hydrolytically remove the RNA primer. [Note: These activities are *exonucleases* because they remove nucleotides from the end of the DNA chain, rather than cleaving the chain internally as do the *endonucleases* (Figure 29.18).] First, *DNA pol I* locates the space (nick) between the 3'-end of the DNA newly synthesized by *DNA pol III* and the 5'-end of the adjacent RNA primer. Next, *DNA pol I* hydrolytically removes the RNA nucleotides "ahead" of itself, moving in the 5'→3' direction (*5'→3' exonuclease* activity). As it removes the RNA, *DNA pol I* replaces it with deoxyribonucleotides, synthesizing DNA in the 5'→3' direction (*5'→3' polymerase* activity). As it synthesizes the DNA, it also "proofreads" the new chain using its *3'→5' exonuclease* activity to remove errors. This removal/synthesis/proofreading continues, one nucleotide at a time, until the RNA primer is totally degraded, and the gap is filled with DNA (Figure 29.19). [Note: *DNA pol I* uses its *5'→3' polymerase* activity to fill in gaps generated during DNA repair (see p.410).]

2. **Comparison of 5'→3' and 3'→5' exonucleases:** The *5'→3' exonuclease* activity of *DNA pol I* allows the *polymerase*, moving 5'→3', to hydrolytically remove one or more nucleotides at a time from the 5' end of the 20 to 30 nucleotide–long RNA primer. In contrast, the *3'→5' exonuclease* activity of *DNA pol I*, as well as *DNA pol II* and *III*, allows these *polymerases*, moving 3'→5', to hydrolytically remove one misplaced nucleotide at a time from the 3' end of a growing DNA strand, increasing the fidelity of replication such that newly replicated DNA has one error per 10^7 nucleotides.

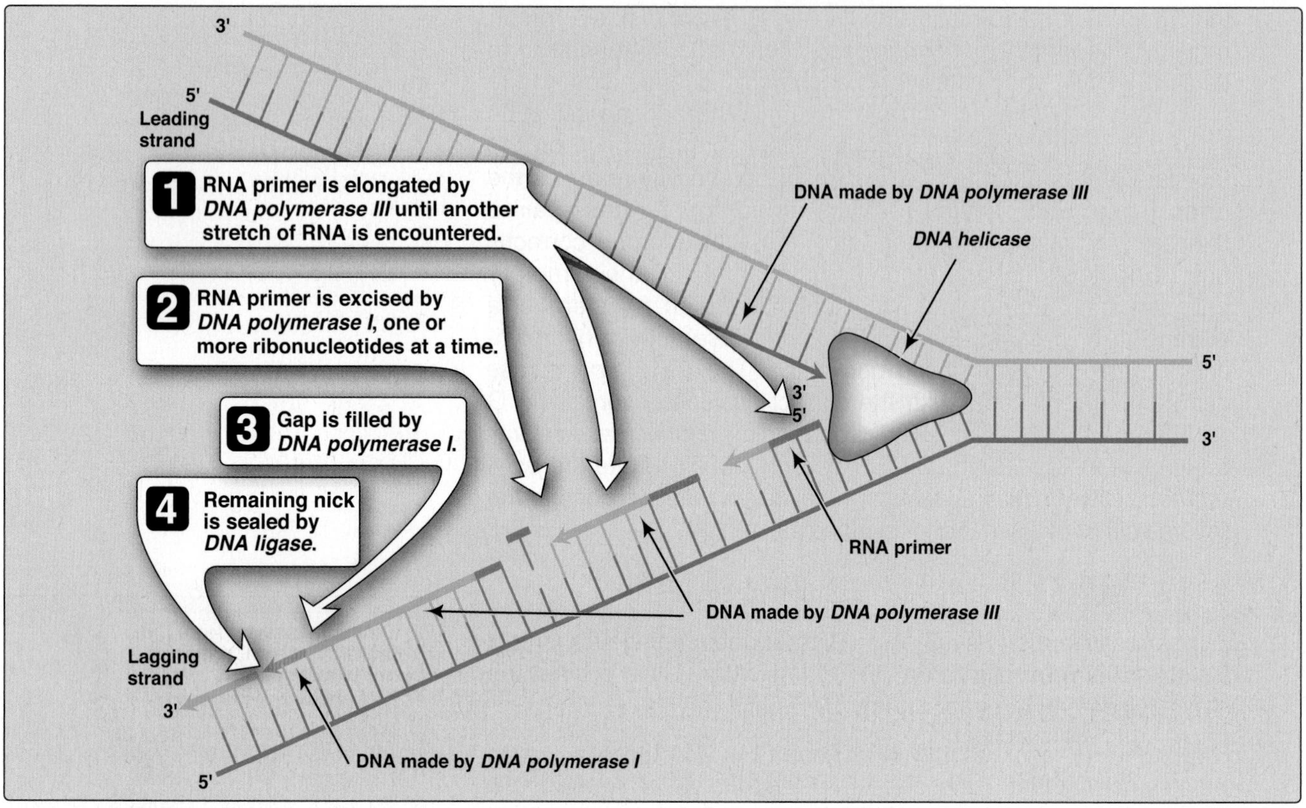

Figure 29.19
Removal of RNA primer and filling of the resulting "gaps" by *DNA polymerase I.*

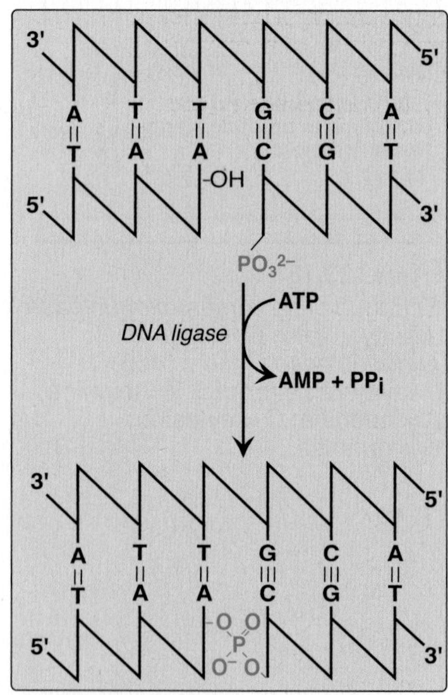

Figure 29.20
Formation of a phosphodiester bond by *DNA ligase.* [Note: AMP is first linked to *ligase,* then to the 5' phosphate, and then released.]

G. DNA ligase

The final phosphodiester linkage between the 5'-phosphate group on the DNA chain synthesized by *DNA pol III* and the 3'-hydroxyl group on the chain made by *DNA pol I* is catalyzed by *DNA ligase* (Figure 29.20). The joining of these two stretches of DNA requires energy, which in most organisms is provided by the cleavage of ATP to AMP + PP_i.

H. Termination

Replication termination in E. coli is mediated by sequence-specific binding of the protein, Tus (terminus utilization substance) to replication termination sites (ter sites) on the DNA, stopping the movement of *DNA polymerase.*

IV. EUKARYOTIC DNA REPLICATION

The process of eukaryotic DNA replication closely follows that of prokaryotic DNA synthesis. Some differences, such as the multiple origins of replication in eukaryotic cells versus single origins of replication in prokaryotes, have already been noted. Eukaryotic single-stranded DNA-binding proteins and ATP-dependent *DNA helicases* have been identified, whose functions are analogous to those of the prokaryotic enzymes previously discussed. In contrast, RNA primers are removed by *RNase H* and *flap endonuclease-1* (*FEN1*) rather than by a *DNA polymerase* (Figure 29.21).

A. Eukaryotic cell cycle

The events surrounding eukaryotic DNA replication and cell division (mitosis) are coordinated to produce the cell cycle (Figure 29.22). The period preceding replication is called the G_1 phase (Gap 1). DNA replication occurs during the S (synthesis) phase. Following DNA synthesis, there is another period (G_2 phase, or Gap 2) before mitosis (M). Cells that have stopped dividing, such as mature T lymphocytes, are said to have gone out of the cell cycle into the G_0 phase. Such quiescent cells can be stimulated to reenter the G_1 phase to resume division. [Note: The cell cycle is controlled at a series of "checkpoints" that prevent entry into the next phase of the cycle until the preceding phase has been completed. Two key classes of proteins that control the progress of a cell through the cell cycle are the cyclins and *cyclin-dependent kinases* (*Cdks*).]

FUNCTION	PROTEIN (s)
Origin recognition	ORC
Helicase activity	*MCM*
ssDNA protection	RPA
Primer synthesis	*Pol a/primase*
Sliding clamp	PCNA
Primer removal	*RNase H, FEN 1*

Figure 29.21
Proteins and their function in eukaryotic replication. ORC = origin recognition complex, MCM = minichromosome maintenance (complex), RPA = replication protein A, PCNA = proliferating cell nuclear antigen.

B. Eukaryotic DNA polymerases

At least five high-fidelity eukaryotic *DNA polymerases* (*pol*) have been identified and categorized on the basis of molecular weight, cellular location, sensitivity to inhibitors, and the templates or substrates on which they act. They are designated by Greek letters rather than by Roman numerals (Figure 29.23).

1. **Pol α:** *Pol* α is a multisubunit enzyme. One subunit has *primase* activity, which initiates strand synthesis on the leading strand and at the beginning of each Okazaki fragment on the lagging strand. The *primase* subunit synthesizes a short RNA primer that is extended by the *5'→3' polymerase* activity of *pol* α, generating a short piece of DNA. [Note: *Pol* α is also referred to as *pol* α/*primase.*]

2. **Pol ε and pol δ:** *Pol* ε is recruited to complete DNA synthesis on the leading strand, whereas *pol* δ elongates the Okazaki fragments of the lagging strand, each using *3'→5' exonuclease* activity to proofread the newly synthesized DNA. [Note: *DNA pol* ε associates with proliferating cell nuclear antigen (PCNA), a protein that serves as a sliding DNA clamp in much the same way the β subunit of *DNA pol III* does in E. coli, thus ensuring high processivity.]

3. **Pol β and pol γ:** *Pol* β is involved in "gap filling" in DNA repair (see below). *Pol* γ replicates mitochondrial DNA.

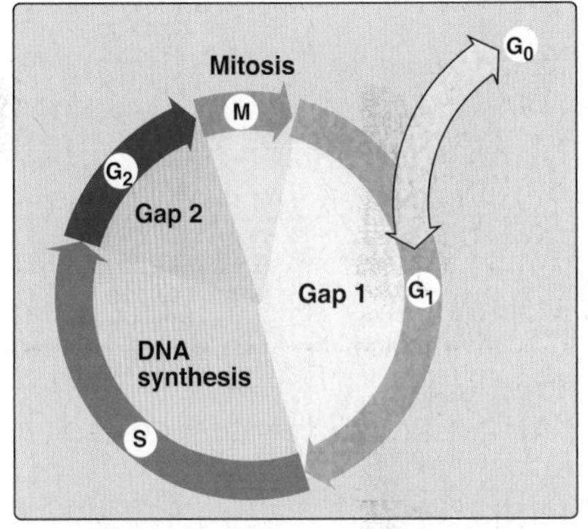

Figure 29.22
The eukaryotic cell cycle. [Note: Cells can leave the cell cycle and enter a reversible quiescent state called G_0.]

POLY-MERASE	FUNCTION	PROOF-READING*
Pol α (alpha)	• Contains primase • Initiates DNA synthesis	–
Pol β (beta)	• Repair	–
Pol γ (gamma)	• Replicates mitochondrial DNA	+
Pol δ (delta)	• Elongates Okazaki fragments of the lagging strand	+
Pol ε (epsilon)	• Elongates the leading strand	+

Figure 29.23
Activities of eukaryotic *DNA polymerase* (*pol*) **3'→5' exonuclease* activity.

C. Telomeres

Telomeres are complexes of noncoding DNA plus proteins (collectively known as shelterin) located at the ends of linear chromosomes. They maintain the structural integrity of the chromosome, preventing attack by *nucleases*, and allow repair systems to distinguish a true end from a break in dsDNA. In humans, telomeric DNA consists of several thousand tandem repeats of a noncoding hexameric sequence, AGGGTT, base-paired to a complementary region of Cs and As. The GT-rich strand is longer than its CA complement, leaving ssDNA a few hundred nucleotides in length at the 3'-end. The single-stranded region is thought to fold back on itself, forming a loop structure that is stabilized by protein.

1. **Telomere shortening:** Eukaryotic cells face a special problem in replicating the ends of their linear DNA molecules. Following

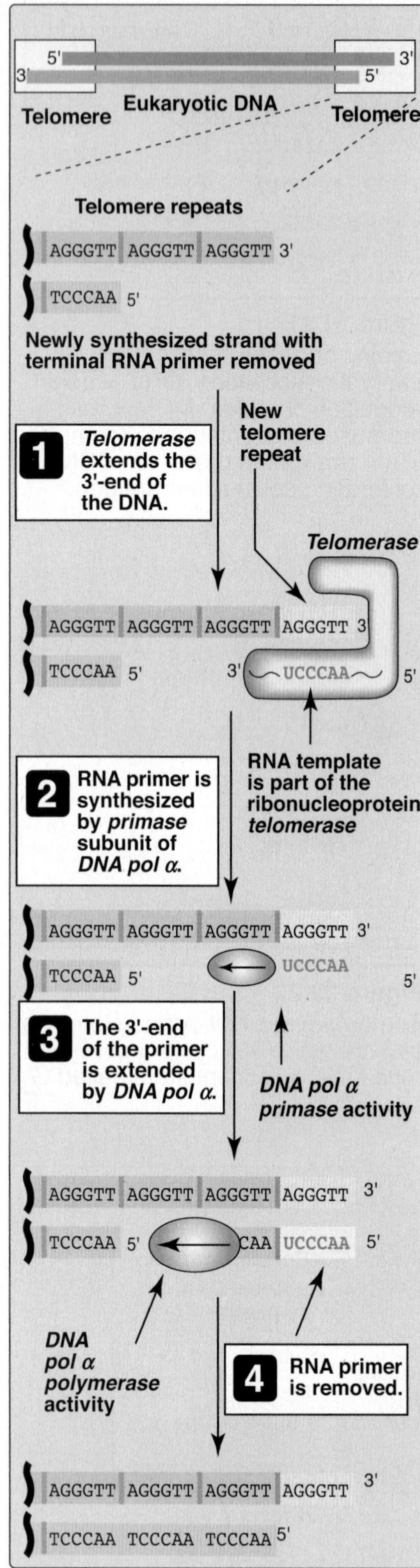

Figure 29.24
Mechanism of action of *telomerase.* T= thymine; A = adenine; C = cytosine; G = guanine; *pol* = *polymerase.*

removal of the RNA primer from the extreme 5'-end of the lagging strand, there is no way to fill in the remaining gap with DNA. Consequently, in most normal human somatic cells, telomeres shorten with each successive cell division. Once telomeres are shortened beyond some critical length, the cell is no longer able to divide and is said to be senescent. In germ cells and other stem cells, as well as in cancer cells, telomeres do not shorten and the cells do not senesce. This is a result of the presence of a ribonucleoprotein, *telomerase*, which maintains telomeric length in these cells.

2. **Telomerase:** This complex contains a protein (Tert) that acts as a *reverse transcriptase* and a short piece of RNA (Terc) that acts as a template. The CA-rich RNA template base-pairs with the GT-rich, single-stranded 3'-end of telomeric DNA (Figure 29.24). The *reverse transcriptase* uses the RNA template to synthesize DNA in the usual 5'$\rightarrow$3' direction, extending the already longer 3'-end. *Telomerase* then translocates to the newly synthesized end, and the process is repeated. Once the GT-rich strand has been lengthened, *primase* activity of *DNA pol* α can use it as a template to synthesize an RNA primer. The RNA primer is extended by *DNA pol* α, and then removed.

> Telomeres may be viewed as mitotic clocks in that their length in most cells is inversely related to the number of times the cells have divided. The study of telomeres provides insight into the biology of aging and cancer.

D. Reverse transcriptases

As seen with *telomerase, reverse transcriptases* are RNA-directed *DNA polymerases.* A *reverse transcriptase* is involved in the replication of retroviruses, such as human immunodeficiency virus (HIV). These viruses carry their genome in the form of ssRNA molecules. Following infection of a host cell, the viral enzyme *reverse transcriptase* uses the viral RNA as a template for the 5'$\rightarrow$3' synthesis of viral DNA, which then becomes integrated into host chromosomes. *Reverse transcriptase* activity is also seen with transposons, DNA elements that can move about the genome (see p. 461). In eukaryotes, such elements are transcribed to RNA, the RNA is used as a template for DNA synthesis by a *reverse transcriptase* encoded by the transposon, and the DNA is randomly inserted into the genome. [Note: Transposons that involve an RNA intermediate are called retrotransposons or retroposons.]

E. Inhibition of DNA synthesis by nucleoside analogs

DNA chain growth can be blocked by the incorporation of certain nucleoside analogs that have been modified on the sugar portion (Figure 29.25). For example, removal of the hydroxyl group from the 3'-carbon of the deoxyribose ring as in 2',3'-dideoxyinosine ([ddI] also known as didanosine), or conversion of the deoxyribose to another sugar, such as arabinose, prevents further chain elongation. By blocking DNA replication, these compounds slow the division of rapidly growing cells and viruses. Cytosine arabinoside (cytarabine, or araC) has been used in anticancer chemotherapy, whereas adenine arabinoside (vidarabine, or araA) is an antiviral agent. Substitution on the sugar moiety, as seen in zidovudine (AZT, ZDV), also terminates DNA chain elongation. [Note: These drugs are generally supplied as nucleosides, which are then converted to the active nucleotides by cellular *kinases*.

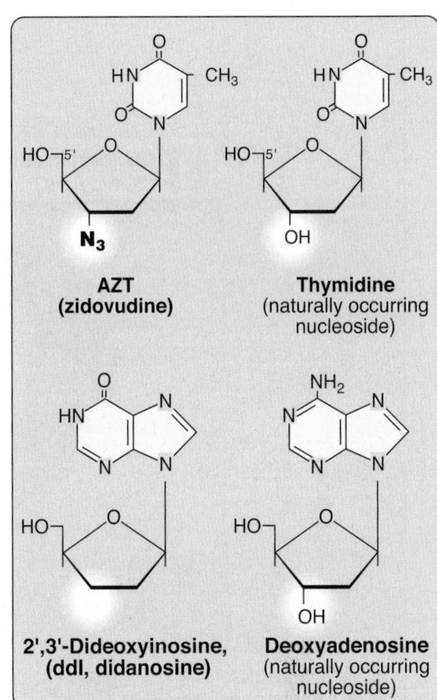

Figure 29.25
Examples of nucleoside analogs that lack a 3'-hydroxyl group. [Note: ddI is converted to its active form (ddATP).]

V. ORGANIZATION OF EUKARYOTIC DNA

A typical (diploid) human cell contains 46 chromosomes, whose total DNA is approximately 2 m long! It is difficult to imagine how such a large amount of genetic material can be effectively packaged into a volume the size of a cell nucleus so that it can be efficiently replicated, and its genetic information expressed. To do so requires the interaction of DNA with a large number of proteins, each of which performs a specific function in the ordered packaging of these long molecules of DNA. Eukaryotic DNA is associated with tightly bound basic proteins, called histones. These serve to order the DNA into fundamental structural units, called nucleosomes, which resemble beads on a string. Nucleosomes are further arranged into increasingly more complex structures that organize and condense the long DNA molecules into chromosomes that can be segregated during cell division. [Note: The complex of DNA and protein found inside the nuclei of eukaryotic cells is called chromatin.]

A. Histones and the formation of nucleosomes

There are five classes of histones, designated H1, H2A, H2B, H3, and H4. These small, evolutionally conserved proteins are positively charged at physiologic pH as a result of their high content of lysine and arginine. Because of their positive charge, they form ionic bonds with negatively charged DNA. Histones, along with ions such as Mg^{2+}, help neutralize the negatively charged DNA phosphate groups.

1. **Nucleosomes:** Two molecules each of H2A, H2B, H3, and H4 form the octameric core of the individual nucleosome "beads." Around this structural core, a segment of dsDNA is wound nearly twice, causing supercoiling (Figure 29.26). [Note: The N-terminal ends of these histones can be acetylated, methylated, or phosphorylated. These reversible covalent modifications influence how tightly the histones bind to the DNA, thereby affecting the expression of specific genes (see p. 422). Histone modification is an example of "epigenetics" or heritable changes in gene expression without alteration of the nucleotide sequence.] Neighboring nucleosomes are joined by "linker" DNA approximately 50 base pairs long. H1, of which there are several related species, is not found in the nucleosome core, but instead binds to the linker DNA chain between the nucleosome beads. H1 is the most tissue specific and species specific of the histones. It facilitates the packing of nucleosomes into more compact structures.

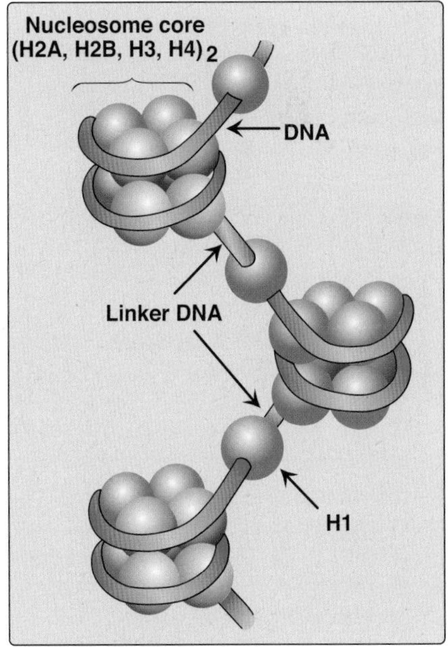

Figure 29.26
Organization of human DNA, illustrating the structure of nucleosomes. H = histone.

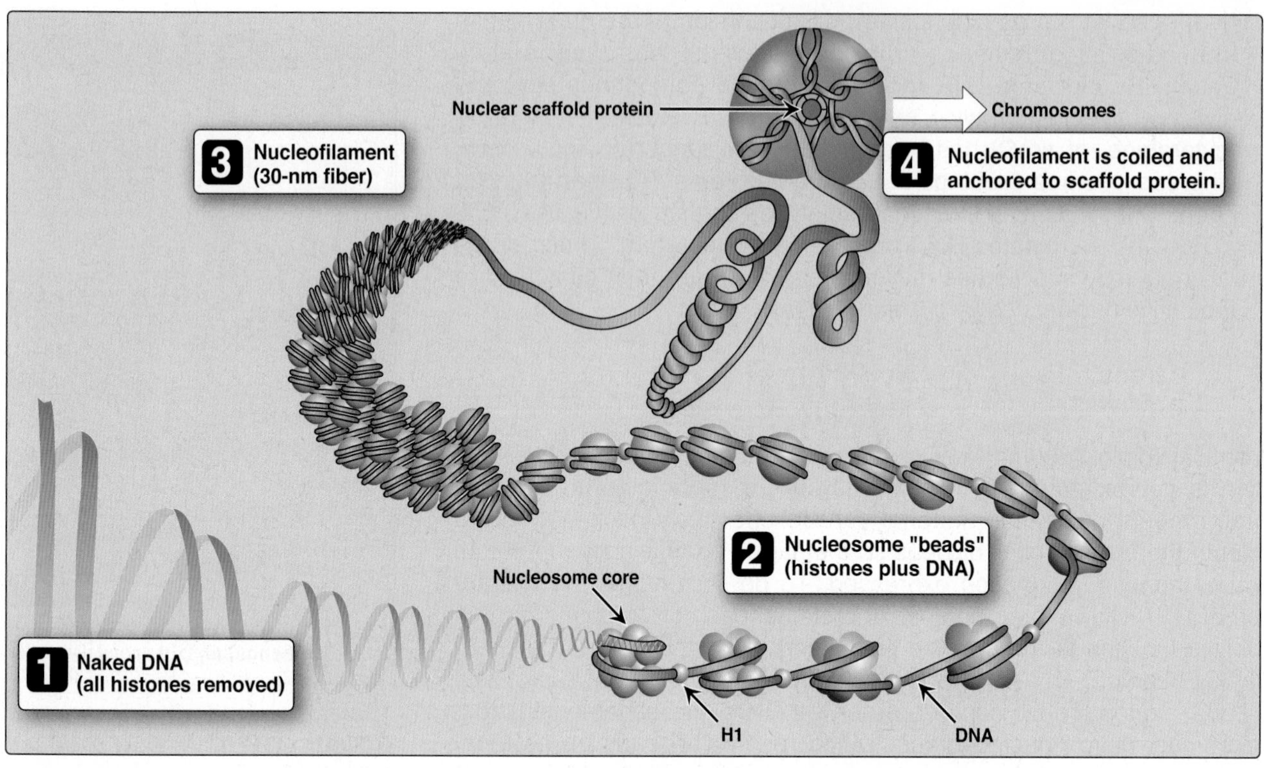

Figure 29.27
Structural organization of eukaryotic DNA. [Note: A 10^4 compaction is seen from 1 to 4.] H = histone.

2. **Higher levels of organization:** Nucleosomes can be packed more tightly to form a polynucleosome (also called a nucleofilament). This structure assumes the shape of a coil, often referred to as a 30-nm fiber. The fiber is organized into loops that are anchored by a nuclear scaffold containing several proteins. Additional levels of organization lead to the final chromosomal structure (Figure 29.27).

B. Fate of nucleosomes during DNA replication

Parental nucleosomes are disassembled to allow access to DNA during replication. Once DNA is synthesized, nucleosomes form rapidly. Their histone proteins come both from new synthesis and from the transfer of intact parental histone octamers.

VI. DNA REPAIR

Despite the elaborate proofreading system employed during DNA synthesis, errors (including incorrect base-pairing or insertion of one to a few extra nucleotides) can occur. In addition, DNA is constantly being subjected to environmental insults that cause the alteration or removal of nucleotide bases. The damaging agents can be either chemicals (for example, nitrous acid, which can deaminate bases), or radiation (for example, non-ionizing ultraviolet light, which can fuse two pyrimidines adjacent to each other in the DNA, and high-energy ionizing radiation, which can cause double-strand breaks). Bases are also altered or lost spontaneously from mammalian DNA at a rate of many thousands per cell per day. If the damage is not repaired, a permanent change (mutation) is introduced that can result in any of a number of deleterious effects, including loss of control over the proliferation of the mutated cell, leading to cancer. Luckily, cells are remarkably efficient at repairing damage done to their DNA. Most of the repair systems involve recognition of the damage (lesion) on the DNA, removal or excision of the damage, replacement or filling the gap left by excision using the sister strand as a template for DNA synthesis, and ligation. These excision repair systems remove one to tens of nucleotides. [Note: Repair synthesis of DNA can occur outside of the S phase.]

A. Repair of mismatched bases (mismatch repair)

Sometimes replication errors escape the proofreading function during DNA synthesis, causing a mismatch of one to several bases. In E. coli, mismatch repair (MMR) is mediated by a group of proteins known as the Mut proteins (Figure 29.28). Homologous proteins are present in humans. [Note: MMR reduces the error rate of replication from one in ten million to one in a billion.]

1. **Identification of the mismatched strand:** When a mismatch occurs, the Mut proteins that identify the mispaired nucleotide(s) must be able to discriminate between the correct strand and the strand with the mismatch. Discrimination is based on the degree of methylation. GATC sequences, which are found approximately once every thousand nucleotides, are methylated on the adenine (A) residue. This methylation is not done immediately after synthesis, so the newly synthesized DNA is hemimethylated (that is, the parental strand is methylated, but the daughter strand is not). The methylated parental strand is assumed to be correct, and it is the daughter strand that gets repaired. [Note: The exact mechanism by which the daughter strand is identified in eukaryotes is not yet known.]

2. **Repair of damaged DNA:** When the strand containing the mismatch is identified, an *endonuclease* nicks the strand, and the mismatched nucleotide(s) is/are removed by an *exonuclease*. Additional nucleotides at the 5'- and 3'-ends of the mismatch are also removed. The gap left by removal of the nucleotides is filled, using the sister strand as a template, by a *DNA polymerase*, typically *DNA pol I*. The 3'-hydroxyl of the newly synthesized DNA is joined to the 5'-phosphate of the remaining stretch of the original DNA strand by *DNA ligase* (see p. 406).

> Mutation to the proteins involved in mismatch repair in humans is associated with hereditary nonpolyposis colorectal cancer (HNPCC), also known as Lynch syndrome. With HNPCC, there is an increased risk for developing colon cancer (as well as other cancers); however, only about 5% of all colon cancer is the result of mutations in mismatch repair.

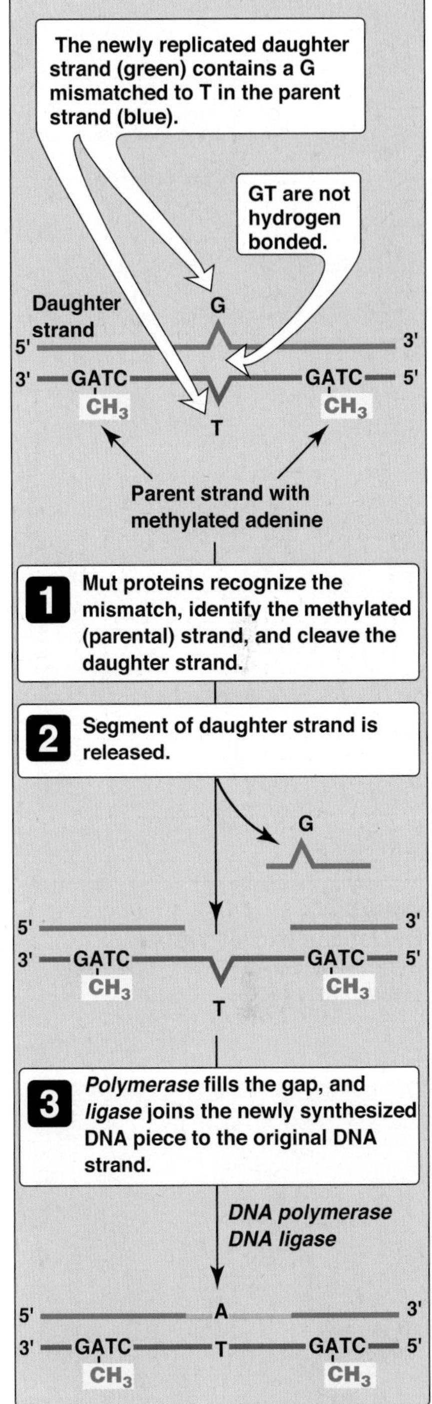

Figure 29.28
Methyl-directed mismatch repair in E. coli. [Note: The Mut proteins, S and L, recognize the mismatch and identify the parental (methylated) strand, and Mut H cleaves the daughter strand.] A = adenine; C= cytosine; G = guanine; T = thymine.

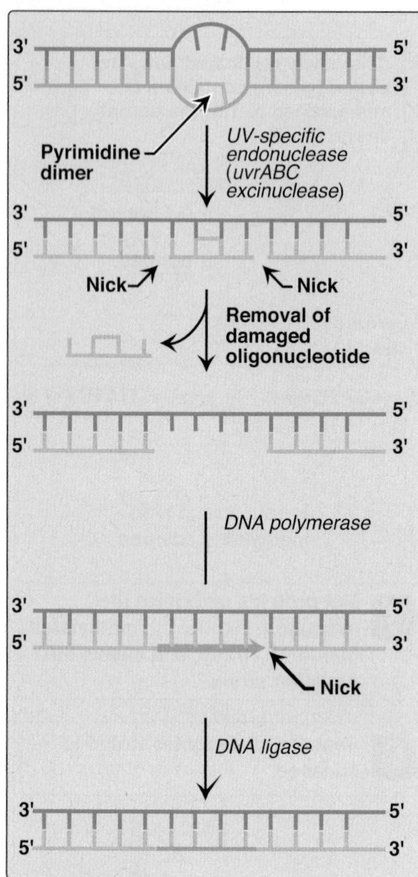

Figure 29.29
Nucleotide excision repair of pyrimidine dimers in E. coli DNA. UV = ultraviolet.

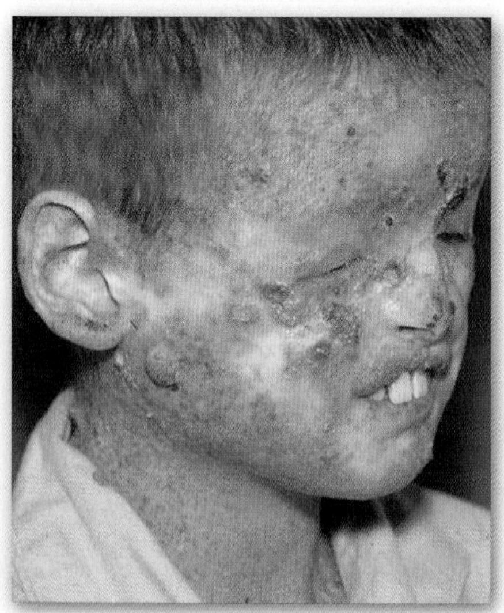

Figure 29.30
Patient with xeroderma pigmentosum.

B. Repair of damage caused by ultraviolet light (nucleotide excision repair)

Exposure of a cell to ultrtaviolet (UV) light can result in the covalent joining of two adjacent pyrimidines (usually thymines), producing a dimer. These thymine dimers prevent *DNA pol* from replicating the DNA strand beyond the site of dimer formation. Thymine dimers are excised in bacteria by UvrABC proteins in a process known as nucleotide excision repair (NER) as illustrated in Figure 29.29. A related pathway is present in humans (see below).

1. **Recognition and excision of dimers by UV-specific endonuclease:** First, a *UV-specific endonuclease* (called *uvrABC excinuclease*) recognizes the dimer and cleaves the damaged strand on both the 5'-side and 3'-side of the dimer. A short oligonucleotide containing the dimer is released, leaving a gap in the DNA strand that formerly contained the dimer. This gap is filled in using a *DNA polymerase* and *DNA ligase.*

2. **UV radiation and cancer:** Pyrimidine dimers can be formed in the skin cells of humans exposed to unfiltered sunlight. In the rare genetic disease xeroderma pigmentosum (XP), the cells cannot repair the damaged DNA, resulting in extensive accumulation of mutations and, consequently, early and numerous skin cancers (Figure 29.30). XP can be caused by defects in any of the several genes that code for the XP proteins required for nucleotide excision repair of UV damage in humans.

C. Repair of base alterations (base excision repair)

The bases of DNA can be altered, either spontaneously, as is the case with cytosine, which slowly undergoes deamination (the loss of its amino group) to form uracil, or by the action of deaminating or alkylating compounds. For example, nitrous acid, which is formed by the cell from precursors such as the nitrosamines, nitrites, and nitrates, is a potent compound that deaminates cytosine, adenine (to hypoxanthine), and guanine (to xanthine). Bases can also be lost spontaneously. For example, approximately 10,000 purine bases are lost this way per cell per day. Lesions involving base alterations or loss can be corrected by base excision repair ([BER] Figure 29.31).

1. **Removal of abnormal bases:** In BER, abnormal bases, such as uracil, which can occur in DNA either by deamination of cytosine or improper use of dUTP instead of dTTP during DNA synthesis, are recognized by specific *glycosylases* that hydrolytically cleave them from the deoxyribose–phosphate backbone of the strand. This leaves an apyrimidinic site (or apurinic, if a purine was removed), both referred to as AP sites.

2. **Recognition and repair of an AP site:** Specific *AP-endonucleases* recognize that a base is missing and initiate the process of excision and gap-filling by making an endonucleolytic cut just to the 5'-side of the AP site. A *deoxyribose phosphate lyase* removes the single, base-free, sugar phosphate residue. *DNA polymerase* and *DNA ligase* complete the repair process.

D. Repair of double-strand breaks

Ionizing radiation or oxidative free radicals (see p. 148) can cause double-strand breaks in DNA that are potentially lethal to the cell. Such breaks also occur naturally during gene rearrangements. dsDNA breaks cannot be corrected by the previously described strategy of excising the damage on one strand and using the remaining strand as a template for replacing the missing nucleotide(s). Instead, they are repaired by one of two systems. The first is nonhomologous end-joining (NHEJ), in which a group of proteins mediates the recognition, processing, and ligation of the ends of two DNA fragments. However, some DNA is lost in the process. Consequently, this mechanism of repair is error prone and mutagenic. Defects in this repair system are associated with a predisposition to cancer and immunodeficiency syndromes. The second repair system, homologous recombination (HR), uses the enzymes that normally perform genetic recombination between homologous chromosomes during meiosis. This system is much less error prone than NHEJ because any DNA that was lost is replaced using homologous DNA as a template. [Note: Mutations to the proteins, BRCA1 or 2 (breast cancer 1 or 2), which are involved in HR, increase the risk for developing breast cancer.]

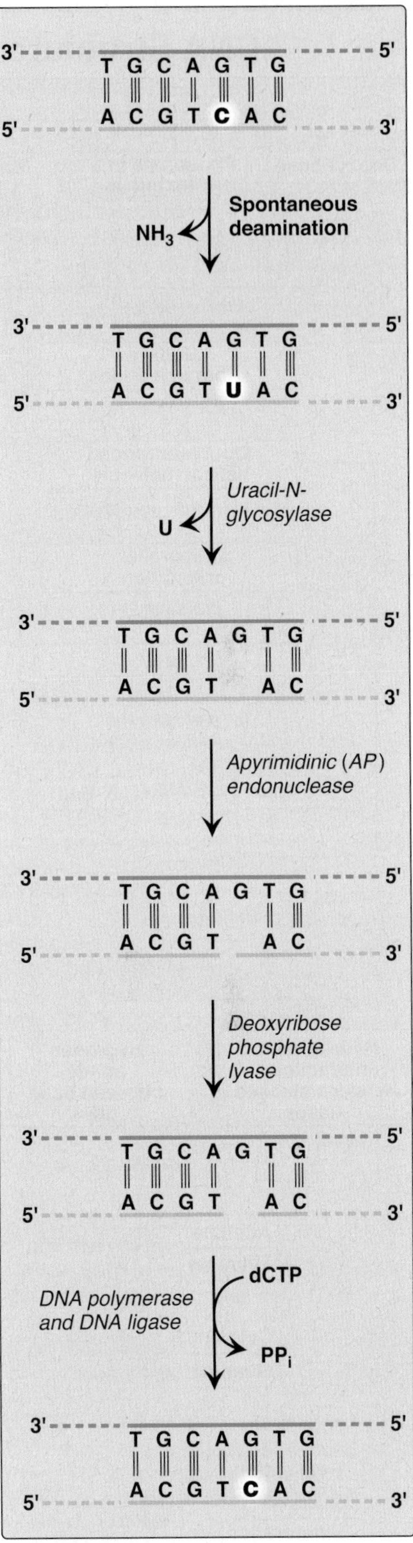

Figure 29.31
Correction of base alterations by base excision repair. T= thymine; A = adenine; C = cytosine; G = guanine; PP_i = pyrophosphate.

VII. CHAPTER SUMMARY

DNA is a polymer of deoxyribonucleoside monophosphates covalently linked by **3'→5'-phosphodiester bonds** (Figure 29.32). The resulting long, unbranched chain has **polarity**, with both a 5'-end and a 3'-end. The sequence of nucleotides is read 5'→3'. DNA exists as a **double-stranded** molecule, in which the two chains are paired in an **antiparallel** manner, and wind around each other, forming a **double helix**. **Adenine** pairs with **thymine**, and **cytosine** pairs with **guanine**. Each strand of the double helix serves as a **template** for constructing a **complementary** daughter strand (**semiconservative replication**). DNA replication occurs in the **S phase** of the cell cycle and begins at the **origin of replication**. As the two strands unwind and separate, synthesis occurs at two replication forks that move away from the origin in opposite directions (bidirectionally). ***Helicase*** unwinds the double helix. As the two strands of the double helix are separated, **positive supercoils** are produced in the region of DNA ahead of the replication fork and negative supercoils behind the fork. **DNA *topoisomerases* types I and II** remove supercoils. ***DNA polymerases* (*pol*)** synthesize **n**ew DNA strands only in the **5'→3'** direction. Therefore, one of the newly synthesized stretches of nucleotide chains must grow in the 5'→3' direction toward the replication fork (**leading strand**) and one in the 5'→3' direction away from the replication fork (**lagging strand**). *DNA pols* require a **primer**. The primer for de novo DNA synthesis is a short stretch of RNA synthesized by ***primase***. The leading strand only needs one RNA primer, whereas the lagging strand needs many. In E. coli, DNA chain elongation is catalyzed by ***DNA pol III***, using **5'-deoxyribonucleoside triphosphates** as substrates. The enzyme **"proofreads"** the newly

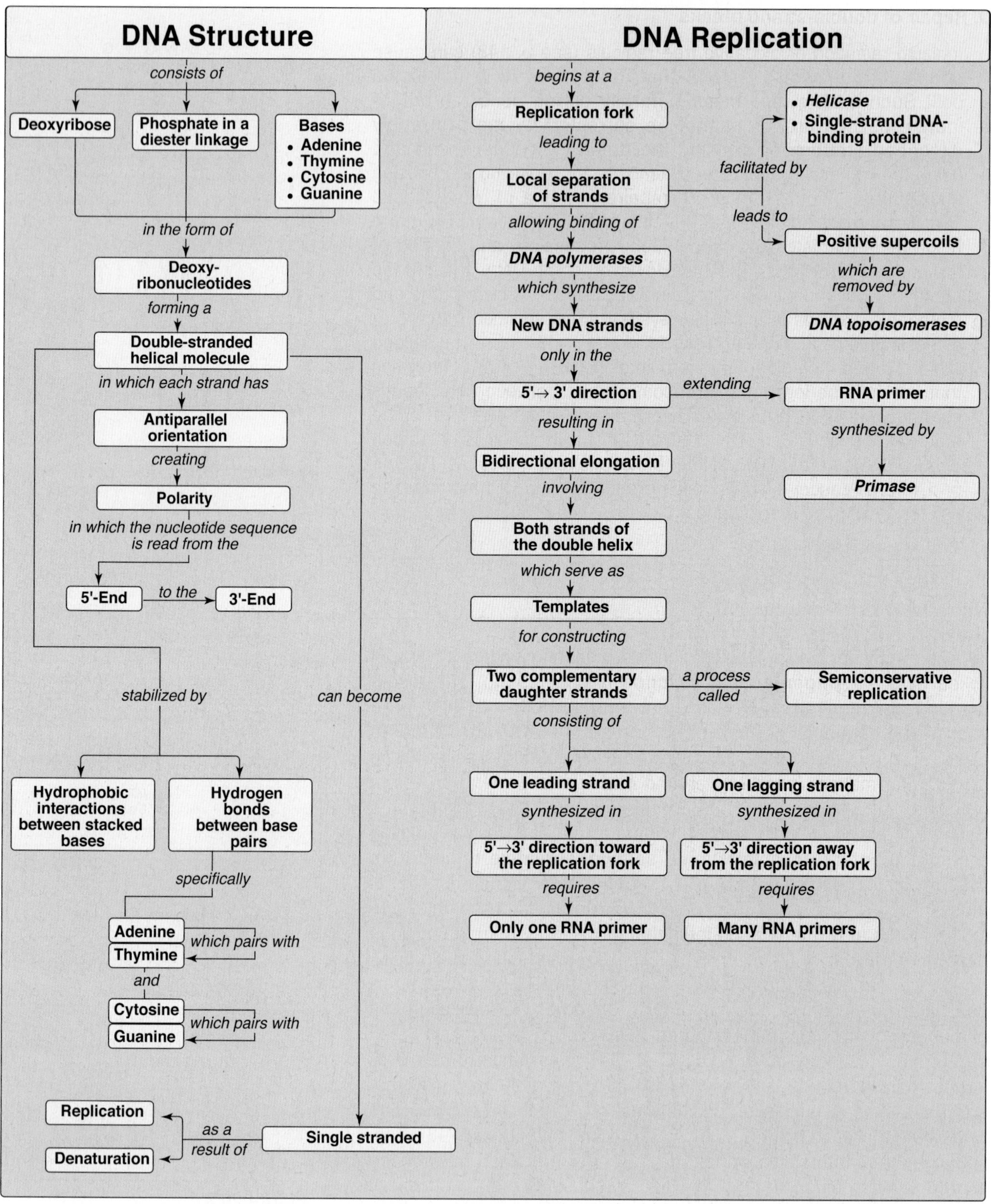

Figure 29.32 (continued on next page)
Key concept map for DNA structure, replication, and repair.

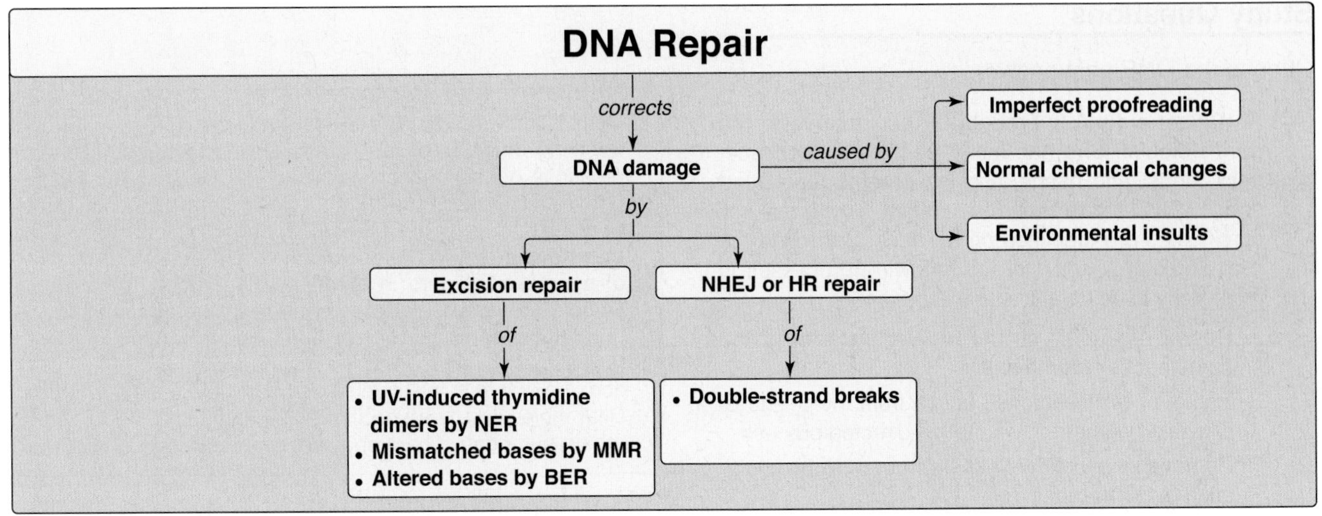

Figure 29.32 (continued from previous page)
Key concept map for DNA structure, replication, and repair. NHEJ = nonhomologous end-joining; HR = homologous recombination; NER = nucleotide excision repair; MMR = mismatch repair; BER = base excision repair; UV = ultraviolet light.

synthesized DNA, removing terminal mismatched nucleotides with its ***3'→5' exonuclease*** activity. RNA primers are removed by ***DNA pol I***, using its ***5'→3' exonuclease*** activity. This enzyme fills the gaps with DNA, proofreading as it synthesizes. The final phosphodiester linkage is catalyzed by ***DNA ligase***. There are at least five high-fidelity **eukaryotic *DNA polymerases***. ***Pol α*** is a multisubunit enzyme, one subunit of which is a ***primase***. *Pol α 5'→3' polymerase* activity adds a short piece of DNA to the RNA primer. ***Pol ε*** completes DNA synthesis on the leading strand, whereas ***pol δ*** elongates each lagging strand fragment. ***Pol β*** is involved with DNA repair, and ***pol γ*** replicates mitochondrial DNA. *Pols ε, δ,* and *γ* use *3'→5' exonuclease* activity to proofread. **Nucleoside analogs** containing modified sugars can be used to block DNA chain growth. They are useful in anticancer and antiviral chemotherapy. **Telomeres** are stretches of **highly repetitive DNA** complexed with protein that protect the **ends** of linear chromosomes. As most cells divide and age, these sequences are shortened, contributing to senescence. In cells that do not senesce (for example, germline and cancer cells), **telomerase** employs its enzyme component ***reverse transcriptase*** to extend the telomeres, using its **RNA** as a **template**. There are five classes of **positively charged histone** (**H**) **proteins**. Two each of histones H2A, H2B, H3, and H4 form an octameric structural core around which DNA is wrapped creating a **nucleosome**. The DNA connecting the nucleosomes, called **linker DNA**, is bound to H1. Nucleosomes can be packed more tightly to form a nucleofilament. Additional levels of organization create a chromosome. Most DNA damage can be corrected by **excision repair** involving recognition and removal of the damage by repair proteins, followed by replacement in E. coli by *DNA pol* and joining by *ligase*. **Ultraviolet light** can cause thymine dimers that are recognized and removed by **uvrABC proteins of nucleotide excision repair.** Defects in the **XP proteins** needed for thymine dimer repair in humans result in **xeroderma pigmentosum**. **Mismatched** bases are repaired by a similar process of recognition and removal by **Mut proteins** in E. coli. The extent of **methylation** is used for strand identification in prokaryotes. Defective mismatch repair by homologous proteins in humans is associated with **hereditary nonpolyposis colorectal cancer**. Abnormal bases (such as uracil) are removed by ***glycosylases*** in **base excision repair**, and the sugar phosphate at the apyrimidinic or apurinic (AP) site is cut out. Double-strand breaks in DNA are repaired by **nonhomologous end-joining** (error prone) and **homologous recombination**.

Study Questions

Choose the ONE best answer.

29.1 A 10-year-old girl is brought by her parents to the dermatologist. She has many freckles on her face, neck, arms, and hands, and the parents report that she is unusually sensitive to sunlight. Two basal cell carcinomas are identified on her face. Based on the clinical picture, which of the following processes is most likely to be defective in this patient?

A. Repair of double-strand breaks by error-prone homologous recombination
B. Removal of mismatched bases from the 3'-end of Okazaki fragments by a methyl-directed process
C. Removal of pyrimidine dimers from DNA by nucleotide excision repair
D. Removal of uracil from DNA by base excision repair

Correct answer = C. The sensitivity to sunlight, extensive freckling on parts of the body exposed to the sun, and presence of skin cancer at a young age indicate that the patient most likely suffers from xeroderma pigmentosum (XP). These patients are deficient in any one of several XP proteins required for nucleotide excision repair of pyrimidine dimers in ultraviolet light–damaged DNA. Double-strand breaks are repaired by nonhomologous end-joining (error prone) or homologous recombination (error free). Methylation is not used for strand discrimination in eukaryotic mismatch repair. Uracil is removed from DNA molecules by a specific glycosylase in base excision repair, but a defect here does not cause XP.

29.2 Telomeres are complexes of DNA and protein that protect the ends of linear chromosomes. In most normal human somatic cells, telomeres shorten with each division. In stem cells and in cancer cells, however, telomeric length is maintained. In the synthesis of telomeres:

A. telomerase, a ribonucleoprotein, provides both the RNA and the protein needed for synthesis.
B. the RNA of telomerase serves as a primer.
C. the RNA of telomerase is a ribozyme.
D. the protein of telomerase is a DNA-directed DNA polymerase.
E. the shorter 3'→5' strand gets extended.
F. the direction of synthesis is 3'→5'.

Correct answer = A. Telomerase is a ribonucleoprotein particle required for telomere maintenance. Telomerase contains an RNA that serves as the template, not the primer, for the synthesis of telomeric DNA by the reverse transcriptase of telomerase. Telomeric RNA has no catalytic activity. As a reverse transcriptase, telomerase synthesizes DNA using its RNA template and so is an RNA-directed DNA polymerase. The direction of synthesis, as with all DNA synthesis, is 5'→3', and it is the 3'-end of the already longer 5'→3' strand that gets extended.

29.3 While studying the structure of a small gene that was sequenced during the Human Genome Project, an investigator notices that one strand of the DNA molecule contains 20 As, 25 Gs, 30 Cs, and 22 Ts. How many of each base is found in the complete double-stranded molecule?

A. A = 40, G = 50, C = 60, T = 44
B. A = 44, G = 60, C = 50, T = 40
C. A = 45, G = 45, C = 52, T = 52
D. A = 50, G = 47, C = 50, T = 47
E. A = 42, G = 55, C = 55, T = 42

Correct answer = E. The two DNA strands are complementary to each other, with A base-paired with T and G base-paired with C. So, for example, the 20 As on the first strand would be paired with 20 Ts on the second strand, the 25 Gs on the first strand would be paired with 25 Cs on the second strand, and so forth. When these are all added together, the correct numbers of each base are indicated in choice E. Notice that, in the correct answer, A = T and G = C.

29.4 List the order in which the following enzymes participate in prokaryotic replication.

A. Ligase
B. Polymerase I (3'→5' exonuclease activity)
C. Polymerase I (5'→3' exonuclease activity)
D. Polymerase I (5'→3' polymerase activity)
E. Polymerase III
F. Primase

Correct answer: F, E, C, D, B, A. Primase makes the RNA primer; Polymerase III extends the primer with DNA (and proofreads); polymerase I removes the primer with its 5'→3' exonuclease activity, fills in the gap with its 5'→3' polymerase activity, and removes errors with its 3'→5' exonuclease activity; and ligase makes the 5'→3' phosphodiester bond that links the DNA made by polymerase I and polymerase III.

29.5 Dideoxynucleotides lack a 3'-hydroxyl group. Why would incorporation of a dideoxynucleotide into DNA stop replication?

The lack of the 3'-OH group prevents formation of the 3'-hydroxyl → 5'-phosphate bond that links one nucleotide to the next in DNA.

RNA Structure, Synthesis, and Processing

30

I. OVERVIEW

The genetic master plan of an organism is contained in the sequence of deoxyribonucleotides in its deoxyribonucleic acid (DNA). However, it is through the ribonucleic acid (RNA), the "working copies" of the DNA, that the master plan is expressed (Figure 30.1). The copying process, during which a DNA strand serves as a template for the synthesis of RNA, is called transcription. Transcription produces messenger RNAs (mRNAs) that are translated into sequences of amino acids (polypeptide chains or proteins) and ribosomal RNAs (rRNAs), transfer RNAs (tRNAs), and additional small RNA molecules that perform specialized structural, catalytic, and regulatory functions and are not translated. That is, they are noncoding RNAs (ncRNAs). [Note: Only about 2% of the genome codes for proteins.] The final product of gene expression, therefore, can be RNA or protein, depending upon the gene. A central feature of transcription is that it is highly selective. For example, many transcripts are made of some regions of the DNA. In other regions, few or no transcripts are made. This selectivity is due, at least in part, to signals embedded in the nucleotide sequence of the DNA. These signals instruct the *RNA polymerase* where to start, how often to start, and where to stop transcription. A variety of regulatory proteins is also involved in this selection process. The biochemical differentiation of an organism's tissues is ultimately a result of the selectivity of the transcription process. [Note: This selectivity of transcription is in contrast to the "all-or-none" nature of genomic replication.] Another important feature of transcription is that many RNA transcripts that initially are faithful copies of one of the two DNA strands may undergo various modifications, such as terminal additions, base modifications, trimming, and internal segment removal, which convert the inactive primary transcript into a functional molecule.

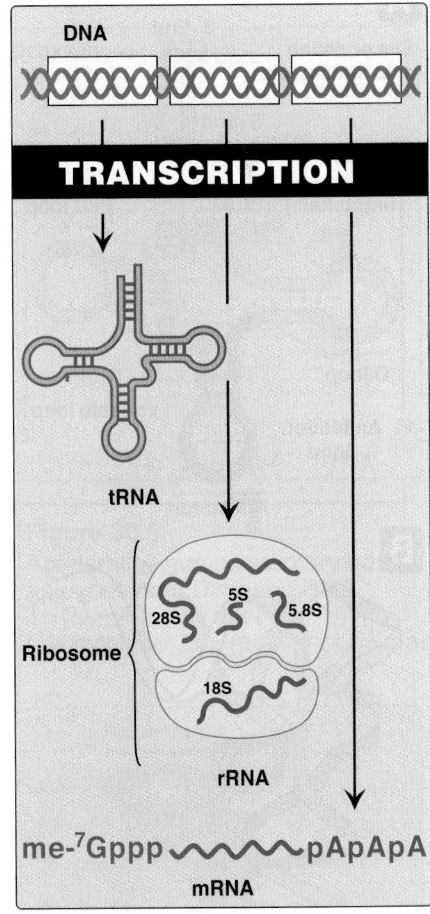

Figure 30.1
Expression of genetic information by transcription. [Note: RNAs shown are eukaryotic.] tRNA = transfer RNA; rRNA = ribosomal RNA; mRNA = messenger RNA; me-^{7}Gppp = 7-methylguanosine triphosphate "cap;" AAA = poly-A "tail," each described on p. 418.

II. STRUCTURE OF RNA

There are three major types of RNA that participate in the process of protein synthesis: rRNA, tRNA, and mRNA. Like DNA, these three types of RNA are unbranched polymeric molecules composed of nucleoside monophosphates joined together by 3'→5'-phosphodiester bonds (see

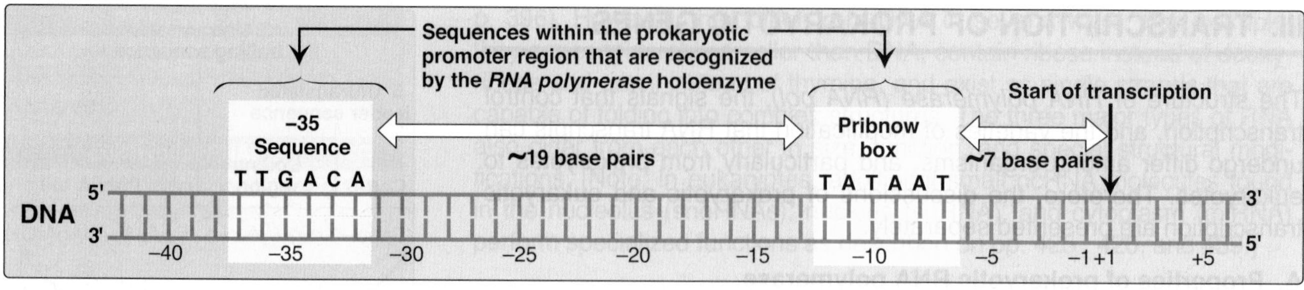

Figure 30.7
Structure of the prokaryotic promoter region. T = thymine; G = guanine; A = adenine; C = cytosine.

at each position is the base most frequently (but not necessarily always) encountered at that position.] Those that are recognized by prokaryotic *RNA polymerase* σ factors include:

a. –35 Sequence: A consensus sequence (5'-TTGACA-3'), centered about 35 bases to the left of the transcription start site (see Figure 30.7), is the initial point of contact for the holoenzyme, and a closed complex is formed. [Note: The regulatory sequences that control transcription are, by convention, designated by the 5'→3' nucleotide sequence on the coding strand. A base in the promoter region is assigned a negative number if it occurs prior to (to the left of, toward the 5'-end of, or "upstream" of) the transcription start site. Therefore, the TTGACA sequence is centered at approximately base –35. The first base at the transcription start site is assigned a position of +1. There is no base designated "0".]

b. Pribnow box: The holoenzyme moves and covers a second consensus sequence (5'-TATAAT-3'), centered at about –10 (see Figure 30.7), which is the site of initial DNA melting (unwinding). Melting of a short stretch (about 14 bases) converts the closed complex to an open complex known as a transcription bubble. [Note: A mutation in either the –10 or the –35 sequence can affect the transcription of the gene controlled by the mutant promoter.]

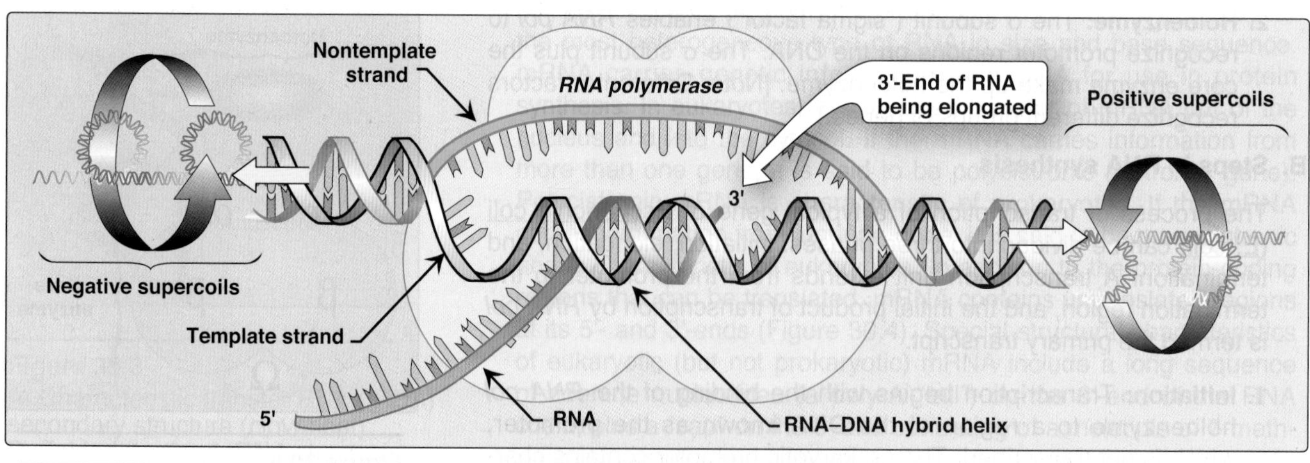

Figure 30.8
Local unwinding of DNA caused by *RNA polymerase* and formation of an open initiation complex.

2. **Elongation:** Once the promoter region has been recognized and bound by the holoenzyme, local unwinding of the DNA helix continues (Figure 30.8), mediated by the *polymerase*. [Note: Unwinding generates supercoils in the DNA that can be relieved by *DNA topoisomerases* (see p. 401.] *RNA pol* begins to synthesize a transcript of the DNA sequence, and several short pieces of RNA are made and discarded. The elongation phase is said to begin when the transcript (typically starting with a purine) exceeds ten nucleotides in length. Sigma is then released, and the core enzyme is able to leave ("clear") the promoter and move along the template strand in a processive manner, serving as its own sliding clamp. During transcription, a short DNA–RNA hybrid helix is formed (see Figure 30.8). Like *DNA pol*, *RNA pol* uses nucleoside triphosphates as substrates and releases pyrophosphate each time a nucleoside monophosphate is added to the growing chain. As with replication, transcription is always in the 5'→3' direction. In contrast to *DNA pol*, *RNA pol* does not require a primer and does not appear to have *3'→5' exonuclease* (proofreading) activity.

3. **Termination:** The elongation of the single-stranded RNA chain continues until a termination signal is reached. Termination can be intrinsic (spontaneous) or dependent upon the participation of a protein known as the ρ (rho) factor.

   a. **ρ-Independent termination**: Seen with most prokaryotic genes, this requires that a sequence in the DNA template generates a sequence in the nascent (newly made) RNA that is self-complementary (Figure 30.9). This allows the RNA to fold back on itself, forming a GC-rich stem (stabilized by hydrogen bonds) plus a loop. This structure is known as a "hairpin." Additionally, just beyond the hairpin, the RNA transcript contains a string of Us at the 3'-end. The bonding of these Us to the complementary As of the DNA template is weak. This facilitates the separation of the newly synthesized RNA from its DNA template, as the double helix "zips up" behind the *RNA polymerase*.

   b. **ρ-Dependent termination:** This requires the participation of an additional protein, rho (ρ), which is a hexameric *ATPase* with *helicase* activity. Rho binds a C-rich "rho recognition site" near the 5'-end of the nascent RNA and, using its *ATPase* activity, moves along the RNA until it reaches the *RNA pol* paused at the termination site. The *ATP-dependent helicase* activity of ρ separates the RNA–DNA hybrid helix, causing the release of the RNA.

4. **Action of antibiotics:** Some antibiotics prevent bacterial cell growth by inhibiting RNA synthesis. For example, rifampin (rifampicin) inhibits transcription by binding to the β subunit of prokaryotic *RNA pol*, and preventing chain extension beyond three nucleotides (Figure 30.10). Rifampin is important in the treatment of tuberculosis. Dactinomycin (known to biochemists as actinomycin D) was the first antibiotic to find therapeutic application in tumor chemotherapy. It binds to the DNA template and interferes with the movement of *RNA pol* along the DNA.

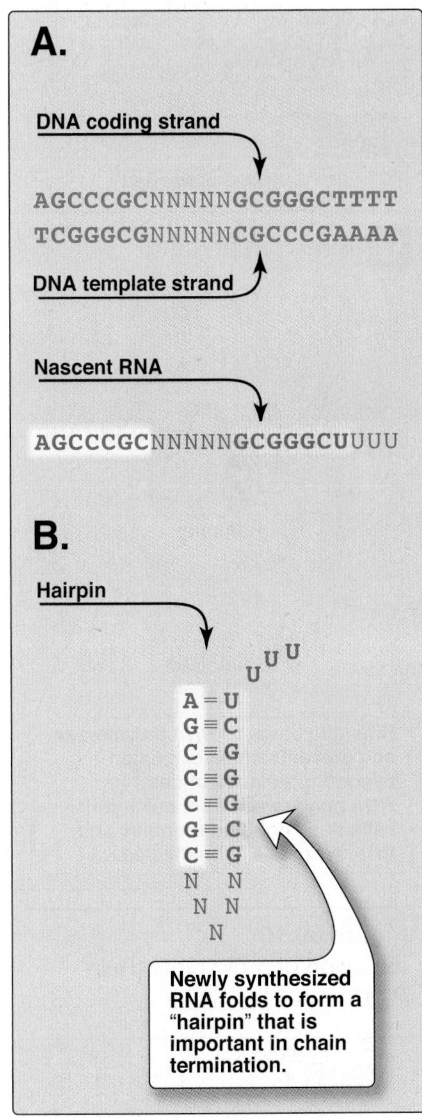

Figure 30.9
Rho-independent termination of prokaryotic transcription. A. DNA template sequence generates a self-complementary sequence in the nascent RNA. B. Hairpin structure formed by the RNA. "N" represents a noncomplementary base; A = adenine, T = thymine; G = guanine; C = cytosine; U = uracil. [Note: Termination of eukaryotic transcription is not well understood.]

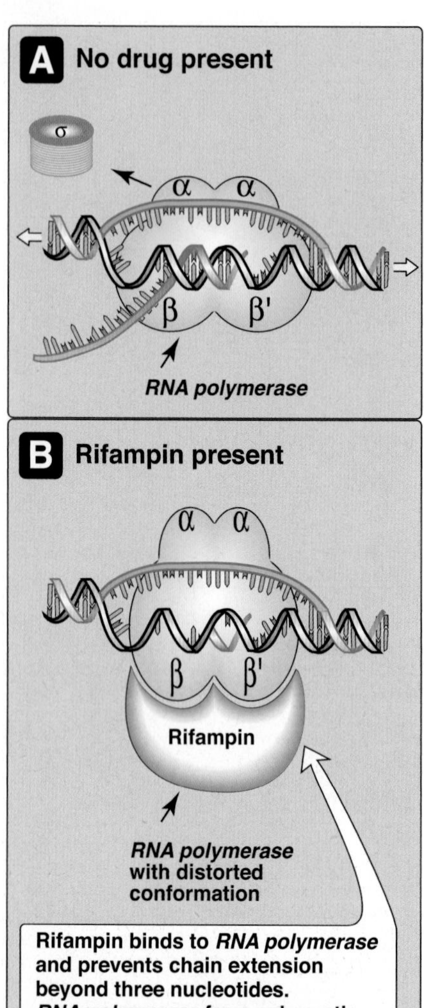

Figure 30.10
Inhibition of prokaryotic *RNA polymerase* by rifampin.

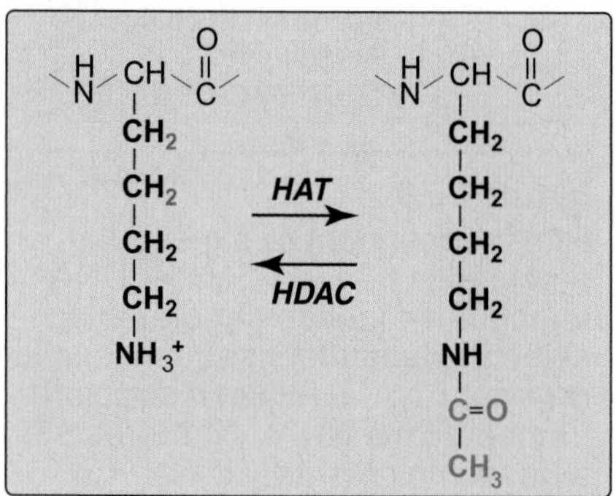

Figure 30.11
Acetylation/deacetylation of a lysine residue in a histone protein. *HAT* = *histone acetyltransferase*; *HDAC* = *histone deacetylase.*

IV. TRANSCRIPTION OF EUKARYOTIC GENES

The transcription of eukaryotic genes is a far more complicated process than transcription in prokaryotes. Eukaryotic transcription involves separate *polymerases* for the synthesis of rRNA, tRNA, and mRNA. In addition, a large number of proteins called transcription factors (TFs) are involved. TFs bind to distinct sites on the DNA either within the core promoter region, close (proximal) to it, or some distance away (distal). They are required both for the assembly of a transcription complex at the promoter and the determination of which genes are to be transcribed. [Note: Each eukaryotic *RNA pol* has its own promoters and TFs that bind core promoter sequences.] For TFs to recognize and bind to their specific DNA sequences, the chromatin structure in that region must be altered (relaxed) to allow access to the DNA. The role of transcription in the regulation of gene expression is discussed in Chapter 32.

A. Chromatin structure and gene expression

The association of DNA with histones to form nucleosomes (see p. 409) affects the ability of the transcription machinery to access the DNA to be transcribed. Most actively transcribed genes are found in a relatively relaxed form of chromatin called euchromatin, whereas most inactive segments of DNA are found in highly condensed heterochromatin. [Note: The interconversion of these forms is called chromatin remodeling.] A major component of chromatin remodeling is the covalent modification of histones (for example, the acetylation of lysine residues at the amino terminus of histone proteins) as shown in Figure 30.11. Acetylation, mediated by *histone acetyltransferases* (*HATs*), eliminates the positive charge on the lysine, thereby decreasing the interaction of the histone with the negatively charged DNA. Removal of the acetyl group by *histone deacetylases* (*HDACs*) restores the positive charge and fosters stronger interactions between histones and DNA. [Note: The ATP-dependent repositioning of nucleosomes is also required to access DNA.]

B. Nuclear RNA polymerases of eukaryotic cells

There are three distinct classes of *RNA pol* in the nucleus of eukaryotic cells. All are large enzymes with multiple subunits. Each class of *RNA pol* recognizes particular types of genes.

1. **RNA polymerase I:** This enzyme synthesizes the precursor of the 28S, 18S, and 5.8S rRNA in the nucleolus.

2. **RNA polymerase II:** This enzyme synthesizes the nuclear precursors of mRNA that are subsequently translated to produce proteins. *RNA pol II* also synthesizes certain small ncRNAs, such as snoRNA (see p. 425), snRNA (see p. 426) and miRNA (see p. 459).

   a. **Promoters for RNA polymerase II:** In some genes transcribed by *RNA pol II*, a sequence of nucleotides (TATAAA) that is nearly identical to that of the Pribnow box (see p. 420) is found centered about 25 nucleotides upstream of the transcription start site. This core promoter consensus sequence is called the TATA, or Hogness, box. In the majority of genes, however, no TATA box is present. Instead, different core promoter elements

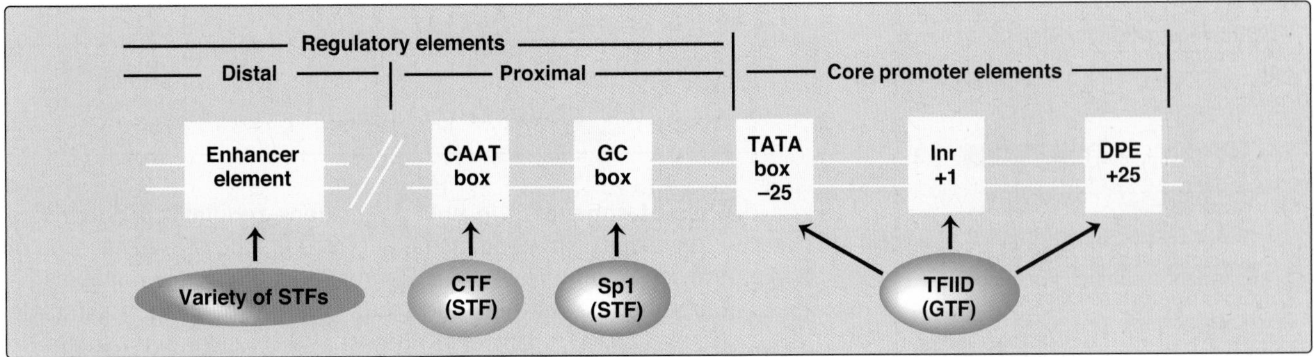

Figure 30.12
Eukaryotic gene cis-acting promoter and regulatory elements and their trans-acting general and specific transcription factors (GTF and STF, respectively). Inr = initiator; DPE = downstream promoter element.

such as Inr (initiator) or DPE (downstream promoter element) are present (Figure 30.12). [Note: No one consensus sequence is found in all core promoters.] Because these sequences are on the same molecule of DNA as the gene being transcribed, they are cis-acting. The sequences serve as binding sites for proteins known as general transcription factors (GTFs), which in turn interact with each other and with *RNA pol II*.

b. **General transcription factors:** These are the minimal requirements for recognition of the promoter, recruitment of *RNA pol II* to the promoter, and initiation of transcription at a basal level (Figure 30.13A). GTFs are encoded by different genes, synthesized in the cytosol, and transit to their sites of action, and so are trans-acting. [Note: In contrast to the prokaryotic holoenzyme, eukaryotic *RNA pol II* does not itself recognize and bind the promoter. Instead, TFIID, a GTF containing TATA-binding protein and TATA-associated factors, recognizes and binds the TATA box (and other core promoter elements). TFIIF, another GTF, brings the *polymerase* to the promoter. The *helicase* activity of TFIIH melts the DNA, and its *kinase* activity phosphorylates *polymerase*, allowing it to clear the promoter.]

c. **Regulatory elements and transcriptional activators:** Upstream of the core promoter are additional consensus sequences (see Figure 30.12). Those close to the core promoter (within 200 nucleotides) are the proximal regulatory elements, such as the CAAT and GC boxes. Those farther away are the distal regulatory elements such as enhancers (see p. 424). Proteins known as transcriptional activators or specific transcription factors (STFs) bind these regulatory elements. STFs bind to promoter proximal elements to regulate the frequency of transcription initiation, and to distal elements to mediate the response to signals such as hormones (see p. 456) and regulate which genes are expressed at a given point in time. A typical protein-coding eukaryotic gene has binding sites for many such factors. [Note: STFs have two binding domains. One is a DNA-binding domain, the other is a transcription activation domain that recruits the GTFs to the core promoter as well as "coactivator" proteins such as the *HAT* enzymes involved in chromatin modification.]

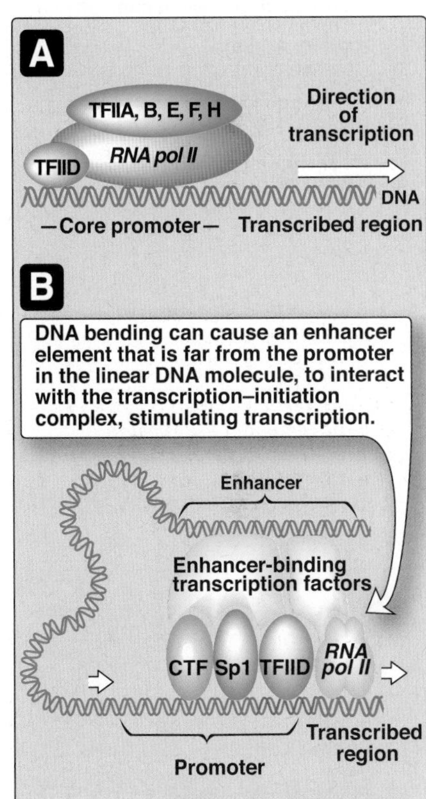

Figure 30.13
A. Association of the general transcription factors (TFIIs) and *RNA polymerase II (RNA pol II)* at the core promoters. [Note: The Roman numeral II denotes the TFs for *RNA pol II*.] B. Enhancer stimulation of transcription. CTF = CAAT box transcription factor; Sp1 = specificity factor-1.

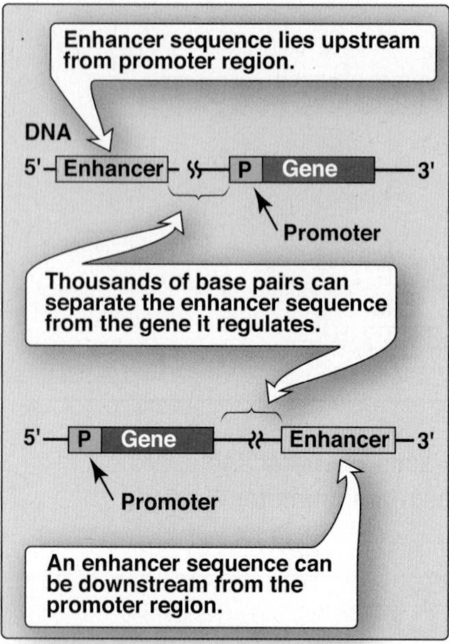

Figure 30.14
Some possible locations of enhancer sequences.

> Transcriptional activators bind DNA through a variety of motifs, such as the helix-loop-helix, zinc finger, and leucine zipper (see p. 18).

d. **Role of enhancers in eukaryotic gene regulation:** Enhancers are special DNA sequences that increase the rate of initiation of transcription by *RNA pol II*. Enhancers are typically on the same chromosome as the gene whose transcription they stimulate (Figure 30.13B). However, they can 1) be located upstream (to the 5'-side) or downstream (to the 3'-side) of the transcription start site, 2) be close to or thousands of base pairs away from the promoter (Figure 30.14), and 3) occur on either strand of the DNA. Enhancers contain DNA sequences called "response elements" that bind STFs (transcriptional activators). By bending or looping the DNA, these enhancer-binding proteins can interact with other transcription factors bound to a promoter and with *RNA pol II*, thereby stimulating transcription (see Figure 30.13B). [Note: Although silencers are similar to enhancers in that they also can act over long distances, they reduce gene expression.]

e. **Inhibitors of RNA polymerase II:** α-Amanitin, a potent toxin produced by the poisonous mushroom Amanita phalloides (sometimes called "the death cap"), forms a tight complex with *RNA pol II*, thereby inhibiting mRNA synthesis.

3. **RNA polymerase III:** This enzyme synthesizes tRNA, 5S rRNA, and some snRNA and snoRNA.

C. Mitochondrial RNA polymerase

Mitochondria contain a single *RNA pol* that more closely resembles bacterial *RNA pol* than the eukaryotic nuclear enzymes.

V. POSTTRANSCRIPTIONAL MODIFICATION OF RNA

A primary transcript is the initial, linear, RNA copy of a transcription unit (the segment of DNA between specific initiation and termination sequences). The primary transcripts of both prokaryotic and eukaryotic tRNA and rRNA are posttranscriptionally modified by cleavage of the original transcripts by *ribonucleases*. tRNAs are then further modified to help give each species its unique identity. In contrast, prokaryotic mRNA is generally identical to its primary transcript, whereas eukaryotic mRNA is extensively modified both co- and posttranscriptionally.

A. Ribosomal RNA

rRNAs of both prokaryotic and eukaryotic cells are generated from long precursor molecules called pre-rRNAs. The 23S, 16S, and 5S rRNA of prokaryotes are produced from a single pre-rRNA molecule, as are the 28S, 18S, and 5.8S rRNA of eukaryotes (Figure 30.15). [Note: Eukaryotic 5S rRNA is synthesized by *RNA pol III* and modified separately.] The pre-rRNAs are cleaved by *ribonucleases* to yield intermediate-sized pieces of rRNA, which are further processed (trimmed by *exonucleases* and modified at some bases and riboses)

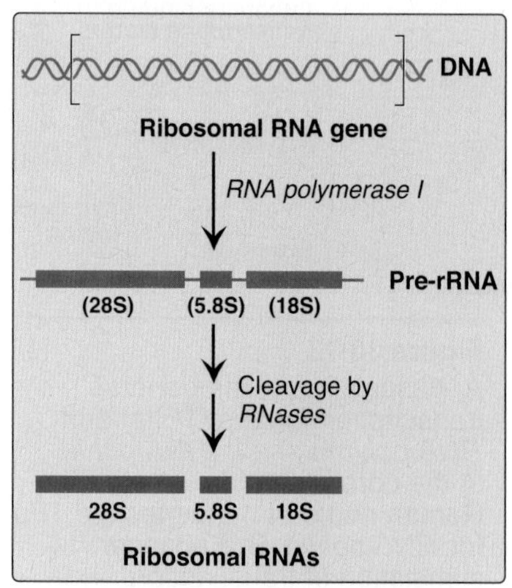

Figure 30.15
Posttranscriptional processing of eukaryotic ribosomal RNA by *ribonucleases* (*RNases*).
S = Svedberg unit.

to produce the required RNA species. [Note: In eukaryotes, rRNA genes are found in long, tandem arrays. rRNA synthesis and processing occur in the nucleolus, with base and sugar modifications facilitated by snoRNA. Some of the proteins destined to become components of the ribosome associate with pre-rRNA prior to and during its modification.]

B. Transfer RNA

Both eukaryotic and prokaryotic tRNAs are also made from longer precursor molecules that must be modified (Figure 30.16). Sequences at both ends of the molecule are removed, and, if present, an intron is removed from the anticodon loop by *nucleases*. Other posttranscriptional modifications include addition of a –CCA sequence by *nucleotidyltransferase* to the 3'-terminal end of tRNA, and modification of bases at specific positions to produce the "unusual bases" characteristic of tRNA (see p. 292).

C. Eukaryotic mRNA

The collection of all the primary transcripts synthesized in the nucleus by *RNA pol II* is known as heterogeneous nuclear RNA (hnRNA). The pre-mRNA components of hnRNA undergo extensive co- and posttranscriptional modification in the nucleus. These modifications usually include the following.

1. **5' "Capping":** This is the first of the processing reactions for pre-mRNA (Figure 30.17). The cap is a 7-methylguanosine attached to the 5'-terminal end of the mRNA through an unusual 5'→5' triphosphate linkage that is resistant to most nucleases. Creation of the cap requires removal of the γ phosphoryl group from the 5'-triphosphate of the pre-mRNA, followed by addition of guanosine

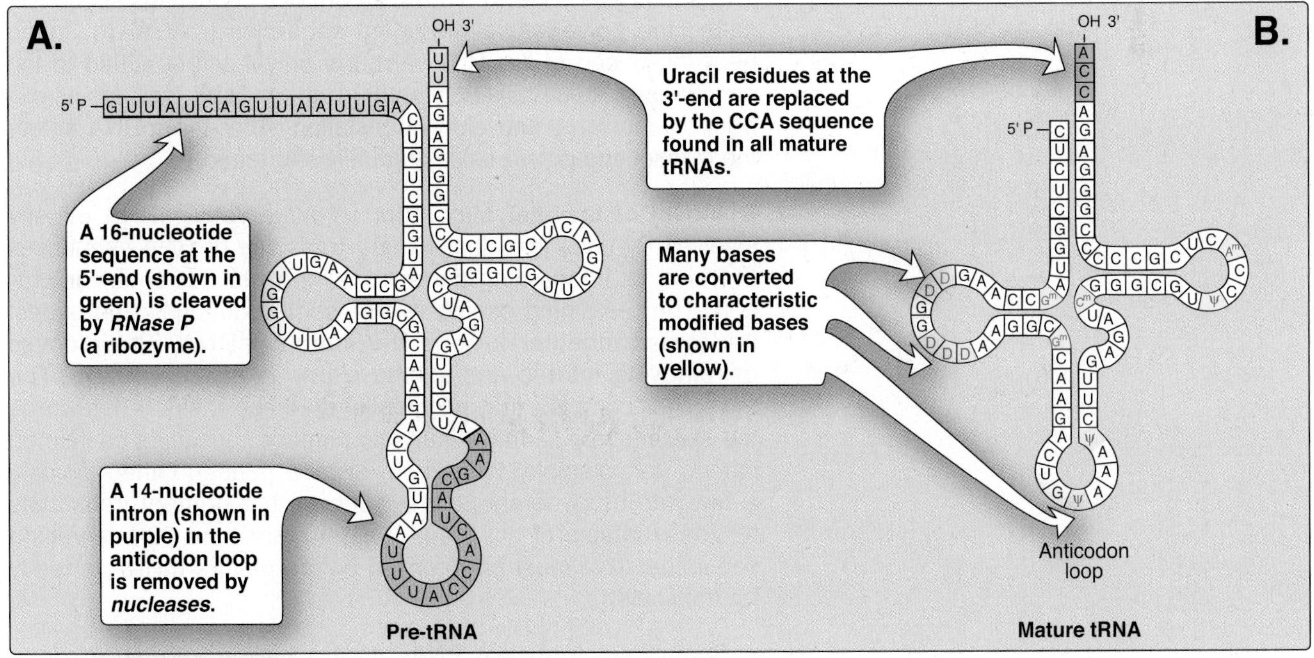

Figure 30.16
A. Primary transfer RNA (tRNA) transcript. B. Functional tRNA after posttranscriptional modification. Modified bases include D (dihydrouracil); ψ (pseudouracil); and ^{m}, which means that the base has been methylated.

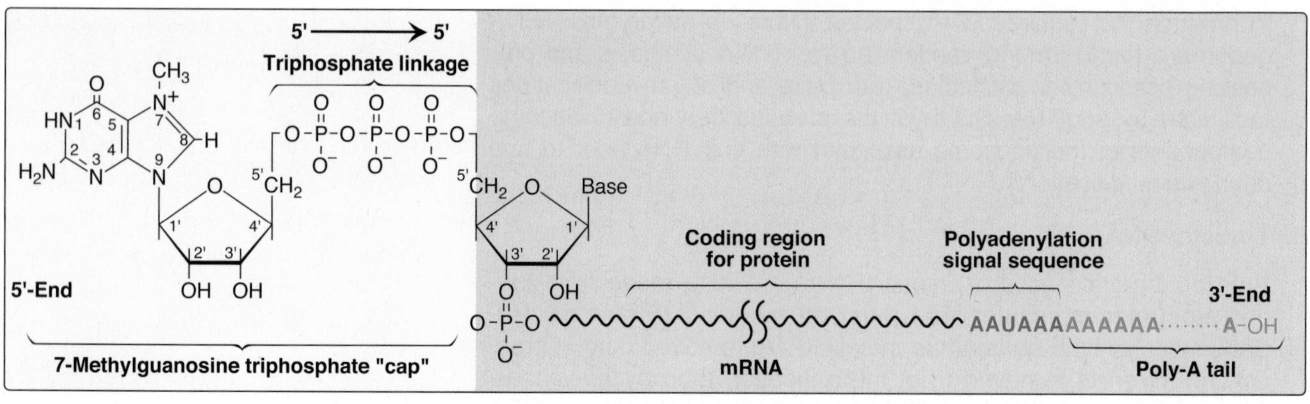

Figure 30.17
Posttranscriptional modification of messenger RNA (mRNA) showing the 7-methylguanosine cap and poly-A tail.

monophosphate (GMP) (from GTP) by the nuclear enzyme *guanylyltransferase*. Methylation of this terminal guanine occurs in the cytosol and is catalyzed by *guanine-7-methyltransferase*. S-adenosylmethionine is the source of the methyl group (see p. 263). Additional methylation steps may occur. The addition of this 7-methylguanosine cap helps stabilize the mRNA and permits efficient initiation of translation (see p. 439).

2. **Addition of a poly-A tail:** Most eukaryotic mRNA (with several notable exceptions, including those coding for the histones) have a chain of 40–250 adenine nucleotides attached to the 3'-end (see Figure 30.17). This poly-A tail is not transcribed from the DNA, but rather is added after transcription by the nuclear enzyme, *polyadenylate polymerase*, using ATP as the substrate. The pre-mRNA is cleaved downstream of a consensus sequence, called the polyadenylation signal sequence (AAUAAA), found near the 3'-end of the RNA, and the poly-A tail is added to the new 3'-end. These tails help stabilize the mRNA, facilitate its exit from the nucleus, and aid in translation. After the mRNA enters the cytosol, the poly-A tail is gradually shortened.

3. **Removal of introns:** Maturation of eukaryotic mRNA usually involves removal from the primary transcript of RNA sequences (introns, or intervening sequences) that do not code for protein. The remaining coding (expressed) sequences, the exons, are joined together to form the mature mRNA. The process of removing introns and joining exons is called splicing. The molecular complex that accomplishes these tasks is known as the spliceosome. A few eukaryotic primary transcripts contain no introns (for example, those from histone genes). Others contain a few introns, whereas some, such as the primary transcripts for the α chains of collagen, contain more than 50 intervening sequences that must be removed before mature mRNA is ready for translation.

   a. **Role of small nuclear RNAs:** In association with multiple proteins, uracil-rich snRNAs form small nuclear ribonucleoprotein particles (snRNPs, or "snurps," designated as U1, U2, U4, U5, and U6) that mediate splicing. They facilitate the removal of introns by forming base pairs with the consensus sequences at each end of the intron (Figure 30.18). [Note: In systemic lupus erythematosus, an autoimmune disease, patients produce antibodies against their own nuclear proteins such as snRNPs.]

b. **Mechanism of splicing:** The binding of snRNPs brings the sequences of the neighboring exons into the correct alignment for splicing, allowing two transesterification reactions to occur. The 2'-OH group of an adenine nucleotide (known as the branch site A) in the intron attacks the phosphate at the 5'-end of the intron (splice donor site), forming an unusual 2'→5' phosphodiester bond and creating a "lariat" structure (see Figure 30.18). The newly freed 3'-OH of exon 1 attacks the 5'-phosphate at the splice acceptor site, forming a phosphodiester bond that joins exons 1 and 2. The excised intron is released as a lariat, which is typically degraded. [Note: The GU and AG sequences at the beginning and end, respectively, of introns are invariant.] After introns have been removed and exons joined, the mature mRNA molecules leave the nucleus and pass into the cytosol through pores in the nuclear membrane. [Note: The introns in tRNA (see Figure 30.16) are removed by a different mechanism.]

c. **Effect of splice site mutations:** Mutations at splice sites can lead to improper splicing and the production of aberrant proteins. It is estimated that over 15% of all genetic diseases are a result of mutations that affect RNA splicing. For example, mutations that cause the incorrect splicing of β-globin mRNA are responsible for some cases of β-thalassemia, a disease in which the production of the β-globin protein is defective (see p. 38). Splice site mutations can result in exons being skipped (removed) or introns retained. They can also activate cryptic splice sites, which are sites that contain the 5' or 3' consensus sequence but aren't normally used.

4. **Alternative splicing of mRNA molecules:** The pre-mRNA molecules from over 50% of human genes can be spliced in alternative ways in different tissues. This produces multiple variations of the mRNA and, therefore, of its protein product (Figure 30.19), and thus is a mechanism for producing a large, diverse set of proteins from a limited set of genes. For example, in eukaryotic cells, the mRNA for tropomyosin, an actin filament–binding protein of the cytoskeleton (and of the contractile apparatus in muscle cells), undergoes extensive tissue-specific alternative splicing with production of multiple isoforms of the tropomyosin protein.

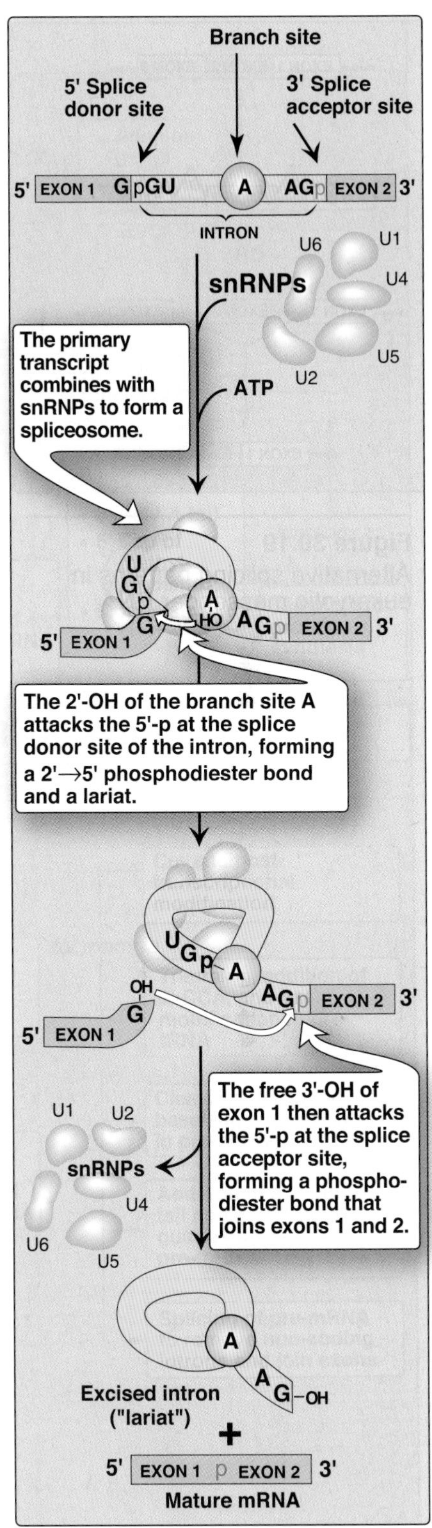

Figure 30.18
Splicing. snRNP = small nuclear ribonucleoprotein particle; mRNA = messenger RNA. [Note: U1 binds the 5' donor site, U2 binds the branch A, and addition of U4–U6 completes the complex.]

VI. CHAPTER SUMMARY

There are three major types of RNA that participate in the process of protein synthesis: **ribosomal RNA (rRNA)**, **transfer RNA (tRNA)**, and **messenger RNA (mRNA)** (Figure 30.20). They are unbranched polymers of nucleotides but differ from DNA by containing **ribose** instead of deoxyribose and **uracil** instead of thymine. **rRNA** is a component of the **ribosomes**. **tRNA** serves as an "adaptor" molecule that carries a

Study Questions

Choose the ONE correct answer.

30.1 An 8-month-old male with severe anemia is found to have β-thalassemia. Genetic analysis shows that one of his β-globin genes has a mutation that creates a new splice acceptor site 19 nucleotides upstream of the normal splice acceptor site of the first intron. Which of the following best describes the new messenger RNA molecule that can be produced from this mutant gene?

A. Exon 1 will be too short.
B. Exon 1 will be too long.
C. Exon 2 will be too short.
D. Exon 2 will be too long.
E. Exon 2 will be missing.

Correct answer = D. Because the mutation creates an additional splice acceptor site (the 3'-end) upstream of the normal acceptor site of intron 1, the 19 nucleotides that are usually found at the 3'-end of the excised intron 1 lariat can remain behind as part of exon 2. Exon 2 can, therefore, have these extra 19 nucleotides at its 5'-end. The presence of these extra nucleotides in the coding region of the mutant messenger RNA (mRNA) molecule will prevent the ribosome from translating the message into a normal β-globin protein molecule. Those mRNAs for which the normal splice site is used to remove the first intron will be normal, and their translation will produce normal β-globin protein.

30.2 A 4-year-old child who easily tires and has trouble walking is diagnosed with Duchenne muscular dystrophy, an X-linked recessive disorder. Genetic analysis shows that the patient's gene for the muscle protein dystrophin contains a mutation in its promoter region. Of the choices listed, which would be the most likely effect of this mutation?

A. Initiation of dystrophin transcription will be defective.
B. Termination of dystrophin transcription will be defective.
C. Capping of dystrophin messenger RNA will be defective.
D. Splicing of dystrophin messenger RNA will be defective.
E. Tailing of dystrophin messenger RNA will be defective.

Correct answer = A. Mutations in the promoter typically prevent formation of the RNA polymerase II transcription complex, resulting in a decrease in the initiation of messenger RNA (mRNA) synthesis. A deficiency of dystrophin mRNA will result in a deficiency in the production of the dystrophin protein. Capping, splicing, and tailing defects are not a consequence of promoter mutations. They can, however, result in mRNA with decreased stability (capping and tailing defects), or a mRNA in which too many or too few introns have been removed (splicing defects).

30.3 A mutation to this sequence in eukaryotic messenger RNA (RNA) will affect the process by which the 3'-end poly-A tail is added to the mRNA.

A. AAUAAA
B. CAAT
C. CCA
D. GU. . . A . . . AG
E. TATAAA

Correct answer = A. An endonuclease cleaves messenger RNA just downstream of this polyadenylation signal, creating a new 3'-end to which the poly A polymerase adds the poly-A tail using ATP as the substrate in a template-independent process. CAAT and TATAAA are sequences found in promoters for RNA polymerase II. CCA is added to the 3'-end of transfer RNA by nucleotidyltransferase. GU...A...AG denotes an intron.

30.4. This protein factor identifies the promoter of protein-coding genes in eukaryotes.

A. Pribnow box
B. Rho
C. Sigma
D. TFIID
E. U1

Correct answer = D. The general transcription factor, TFIID, recognizes and binds core promoter elements such as the TATA-like box in eukaryotic protein-coding genes. These genes are transcribed by RNA polymerase II. The Pribnow box is a cis-acting element in prokaryotic promoters. Rho is involved in the termination of prokaryotic transcription. Sigma is the subunit of prokaryotic RNA polymerase that recognizes and binds the prokaryotic promoter. U1 is a ribonucleoprotein involved in splicing of eukaryotic pre-messenger RNA.

30.5 What is the sequence (conventionally written) of the RNA product of the DNA template sequence, GATCTAC?

Correct answer = 5'-GUAGAUC-3'. The RNA product has a sequence that is complementary to the template strand, with U replacing T.

Protein Synthesis

31

I. OVERVIEW

Genetic information, stored in the chromosomes and transmitted to daughter cells through DNA replication, is expressed through transcription to RNA and, in the case of messenger RNA (mRNA), subsequent translation into proteins (polypeptide chains) as shown in Figure 31.1. The process of protein synthesis is called translation because the "language" of the nucleotide sequence on the mRNA is translated into the language of an amino acid sequence. Translation requires a genetic code, through which the information contained in the nucleic acid sequence is expressed to produce a specific sequence of amino acids. Any alteration in the nucleic acid sequence may result in an incorrect amino acid being inserted into the polypeptide chain, potentially causing disease or even death of the organism. Newly made (nascent) proteins undergo a number of processes to achieve their functional form. They must fold properly, and misfolding can result in aggregation or degradation of the protein. Many proteins are covalently modified to activate them or alter their activities. Finally, proteins are targeted to their final intra- or extracellular destinations by signals present in the proteins themselves.

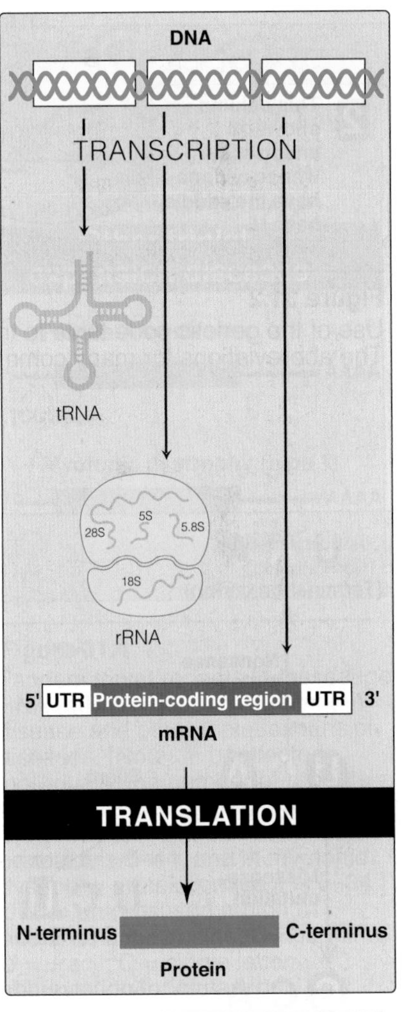

Figure 31.1
Protein synthesis or translation. tRNA = transfer RNA; rRNA = ribosomal RNA; mRNA = messenger RNA; UTR = untranslated region.

II. THE GENETIC CODE

The genetic code is a dictionary that identifies the correspondence between a sequence of nucleotide bases and a sequence of amino acids. Each individual "word" in the code is composed of three nucleotide bases. These genetic words are called codons.

A. Codons

Codons are presented in the mRNA language of adenine (A), guanine (G), cytosine (C), and uracil (U). Their nucleotide sequences are always written from the 5'-end to the 3'-end. The four nucleotide bases are used to produce the three-base codons. There are, therefore, 64 different combinations of bases, taken three at a time (a triplet code) as shown in the table in Figure 31.2.

1. **How to translate a codon:** This table (or "dictionary") can be used to translate any codon and, thus, to determine which amino acids are coded for by an mRNA sequence. For example, the codon 5'-AUG-3' codes for methionine ([Met] see Figure 31.2). [Note:

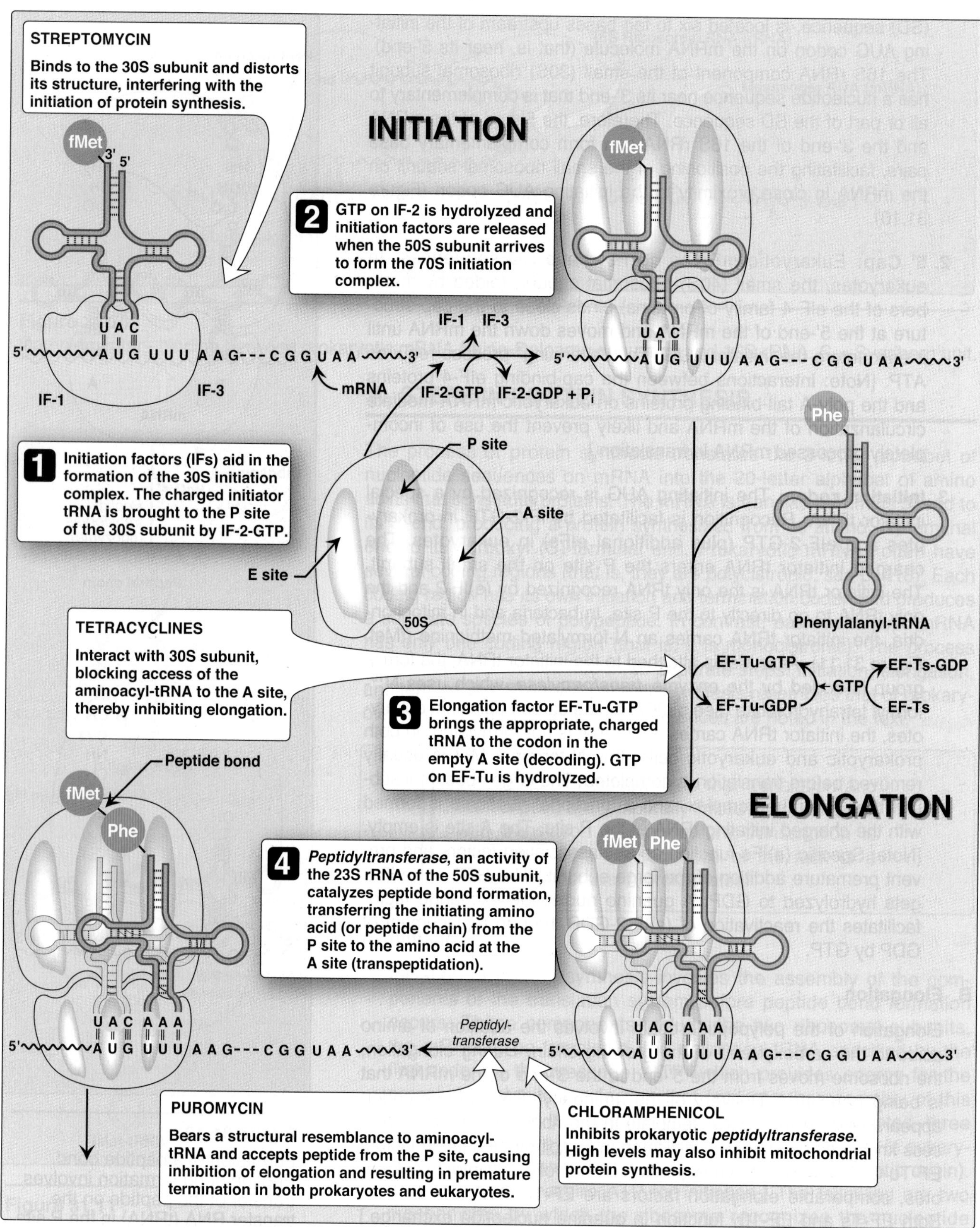

Figure 31.13 (*continued on the next page*)
Steps in prokaryotic protein synthesis (translation), and their inhibition by antibiotics. [Note: EF-Ts is a guanine nucleotide exchange factor. It facilitates the removal of GDP, allowing its replacement by GTP. The eukaryotic equivalent is EF-1βγ.] fMet = formylated methionine; S = Svedberg unit; GTP = guanine nucleoside triphosphate; Phe = phenylalanine.

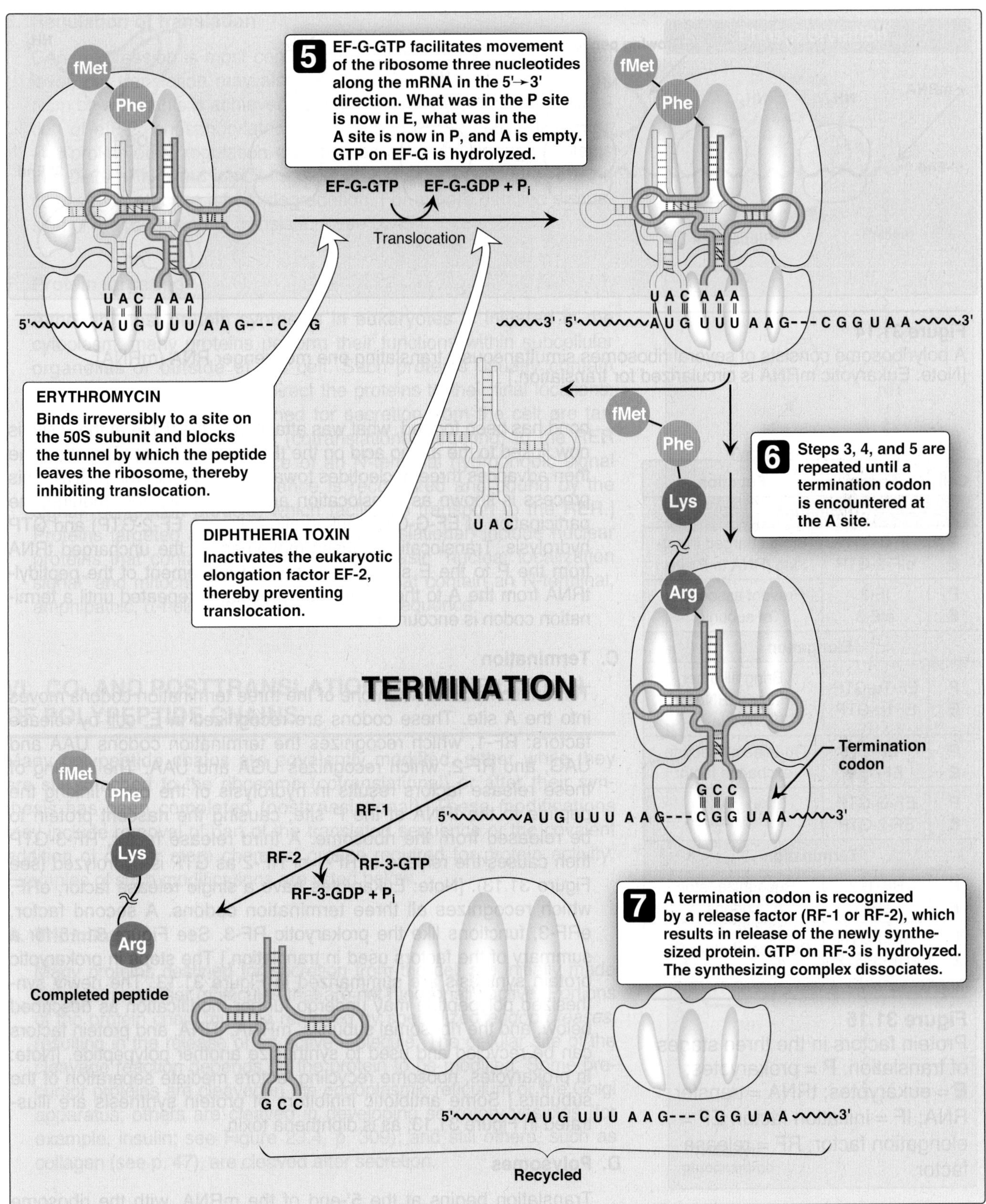

Figure 31.13 (*Continued from the previous page*)
[Note: Ricin, a toxin from castor beans, removes an A from the 28 S rRNA in the large subunit of eukaryotic ribosomes, thereby inhibiting their function.] Lys = lysine; Arg = arginine.

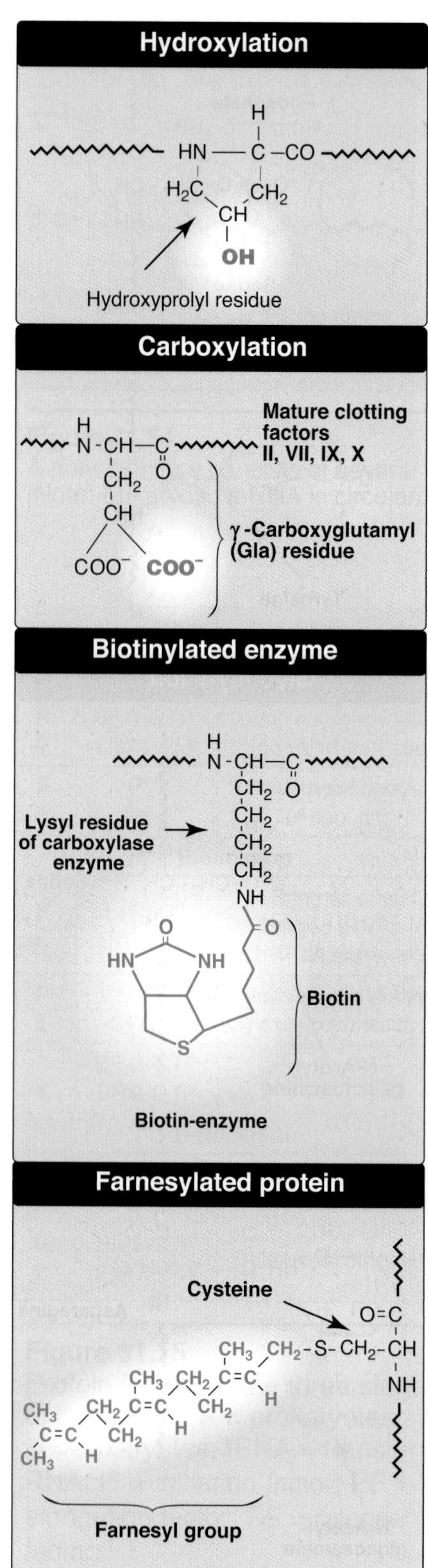

Figure 31.16 *(continued from previous page)* Covalent modifications of some amino acid residues.

1. **Phosphorylation:** Phosphorylation occurs on the hydroxyl groups of serine; threonine; or, less frequently, tyrosine residues in a protein. This phosphorylation is catalyzed by one of a family of protein *kinases* and may be reversed by the action of cellular protein *phosphatases*. The phosphorylation may increase or decrease the functional activity of the protein. Several examples of phosphorylation reactions have been previously discussed (for example, see Chapter 11, p. 131, for the regulation of glycogen synthesis and degradation).

2. **Glycosylation:** Many of the proteins that are destined to become part of a plasma membrane or to be secreted from a cell have carbohydrate chains added en bloc to the amide nitrogen of asparagine (N-linked) or built sequentially on the hydroxyl groups of serine, threonine, or hydroxylysine (O-linked). N-glycosylation occurs in the endoplasmic reticulum and O-glycosyation in the Golgi. (The process of producing such glycoproteins was discussed on p. 165.) Glycosylation is also used to target proteins to the matrix of lysosomes. Lysosomal acid *hydrolases* are modified by the phosphorylation of mannose residues at carbon 6 (see p. 169).

3. **Hydroxylation:** Proline and lysine residues of the α chains of collagen are extensively hydroxylated by vitamin C–dependent *hydroxylases* in the endoplasmic reticulum (see p. 47).

4. **Other covalent modifications:** These may be required for the functional activity of a protein. For example, additional carboxyl groups can be added to glutamate residues by vitamin K–dependent carboxylation (see p. 389). The resulting γ-carboxyglutamate (Gla) residues are essential for the activity of several of the blood-clotting proteins. (See online Chapter 34.) Biotin is covalently bound to the ε-amino groups of lysine residues of biotin-dependent enzymes that catalyze carboxylation reactions such as *pyruvate carboxylase* (see p. 119). Attachment of lipids, such as farnesyl groups, can help anchor proteins to membranes. Many eukaryotic proteins are cotranslationally acetylated at the N-end. [Note: Reversible acetylation of histone proteins influences gene expression (see p. 409).]

C. Protein folding

Proteins must fold to assume their functional, native state. Folding can be spontaneous (as a result of the primary structure) or facilitated by proteins known as chaperones (see p. 20).

D. Protein degradation

Proteins that are defective (for example, misfolded) or destined for rapid turnover are often marked for destruction by ubiquitination, the attachment of chains of a small, highly conserved protein, called ubiquitin (see Figure 19.3 on p. 247). Proteins marked in this way are rapidly degraded by a cellular component known as the proteasome, which is a macromolecular, ATP-dependent, proteolytic system located in the cytosol. [Note: The ΔF508 mutation seen in CF causes misfolding of the CFTR protein, resulting in its proteasomal degradation.]

VII. CHAPTER SUMMARY

Codons are composed of three nucleotide bases presented in the messenger (mRNA) language of **adenine (A), guanine** (G), **cytosine (C),** and **uracil (U).** They are always written **5'→3'**. Of the 64 possible three-base combinations, 61 code for the 20 common amino acids and 3 signal termination of protein synthesis (**translation**). Altering the nucleotide sequence in a codon can cause **silent mutations** (the altered codon codes for the original amino acid), **missense mutations** (the altered codon codes for a different amino acid), or **nonsense mutations** (the altered codon is a termination codon). Characteristics of the genetic code include **specificity**, **universality**, and **degeneracy**, and it is **nonoverlapping** and **commaless** (Figure 31.17). Requirements for protein synthesis include all the amino acids that eventually appear in the finished protein, at least one specific type of transfer RNA (tRNA) for each amino acid, one ***aminoacyl-tRNA synthetase*** for each amino acid, the mRNA coding for the protein to be synthesized, fully competent **ribosomes**, **protein factors** needed for initiation, elongation, and termination of protein synthesis, and **ATP** and **GTP** as energy sources. tRNA has an attachment site for a specific amino acid at its 3'-end, and an anticodon region that can recognize the codon specifying the amino acid the tRNA is carrying. **Ribosomes** are large complexes of protein and ribosomal (rRNA). They consist of **two subunits**. Each ribosome has three binding sites for tRNA molecules: the A, P, and E sites that cover three neighboring codons. The **A-site** codon binds an **incoming aminoacyl-tRNA**, the **P-site** codon is occupied by **peptidyl-tRNA**, and the **E site** is occupied by the **empty tRNA** as it is about to exit the ribosome. Recognition of an mRNA codon is accomplished by the tRNA **anticodon**. The anticodon binds to the codon following the rules of **complementarity** and **antiparallel** binding. (Nucleotide sequences are always assumed to be written in the 5' to 3' direction unless otherwise noted.) The **"wobble" hypothesis** states that the first (5') base of the anticodon is not as spatially defined as the other two bases. Movement of that first base allows nontraditional base-pairing with the last (3') base of the codon, thus allowing a single tRNA to recognize more than one codon for a specific amino acid. For **initiation of protein synthesis**, the components of the translation system are assembled, and mRNA associates with the small ribosomal subunit. The process requires **initiation factors**. In **prokaryotes**, a purine-rich region of the mRNA (the **Shine-Dalgarno sequence**) base-pairs with a complementary sequence on 16S rRNA, resulting in the positioning of the small subunit on the mRNA so that translation can begin. The **5'-cap** (bound by proteins of the eIF-4 family) on **eukaryotic mRNA** is used to position the small subunit on the mRNA. The **initiation codon** is **AUG**, and **N-formylmethionine** is the initiating amino acid in prokaryotes, whereas methionine is used in eukaryotes. The polypeptide chain is elongated by the addition of amino acids to the carboxyl end of its growing chain. The process requires **elongation factors** that facilitate the binding of the aminoacyl-tRNA to the A site as well as the movement of the ribosome along the mRNA. The formation of the peptide bond is catalyzed by ***peptidyltransferase***, which is an activity intrinsic to the rRNA of the large subunit and, therefore, is a **ribozyme**. Following peptide bond formation, the ribosome advances along the mRNA in the **5'→3' direction** to the next codon (translocation). Because of the length of most mRNAs, more than one ribosome at a time can translate a message, forming a **polysome**. Termination begins when one of the three termination codons moves into the A site. These codons are recognized by **release factors**. The newly synthesized protein is released from the ribosomal complex, and the ribosome is dissociated from the mRNA. Initiation, elongation, and termination are driven by the hydrolysis of **GTP**. Initiation in eukaryotes also requires **ATP** for scanning. Numerous **antibiotics** interfere with the process of protein synthesis. Many polypeptide chains are covalently modified during or after translation. Such modifications include **removal of amino acids**; **phosphorylation,** which may activate or inactivate the protein; **glycosylation**, which plays a role in protein targeting; and **hydroxylation** such as that seen in collagen. Proteins must fold to achieve their functional form. Folding can be spontaneous or facilitated by **chaperones**. Proteins that are defective (for example misfolded) or destined for rapid turnover are marked for destruction by the attachment of chains of a small, highly conserved protein called **ubiquitin**. Ubiquitinated proteins are rapidly degraded by a cytosolic complex known as the **proteasome**.

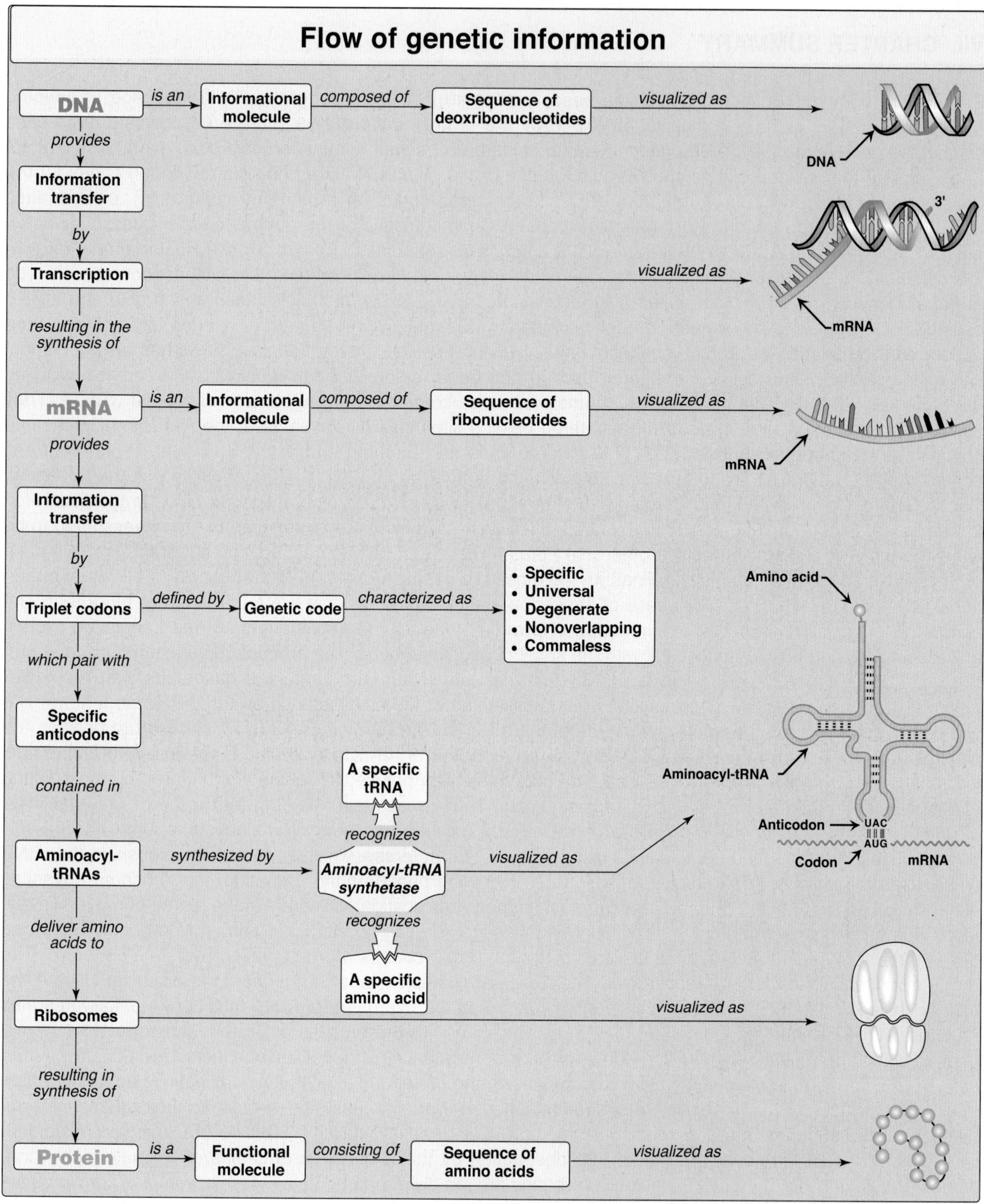

Figure 31.17
Key concept map for protein synthesis. mRNA = messenger RNA; tRNA = transfer RNA; A = adenine; G = guanine; C = cytosine; U = uracil.

Study Questions

Choose the ONE best answer.

31.1 A 20-year-old man with a microcytic anemia is found to have an abnormal form of β-globin (Hemoglobin Constant Spring) that is 172 amino acids long, rather than the 141 found in the normal protein. Which of the following point mutations is consistent with this abnormality?

A. CGA → UGA
B. GAU → GAC
C. GCA → GAA
D. UAA → CAA
E. UAA → UAG

Correct answer = D. Mutating the normal termination (stop) codon for β-globin from UAA to CAA causes the ribosome to insert a glutamine at that point. It will continue extending the protein chain until it comes upon the next stop codon further down the message, resulting in an abnormally long protein. The replacement of CGA (arginine) with UGA (stop) would cause the protein to be too short. GAU and GAC both encode aspartate and would cause no change in the protein. Changing GCA (alanine) to GAA (glutamate) would not change the size of the protein product. A change from UAA to UAG would simply change one termination codon for another, and would have no effect on the protein

31.2 A pharmaceutical company is studying a new antibiotic that inhibits bacterial protein synthesis. When this antibiotic is added to an in vitro protein synthesis system that is translating the messenger RNA sequence AUGUUUUUUUAG, the only product formed is the dipeptide fMet-Phe. What step in protein synthesis is most likely inhibited by the antibiotic?

A. Initiation
B. Binding of charged transfer RNA to the ribosomal A site
C. Peptidyltransferase activity
D. Ribosomal translocation
E. Termination

Correct answer = D. Because fMet-Phe is made, the ribosomes must be able to complete initiation, bind Phe-tRNA to the A site, and use peptidyltransferase activity to form the first peptide bond. Because the ribosome is not able to proceed any further, ribosomal movement (translocation) is most likely the inhibited step. The ribosome is, therefore, frozen before it reaches the termination codon of this message.

31.3 A transfer RNA (tRNA) molecule that is supposed to carry cysteine ($tRNA^{cys}$) is mischarged, so that it actually carries alanine ($ala\text{-}tRNA^{cys}$). Assuming no correction occurs, what will be the fate of this alanine residue during protein synthesis?

A. It will be incorporated into a protein in response to a codon for alanine.
B. It will be incorporated into a protein in response to a codon for cysteine.
C. It will be incorporated randomly at any codon.
D. It will remain attached to the tRNA because it cannot be used for protein synthesis.
E. It will be chemically converted to cysteine by cellular enzymes.

Correct answer = B. Once an amino acid is attached to a transfer (tRNA) molecule, only the anticodon of that tRNA determines the specificity of incorporation. The mischarged alanine will, therefore, be incorporated into the protein at a position determined by a cysteine codon.

31.4 In a patient with cystic fibrosis caused by the ΔF508 mutation, the mutant cystic fibrosis transmembrane conductance regulator (CFTR) protein folds incorrectly. The patient's cells modify this abnormal protein by attaching ubiquitin molecules to it. What is the fate of this modified CFTR protein?

A. It performs its normal function because the ubiquitin largely corrects for the effect of the mutation.
B. It is secreted from the cell.
C. It is placed into storage vesicles.
D. It is degraded by the proteasome.
E. It is repaired by cellular enzymes.

Correct answer = D. Ubiquitination usually marks old, damaged, or misfolded proteins for destruction by the cytosolic proteasome. There is no known cellular mechanism for repair of damaged proteins.

31.5 Many antimicrobials inhibit protein translation. Which of the following antimicrobials is correctly paired with its mechanism of action?

A. Erythromycin binds to the 60S ribosomal subunit.
B. Puromycin inactivates EF-2.
C. Streptomycin binds to the 30S ribosomal subunit.
D. Tetracyclines inhibit peptidyltransferase.

Correct answer = C. Streptomycin binds the 30S subunit and inhibits translation initiation. Erythromycin binds the 50S ribosomal subunit (60S denotes a eukaryote) and blocks the tunnel through which the peptide leaves the ribosome. Puromycin has structural similarity to aminoacyl-tRNA. It is incorporated into the growing chain, inhibits elongation, and results in premature termination in both prokaryotes and eukaryotes. Tetracyclines bind the 30S ribosomal subunit and block access to the A site, inhibiting elongation.

31.6 Translation of a synthetic polyribonucleotide containing the repeating sequence CAA in a cell-free protein-synthesizing system produces three homopolypeptides: polyglutamine, polyasparagine, and polythreonine. If the codons for glutamine and asparagine are CAA and AAC, respectively, which of the following triplets is the codon for threonine?

A. AAC
B. ACA
C. CAA
D. CAC
E. CCA

Correct answer = B. The synthetic polynucleotide sequence of CAACAACAACAA . . could be read by the in vitro protein synthesizing system starting at the first C, the first A, or the second A. In the first case, the first triplet codon would be CAA, which codes glutamine; in the second case, the first triplet codon would be AAC, which codes for asparagine; in the last case, the first triplet codon would be ACA, which codes for threonine.

31.7 Which of the following is required for both prokaryotic and eukaryotic protein synthesis?

A. Binding of the small ribosomal subunit to the Shine-Dalgarno sequence
B. fMet-tRNA
C. Movement of the messenger RNA out of the nucleus and into the cytoplasm
D. Recognition of the 5'-cap by initiation factors.
E. Translocation of the peptidyl-tRNA from the A site to the P site

Correct answer = E. In both prokaryotes and eukaryotes, continued translation (elongation) requires movement of the peptidyl-tRNA from the A to the P site to allow the next aminoacyl-tRNA to enter the A site. Only prokaryotes have a Shine-Dalgarno sequence and use fMet, and only eukaryotes have a nucleus and co- and posttranscriptionally process their mRNA.

31.8 α1-Antitrypsin (AAT) deficiency can result in emphysema, a lung pathology, because the action of elastase, a serine protease, is unopposed. Deficiency of AAT in the lungs is the consequence of impaired secretion from the liver, the site of its synthesis. Proteins such as AAT that are destined to be secreted are best characterized by which of the following statements?

A. Their synthesis is initiated on the smooth endoplasmic reticulum.
B. They contain a mannose 6-phosphate targeting signal.
C. They always contain methionine as the N-terminal amino acid.
D. They are produced from translation products that have an N-terminal hydrophobic signal sequence.
E. They contain no sugars with O-glycosidic linkages because their synthesis does not involve the Golgi apparatus.

Correct answer = D. Synthesis of secreted proteins is begun on free (cytosolic) ribosomes. As the N-terminal signal sequence of the peptide emerges from the ribosome, it is bound by the signal recognition particle, taken to the rough endoplasmic reticulum (RER), threaded into the lumen, and removed as translation continues. The proteins move through the RER and the Golgi, and undergo processing such as N-glycosylation (RER) and O-glycosylation (Golgi). In the Golgi, they are packaged in secretory vesicles and released from the cell. The smooth endoplasmic reticulum is associated with synthesis of lipids, not proteins, and has no ribosomes attached. Phosphorylation at carbon 6 of terminal mannose residues in glycoproteins targets these proteins (acid hydrolases) to lysosomes. The N-terminal methionine is removed from most proteins during processing.

31.9 Why is the genetic code described both as degenerate and unambiguous?

A given amino acid can be coded for by more than one codon (degenerate code), but a given codon codes for just one particular amino acid (unambiguous code).

Regulation of Gene Expression

32

I. OVERVIEW

Gene expression refers to the multistep process that ultimately results in the production of a functional gene product, either ribonucleic acid (RNA) or protein. The first step in gene expression, the use of deoxyribonucleic acid (DNA) for the synthesis of RNA (transcription), is the primary site of regulation in both prokaryotes and eukaryotes. In eukaryotes, however, gene expression also involves extensive posttranscriptional and posttranslational processes as well as actions that influence access to particular regions of the DNA. Each of these steps can be regulated to provide additional control over the kinds and amounts of functional products that are produced.

Not all genes are regulated. For example, genes described as constitutive encode products required for basic cellular functions and so are continually expressed. They are also known as "housekeeping" genes. Regulated genes, however, are expressed only under certain conditions. They may be expressed in all cells or in only a subset of cells, for example, hepatocytes. The ability to regulate gene expression (that is, to determine if, how much, and when particular gene products will be made) gives the cell control over structure and function. It is the basis for cellular differentiation, morphogenesis, and adaptability of any organism. Control of gene expression is best understood in prokaryotes, but many themes are repeated in eukaryotes. Figure 32.1 lists some common strategies employed in gene regulation.

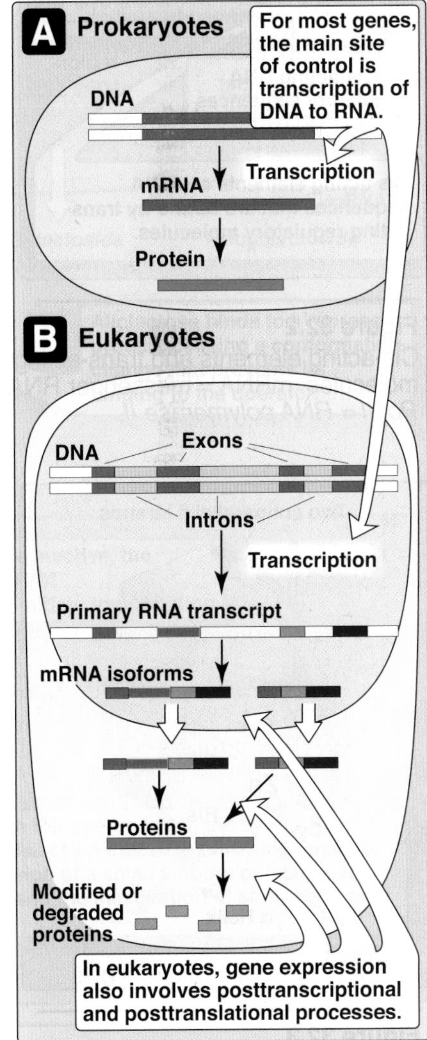

Figure 32.1
Control of gene expression. mRNA = messenger RNA.

II. REGULATORY SEQUENCES AND MOLECULES

Regulation of transcription, the initial step in all gene expression, is controlled by regulatory sequences of DNA, usually embedded in the noncoding regions of the genome. The interaction between these DNA segments and regulatory molecules, such as transcription factors, can engage or repress the transcriptional machinery, influencing the kinds and amounts of products that are produced. These DNA sequences flanking a gene are called cis-acting because they influence expression of genes only on the same chromosome (see p. 423). A trans-acting

[Note: The physiologic function of this acetylation is unknown.] All of these proteins are maximally produced only when lactose is available to the cell and glucose is not. [Note: Bacteria use glucose, if available, as a fuel in preference to any other sugar.] The regulatory portion of the operon is upstream of the three structural genes and consists of the promoter region where *RNA polymerase* binds and two additional sites, the operator (O) site and the CAP site, where regulatory proteins bind. The lacZ, lacY, and lacA genes are expressed only when the O site is empty, and the CAP site is bound by a complex of cyclic adenosine monophosphate ([cAMP] see p. 94) and the catabolite activator protein (CAP), sometimes called the cAMP regulatory protein (CRP). A regulatory gene, the lacI gene, codes for the repressor protein (a trans-acting factor) that binds to the O site with high affinity. [Note: The lacI gene has its own promoter.]

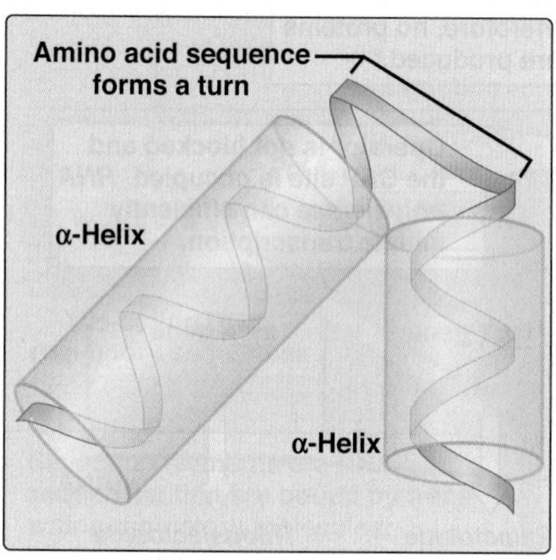

Figure 32.5
Helix-turn-helix motif of the lac repressor protein.

1. **When only glucose is available:** In this case, the lac operon is repressed (turned off). Repression is mediated by the repressor protein binding via a helix-turn-helix motif (Figure 32.5) to the operator site, which is downstream of the promoter region (see Figure 32.4A). Binding of the repressor interferes with the progress of *RNA polymerase* and blocks transcription of the structural genes. This is an example of negative regulation.

2. **When only lactose is available:** In this case, the lac operon is induced (maximally expressed, or turned on). A small amount of lactose is converted to an isomer, allolactose. This compound is an inducer that binds to the repressor protein, changing its conformation so that it can no longer bind to the operator. In the absence of glucose, *adenylyl cyclase* is active, and sufficient quantities of cAMP are made and bind to the CAP protein. The cAMP–CAP trans-acting complex binds to the CAP site, causing *RNA polymerase* to more efficiently initiate transcription at the promoter site (see Figure 32.4B). This is an example of positive regulation. The transcript is a single polycistronic mRNA molecule that contains three sets of start and stop codons. Translation of the mRNA produces the three proteins that allow lactose to be used for energy production by the cell. [Note: In contrast to the inducible lacZ, lacY, and lacA genes, whose expression is regulated, the lacI gene is constitutive. Its gene product, the repressor protein, is always made and is active unless the inducer is present.]

3. **When both glucose and lactose are available:** In this case, transcription of the lac operon is negligible, even if lactose is present at a high concentration. *Adenylyl cyclase* is inhibited in the presence of glucose (a process known as catabolite repression) so no cAMP–CAP complex forms, and the CAP site remains empty. *RNA polymerase* is, therefore, unable to effectively initiate transcription, even though the repressor may not be bound to the operator region. Consequently, the three structural genes of the operon are not expressed (see Figure 32.4C).

D. Tryptophan operon

The tryptophan (trp) operon contains five structural genes that code for enzymes required for the synthesis of the amino acid, tryptophan.

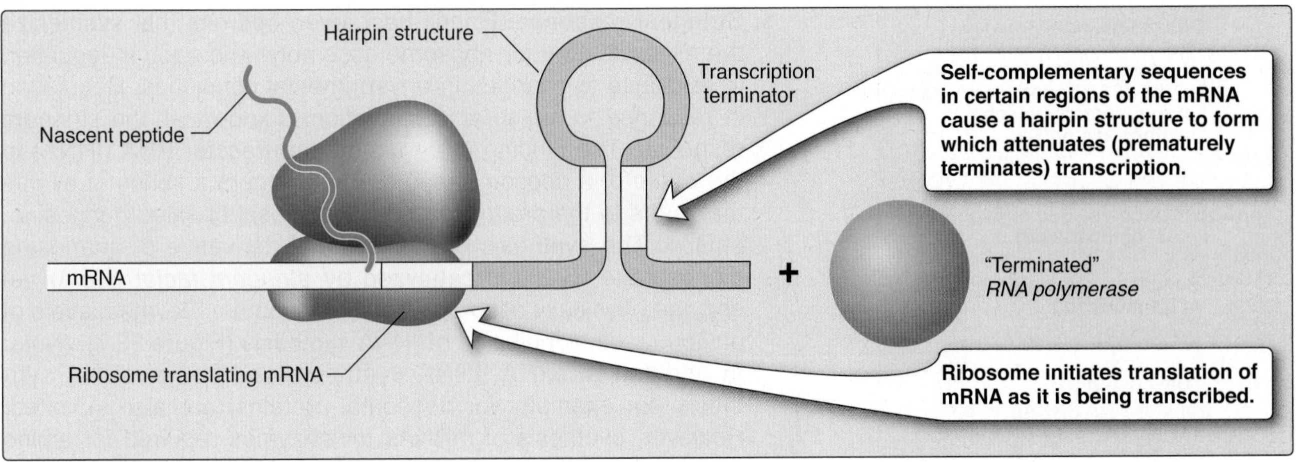

Figure 32.6
Attenuation of transcription of the trp operon when tryptophan is plentiful. mRNA = messenger RNA.

As with the lac operon, the trp operon is subject to negative control. However, for the repressible trp operon, negative control includes Trp itself binding to a repressor protein and facilitating the binding of the repressor to the operator: Trp is a corepressor. Because repression by Trp is not always complete, unlike the lac operon, the trp operon is also regulated by a process known as attenuation. With attenuation, transcription is initiated but is terminated well before completion (Figure 32.6). If Trp is plentiful, transcription initiation that escaped repression by Trp is attenuated (stopped) by the formation at the 5'-end of the mRNA of a hairpin (stem–loop) structure like that seen in rho-independent termination (see p. 421). [Note: Transcription and translation are temporally linked in prokaryotes (see p. 438), and, therefore, attenuation also results in the formation of a truncated, nonfunctional peptide product that is rapidly degraded.] If Trp becomes scarce, the operon is expressed. The 5'-end of the mRNA contains two adjacent codons for Trp. The lack of Trp causes ribosomes to stall at these codons, covering regions of the mRNA required for formation of the attenuation hairpin. This prevents attenuation and allows transcription to continue.

> Transcriptional attenuation can occur in prokaryotes because translation of an mRNA begins before its synthesis is complete. This does not occur in eukaryotes because the presence of a membrane-bound nucleus spatially and temporally separates transcription and translation.

E. Coordination of transcription and translation in prokaryotes

Whereas transcriptional regulation of mRNA production is primary in bacteria, regulation at the level of ribosomal RNA (rRNA) and protein synthesis also occurs and plays important roles in the microbe's ability to adapt to environmental stress.

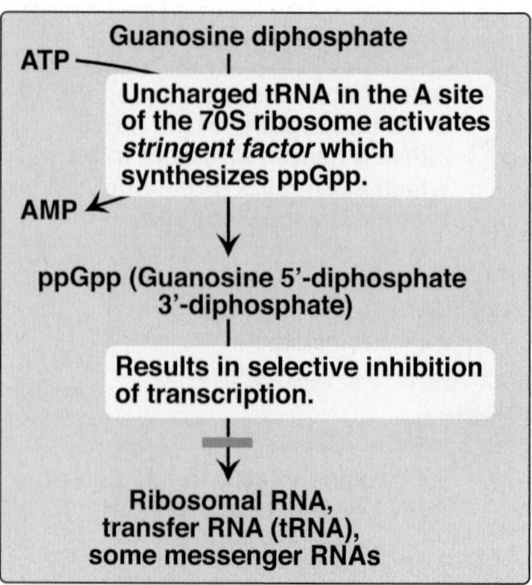

Figure 32.7
Regulation of transcription by the stringent response to amino acid starvation. S = Svedberg unit.

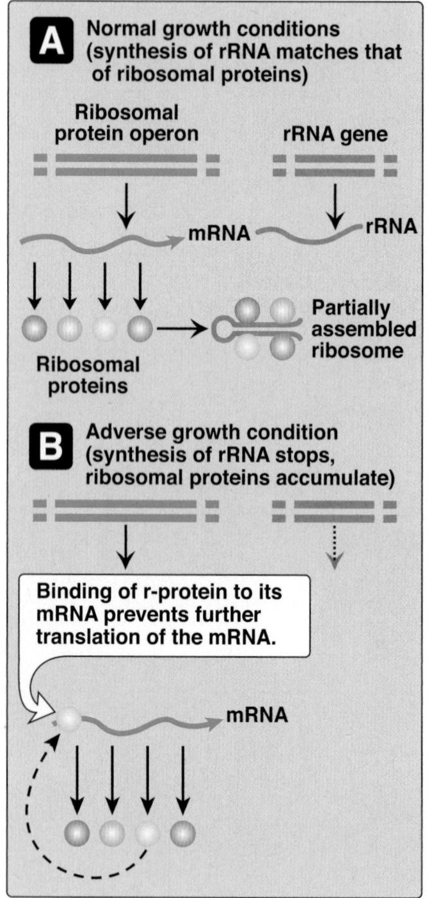

Figure 32.8
Regulation of translation by an excess of ribosomal proteins. mRNA = messenger RNA; rRNA = ribosomal RNA; r-protein = ribosomal protein.

1. **Stringent response:** E. coli has seven operons that synthesize the rRNA needed for ribosome assembly, and each is regulated in response to changes in environmental conditions. Regulation in response to amino acid starvation is known as the stringent response. The binding of an uncharged transfer RNA (tRNA) to the A site of a ribosome (see p. 436) triggers a series of events that leads to the production of a polyphosphorylated guanosine, ppGpp. The synthesis of this unusual derivative of guanosine diphosphate (GDP) is catalyzed by *stringent factor* (*RelA*), an enzyme physically associated with ribosomes. Elevated levels of ppGpp result in inhibition of rRNA synthesis (Figure 32.7). [Note: In addition to rRNA, tRNA synthesis and some mRNA synthesis (for example, for ribosomal proteins) are also inhibited. However, synthesis of mRNAs for enzymes required for amino acid biosynthesis is not inhibited. ppGpp appears to alter promoter selection through use of different sigma-factors for *RNA polymerase* (see p.419.]

2. **Regulatory ribosomal proteins:** Operons for ribosomal proteins (r-proteins) can be inhibited by an excess of their own protein products. For each operon, one specific r-protein functions in the repression of translation of the polycistronic mRNA from that operon (Figure 32.8). The r-protein does so by binding to the Shine-Dalgarno (SD) sequence located on the mRNA just upstream of the first initiating AUG codon (see p. 439) and acting as a physical impediment to the binding of the small ribosomal subunit to the SD sequence. One r-protein thus inhibits synthesis of all the r-proteins of the operon. This same r-protein also binds to rRNA and with a higher affinity than for mRNA. If the concentration of rRNA falls, the r-protein then is available to bind its own mRNA and inhibit its translation. This coordinated regulation keeps the synthesis of r-proteins in balance with the transcription of rRNA, so that each is present in appropriate amounts for the formation of ribosomes.

IV. REGULATION OF EUKARYOTIC GENE EXPRESSION

The higher degree of complexity of eukaryotic genomes, as well as the presence of a nuclear membrane, necessitates a wider range of regulatory processes. As with the prokaryotes, the primary site of regulation is at the level of transcription. Again, the theme of trans-acting molecules binding to cis-acting elements is seen. Operons, however, are generally not found in eukaryotes, which must use alternative strategies to solve the problem of how to coordinately regulate all the genes required for a specific response. In eukaryotes, gene expression is also regulated at multiple levels other than transcription. For example, the major modes of posttranscriptional regulation at the mRNA level are alternative mRNA splicing, control of mRNA stability, and control of translational efficiency. Additional regulation at the protein level occurs by mechanisms that modulate stability, processing, or targeting of the protein.

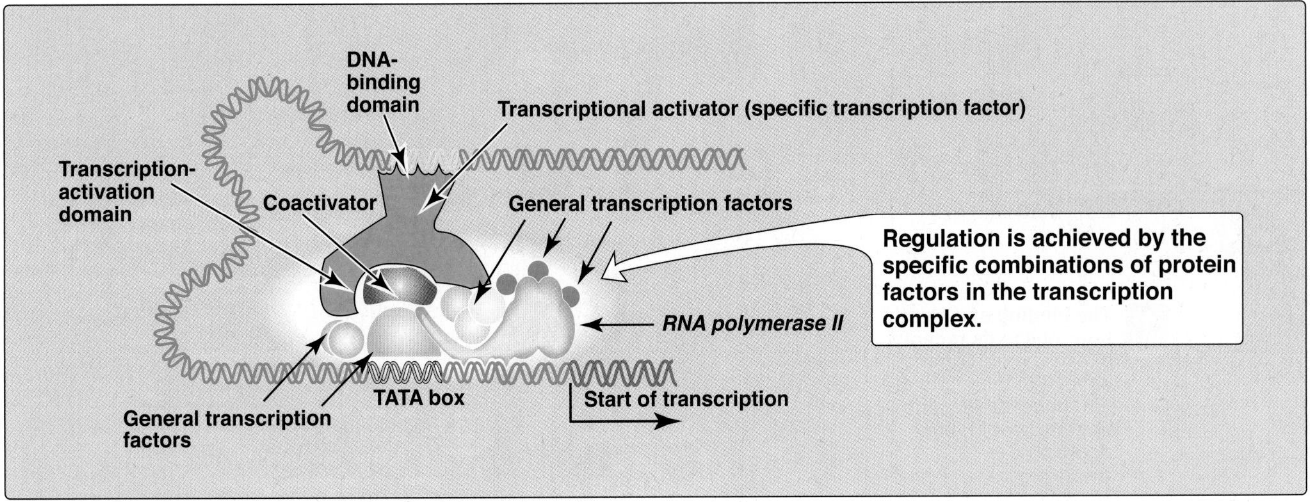

Figure 32.9
Combinatorial control of transcription.

A. Trans-acting molecules

Specific transcription factors are trans-acting DNA-binding proteins that function as transcriptional activators. They have at least two binding domains: the DNA-binding domain, and the transcription-activation domain. The DNA-binding domain contains specific structural motifs, such as zinc fingers (see p. 450), that bind consensus sequences in DNA. The transcription-activation domain recruits other proteins, such as the general transcription factors ([GTFs] see p.423) and coactivators (for example, *histone acetyltransferases* [*HATs*]; see p. 422). These facilitate formation of the transcription initiation complex (*RNA polymerase II* plus the GTFs) at the promoter, and, thus, activate transcription (Figure 32.9). Regulation is achieved by the formation of a multiprotein complex bound to DNA, with protein–protein and protein–DNA interactions controlling assembly of the complex. Although activation domains recruit a variety of proteins, the specific effect of any one of them is dependent upon the protein composition of the complex. This is known as combinatorial control. [Note: DNA-binding proteins can also inhibit transcription.]

B. Cis-acting regulatory elements

The need to coordinately regulate a group of genes to cause a particular response is of key importance in multicellular organisms including humans. An underlying theme occurs repeatedly: A protein binds to a regulatory consensus element on each of the genes in the group and coordinately affects the expression of those genes, even if they are on different chromosomes. For example, hormone-response elements (HREs) are cis-acting DNA sequences that bind trans-acting protein factors and regulate gene expression in response to hormonal signals. In general, hormones bind either to intracellular receptors (steroid hormones are an example; see p. 240) or to cell-surface receptors (the peptide hormone glucagon is an example; see p. 314).

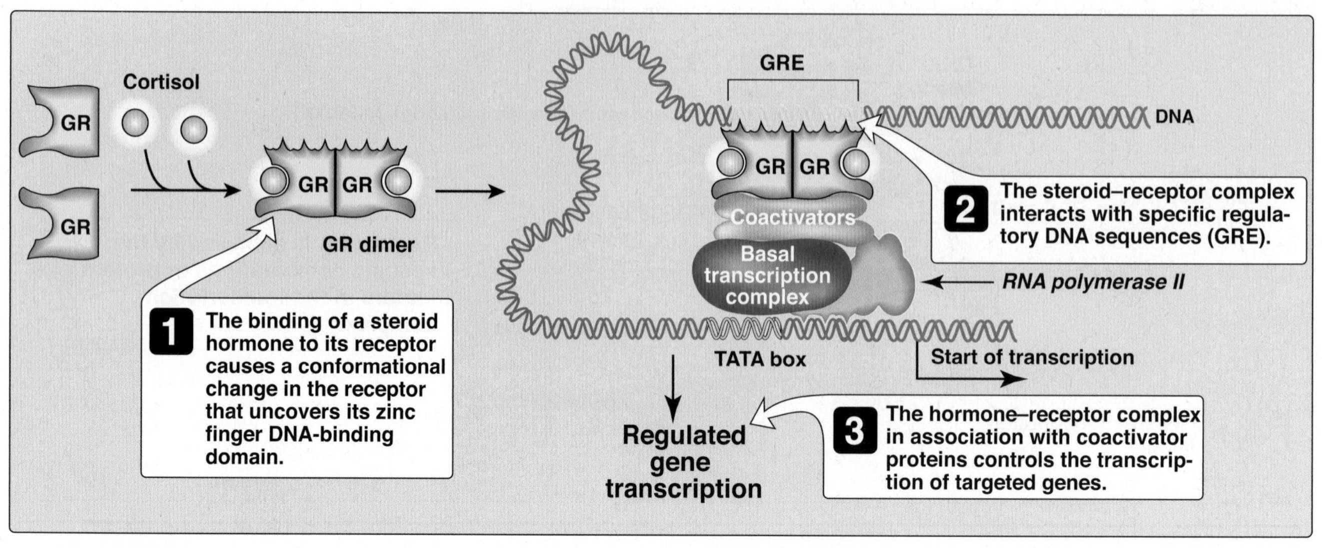

Figure 32.10
Transcriptional regulation by intracellular steroid hormone receptors. GRE = glucocorticoid-response element (an example of a hormone-response element); GR = glucocorticoid receptor.

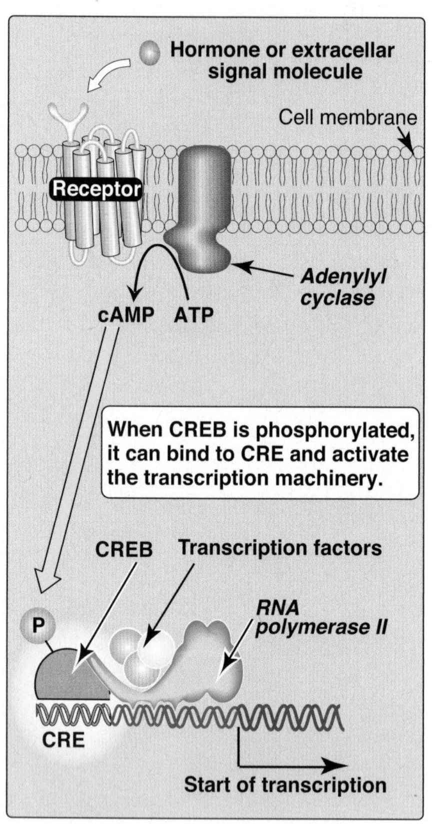

Figure 32.11
Transcriptional regulation by receptors located in the cell membrane. [Note: Cyclic AMP activates *protein kinase A* that phosphorylates cAMP response element–binding (CREB) protein.] CRE = cAMP response element.

1. **Regulatory signals mediated by intracellular receptors:** Members of the nuclear receptor superfamily, which includes the steroid hormone (glucocorticoids, mineralocorticoids, androgens, and estrogens), vitamin D, retinoic acid, and thyroid hormone receptors, all directly influence gene expression by functioning as specific transcription factors. These receptors, therefore, contain a DNA-binding domain and an activation domain. They also contain a ligand-binding domain. For example, steroid hormones such as cortisol (a glucocorticoid) bind to soluble, intracellular receptors at the ligand-binding domain (Figure 32.10). Binding causes a conformational change in the receptor that activates it. The receptor–ligand complex enters the nucleus, dimerizes, and binds via a zinc finger motif to nuclear DNA at a cis-acting regulatory element, the glucocorticoid-response element (GRE), an example of an HRE. Binding allows recruitement of coactivators to the activation domain and results in increased expression of cortisol-responsive genes, each of which is under the control of its own GRE. Binding of the receptor–hormone complex to the GRE allows coordinate expression of a group of target genes, even when these genes are located on different chromosomes. The GRE can be located upstream or downstream of the genes it regulates and is able to function at great distances from those genes. The GRE, then, can function as a true enhancer (see p. 424). [Note: If associated with corepressors, hormone–receptor complexes inhibit transcription.]

2. **Regulatory signals mediated by cell-surface receptors:** Cell-surface receptors include those for insulin, epinephrine, and glucagon. Glucagon, for example, is a peptide hormone that binds its G protein–coupled plasma membrane receptor on glucagon-responsive cells. This extracellular signal is then transduced to intracellular cAMP (Figure 32.11; also see Figure 8.7 on p. 95), which can affect protein expression (and activity) through *protein kinase A*–mediated phosphorylation. In response to a rise

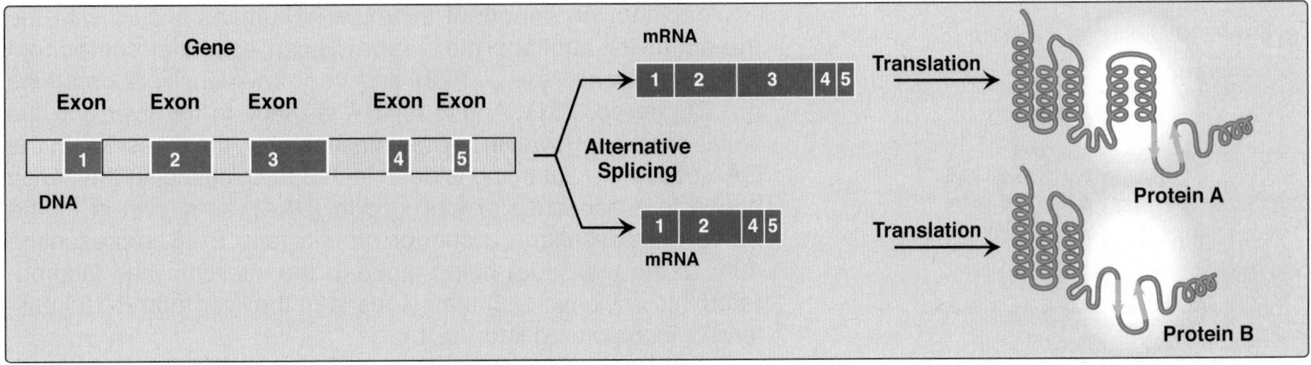

Figure 32.12
Tissue-specific alternative splicing produces multiple related proteins, or isoforms, from a single gene.

in cAMP, a trans-acting factor (cAMP response element–binding [CREB] protein) is phosphorylated and activated. Active CREB protein binds via a leucine zipper motif to a cis-acting regulatory element, the cAMP response element (CRE), resulting in transcription of target genes with CREs in their promoters. [Note: The genes for *phosphoenolpyruvate carboxykinase* and *glucose 6-phosphatase*, key enzymes of gluconeogenesis (see p. 117), are examples of genes upregulated by the cAMP/CRE/CREB system.]

C. Regulation by processing of messenger RNA

Eukaryotic mRNA undergoes several modifications before it is exported from the nucleus to the cytoplasm for use in protein synthesis (see p. 418). Capping at the 5'-end, polyadenylation at the 3'-end, and splicing are essential processing events for the production of a functional eukaryotic messenger from most pre-mRNA (see p. 425), and variations in these events can affect gene expression. In addition, messenger stability also affects gene expression.

1. **Splice-site choice:** Tissue-specific protein isoforms can be made from the same pre-mRNA through differential cotranscriptional processing, particularly the use of alternative splice sites (Figure 32.12). For example, tropomyosin (TM) is an actin filament–binding protein that regulates the functions of actin in both muscle and nonmuscle cells. Its pre-mRNA undergoes tissue-specific differential splicing to yield a number of TM isoforms (see p. 427).

> Over 60% percent of the approximately 25,000 genes in the human genome undergo differential splicing. The use of alternative polyadenylation and transcription start sites is also seen in many genes. This explains, at least in part, how 25,000 genes can give rise to hundreds of thousands of proteins.

2. **Messenger RNA editing:** Even after mRNA has been fully processed, it may undergo additional posttranscriptional modification in which a base in the mRNA is altered. This is known as

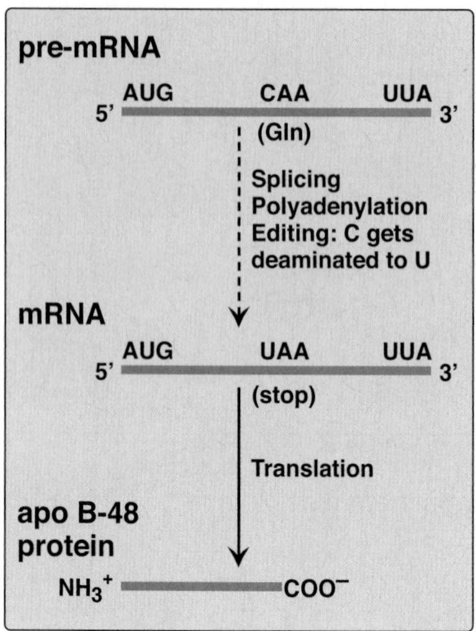

Figure 32.13
RNA editing of apolipoprotein (apo) B in the intestine and generation of the apo B-48 protein needed for chylomicron synthesis. Gln = glutamine; mRNA = messenger RNA.

RNA editing. An important example in humans occurs with the transcript for apolipoprotein (apo) B, an essential component of chylomicrons (see p. 228) and very low density lipoproteins ([VLDL] see p. 231). Apo B mRNA is made in the liver and the small intestine. However, in the intestine only, the C residue in the CAA codon for glutamine is deaminated to U, changing the sense codon to a nonsense or stop codon (UAA), as shown in Figure 32.13. This results in a shorter protein (apo B-48, representing 48% of the message) being made in the intestine (and incorporated into chylomicrons) than is made in the liver (apo B-100, full-length, incorporated into VLDL).

3. **Messenger RNA stability:** How long an mRNA remains in the cytosol before it is degraded influences how much protein product can be produced from it. Regulation of iron metabolism and the gene-silencing process of RNA interference illustrate the importance of mRNA stability in the regulation of gene expression.

   a. **Iron metabolism:** Transferrin is a plasma protein that transports iron. Transferrin binds to cell-surface receptors (transferrin receptors [TfRs]) that get internalized and provide cells, such as erythroblasts, with iron. The mRNA for the TfR has several cis-acting iron-responsive elements (IREs) at its 3'-end. IREs have a short stem–loop structure that can be bound by trans-acting iron regulatory proteins ([IRPs] Figure 32.14). When the iron concentration in the cell is low, the IRPs bind to the 3'-IREs and stabilize the mRNA for TfR, allowing TfR synthesis. When intracellular iron levels are high, the IRPs are degraded. The lack of IRPs bound to the mRNA hastens its destruction, resulting in decreased TfR synthesis. [Note: The mRNA for apoferritin, an intracellular protein of iron storage, has a single IRE at its 5'-end. When iron levels in the cell are low, IRPs bind the 5'-IRE and prevent the use of the

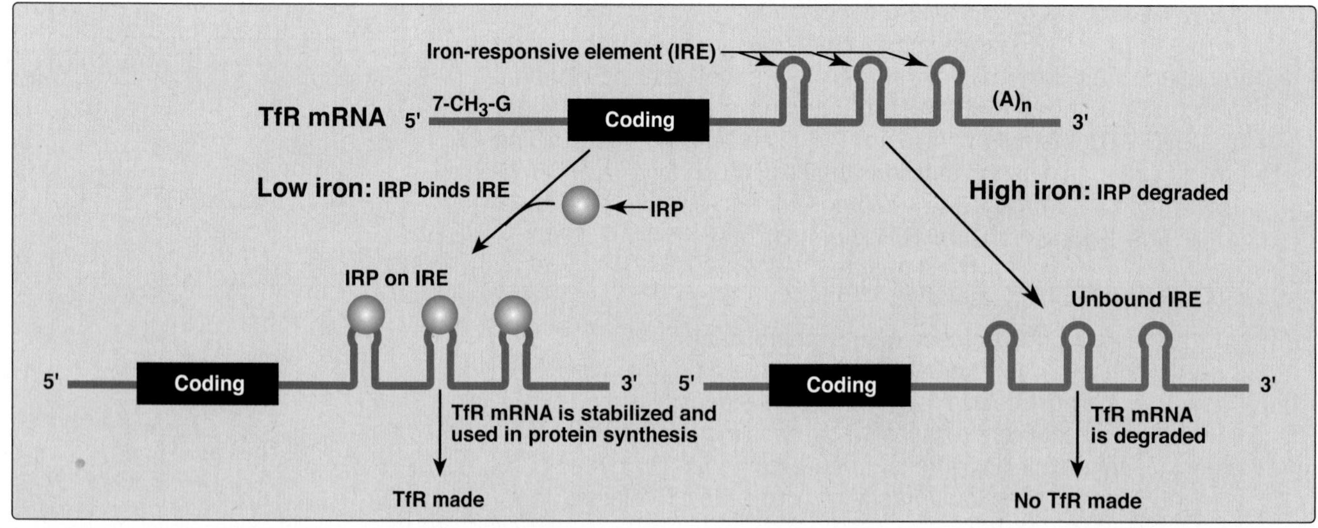

Figure 32.14
Regulation of transferrin receptor (TfR) synthesis. IRP = iron regulatory protein. [Note: The IREs are located in the 3' UTR (untranslated region) of the TfR mRNA.]

mRNA, and less apoferritin is made. When iron accumulates in the cell, the IRP is degraded, allowing synthesis of apoferritin molecules to store the excess iron. *ALAS2*, the regulated enzyme of heme synthesis (see p. 279) in erythroblasts, also contains a 5'-IRE.]

b. RNA interference: RNA interference (RNAi) is a mechanism of gene silencing through decreased expression of mRNA, either by repression of translation or by increased degradation. It is thought to play a key role in such fundamental processes as cell proliferation, differentiation, and apoptosis. RNAi is mediated by short (~22 bp), noncoding RNAs called microRNAs (miRNAs), which arise from far longer, genomically encoded nuclear transcripts, primary miRNA (pri-miRNA) that are partially processed in the nucleus to pre-miRNA by an *endonuclease* (*Drosha*) then transported to the cytoplasm. There, an *endonuclease* (*Dicer*) completes the processing and generates short, double-stranded miRNA. A single strand (the guide, or antisense strand) of the miRNA associates with a cytosolic protein complex known as the RNA-induced silencing complex (RISC). The guide strand hybridizes with a complementary sequence on a full length target mRNA, bringing RISC to the mRNA. This can result in repression of translation of the mRNA or its degradation by an *endonuclease* (*Argonaute/Ago/Slicer*) of the RISC. The extent of complementarity appears to be the determining factor (Figure 32.15). RNAi can also be triggered by double-stranded short interfering RNAs (siRNAs) introduced into a cell from exogenous sources. [Note: In vertebrates, the function of siRNAs that may arise from endogenous sources is unclear.]

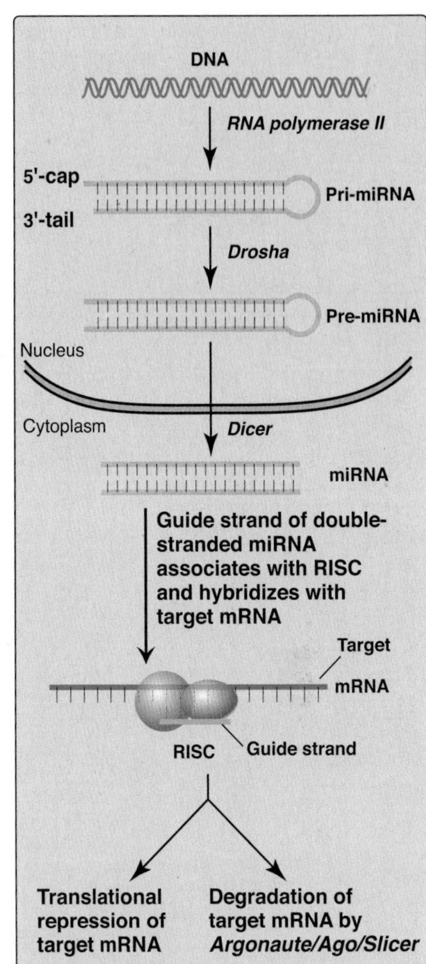

Figure 32.15
Biogenesis and actions of miRNA. [Note: The extent of complementarity between the target messenger RNA (mRNA) and the microRNA (miRNA) determines the final outcome.] RISC = RNA-induced silencing complex.

1) RNA-interference–based therapeutics: Modulation of gene expression by providing siRNA to trigger RNAi has enormous therapeutic potential. The first clinical trial of RNAi-based therapy involved patients with the neovascular form of age-related macular degeneration (AMD), a leading form of adult blindness. Neovascular AMD is triggered by overproduction of vascular endothelial growth factor (VEGF), leading to the sprouting of excess blood vessels behind the retina. The vessels leak, clouding and often entirely destroying vision (therefore, neovascular AMD is also referred to as "wet" macular degeneration). An siRNA designed to target the mRNA of VEGF and promote its degradation went to clinical trials. Although considerable effort and resources have been expended to develop RNAi-based therapeutics, especially for the treatment of cancer, no products have gone from trials to the market. Development has been hindered by the problems of targeted delivery and stability. The use of nano-sized vectors such as liposomes may eliminate these issues. The research applications of RNAi, however, have grown rapidly.

4. Translation of messenger RNA: Regulation of gene expression can also occur at the level of translation. One mechanism by which translation is regulated is through phosphorylation of the eukaryotic

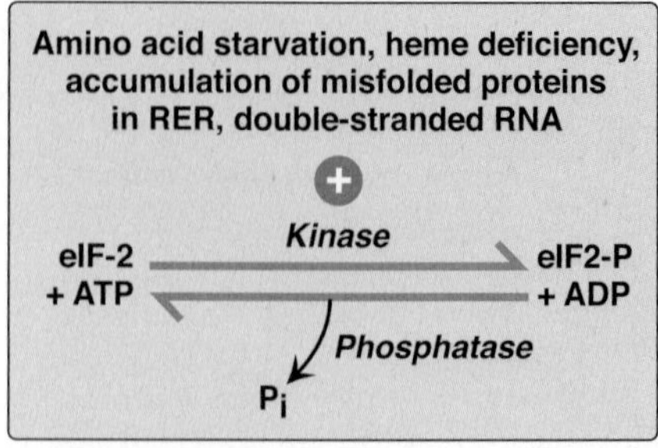

Figure 32.16
Regulation of translation initiation in eukaryotes by phosphorylation of eukaryotic translation initiation factor, eIF-2. RER = rough endoplasmic reticulum; ADP = adenosine diphosphate; P_i = inorganic phosphate.

translation initiation factor, eIF-2 (Figure 32.16). Phosphorylation of eIF-2 inhibits its function and so inhibits translation at the initiation step (see p. 443). [Note: Phosphorylation of eIF-2 prevents its reactivation by inhibiting GDP–GTP exchange.] Phosphorylation is catalyzed by *kinases* that are activated in response to environmental conditions, such as amino acid starvation, heme deficiency in erythroblasts, the presence of double-stranded RNA (signaling viral infection), and the accumulation of misfolded proteins in the rough endoplasmic reticulum.

D. Regulation through modifications to DNA

Gene expression in eukaryotes is also influenced by the availability of DNA to the transcriptional apparatus, the amount of DNA, and the arrangement of DNA. [Note: Localized transitions between the B and Z forms of DNA (see p. 398) can also affect gene expression.]

1. **Access to DNA:** In eukaryotes, DNA is found complexed with histone and nonhistone proteins to form chromatin (see p. 409). Transcriptionally active, decondensed chromatin (euchromatin) differs from the more condensed, inactive form (heterochromatin) in a number of ways. Active chromatin contains histone proteins that have been covalently modified at their amino terminal ends by acetylation or phosphorylation (see p. 422 for a discussion of histone acetylation/deacetylation by the *histone acetyltransferase* and *histone deacetylase* enzymes). Such modifications decrease the positive charge of these basic proteins, thereby decreasing the strength of their association with negatively charged DNA. This relaxes the nucleosome (see p. 409), allowing transcription factors access to specific regions on the DNA. Nucleosomes can also be repositioned, an ATP-requiring process called chromatin remodeling. Another difference between transcriptionally active and inactive chromatin is the extent of methylation of cytosine bases in CG-rich regions (CpG islands) in the promoter region of many genes. Methylation is by *methyltransferases* that use S-adenosylmethionine as the methyl donor (Figure 32.17). Transcriptionally active genes are less methylated (hypomethylated) than their inactive counterparts, suggesting that DNA hypermethylation silences gene expression. [Note: Modification of histones and methylation of DNA are epigenetic. They are heritable changes in DNA that alter gene expression without altering the base sequence.]

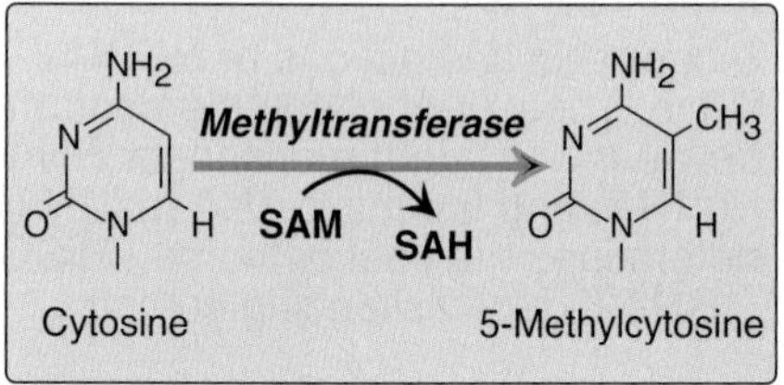

Figure 32.17
The methylation of cytosine in eukaryotic DNA. SAM = S-adenosylmethionine; SAH = S-adenosylhomocysteine.

2. **Amount of DNA:** A change up or down in the number of copies of a gene can affect the amount of gene product produced. An increase in copy number (gene amplification) has contributed to increased genomic complexity and is still a normal developmental process in certain nonmammalian species. In mammals, however, gene amplification is seen with some diseases and in response to particular chemotherapeutic drugs such as methotrexate, an inhibitor of the enzyme *dihydrofolate reductase* (*DHFR*), required for the synthesis of thymidine triphosphate (TTP) in the pyrimidine biosynthetic pathway (see p. 304). TTP is essential for DNA synthesis. Gene amplification results in an increase in the number of *DHFR* genes and resistance to the drug, allowing TTP to be made.

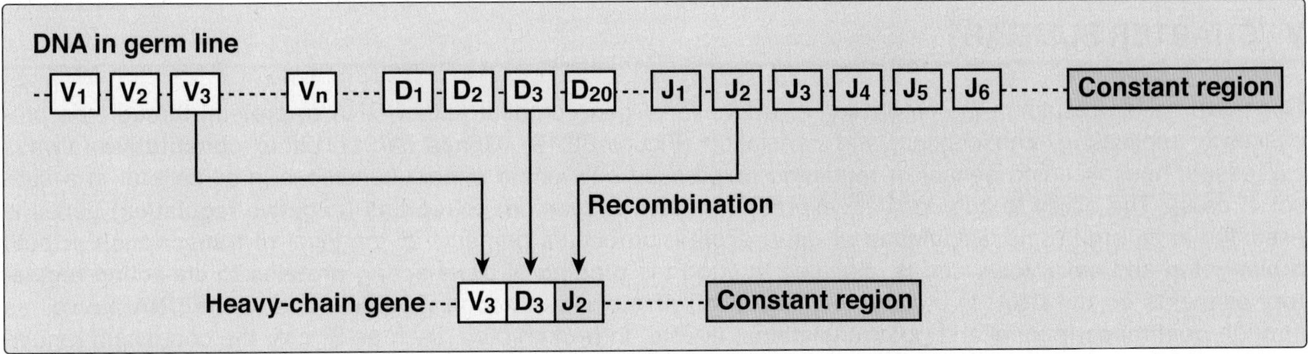

Figure 32.18
DNA rearrangements in the generation of immunoglobulins. V= variable; D = diversity; J = joining.

3. **Arrangement of DNA:** The process by which immunoglobulins (antibodies) are produced by B lymphocytes involves permanent rearrangements of the DNA in these cells. The immunoglobulins (for example, IgG) consist of two light and two heavy chains, with each chain containing regions of variable and constant amino acid sequence. The variable region is the result of somatic recombination of segments within both the light- and the heavy-chain genes. During B-lymphocyte development, single variable (V), diversity (D), and joining (J) gene segments are brought together through gene rearrangement to form a unique variable region (Figure 32.18). This process allows the generation of 10^9–10^{11} different immunoglobulins from a single gene, providing the diversity needed for the recognition of an enormous number of antigens. [Note: The shift from the membrane-bound form to the secreted form of immunoglobulins involves poly-A site choice (see p. 426).]

4. **Mobile DNA elements:** Transposons (Tns) are mobile segments of DNA that move in an essentially random manner from one site to another on the same or a different chromosome. Movement is mediated by *transposase*, an enzyme encoded by the Tn itself. Movement can be direct, in which *transposase* cuts out and then inserts the Tn at a new site, or replicative, in which the Tn is copied and the copy inserted elsewhere while the original remains in place. In eukaryotes, including humans, replicative transposition frequently involves an RNA intermediate, in which case the Tn is called a retrotransposon (see p. 408). Transposition has contributed to structural variation in the genome but also has the potential to alter gene expression and even to cause disease. Although the vast majority of retrotransposons in the human genome have lost the ability to move, some are still active. Their transposition is thought to be the basis for some rare cases of hemophilia A and Duchenne muscular dystrophy. [Note: The growing problem of antibiotic-resistant bacteria is a consequence, at least in part, of the exchange of plasmids among bacterial cells. If the plasmids contain Tns carrying antibiotic resistance genes, the recipient bacteria gain resistance to one or more antimicrobial drugs.]

V. CHAPTER SUMMARY

Gene expression results in the production of a functional gene product (either RNA or protein) through the processes of replication, transcription, and translation (Figure 32.19). **Genes** can be either **constitutive** (always expressed, housekeeping genes) or **regulated** (expressed only under certain conditions in all cells or in a subset of cells). The ability to appropriately **express** (**positive regulation**) or **repress** (**negative regulation**) genes is essential in all organisms. **Regulation** of gene expression occurs primarily at the level of **transcription** in both **prokaryotes** and **eukaryotes** and is mediated through the **binding** of **trans-acting proteins to cis-acting regulatory elements on the DNA**. In **eukaryotes**, regulation also occurs through **modifications to the DNA** as well as through **posttranscriptional** and **posttranslational events**. In **prokaryotes**, such as E. coli, the coordinate regulation of genes whose protein products are required for a particular process is achieved through **operons** (groups of genes sequentially arranged on the chromosome along with the regulatory elements that determine their transcription). The **lac operon** contains the Z, Y, and A structural genes, the protein products of which are needed for the catabolism of lactose. It is subject to negative and positive regulation. When **glucose is available**, the **operon is repressed** by the binding of the **repressor protein** (the product of the lacI gene) to the **operator**, thus preventing transcription. When **only lactose is present**, the **operon is induced** by an isomer of lactose (**allolactose**) that binds the repressor protein, preventing it from binding to the operator. In addition, **cyclic AMP binds the catabolite-activator protein (CAP)**, and the complex **binds the DNA** at the **CAP site**. This **increases promoter efficiency** and results in the expression of the structural genes through the production of a **polycistronic messenger RNA (mRNA)**. When both **glucose and lactose are present**, glucose prevents formation of cAMP and **transcription** of these genes is **negligible**. The **trp operon** contains genes needed for the synthesis of tryptophan (Trp), and, like the lac operon, it is regulated by **negative control**. Unlike the lac operon, it is **also regulated by attenuation**, in which mRNA synthesis that escaped repression by Trp is terminated before completion. **Transcription** of **ribosomal RNA** and **transfer RNA** is selectively **inhibited** in prokaryotes by the **stringent response to amino acid starvation**. **Translation** is also a site of **prokaryotic gene regulation**: Excess ribosomal proteins bind the Shine-Dalgarno sequence on their own polycistronic mRNA, preventing ribosomes from binding. **Gene regulation** is **more complex in eukaryotes**. **Operons** typically are **not present**, but **coordinate regulation** of the transcription of genes located on different chromosomes can be achieved through the **binding of trans-acting proteins to cis-acting elements**. In **multicellular organisms**, **hormones** can **cause coordinated regulation**, either through the **binding** of the **hormone receptor–hormone complex to the DNA** (as with steroid hormones) or through the **binding of a protein** that is activated in **response to a second messenger** (as with glucagon). In each case, binding to DNA is mediated through structural motifs such as the **zinc finger. Co- and posttranscriptional regulation** is also seen in **eukaryotes** and includes **splice-site choice**, **polyA-site choice**, **mRNA editing**, and variations in **mRNA stability** as seen with transferrin receptor synthesis and with **RNA interference**. **Regulation at the translational level** can be caused by the **phosphorylation and inhibition of eukaryotic initiation factor, eIF-2**. Gene expression in eukaryotes is also influenced by availability of DNA to the transcriptional apparatus, the amount of DNA, and the arrangement of the DNA. **Epigenetic changes** to histone proteins and DNA also influence gene expression.

Study Questions

Choose the one best answer.

32.1 Which of the following mutations is most likely to result in reduced expression of the lac operon?

A. cya^- (no adenylyl cyclase made)

B. i^- (no repressor protein made)

C. O^c (operator cannot bind repressor protein)

D. One resulting in functionally impaired glucose transport

Correct answer = A. In the absence of glucose, adenylyl cyclase makes cyclic AMP, which forms a complex with the catabolite activator protein (CAP). The cAMP–CAP complex binds the CAP site on the DNA, causing RNA polymerase to bind more efficiently to the lac operon promoter, thereby increasing expression of the operon. With cya^- mutations, adenylyl cyclase is not made, and so the operon is unable to be turned on even when glucose is absent and lactose is present. The absence of a repressor protein or decreased ability of the repressor to bind the operator results in constitutive (constant) expression of the lac operon.

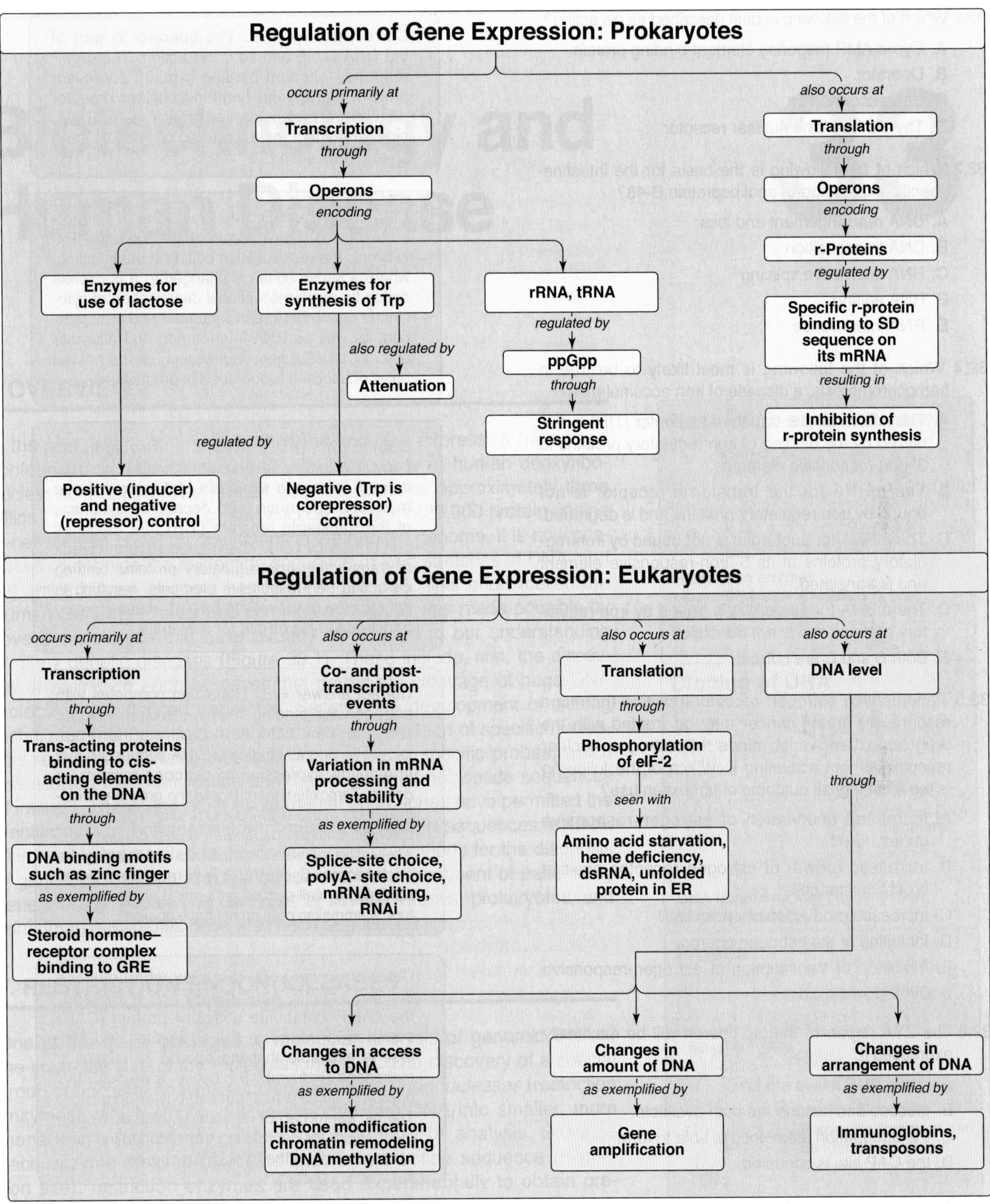

Figure 32.19
Summary of key concepts for the regulation of gene expression. GRE = glucocorticoid-response element; ppGpp = polyphosphorylated guanosine; r-protein = ribosomal protein; SD sequence = Shine-Dalgarno sequence; RNAi = RNA interference; eIF-2 = eukaryotic initiation factor 2.

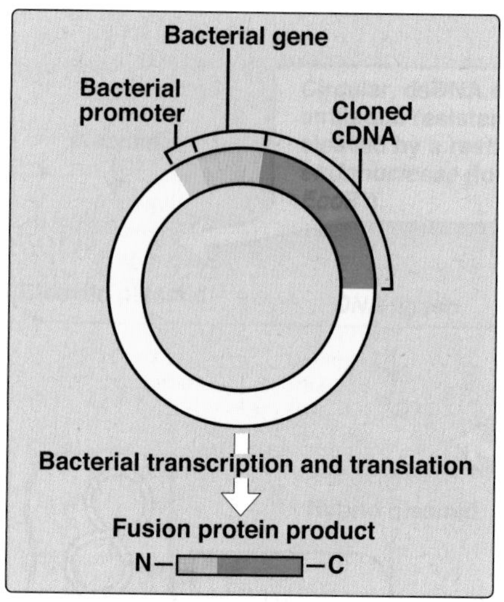

Figure 33.8
An expression vector. The complementary DNA (cDNA) is inserted within a bacterial gene, downstream of the promoter sequence, and the sequences for the messenger RNA Shine-Dalgarno sequence, start codon, and codons for the first few amino acids of the bacterial protein. The product is a fusion protein that contains just some amino acids of the bacterial protein ■ and all the amino acids of the cDNA-encoded protein ■.

the resulting mRNA molecule. The cDNA is inserted downstream of the promoter and within a gene for a protein that is expressed in the bacterium (for example, lacZ; see p.450), such that the mRNA produced contains an SD sequence, a few codons for the bacterial protein, and all the codons for the eukaryotic protein. This allows for more efficient expression and results in the production of a fusion protein. [Note: Therapeutic human insulin is made in bacteria through this technology. However, the extensive co- and posttranslational modifications (see p. 443) required for most other human proteins (for example, blood clotting factors) necessitates the use of eukaryotic, even mammalian, hosts.]

C. Sequencing of cloned DNA fragments

The base sequence of DNA fragments that have been cloned can be determined. The original procedure for this purpose was the Sanger dideoxy method illustrated in Figure 33.9. In this method, the single-stranded DNA (ssDNA) to be sequenced is used as the template for DNA synthesis by *DNA polymerase*. A radiolabeled primer complementary to the 3'-end of the target DNA is added, along with the four deoxyribonucleoside triphosphates (dNTPs). The sample is divided into four reaction tubes, and a small amount of one of the four dideoxyribonucleoside triphosphates (ddNTPs) is added to each tube. Because it contains no 3'-hydroxyl group, incorporation of a ddNMP terminates elongation at that point. The products of this reaction, then, consist of a mixture of DNA strands of different lengths, each terminating at a specific base. Separation of the various DNA products by size using polyacrylamide gel electrophoresis, followed by autoradiography, yields a pattern of bands from which the DNA base sequence can be read. [Note: The shorter the fragment, the farther it travels on the gel, with the shortest fragment representing that which was made first (that is, the 5'-end).] In place of a labeled primer, a mixture of the four ddNTPs linked to different fluorescent dyes and in a single reaction tube is now commonly used. [Note: The Human Genome Project used highly automated variations of this technique to determine the base sequence of the human genome.] Advances in sequencing technology, so-called next generation, or deep sequencing, now allow the sequencing of longer segments in a shorter time with increased fidelity and decreased cost through the simultaneous (parallel) sequencing of many DNA pieces.

IV. PROBES

Cleavage of large DNA molecules by restriction enzymes produces a bewildering array of fragments. How can the DNA sequence of interest be picked out of a mixture of thousands or even millions of irrelevant DNA fragments? The answer lies in the use of a probe, a short piece of ssDNA or RNA, labeled with a radioisotope, such as ^{32}P, or with a nonradioactive molecule, such as biotin or a fluorescent dye. The sequence of a probe is complementary to a sequence in the DNA of interest, called the target DNA. Probes are used to identify which band on a gel or which clone in a library contains the target DNA, a process called screening.

A. Hybridization of a probe to DNA fragments

The utility of probes hinges on the phenomenon of hybridization (or annealing) in which a probe containing a complementary sequence binds a single-stranded sequence of a target DNA. ssDNA, produced by alkaline denaturation of dsDNA, is first bound to a solid support, such as a nitrocellulose membrane. The immobilized DNA strands are prevented from self-annealing but are available for hybridization to the exogenous, radiolabeled, ssDNA probe. The extent of hybridization is measured by the retention of radioactivity on the membrane. Excess probe molecules that do not hybridize are removed by washing the membrane.

B. Synthetic oligonucleotide probes

If the sequence of all or part of the target DNA is known, short, single-stranded oligonucleotide probes can be synthesized that

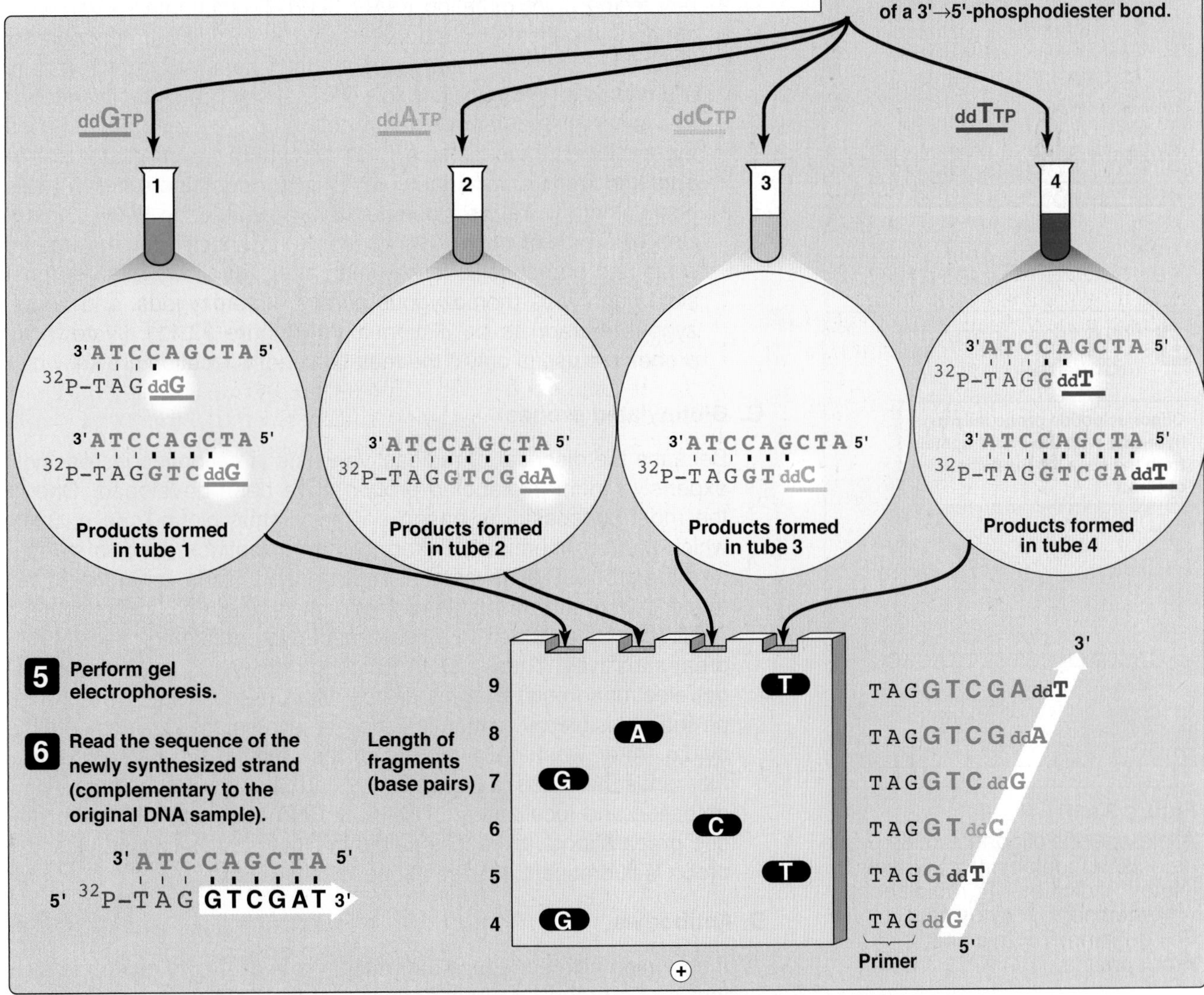

Figure 33.9
DNA sequencing by the Sanger dideoxy method. [Note: The original method utilized a radiolabeled primer. Fluorescent dye-labeled ddNTPs are now commonly used.] A = adenine; C = cytosine; G = guanine; T = thymine; d = deoxy; dd = dideoxy.

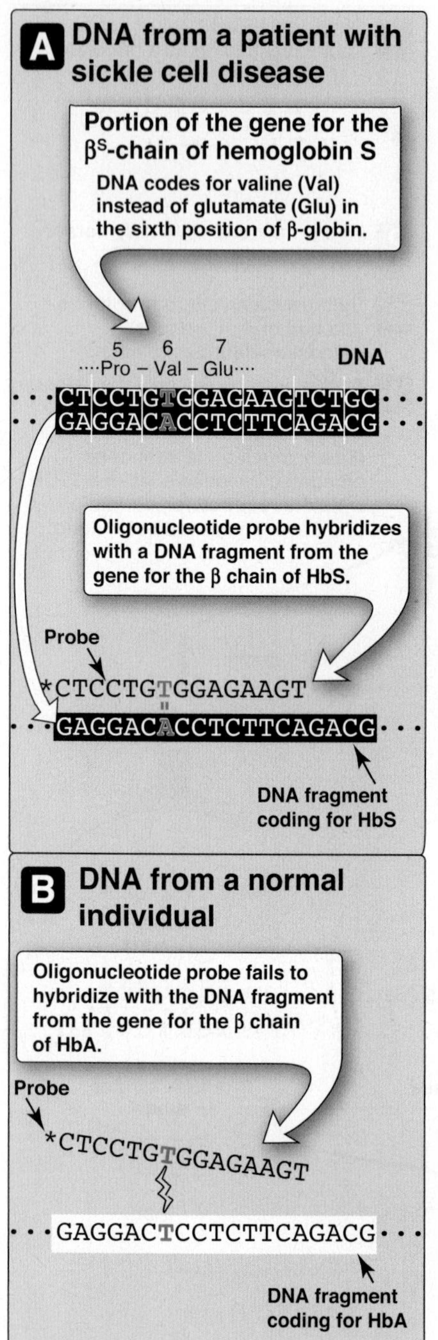

Figure 33.10
Allele-specific oligonucleotide probe detects hemoglobin (Hb) S allele. [Note: * indicates ^{32}P radiolabel.] A = adenine; C = cytosine; G = guanine; T = thymine; Pro = proline.

are complementary to a small region of the gene of interest. If the sequence of the gene is unknown, the amino acid sequence of the protein, the final gene product, may be used to construct a nucleic acid probe using the genetic code as a guide. Because of the degeneracy of the genetic code, it is necessary to synthesize several oligonucleotides. [Note: Oligonucleotides can be used to detect single-base changes in the sequence to which they are complementary. In contrast, cDNA probes contain many thousands of bases, and their binding to a target DNA with a single-base change is unaffected.]

1. **Detecting the β^S-globin mutation:** A synthetic allele-specific oligonucleotide (ASO) probe can be used to detect the presence of the sickle cell mutation in the β-globin gene (Figure 33.10). DNA, isolated from leukocytes and amplified, is denatured and applied to a membrane. A radiolabeled oligonucleotide probe, complementary to the point mutation (GAG $\rightarrow$ GTG, glutamate $\rightarrow$ valine) at codon 6 in patients with the β^S gene, is applied to the membrane. DNA isolated from a heterozygous individual (sickle cell trait) or a homozygous patient (sickle cell disease) contains a sequence that is complementary to the probe, and a double-stranded hybrid forms that can be detected by electrophoresis. In contrast, DNA obtained from normal individuals is not complementary at this positon and, therefore, does not form a hybrid (see Figure 33.10). Use of a pair of such ASO probes (one specific for the normal allele and one specific for the mutant allele) allows all three possible genotypes (homozygous normal, heterozygous, and homozygous mutant) to be distinguished (Figure 33.11). [Note: ASO probes are useful only if the mutation and its location are known.]

C. Biotinylated probes

Because the disposal of radioactive waste is becoming increasingly expensive, nonradiolabeled probes have been developed. One of the most successful is based on the vitamin biotin (see p. 381), which can be chemically linked to the nucleotides used to synthesize the probe. Biotin was chosen because it binds very tenaciously to avidin, a readily available protein contained in chicken egg whites. Avidin can be attached to a fluorescent dye detectable optically with great sensitivity. Thus, a DNA fragment (displayed, for example, by gel electrophoresis) that hybridizes with the biotinylated probe can be made visible by immersing the gel in a solution of dye-coupled avidin. After washing away the excess avidin, the DNA fragment that binds the probe is fluorescent. [Note: Labeled probes can allow detection and localization of DNA or RNA sequences in cell or tissue preparations, a process called in situ hybridization (ISH). If the probe is fluorescent, the technique is called FISH.]

D. Antibodies

If no amino acid sequence information is available to guide the synthesis of a probe for direct detection of the DNA of interest, a gene can be identified indirectly by cloning cDNA in an expression vector that allows the cloned cDNA to be transcribed and translated. A labeled antibody is used to identify which bacterial colony produces the protein and, therefore, contains the cDNA of interest.

V. SOUTHERN BLOTTING

Southern blotting is a technique that combines the use of restriction enzymes, electrophoresis, and DNA probes to generate, separate, and detect pieces of DNA.

A. Experimental procedure

This method, named after its inventor, Edward Southern, involves the following steps (Figure 33.12). First, DNA is extracted from cells, for example, a patient's leukocytes. Second, the DNA is cleaved into many fragments using a restriction enzyme. Third, the resulting fragments are separated on the basis of size by electrophoresis. [Note: Because the large fragments move more slowly than the smaller ones, the lengths of the fragments, usually expressed as the number of base pairs, can be calculated from comparison of the position of the band relative to standard fragments of known size.] The DNA fragments in the gel are denatured and transferred (blotted) to a nitrocellulose membrane for analysis. If the original DNA represents the individual's entire genome, the enzymic digest contains a million or more fragments. The gene of interest is on only one (or a few if the gene itself was fragmented) of these pieces of DNA. If all the DNA segments were visualized by a nonspecific technique, they would appear as an unresolved blur of overlapping bands. To avoid this, the last step in Southern blotting uses a probe to identify the DNA fragments of interest. The patterns observed on Southern blot analysis depend both on the specific *restriction endonuclease* and on the probe used to visualize the restriction fragments. [Note: Variants of the Southern blot have been facetiously named "Northern" (electrophoresis of mRNA followed by hybridization with a specific probe), and "Western" (electrophoresis of protein followed by detection with an antibody directed against the protein of interest), neither of which relates to anyone's name or to points of the compass.]

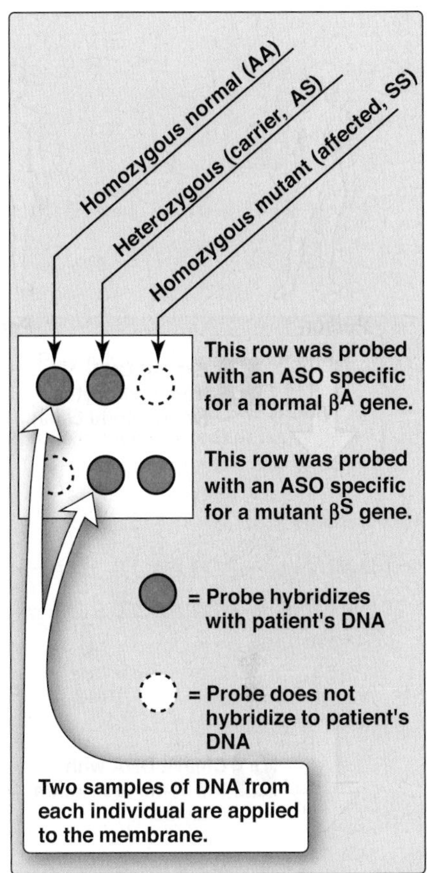

Figure 33.11
Allele-specific oligonucleotide (ASO) probes used to detect the sickle cell mutation and differentiate between sickle cell trait and disease.

B. Detection of mutations

Southern blotting can detect DNA mutations such as large insertions, deletions, or rearrangements of nucleotides. It can also detect point mutations (replacement of one nucleotide by another; see p. 433) that cause the loss or gain of restriction sites. Such mutations cause the pattern of bands to differ from those seen with a normal gene. Longer fragments are generated if a restriction site is lost. For example, in Figure 33.12, Person 2 lacks a restriction site present in Person 1. Alternatively, the point mutation may create a new cleavage site with the production of shorter fragments. [Note: Most sequence differences at restriction sites are harmless variations in the DNA.]

VI. RESTRICTION FRAGMENT LENGTH POLYMORPHISM

It has been estimated that the genomes of any two unrelated people are 99.5% identical. With 6 billion bp in the diploid human genome, that represents variation in about 30 million bp. These genome variations are the result of mutations that lead to polymorphisms. A polymorphism is a change in genotype that can result in no change in phenotype or a change in phenotype that is harmless; causes increased susceptibility

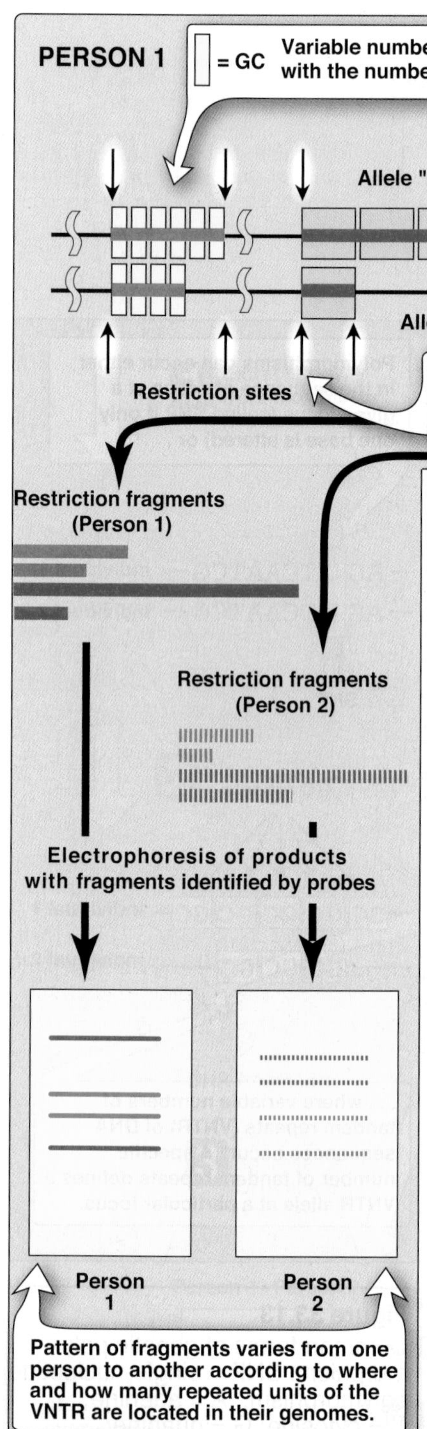

Figure 33.14
Restriction fragment length polymorphism of variable number tandem repeats (VNTR). For each person, a pair of homologous chromosomes is shown.

fewer fragments are produced by enzymic cleavage. An individual who is heterozygous for a polymorphism has a sequence variation in the DNA of one chromosome and not in the homologous chromosome. In such individuals, each chromosome can be traced from parent to offspring by determining the presence or absence of the polymorphism.

C. Prenatal diagnosis

Families with a history of severe genetic disease, such as an affected previous child or near relative, may wish to determine the presence of the disorder in a developing fetus. Prenatal diagnosis, in association with genetic counseling, allows for an informed reproductive decision if the fetus is affected.

1. **Methods available:** The available diagnostic methods vary in sensitivity and specificity. Visualization of the fetus, for example, by ultrasound or fiberoptic devices (fetoscopy), is useful only if the genetic abnormality results in gross anatomic defects (for example, neural tube defects). The chemical composition of the amniotic fluid can also provide diagnostic clues. For example, the presence of high levels of α-fetoprotein is associated with neural tube defects. Fetal cells obtained from amniotic fluid or from biopsy of the chorionic villi can be used for karyotyping, which assesses the morphology of metaphase chromosomes. Staining and cell sorting techniques permit the rapid identification of trisomies and translocations that produce an extra chromosome or chromosomes of abnormal lengths. However, molecular analysis of fetal DNA provides the most detailed genetic picture.

2. **Sources of DNA:** DNA may be obtained from white blood cells, amniotic fluid, or chorionic villi (Figure 33.15). For amniotic fluid, it used to be necessary to grow cells in culture for two to three weeks in order to have sufficient DNA for analysis. The ability to amplify DNA by PCR (see p. 479) has dramatically shortened the time needed for a DNA analysis.

3. **Direct diagnosis of sickle cell anemia using RFLP:** The genetic disorders of hemoglobin (Hb) are the most common genetic diseases in humans. In the case of sickle cell anemia (Figure 33.16),

the mutation that gives rise to the disease is actually one and the same mutation that gives rise to the polymorphism. Direct detection by RFLP of diseases that result from point mutations is, however, limited to only a few genetic diseases.

a. **Early efforts to diagnose sickle cell anemia:** In the past, prenatal diagnosis of hemoglobinopathies involved the determination of the amount and kinds of Hb synthesized in red cells obtained from fetal blood. However, the invasive procedures to obtain fetal blood have a high mortality rate (approximately 5%), and diagnosis cannot be carried out until late in the second trimester of pregnancy when HbS begins to be produced.

b. **RFLP analysis:** Sickle cell anemia is an example of a genetic disease caused by a point mutation (see p. 35). The sequence altered by the mutation abolishes the recognition site of the *restriction endonuclease Mst*II: CCTNAGG (where N is any nucleotide; see Figure 33.16). Thus, the A-to-T mutation in codon 6 of the β^S-globin gene eliminates a cleavage site for the enzyme. Normal DNA digested with *Mst*II yields a 1.15-kb fragment, whereas a 1.35-kb fragment is generated from the β^S gene as a result of the loss of one *Mst*II cleavage site. Diagnostic techniques that allow analysis of fetal DNA from amniotic cells or chorionic villus sampling rather than fetal blood have proved valuable because they provide safe, early detection of sickle cell anemia as well as other genetic diseases. [Note: Genetic disorders caused by insertions or deletions between two restriction sites, rather than by the creation or loss of cleavage sites, will also display RFLP.]

4. **Indirect, prenatal diagnosis of phenylketonuria using RFLP:** The gene for *phenylalanine hydroxylase* (*PAH*), deficient in phenylketonuria ([PKU] see p. 270), is located on chromosome 12. It spans about 90 kb of genomic DNA and contains 13 exons separated by introns (Figure 33.17; see p. 426 for a description of exons and introns). Mutations in *PAH* usually do not directly affect any *restriction endonuclease* recognition site. To establish a diagnostic protocol for this disease, DNA of family members of the affected individual must be analyzed. The goal is to identify genetic markers (RFLPs) that are tightly linked to the disease trait. Once these markers are identified, RFLP analysis can be used to carry out prenatal diagnosis.

a. **Identification of the gene:** Determinining the presence of the mutant gene by identifying the polymorphism marker can be done if two conditions are satisfied. First, if the polymorphism is closely linked to a disease-producing mutation, the defective gene can be traced by detection of the RFLP. For example, if DNA from a family carrying a disease-causing gene is examined by restriction enzyme cleavage and Southern blotting, it is sometimes possible to find an RFLP that is consistently associated with that gene (that is, they show close linkage and are coinherited). It is then possible to trace the inheritance of the gene within a family without knowledge of the nature of the genetic defect or its precise location in the genome. [Note: The

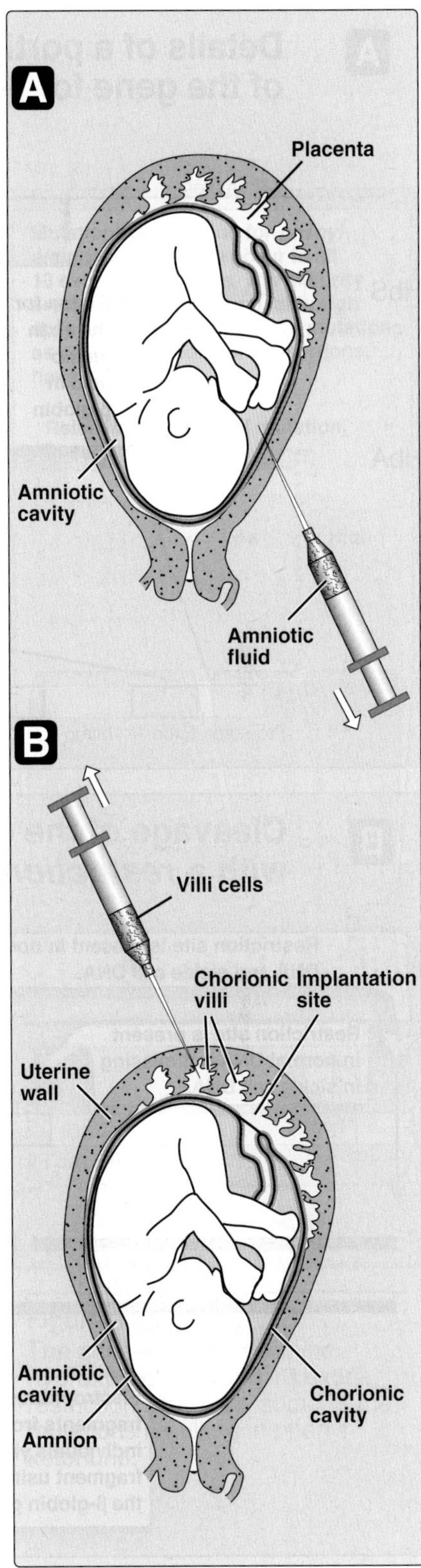

Figure 33.15
Sampling of fetal cells. A. Amniotic fluid. B. Chorionic villus.

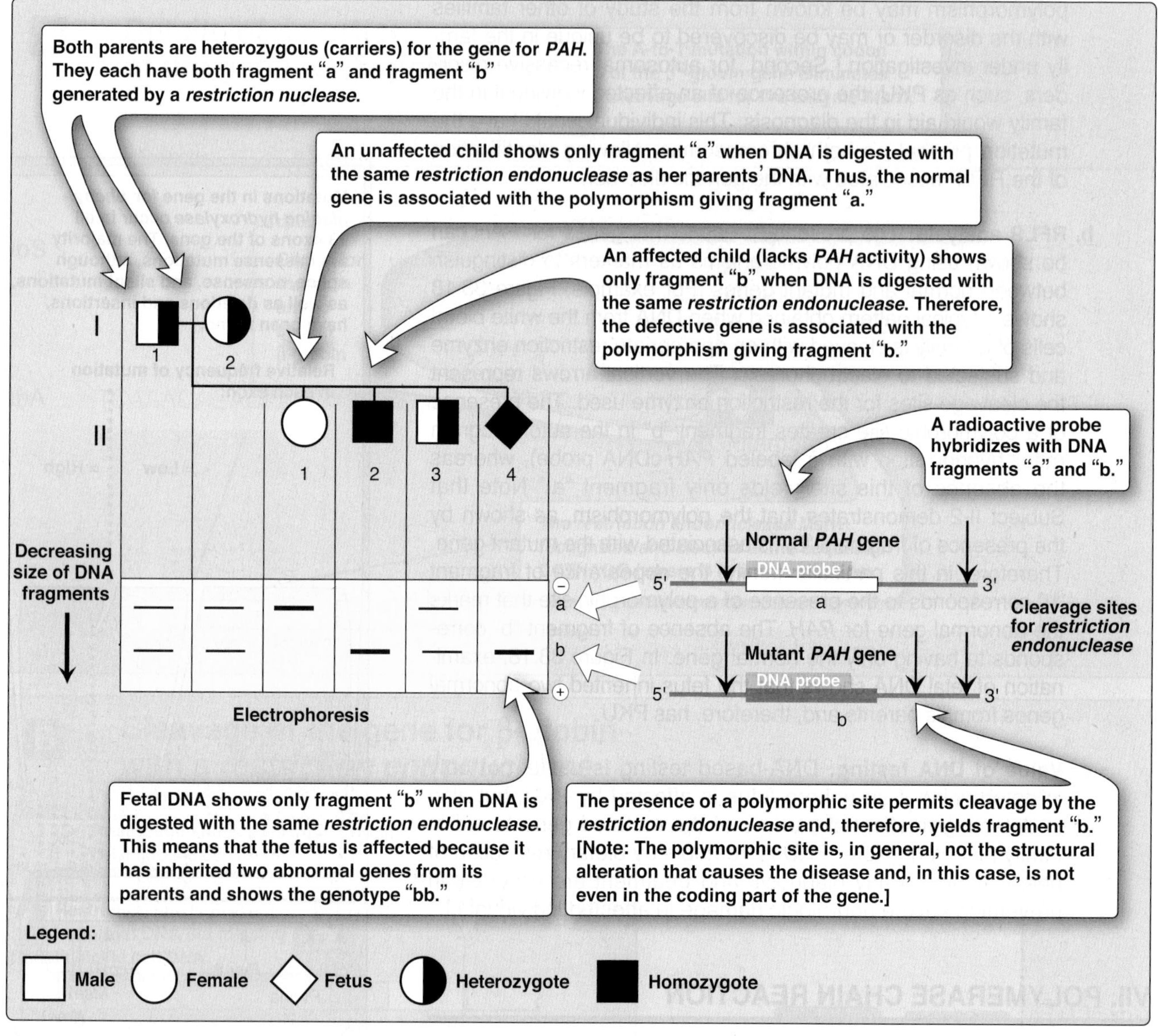

Figure 33.18
Analysis of restriction fragment length polymorphism in a family with a child affected by phenylketonuria (PKU), an autosomal recessive disease. The molecular defect in the gene for *phenylalanine hydroxylase* (*PAH*) in the family is not known. The family wanted to know if the current pregnancy would be affected by PKU.

1. **Primer construction:** It is not necessary to know the nucleotide sequence of the target DNA in the PCR method. However, it is necessary to know the nucleotide sequence of short segments on each side of the target DNA. These stretches, called flanking sequences, bracket the DNA sequence of interest. The nucleotide sequences of the flanking regions are used to construct two, single-stranded oligonucleotides, usually 20–35 nucleotides long, which are complementary to the respective flanking sequences. The 3'-hydroxyl end of each oligonucleotide points toward the target sequence (see Figure 33.19). These synthetic oligonucleotides function as primers in PCR reactions.

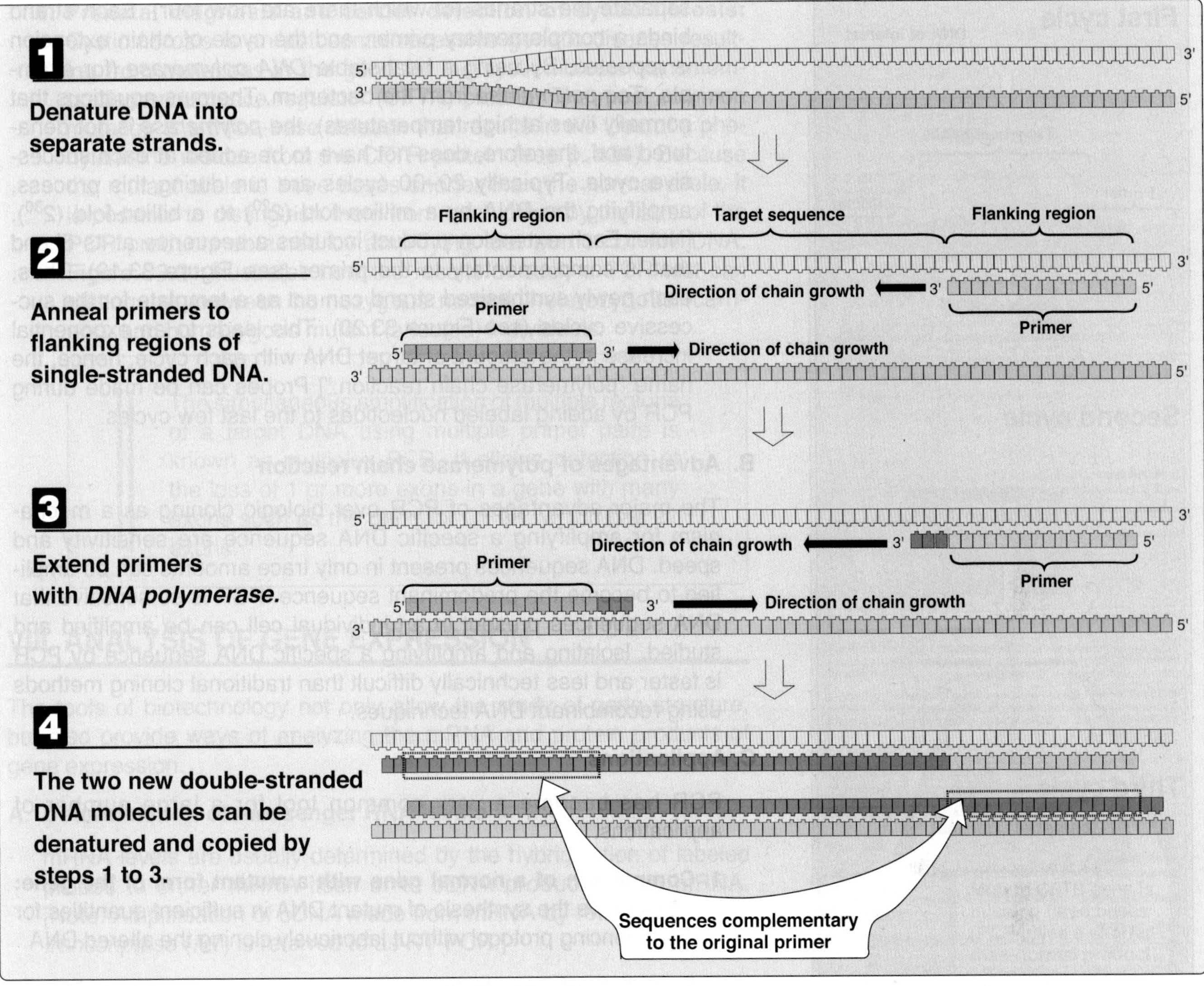

Figure 33.19
Steps in one cycle of the polymerase chain reaction.

2. **Denature the DNA:** The DNA to be amplified is heated to separate the double-stranded target DNA into single strands.

3. **Annealing of primers to single-stranded DNA:** The separated strands are cooled and allowed to anneal to the two primers (one for each strand).

4. **Chain extension:** *DNA polymerase* and deoxyribonucleoside triphosphates (in excess) are added to the mixture to initiate the synthesis of two new strands complementary to the original DNA strands. *DNA polymerase* adds nucleotides to the 3'-hydroxyl end of the primer, and strand growth extends across the target DNA, making complementary copies of the target. [Note: PCR products can be several thousand bp long.] At the completion of one cycle of replication, the reaction mixture is heated again to

33.2 An Ashkenazi Jewish couple brings their 6-month-old son to you for evaluation of listlessness, poor head control, and a fixed gaze. You determine that he has Tay-Sachs disease, an autosomal recessive disorder. The couple also has a daughter. The family's pedigree is shown to the right, along with Southern blots of a restriction fragment length polymorphism very closely linked to the gene for hexosaminidase A, which is defective in Tay-Sachs. Which of the statements below is most accurate with respect to the daughter?

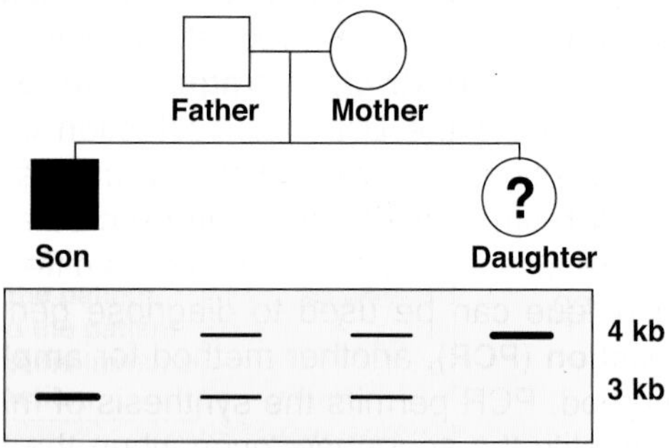

A. She has a 25% chance of having Tay-Sachs disease.
B. She has a 50% chance of having Tay-Sachs disease.
C. She has Tay-Sachs disease.
D. She is a carrier for Tay-Sachs disease.
E. She is homozygous normal.

Correct answer = E. Because they have an affected son, both the biological father and mother must be carriers for this disease. The affected son must have inherited a mutant allele from each parent. Because he shows only the 3-kilobase (kb) band on the Southern blot, the mutant allele for this disease must be linked to the 3-kb band. The normal allele must be linked to the 4-kb band, and, because the daughter inherited only the 4-kb band, she must be homozygous normal for the hexosaminidase A gene.

33.3 A physician would like to determine the global patterns of gene expression in two different types of tumor cells in order to develop the most appropriate form of chemotherapy for each patient. Which of the following techniques would be most appropriate for this purpose?

A. Enzyme-linked immunosorbent assay
B. Microarray
C. Northern blot
D. Southern blot
E. Western blot

Correct answer = B. Microarray analysis allows the determination of messenger RNA (mRNA) production (gene expression) from thousands of genes at once. A Northern blot only measures mRNA production from one gene at a time. Western blots and enzyme-linked immunosorbent assay measure protein production (also gene expression) but only from one gene at a time. Southern blots are used to analyze DNA, not DNA expression.

33.4 A 2-week-old infant is diagnosed with a urea cycle defect. Enzymic analysis showed no activity for ornithine transcarbamoylase (OTC), an enzyme of the cycle. Molecular analysis revealed that the messenger RNA (mRNA) product of the gene for OTC was identical to that of a control. Which of the techniques listed below was most likely used to analyze mRNA?

A. Dideoxy chain termination
B. Northern blot
C. Polymerase chain reaction
D. Southern blot
E. Western blot

Correct answer = B. Northern blot allows analysis of the messenger RNA present (expressed) in a particular cell or tissue. Southern blot is used for DNA analysis, whereas Western blot is used for protein analysis. Dideoxy chain termination is used to sequence DNA. Polymerase chain reaction is used to generate multiple, identical copies of a DNA sequence in vitro.

33.5 For the patient above, which phase of the central dogma was most likely affected?

Correct answer = Translation. The gene is present and is able to be expressed as evidenced by messenger RNA production. The lack of enzymic activity means that some aspect of protein synthesis is affected.

APPENDIX
Clinical Cases

I. INTEGRATIVE CASES

Metabolic pathways, initially presented in isolation, are, in fact, linked to form an interconnected network. The following four integrative case studies illustrate how a perturbation in one process can result in perturbations in other processes of the network.

CASE 1: CHEST PAIN

Patient Presentation: A 35-year-old man with severe substernal chest pain of about 2 hours' duration is brought by ambulance to his local hospital at 5 a.m. The pain is accompanied by dyspnea (shortness of breath), diaphoresis (sweating), and nausea.

Focused History: The patient reports episodes of exertional chest pain in the last few months, but they were less severe and of short duration. He smokes (2–3 packs per day), drinks alcohol only rarely, eats a "typical" diet, and walks with his wife most weekends. His blood pressure has been normal. Family history reveals that his father and paternal aunt died of heart disease at age 45 years and 39 years, respectively. His mother and younger (age 31 years) brother are said to be in good health.

Physical Examination (Pertinent Findings): The patient is pale and clammy and is in distress due to chest pain. Blood pressure and respiratory rate are elevated. Lipid deposits are noted on the periphery of his corneas (corneal arcus; see left Image) and under the skin on and around his eyelids (xanthelasmas; see right Image). No deposits on his tendons (xanthomas) are detected.

Corneal arcus

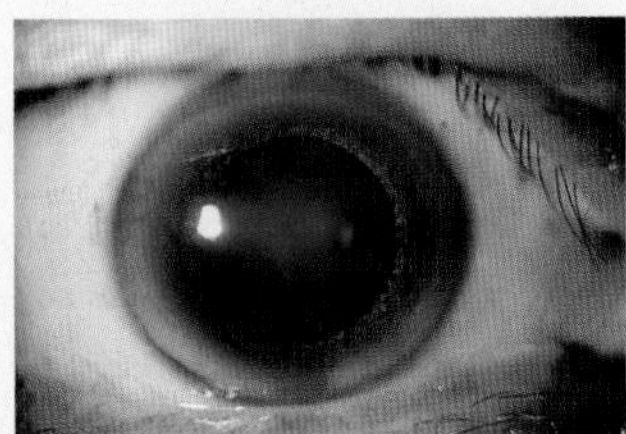

Xanthelasmas

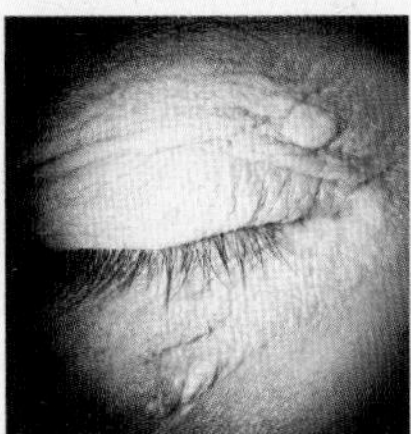

Pertinent Test Results: The patient's electrocardiogram is consistent with a myocardial infarction (MI). Angiography reveals areas of severe stenosis (narrowing) of several coronary arteries. Initial results from the clinical laboratory include:

	Patient	Reference Range
Troponin	+	0
Total cholesterol	365 mg/dl (**H**)	<200
Low-density lipoprotein (LDL)-cholesterol	304 mg/dl (**H**)	<130
High-density lipoprotein (HDL)-cholesterol	38 mg/dl (**L**)	>45
Triglycerides (triacylglycerols)	115 mg/dl	<150

H = High; **L** = Low. [Note: The patient had not eaten for about 8 hours prior to the blood draw.]

Diagnosis: MI, the irreversible necrosis (death) of heart muscle secondary to ischemia (decreased blood supply) is caused by the occlusion (blockage) of a blood vessel most commonly by a blood clot (thrombus). The patient subsequently is determined to have heterozygous familial hypercholesterolemia (FH), also known as type IIa hyperlipidemia.

Immediate Treatment: The patient is given O_2, a vasodilator, pain medication, and drugs to dissolve blood clots (thrombolytics) and reduce clotting (antithrombotics).

Long-term Treatment: Lipid-lowering drugs (for example, high-potency statins, bile acid [BA] sequestrants, and niacin), daily aspirin; β-blockers; and counseling on nutrition, exercise, and smoking cessation would be part of the long-term treatment plan.

Prognosis: Patients with heterozygous FH have ~50% of the normal number of functional LDL receptors and a hypercholesterolemia (two to three times normal) that puts them at high risk (>50% risk) for premature coronary heart disease (CHD). However, less than 5% of patients with hypercholesterolemia have FH.

Nutrition Nugget: Dietary recommendations for individuals with heterozygous FH include limiting saturated fats to <7% of total calories and cholesterol to <200 mg/day; substituting unsaturated fats for saturated fats; and adding soluble fiber (10–20 g/day) and plant sterols (2 g/day) for their hypocholesterolemic effects. Fiber increases BA excretion. This results in increased hepatic uptake of cholesterol-rich LDLs to supply the substrate for BA synthesis. Plant sterols decrease cholesterol absorption in the intestine.

Genetics Gem: FH is caused by hundreds of different mutations in the gene for the LDL receptor (on chromosome 19) that affect receptor amount and/or function. FH is an autosomal-dominant disease in which homozygotes are more seriously affected than heterozygotes. Heterozygous FH has an incidence of ~1:500 in the general population. It is associated with increased risk of cardiovascular disease. Genetic screening of the first-degree relatives of the patient would identify affected individuals to allow their treatment.

REVIEW QUESTIONS: Choose the ONE best answer.

RQ1. Triacylglycerols are glycerol-based lipids. Which of the following is also a glycerol-based lipid?

A. Ganglioside GM_2
B. Phosphatidylcholine
C. Prostaglandin PGI_2
D. Sphingomyelin
E. Vitamin D

RQ2. Statins are of benefit to patients with hypercholesterolemia because they:

A. decrease a rate-limiting and regulated step of de novo cholesterol biosynthesis by inhibiting hydroxymethylglutaryl coenzyme A (HMG CoA) reductase.
B. decrease expression of the gene for the LDL receptor by preventing the movement of the sterol regulatory element–binding protein-2 (SREBP-2) in complex with SREBP cleavage–activating protein (SCAP) from the membrane of the endoplasmic reticulum to the membrane of the Golgi.
C. increase the oxidation of cholesterol to CO_2 + H_2O.
D. interfere with the absorption of bile salts in the enterohepatic circulation, thereby causing the liver to take up cholesterol from the blood for use in bile acid synthesis.
E. reduce cholesterol by increasing steroid hormone and vitamin D synthesis.

RQ3. Statins are competitive inhibitors of HMG CoA reductase. Which of the following statements about competitive inhibitors is correct?

A. Competitive inhibitors are examples of irreversible inhibitors.
B. Competitive inhibitors increase both the apparent Michaelis constant (K_m) and the apparent maximal velocity (V_{max}).
C. Competitive inhibitors increase the apparent K_m and have no effect on the V_{max}.
D. Competitive inhibitors decrease both the apparent K_m and the apparent V_{max}.
E. Competitive inhibitors have no effect on the K_m and decrease the apparent V_{max}.

RQ4. In a myocardial infarction, a blood clot forms as a result of injury to a blood vessel that leads to production of a platelet plug and a meshwork of thrombin. The clot occludes the blood vessel, preventing blood flow and, therefore, delivery of O_2. Destruction of the clot (thrombolysis) restores blood flow. Which one of the following is an example of a thrombolytic agent?

A. Activated protein C complex
B. Antithrombin III
C. Aspirin
D. Factor XIII
E. Heparin
F. Tissue plasminogen activator
G. Vitamin K
H. Warfarin

RQ5. Decreased tissue perfusion results in hypoxia (decreased O_2 availability). Relative to normoxia, in hypoxia the:

A. electron transport will be upregulated to provide protons for adenosine triphosphate synthesis.
B. ratio of the oxidized form of nicotinamide adenine dinucleotide (NAD^+) to the reduced form (NADH) will increase.
C. pyruvate dehydrogenase complex will be active.
D. process of substrate-level phosphorylation will be increased in the cytosol.
E. tricarboxylic acid cycle will be upregulated to provide the reducing equivalents needed for oxidative phosphorylation to occur.

RQ6. Genetic screening of the patient's first-degree relatives would be accomplished by mutation analysis via polymerase chain reaction–based amplification followed by automated sequencing of the promoter region and the 18 exons of the LDL receptor gene. This process would involve the:

A. generation and use of complementary DNA (cDNA).
B. initiation of DNA synthesis with dideoxynucleotides.
C. isolation of genomic DNA from germ cells.
D. use of fluorescently labeled nucleotides.

THOUGHT QUESTIONS

TQ1. Relative to an individual with familial defective LDL receptors, what would be the expected phenotype in an individual with familial defective apolipoprotein B-100? With apolipoprotein E-2, the isoform that only poorly binds its receptor?

TQ2. Why was aspirin prescribed? **Hint**: What pathway of lipid metabolism is affected by aspirin?

TQ3. Heart muscle normally uses aerobic metabolism to meet its energy needs. However, in hypoxia, anaerobic glycolysis is increased. What allosteric activator of glycolysis is responsible for this effect? With hypoxia, what will be the end product of glycolysis?

TQ4. One of the reasons for encouraging smoking cessation and exercise in the patient is that these changes raise the level of HDLs, and elevated HDL reduces the risk for CHD. How does a rise in HDL reduce the risk for CHD?

CASE 2: SEVERE FASTING HYPOGLYCEMIA

Patient Presentation: Jason S. is a 4-month-old boy whose mother is concerned about the "twitching" movements he makes just before feedings. She tells the pediatrician that the movements started about 1 week ago, are most apparent in the morning, and disappear shortly after eating.

Focused History: Jason is the product of a normal pregnancy and delivery. He appeared normal at birth. He has been at the 30th percentile for both weight and length since birth. His immunizations are up to date. Jason last ate a few hours ago.

Physical Examination (Pertinent Findings): Jason appears sleepy and feels clammy to the touch. His respiratory rate is elevated. His temperature is normal. Jason has a protuberant, firm abdomen that appears to be nontender. His liver is palpable 4 cm below the right costal margin and is smooth. His kidneys are enlarged and symmetrical.

Pertinent Test Results:

	Patient	Pediatric Reference Range
Glucose	50 mg/dl (**L**)	60–105
Lactate	3.4 mmol/l (**H**)	0.6–3.2
Urate	5.6 mg/dl (**H**)	2.4–5.4
Total cholesterol	220 mg/dl (**H**)	<170
Triglycerides (triacylglycerols)	280 mg/dl (**H**)	<90
pH	7.30 (**L**)	7.35–7.45
HCO_3^-	12 mEq/l (**L**)	19–25

H = High; **L** = Low

Jason is sent to the regional children's hospital for further evaluation. Ultrasound studies confirm hepatomegaly and renomegaly and show no evidence of tumors. A liver biopsy is performed. The hepatocytes are distended. Staining reveals large amounts of lipid (primarily triacylglycerol) and carbohydrate. Liver glycogen is elevated in amount and normal in structure. Enzyme assay using liver homogenate treated with detergent reveals less than 10% of the normal activity of *glucose 6-phosphatase*, an enzyme of the endoplasmic reticulum (ER) membrane in the liver and the kidneys.

Diagnosis: *Glucose 6-phosphatase* deficiency (glycogen storage disease [GSD] type Ia, von Gierke disease)

Treatment (Immediate): Jason was given glucose intravenously, and his blood glucose level rose into the normal range. However, as the day progressed, it fell to well below normal. Administration of glucagon had no effect on blood glucose levels but increased blood lactate. Jason's blood glucose levels were able to be maintained by constant infusion of glucose.

Prognosis: Individuals with *glucose 6-phosphatase* deficiency develop hepatic adenomas starting in the second decade of life and are at increased risk for hepatic carcinoma. Kidney glomerular function is impaired and can result in kidney failure. Patients are at increased risk for developing gout, but this rarely occurs before puberty.

Nutrition Nugget: Long-term medical nutrition therapy for Jason is designed to maintain his blood glucose levels in the normal range. Frequent (every 2–3 hours) daytime feedings rich in carbohydrate (provided by uncooked cornstarch that is slowly hydrolyzed) and nighttime nasogastric infusion (pump assisted) of glucose are advised. Avoidance of fructose and galactose is recommended because they are metabolized to glycolytic intermediates and lactate and can exacerbate the metabolic problems. Calcium and vitamin D supplements are prescribed.

Genetics Gem: GSD Ia is an autosomal-recessive disorder caused by more than 100 known mutations to the gene for *glucose 6-phosphatase* located on chromosome 17. It has an incidence of 1:100,000 and accounts for approximately 25% of all cases of GSDs in the United States. It is one of the few genetic causes of hypoglycemia in newborns. GSD Ia is not routinely screened for in newborns. [Note: Deficiency of the translocase that moves glucose 6-phosphate out of the cytosol and into the ER is the cause of GSD Ib.]

REVIEW QUESTIONS: Choose the ONE best answer.

RQ1. Jason is hypoglycemic because:

A. free (nonphosphorylated) glucose cannot be produced from either glycogenolysis or gluconeogenesis as a result of the deficiency in glucose 6-phosphatase.

B. glycogen phosphorylase is dephosphorylated and inactive, and glycogen cannot be degraded.

C. hormone-sensitive lipase is dephosphorylated and inactive, and fatty acid substrates for gluconeogenesis cannot be generated.

D. the decrease in the insulin/glucagon ratio upregulates glucose transporters in the liver and kidneys, resulting in increased uptake of blood glucose.

RQ2. Jason was prescribed calcium supplements because chronic acidosis can cause bone demineralization, resulting in osteopenia. Vitamin D was also prescribed because vitamin D:

A. binds G_q protein–coupled membrane receptors and causes a rise in inositol trisphosphate with release of calcium from intracellular stores.

B. cannot be synthesized by humans and, therefore, must be supplied in the diet.

C. is a fat-soluble vitamin that increases intestinal absorption of calcium.

D. is the coenzyme-prosthetic group for calbindin, a calcium transporter in the intestine.

RQ3. The hepatomegaly and renomegaly seen in Jason are primarily the result of an increase in the amount of glycogen stored in these organs. What is the basis for glycogen accumulation in these organs?

A. Glycolysis is downregulated, which pushes glucose to glycogenesis.
B. Increased oxidation of fatty acids spares glucose for glycogenesis.
C. Glucose 6-phosphate is an allosteric activator of glycogen synthase b.
D. The rise in the insulin/glucagon ratio favors glycogenesis.

RQ4. Glucose 6-phosphatase is an integral protein of the membrane of the endoplasmic reticulum. Which of the following statements about such proteins is correct?

A. If glycosylated, the carbohydrate is on the portion of the protein that extends into the cytosol.
B. They are synthesized on ribosomes that are free in the cytosol.
C. The membrane-spanning domain consists of hydrophilic amino acids.
D. The initial targeting signal is an amino terminal hydrophobic signal sequence.

THOUGHT QUESTIONS

TQ1. What is the likely reason for Jason's twitching movements?

TQ2. Why was the liver homogenate treated with detergent? **Hint**: Think about where the enzyme is located.

TQ3. Why is Jason's blood glucose level unaffected by glucagon? **Hint**: What is the role of glucagon in normal individuals who experience a drop in blood glucose?

TQ4. Why are urate and lactate elevated in a disorder of glycogen metabolism? **Hint**: It is the result of a decrease in inorganic phosphate (P_i), but why is P_i decreased?

TQ5. A. Why are triacylglycerols and cholesterol elevated? **Hint**: Glucose is the primary carbon source for their synthesis.

B. Why are ketone bodies not elevated?

CASE 3: HYPERGLYCEMIA AND HYPERKETONEMIA

Patient Presentation: A 40-year-old woman was brought to the hospital in a disoriented, confused state by her husband.

Focused History: As noted on her medical alert bracelet, the patient has had type 1 diabetes (T1D) for the last 24 years. Her husband reports that this is her first medical emergency in 2 years.

Physical Examination (Pertinent Findings): The patient displayed signs of dehydration (such as dry mucous membranes and skin, poor skin turgor, and low blood pressure) and acidosis (such as deep and rapid breathing [Kussmaul respiration]). Her breath had a faintly fruity odor. Her temperature was normal.

Pertinent Test Results: Rapid, bedside tests were strongly positive for glucose and acetoacetate and negative for protein. Results on blood tests performed by the clinical laboratory are shown below:

	Patient	**Reference Range**
Glucose	414 mg/dl (23 mmol/l) (**H**)	70–99 (3.9–5.5)
Blood urea nitrogen	8 mmol/l (**H**)	2.5–6.4
3-Hydroxybutyrate	350 mg/dl (**H**)	0–3
HCO_3^-	12 mmol/l (**L**)	22–28
Na^+	136 mmol/l	138–150
K^+	5.3 mmol/l	3.5–5.0
Cl^-	102 mmol/l	95–105
pH	7.1 (**L**)	7.35–7.45

H = High; **L** = Low

Microscopic examination of her urine revealed a urinary tract infection (UTI).

Diagnosis: The patient is in diabetic ketoacidosis that was precipitated by a UTI. [Note: Diabetes increases the risk for infections such as UTIs.]

Immediate Treatment: The patient was rehydrated with normal saline given intravenously (IV). She also was given insulin IV. Blood glucose, ketone bodies, and electrolytes were measured periodically. The patient was started on an antibiotic for her UTI.

Long-term Treatment: Diabetes increases the risk for macrovascular complications (such as coronary artery disease and stroke) and microvascular complications (such as retinopathy, nephropathy, and neuropathy). Ongoing monitoring for these complications will be continued.

Prognosis: Diabetes is the sixth leading cause of death by disease in the United States. Individuals with diabetes have a reduced life expectancy relative to those without diabetes.

Nutrition Nugget: Monitoring total intake of carbohydrate is primary in blood glucose control. Carbohydrate should come from whole grains, vegetables, legumes, and fruits. Low-fat dairy products and nuts and fish rich in ω-3 fatty acids are encouraged. Intake of saturated and trans fats should be minimized.	Genetics Gem: Autoimmune destruction of pancreatic β cells is characteristic of T1D. Of the genetic loci that confer risk for T1D, the human-leukocyte antigen (HLA) region on chromosome 6 has the strongest association. The majority of genes in the HLA region are involved in the immune response.

REVIEW QUESTIONS: Choose the ONE best answer.

RQ1. Which of the following statements concerning T1D is correct?

A. Diagnosis can be made by measuring the level of glucose or glycosylated hemoglobin (HbA_{1C}) in the blood.

B. During periods of physiologic stress, the urine of an individual with T1D would likely test negative for reducing sugars.

C. T1D is associated with obesity and a sedentary lifestyle.

D. The characteristic metabolic abnormalities seen in T1D result from insensitivity to both insulin and glucagon.

E. Treatment with exogenous insulin allows normalization of blood glucose (euglycemia).

RQ2. Diabetic ketoacidosis occurs when the rate of ketone body production is greater than the rate of utilization. Which of the following statements concerning ketone body metabolism is correct? Ketone bodies:

A. are made in mitochondria from acetyl coenzyme A (CoA) produced by the oxidation of glucose.

B. are utilized by many tissues, particularly the liver, after conversion to acetyl CoA.

C. include acetoacetate, which can impart a fruity odor to the breath.

D. require albumin for transport through the blood.

E. utilized in energy metabolism are organic acids that can add to the proton load of the body.

RQ3. Adipose lipolysis followed by β-oxidation of the fatty acid products is required for the generation of ketone bodies. Which of the following statements concerning the generation and use of fatty acids is correct?

A. Mitochondrial β-oxidation of fatty acids is inhibited by malonyl CoA.

B. Production of fatty acids from adipose lipolysis is upregulated by insulin.

C. The acetyl CoA product of fatty acid β-oxidation favors the use of pyruvate for gluconeogenesis by activating the pyruvate dehydrogenase complex.

D. The β-oxidation of fatty acids utilizes reducing equivalents generated by gluconeogenesis.

E. The fatty acids produced by lipolysis are taken up by the brain and oxidized for energy.

THOUGHT QUESTIONS

TQI. At admission, the patient was hypoinsulinemic, and she was given insulin. Why did the patient's hypoinsulinemia result in hyperglycemia? **Hint**: What is the role of insulin in glucose metabolism?

TQ2. Why is there glucose in the patient's urine (glucosuria)? How is the glucosuria related to her dehydrated state?

TQ3. Why is the majority of the acetyl CoA from fatty acid β-oxidation being used for ketogenesis rather than being oxidized in the tricarboxylic acid cycle?

TQ4. Was the patient in positive or negative nitrogen balance when she was brought to the hospital?

TQ5. What response to the ketoacidosis is apparent in the patient? What response is likely occurring in the kidney? **Hint**: In addition to conversion to urea, how is toxic ammonia removed from the body?

TQ6. What would be true about the levels of ketone bodies and glucose during periods of physiologic stress in individuals with impaired fatty acid oxidation?

CASE 4: HYPOGLYCEMIA, HYPERKETONEMIA, AND LIVER DYSFUNCTION

Patient Presentation: AK, a 59-year-old male with slurred speech, ataxia (loss of skeletal muscle coordination), and abdominal pain, was dropped off at the Emergency Department (ED).

Focused History: AK is known to the ED staff from previous visits. He has a 6-year history of chronic, heavy alcohol consumption. He is not known to take illicit drugs. At this ED visit, AK reports that he has been drinking heavily in the past day or so. He cannot recall having eaten anything in that time. There is evidence of recent vomiting, but no blood is apparent.

Physical Examination (Pertinent Findings): The physical examination was remarkable for the emaciated appearance of the patient. (His body mass index was later determined to be 17.5, which put him in the underweight category.) The cheeks of his face were erythematous (red in color) due to dilated blood vessels in the skin (telangiectasia). Eye movement was normal. Neither icterus (jaundice) nor edema (swelling due to fluid retention) was seen. The liver was slightly enlarged. Bedside tests revealed hypoglycemia and hyperketonemia (as acetoacetate). Blood was drawn and sent to the clinical laboratory.

Pertinent Test Results:

	Patient	Reference Range
Ethanol	180 mg/dl (**H**)	(>80 considered positive for DUI*)
Glucose	58 mg/dl (**L**)	70–99
Lactate	23 mg/dl (**H**)	5–15
Uric acid	7.0 mg/dl	2.5–8.0
3-Hydroxybutyrate	50 mg/dl (**H**)	0–3.0
Total bilirubin	1.5 mg/dl (**H**)	0.3–1.0
Direct bilirubin	0.5 mg/dl (**H**)	0.1–0.3
Albumin	3.0 g/dl (**L**)	3.5–5.8
Aspartate transaminase (AST)	130 U/l (**H**)	0–35
Alanine transaminase (ALT)	75 U/l (**H**)	0–35
Prothrombin time	15.5 sec (**H**)	11.0–13.2
	H = High; **L** = Low	*driving under the influence

Additional Tests: Complete blood count (CBC) and blood smear revealed a macrocytic anemia (right Image). Folate and B_{12} levels were ordered.

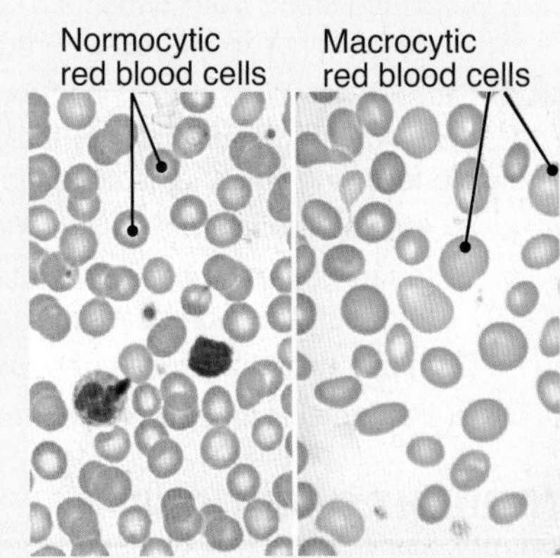

Diagnosis: Alcoholism

Treatment (Immediate): Thiamine and glucose were given intravenously.

Prognosis: Alcoholism (alcohol dependence) is the third most common cause of preventable death in the United States. People with alcoholism are at increased risk for liver cirrhosis, pancreatitis, gastrointestinal bleeding, and some cancers.

Nutrition Nugget: Those with alcoholism are at risk for vitamin deficiencies as a result of decreased intake and absorption. Thiamine (vitamin B_1) deficiency is common and can have serious consequences such as Wernicke-Korsakoff syndrome with its neurologic effects. Thiamine pyrophosphate (TPP), the coenzyme form, is required for the *dehydrogenase*-mediated oxidation of α-keto acids (such as pyruvate) as well as the transfer of two-carbon ketol groups by *transketolase* in the reversible sugar interconversions in the pentose phosphate pathway.

Genetics Gem: Acetaldehyde, the product of ethanol oxidation by the hepatic, cytosolic, nicotinamide adenine dinucleotide (NAD^+)-requiring enzyme *alcohol dehydrogenase* (*ADH*), is oxidized to acetate by the mitochondrial, NAD^+-requiring *aldehyde dehydrogenase* (*ALDH2*). The majority of individuals of East Asian (but not European or African) heritage have a single nucleotide polymorphism (SNP) that renders *ALDH2* essentially inactive. This results in aldehyde-induced facial flushing and mild to moderate intoxication after consumption of small amounts of ethanol.

REVIEW QUESTIONS: Choose the ONE best answer.

RQ1. Many of the metabolic consequences of chronic excessive alcohol consumption seen in the patient are the result of an increase in the ratio of reduced nicotinamide adenine dinucleotide (NADH) to its oxidized form (NAD^+) in both the cytoplasm and mitochondrion. Which of the following statements concerning the effects of the rise in mitochondrial NADH is correct?

A. Fatty acid oxidation is increased.

B. Gluconeogenesis is increased.

C. Lipolysis is inhibited.

D. The tricarboxylic acid cycle is inhibited.

E. The reduction of malate to oxaloacetate in the malate–aspartate shuttle is increased.

RQ2. Ethanol can also be oxidized by cytochrome P450 (CYP) enzymes, and CYP2E1 is an important example. CYP2E1, which is ethanol inducible, generates reactive oxygen species (ROS) in its metabolism of ethanol. Which of the following statements concerning the CYP proteins is correct?

A. CYP proteins are heme-containing dioxygenases.

B. CYP proteins of the inner mitochondrial membrane are involved in detoxification reactions.

C. CYP proteins of the smooth endoplasmic reticulum membrane are involved in the synthesis of steroid hormones, bile acids, and calcitriol.

D. ROS such as hydrogen peroxide generated by CYP2E1 can be oxidized by glutathione peroxidase.

E. The pentose phosphate pathway is an important source of the nicotinamide adenine dinucleotide phosphate (NADPH) that provides the reducing equivalents needed for activity of CYP proteins and the regeneration of functional glutathione.

RQ3. Alcohol is known to modulate the levels of serotonin in the central nervous system, where it functions as a neurotransmitter. Which of the following statements about serotonin is correct? Serotonin is:

A. associated with anxiety and depression.

B. degraded via methylation by monoamine oxidase, which also degrades the catecholamines.

C. released by activated platelets.

D. synthesized from tyrosine in a two-step process that utilizes a tetrahydrobiopterin-requiring hydroxylase and a pyridoxal phosphate-requiring carboxylase.

RQ4. Chronic, excessive consumption of alcohol is a leading cause of acute pancreatitis, a painful inflammatory condition that results from autodigestion of the gland by premature activation of pancreatic enzymes. Which of the following statements concerning the pancreas is correct?

A. Autodigestion of the pancreas would be expected to result in a decrease in pancreatic proteins in the blood.

B. In individuals who progress from acute to chronic pancreatitis, with the characteristic structural changes that result in decreased pancreatic function, diabetes and steatorrhea are expected findings.

C. In response to secretin, the exocrine pancreas secretes protons to lower the pH in the intestinal lumen.

D. Pancreatitis may also be seen in individuals with hypercholesterolemia.

THOUGHT QUESTIONS

TQ1. A. What effect does the rise in cytosolic NADH seen with ethanol metabolism have on glycolysis? **Hint**: What coenzyme is required in glycolysis?

B. How does this relate to the fatty liver (steatosis) commonly seen in alcohol-dependent individuals?

TQ2. Why might individuals with a history of gouty attacks be advised to reduce their consumption of ethanol?

TQ3. Why might prothrombin time be affected in alcohol-dependent individuals?

TQ4. Folate and vitamin B_{12} deficiencies cause a macrocytic anemia that may be seen in those with alcoholism. Why is it advisable to measure vitamin B_{12} levels before supplementing with folate in an individual with macrocytic anemia?

II. INTEGRATIVE CASE ANSWERS

CASE 1: Answers to Review Questions

RQ1. Answer = B. Phosphatidylcholine is a glycerol-based phospholipid derived from diacylglycerol phosphate (phosphatidic acid) and cytidine diphosphate-choline. Gangliosides are derived from ceramides, lipids with a sphingosine backbone. Prostaglandins of the 2 series are derived from the 20-carbon polyunsaturated fatty acid arachadonic acid. Sphingomyelin is a sphingophospholipid derived from ceramide. Vitamin D is derived from an intermediate in the biosynthetic pathway for the sterol cholesterol.

RQ2. Answer = A. Statins inhibit hydroxymethylglutaryl coenzyme A (HMG CoA) reductase, thereby preventing the reduction of HMG CoA to mevalonate and decreasing cholesterol biosynthesis (see Figure). The decrease in cholesterol content caused by statins results in movement of the sterol regulatory element–binding protein-2 (SREBP-2) in complex with SREBP cleavage–activating protein (SCAP) from the endoplasmic reticular membrane to the Golgi membrane, where SREBP-2 is cleaved, generating a transcription factor that moves to the nucleus and binds to the sterol regulatory element upstream of the genes for HMG CoA reductase and the low-density lipoprotein (LDL) receptor, increasing their expression. Humans are unable to degrade the steroid nucleus to CO_2 + H_2O. Bile acid sequestrants, such as cholestyramine, prevent the absorption of bile salts by the liver, thereby increasing their excretion. The liver then takes up cholesterol via the LDL receptor and uses it to make bile acids, thereby reducing blood cholesterol levels. Steroid hormones are synthesized from cholesterol, and vitamin D is synthesized from an intermediate (7-dehydrocholesterol) in the cholesterol biosynthetic pathway. Therefore, inhibition of cholesterol synthesis would be expected to decrease their production as well.

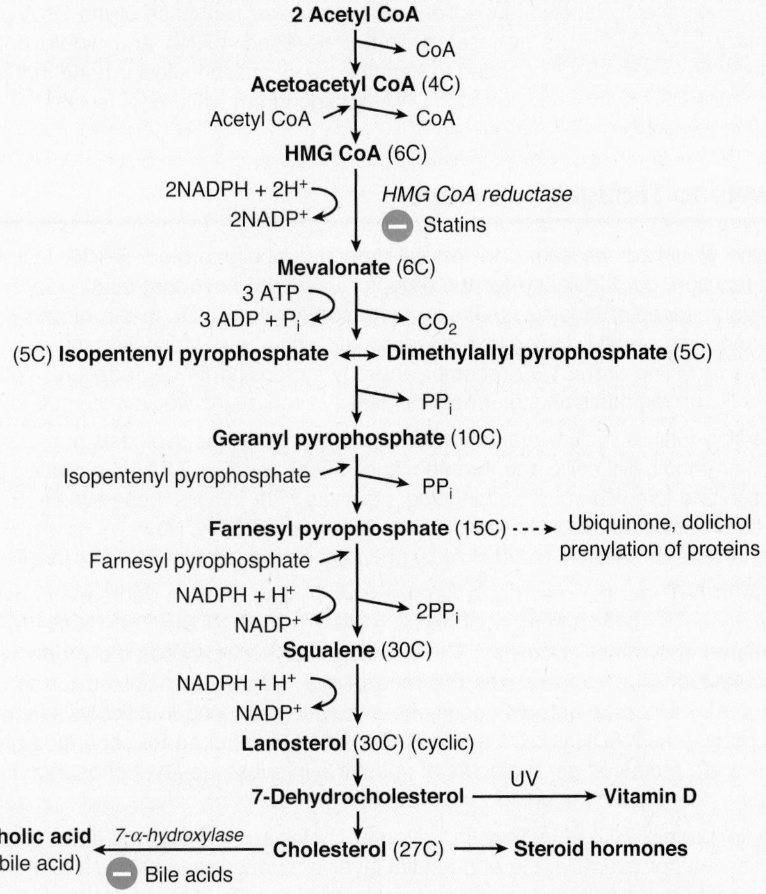

RQ3. Answer = C. Competitive inhibitors bind to the same site as the substrate. Once bound, they prevent the substrate from binding. This results in an increase in the apparent K_m, that substrate concentration that gives one half of the maximal velocity (V_{max}). However, because the inhibition can be reversed by adding additional substrate, the V_{max} is unchanged (see Figure). It is noncompetitive inhibitors that decrease the apparent V_{max} and have no effect on K_m.

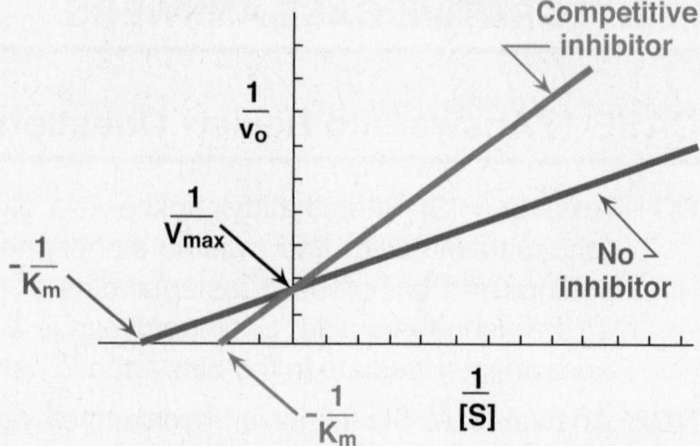

RQ4. Answer = F. Tissue plasminogen activator converts plasminogen to plasmin that degrades fibrin (fibrinolysis), thereby degrading the clot (thrombolysis). Aspirin, an inhibitor of cyclooxygenase, is an antiplatelet drug. Antithrombin III (ATIII) removes thrombin from the blood, and its action is potentiated by heparin. Activated protein C (APC) complex cleaves the accessory proteins factor (F)Va and FVIIIa. ATIII and APC are involved in anticoagulation. FXIII is a transglutaminase that cross-links the fibrin mesh. Vitamin K is a fat-soluble vitamin required for the γ-carboxylation of FII, FVII, FIX, and FX. Warfarin prevents regeneration of the functional, reduced form of vitamin K.

RQ5. Answer = D. In hypoxia, substrate level phosphorylation in glycolysis provides adenosine triphosphate (ATP). Oxidative phosphorylation is inhibited by the lack of O_2. Because the rate of ATP synthesis by oxidative phosphorylation controls the rate of cellular respiration, electron transport is inhibited. The resulting rise in the ratio of the reduced form of nicotinamide adenine dinucleotide (NADH) to the oxidized form (NAD^+) inhibits the tricarboxylic acid cycle and the pyruvate dehydrogenase complex.

RQ6. Answer = D. Fluorescently labeled nucleotides allow the base sequence of the DNA of interest to be detected. Complementary DNA (cDNA) is generated from processed mRNA and would not contain the promoter. Dideoxynucleotides lack the 3'-OH needed to form the 3'→5' phosphodiester bond that joins the nucleotides and, thus, will terminate DNA synthesis. Genomic DNA obtained from white cells isolated from a blood sample would be the source of the DNA.

CASE 1: Answers to Thought Questions

TQ1. The phenotype would be the same. In familial defective apolipoprotein B-100, LDL receptors are normal in number and function, but the ligand for the receptor is altered such that binding to the receptor is decreased. Decreased ligand–receptor binding results in increased levels of LDL in the blood with hypercholesterolemia. [Note: The phenotype would be the same in individuals with a gain-of-function mutation to PCSK9, the protease that decreases recycling of the LDL receptor, thereby increasing its degradation.] With the apolipoprotein E-2 isoform, chylomicron remnants and intermediate-density lipoproteins would accumulate in blood.

TQ2. Aspirin irreversibly inhibits cyclooxygenase (COX) and, therefore, the synthesis of prostaglandins (PGs), such as PGI_2 in vascular endothelial cells, and thromboxanes (TXs), such as TXA_2 in activated platelets. TXA_2 promotes vasoconstriction and formation of a platelet plug, whereas PGI_2 inhibits these events. Because platelets are anucleate, they can't overcome this inhibition by synthesizing more COX. However, endothelial cells have a nucleus. Aspirin, then, inhibits formation of blood clots by preventing production of TXA_2 for the life of the platelet.

TQ3. The decrease in ATP (as the result of a decrease in O_2 and, thus, a decrease in oxidative phosphorylation) causes an increase in adenosine monophosphate (AMP). AMP allosterically activates phosphofructokinase-1, the key regulated enzyme of glycolysis. The rise in glycolysis increases the production of ATP by substrate-level phosphorylation. It also increases the ratio of the reduced to oxidized forms of nicotinamide adenine dinucleotide (NAD). Under anaerobic conditions, pyruvate produced in glycolysis is reduced to lactate by lactate dehydrogenase as NADH is oxidized to NAD^+. NAD^+ is required for continued glycolysis. Because fewer ATP molecules are produced per molecule of substrate in substrate-level phosphorylation relative to oxidative phosphorylation, there is a compensatory increase in the rate of glycolysis under anaerobic conditions.

TQ4. High-density lipoprotein (HDL) functions in "reverse" cholesterol transport. It takes cholesterol from nonhepatic (peripheral) tissues (for example, the endothelial layer of arteries) and brings it to the liver (see Figure below). The ABCA1 transporter mediates the efflux of cholesterol to HDL. The cholesterol is esterified by lecithin-cholesterol acyl transferase (LCAT) that requires apo A-1 as a coenzyme. Some cholesteryl ester is transferred to very-low-density lipoproteins (VLDLs) by cholesteryl-ester transfer protein (CETP) in exchange for triacylglycerol. The remainder is taken up by a scavenger receptor (SR-B1) on the surface of hepatocytes. The liver can use the cholesterol from HDL in the synthesis of bile acids. Removal of cholesterol from endothelial cells prevents its accumulation (as cholesterol or cholesteryl ester), decreasing the risk of heart disease. [Note: In contrast, LDL carries cholesterol from the liver to peripheral tissues.]

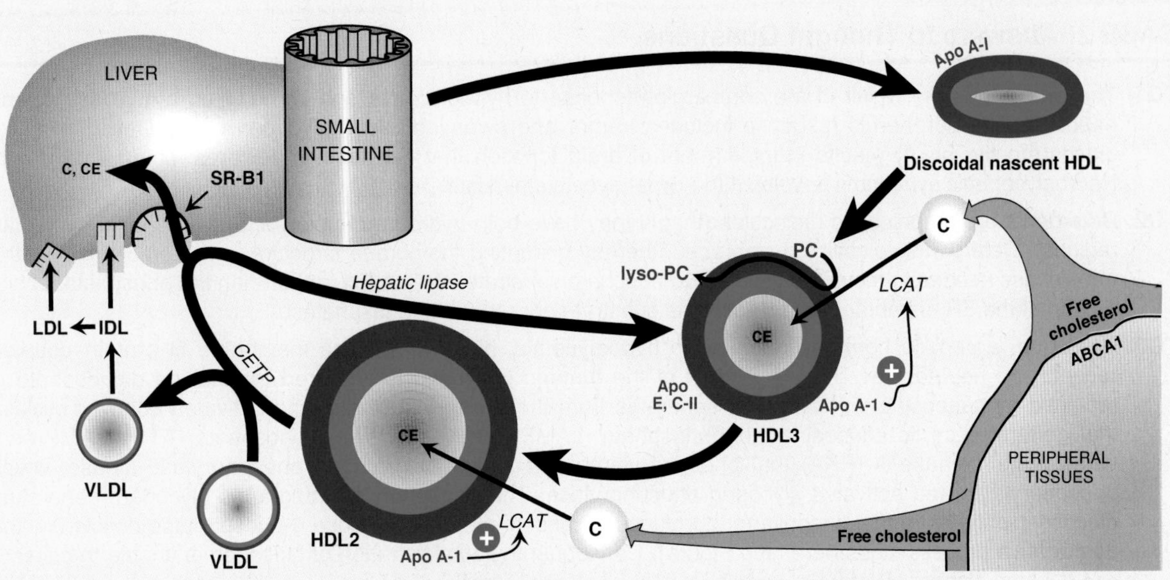

CASE 2: Answers to Review Questions

RQ1. Answer = A. Deficiency of glucose 6-phosphatase prevents the glucose 6-phosphate generated by glycogenolysis and gluconeogenesis from being dephosphorylated and released into the blood (see Figure below). Blood glucose levels fall, and a severe, fasting hypoglycemia results. [Note: Jason's symptoms appeared only recently because, at age 4 months, he is going longer periods between feedings.] Hypoglycemia stimulates release of glucagon, which leads to phosphorylation and activation of glycogen phosphorylase kinase that phosphorylates and activates glycogen phosphorylase. Epinephrine is also released and leads to phosphorylation and activation of hormone-sensitive lipase. However, typical fatty acids cannot serve as substrates for gluconeogenesis. The glucose transporters in the liver and kidneys are insulin insensitive.

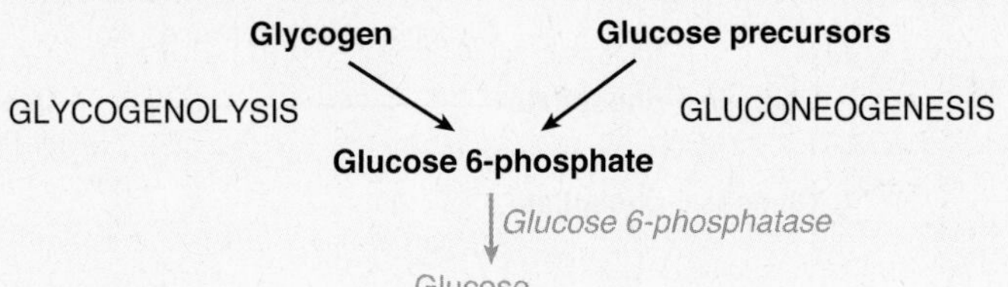

RQ2. Answer = C. Vitamin D is a fat-soluble vitamin that functions as a steroid hormone. In complex with its intracellular nuclear receptor, it increases transcription of the gene for calbindin, a calcium transporter protein in the intestine (see Figure). Vitamin D does not bind to a membrane receptor and does not produce second messengers. It can be synthesized in the skin by the action of ultraviolet light on an intermediate of cholesterol synthesis, 7-dehydrocholesterol. Of the fat-soluble vitamins (A, D, E, and K), only vitamin K functions as a coenzyme.

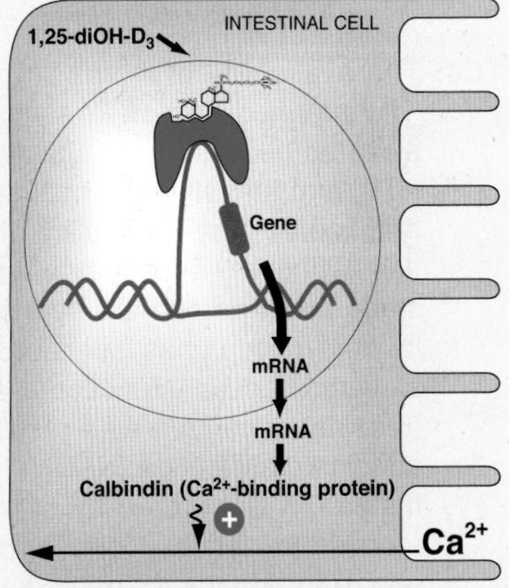

RQ3. Answer = C. Glucose 6-phosphate is a positive allosteric effector of the covalently inhibited (phosphorylated) glycogen synthase b. With the rise in glucose 6-phosphate, glycogen synthesis is activated and glycogen stores are increased in both the liver and kidneys. The increased availability of glucose 6-phosphate also drives glycolysis. The increase in glycolysis provides substrates for lipogenesis, thereby increasing synthesis of fatty acids and triacylglycerols (TAGs). In hypoglycemia, the insulin/glucagon ratio is low, not high.

RQ4. Answer = D. Membrane proteins are initially targeted to the endoplasmic reticulum (ER) by an amino terminal hydrophobic signal sequence. Glycosylation is the most common posttranslational modification found in proteins. The glycosylated portion of membrane proteins is found on the outside face of the membrane. The membrane-spanning domain consists of approximately 22 hydrophobic amino acids. Proteins destined for secretion or for membrane, the ER lumen, Golgi, or lysosomes are synthesized on ribosomes associated with the ER.

CASE 2: Answers to Thought Questions

TQ1. The twitching is the result of the adrenergic response to hypoglycemia and is mediated by the rise in epinephrine. The adrenergic response includes tremor and sweating. Neuroglycopenia (impaired delivery of glucose to the brain) results in impairment of brain function that can lead to seizures, coma, and death. Neuroglycopenic symptoms develop if the hyperglycemia persists.

TQ2. Detergents are amphipathic molecules (that is they have both hydrophilic [polar] and hydrophobic [nonpolar] regions). Detergents solubilize membranes, thereby disrupting membrane structure. If the problem were the translocase needed to move the glucose 6-phosphate substrate into the ER, rather than the phosphatase, disruption of the ER membrane would allow the substrate access to the phosphatase.

TQ3. Glucagon, a peptide hormone released in hypoglycemia, binds its plasma membrane G protein–coupled receptor on hepatocytes. The α_s subunit of the trimeric G protein is activated (guanosine diphosphate is replaced by guanosine triphosphate), separates from the β and γ subunits, and activates adenylyl cyclase that generates cyclic adenosine monophosphate (cAMP) from adenosine triphosphate (ATP). cAMP activates protein kinase A (PKA) that phosphorylates and activates glycogen phosphorylase kinase, which phosphorylates and activates glycogen phosphorylase. The phosphorylase degrades glycogen, generating glucose 1-phosphate that is converted to glucose 6-phosphate. With glucose 6-phosphatase deficiency, the degradative process stops here (see Figure). Consequently, administration of glucagon is unable to cause a rise in blood glucose. [Note: Epinephrine would be similarly ineffective.]

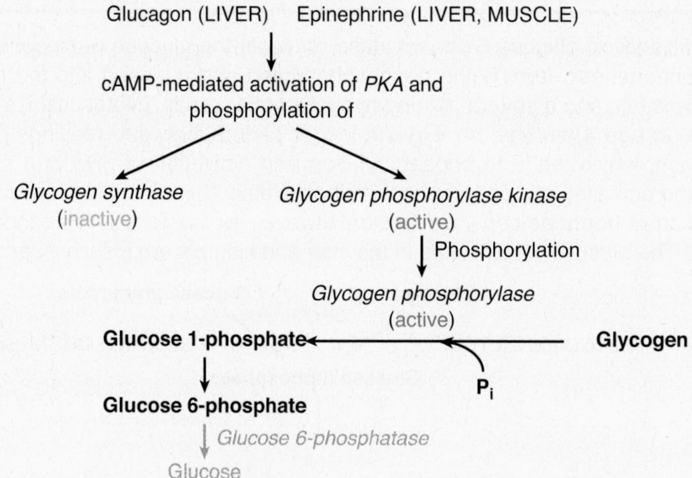

TQ4. The availability of inorganic phosphate (P_i) is decreased because it is trapped as phosphorylated glycolytic intermediates as a result of the upregulation of glycolysis by the rise in glucose 6-phosphate. Urate is elevated because the trapping of P_i decreases the ability to phosphorylate adenosine diphosphate (ADP) to ATP, and the fall in ATP causes a rise in adenosine monophosphate (AMP). The AMP is degraded to urate. Additionally, the availability of glucose 6-phosphate drives the pentose phosphate pathway, resulting in a rise in ribose 5-phosphate (from ribulose 5-phosphate) and, consequently, a rise in purine synthesis. Purines made beyond need are degraded to urate (see Figure below). [Note: The decrease in P_i reduces the activity of glycogen phosphorylase, resulting in increased storage of glycogen with a normal structure.] Lactate is elevated because the decrease in phosphorylation of ADP to ATP results in a decrease in cellular respiration (respiratory control) as a result of these processes being coupled. As a consequence, reduced nicotinamide adenine dinucleotide (NADH) from glycolysis cannot be oxidized by complex I of the electron transport chain. Instead, it is oxidized by cytosolic lactate dehydrogenase (LDH) with its coenzyme NADH as pyruvate is reduced to lactate. [Note: Pyruvate is increased as a result of the increase in glycolysis.] The lactate ionizes, releasing protons (H^+) and leading to a metabolic acidosis (low pH caused here by increased production of acid). Respiratory compensation causes an increased respiratory rate.

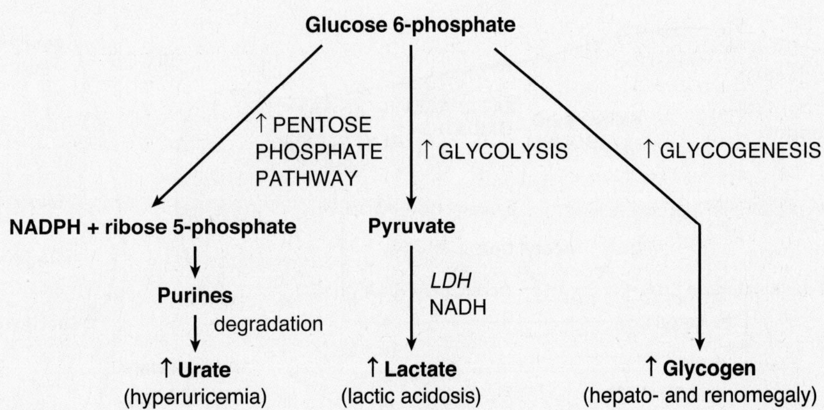

TQ5. Increased glycolysis results in increased availability of glycerol 3-phosphate for hepatic TAG synthesis. Additionally, some of the pyruvate generated in glycolysis will be oxidatively decarboxylated to acetyl coenzyme A (CoA). However, the tricarboxylic acid cycle is inhibited by the rise in NADH, and the acetyl CoA is transported to the cytosol as citrate. The rise of acetyl CoA in the cytosol results in increased fatty acid synthesis. Recall that citrate is an allosteric activator of acetyl CoA carboxylase (ACC). The malonyl product of ACC inhibits fatty acid oxidation at the carnitine palmitoyltransferase I step. Because mitochondrial fatty acid oxidation generates the acetyl CoA substrate for hepatic ketogenesis, ketone body levels do not rise. The fatty acids get esterified to the glycerol backbone, resulting in an increase in TAGs that get sent out of liver as components of very-low-density lipoproteins (VLDLs). [Note: The hypoglycemia results in release of epinephrine and the activation of TAG lipolysis with release of free fatty acids into the blood. The fatty acids are used in hepatic TAG synthesis.] The acetyl CoA is also a substrate for cholesterol synthesis. Thus, the increase in glycolysis results in the hyperlipidemia seen in the patient (see Figure).

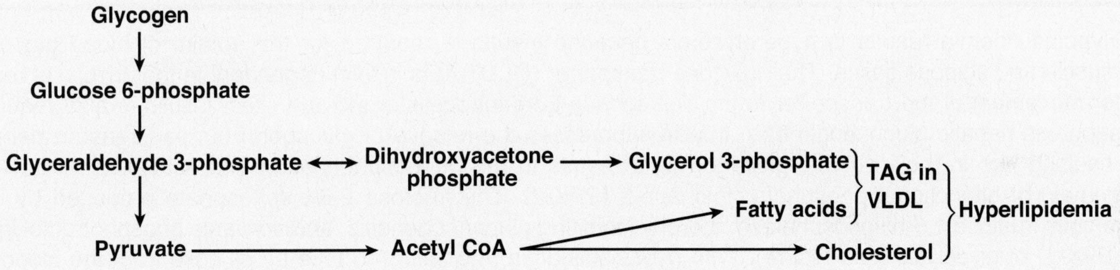

CASE 3: Answers to Review Questions

RQ1. Correct answer = A. Diabetes is characterized by hyperglycemia. Chronic hyperglycemia can result in the nonenzymatic glycosylation (glycation) of hemoglobin (Hb) producing HbA_{1c}. Therefore, measurement of glucose or HbA_{1c} in the blood is used to diagnose diabetes. In response to physiologic stress (for example, a urinary tract infection), secretion of counterregulatory hormones (such as the catecholamines) results in a rise in blood glucose. Glucose is a reducing sugar. It is type 2 diabetes (T2D) that is associated with obesity and a sedentary lifestyle and is caused by insensitivity to insulin (insulin resistance). T1D is caused by lack of insulin as a result of the autoimmune destruction of pancreatic β cells. Even individuals on a program of tight glycemic control do not achieve euglycemia.

RQ2. Correct answer = E. 3-Hydroxybutyrate and acetoacetate are organic acids, and their ionization contributes to the proton load of the body. Ketone bodies are made in the mitochondria of liver cells using acetyl coenzyme A (CoA) generated primarily from the β-oxidation of fatty acids (see Figure below). Because they are water soluble, they do not require a transporter. Liver cannot use them because it lacks the enzyme thiophorase, which moves CoA from succinyl CoA to acetoacetate for conversion to two molecules of acetyl CoA. It is the acetone released in the breath that can impart a fruity odor.

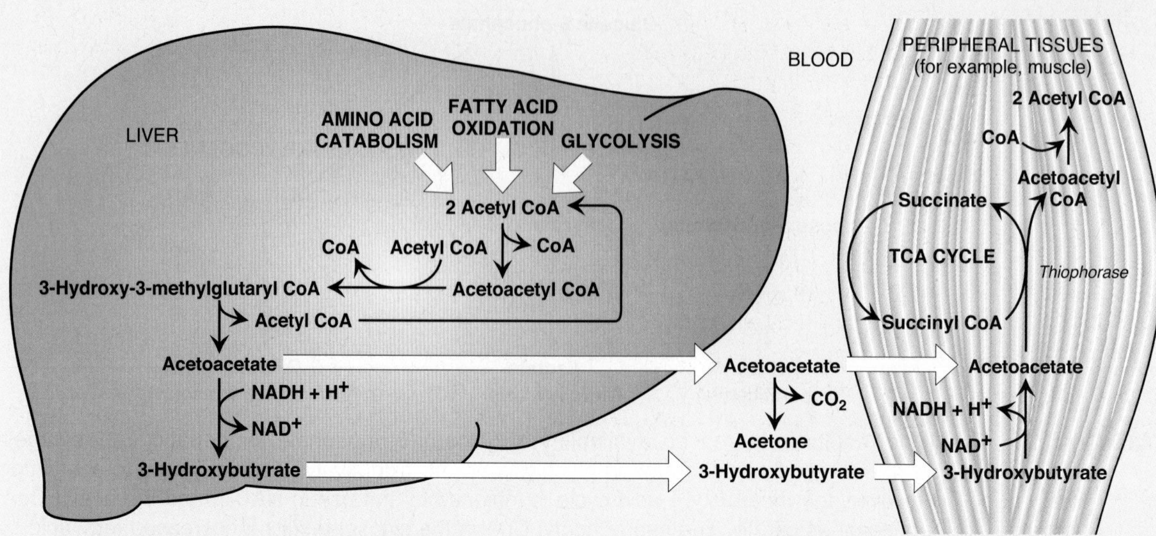

RQ3. Correct answer = A. Malonyl CoA, an intermediate of fatty acid synthesis, inhibits fatty acid β-oxidation through inhibition of carnitine palmitoyltransferase I. Lipolysis occurs when the insulin-to-counterregulatory hormone ratio decreases. Acetyl CoA, the product of fatty acid β-oxidation, inhibits pyruvate dehydrogenase (PDH) through activation of PDH kinase and activates pyruvate carboxylase. Acetyl CoA then pushes pyruvate to gluconeogenesis. β-Oxidation generates reduced nicotinamide adenine dinucleotide (NADH), the reducing equivalent required for gluconeogenesis. The blood–brain barrier inhibits use of fatty acids by the brain.

CASE 3: Answers to Thought Questions

TQ1. Hypoinsulinemia results in hyperglycemia because insulin is required for the uptake of blood glucose by muscle and adipose tissue. Their glucose transporter (GLUT-4) is insulin dependent in that insulin is required for movement of the transporter to the cell surface from intracellular storage sites. Insulin is also required to suppress hepatic gluconeogenesis. Insulin suppresses the release of glucagon from pancreatic α cells. The resulting rise in the insulin-to-glucagon ratio results in the dephosphorylation and activation of the kinase domain of bifunctional phosphofructokinase-2 (PFK-2). The fructose 2,6-bisphosphate produced by PFK-2 inhibits fructose 1,6-bisphosphatase, thereby inhibiting gluconeogenesis, and activates phosphofructokinase-1 (PFK-1) of glycolysis (see Figure). With hypoinsulinemia, the failure to take up glucose from the blood while simultaneously sending it out into the blood results in hyperglycemia.

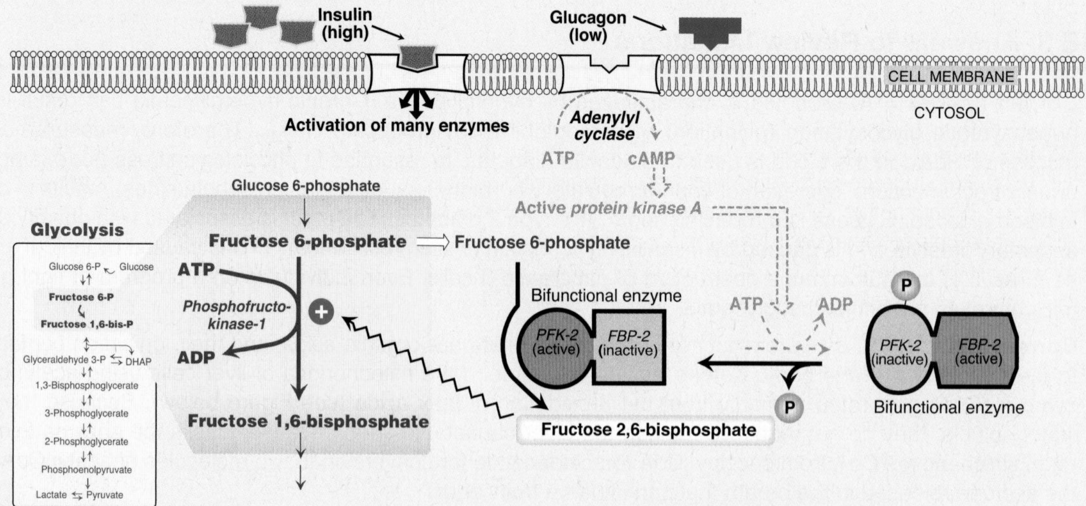

TQ2. The blood glucose level has exceeded the capacity of the kidney to reabsorb glucose (via a sodium-dependent glucose transporter [SGLT]). The high concentration of glucose in the urine osmotically draws water from the body. This causes increased urination (polyuria) with loss of water that results in dehydration.

TQ3. The NADH generated in fatty acid β-oxidation inhibits the tricarboxylic acid (TCA) cycle at the three NADH-producing dehydrogenase steps. This shifts acetyl CoA away from oxidation in the TCA cycle and toward use as a substrate in hepatic ketogenesis.

TQ4. The patient was in negative nitrogen balance: more nitrogen was going out than coming in. This is reflected in the elevated blood urea nitrogen (BUN) level seen in the patient (see Figure). [Note: The BUN value also reflects dehydration.] Muscle proteolysis and amino acid catabolism are occurring as a result of the fall in insulin. (Recall that skeletal muscle does not express the glucagon receptor.) Amino acid catabolism produces ammonia (NH_3), which is converted to urea by the hepatic urea cycle and sent into the blood. [Note: Urea in the urine is reported as urinary urea nitrogen (UUN).]

SKELETAL MUSCLE
Proteolysis
Amino acids
Catabolism
NH_3
Urea cycle
Urea —BLOOD→ **BUN**

TQ5. The Kussmaul respiration seen in the patient is a respiratory response to the metabolic acidosis. Hyperventilation blows off carbon dioxide (CO_2) and water, reducing the concentration of protons (H^+) and bicarbonate (HCO_3^-) as reflected in the following equation:

$$H^+ + HCO_3^- \leftrightarrow H_2CO_3 \text{ (carbonic acid)} \leftrightarrow CO_2 + H_2O.$$

The renal response includes, in part, the excretion of H^+ as ammonium (NH_4^+). Degradation of branched-chain amino acids in skeletal muscle results in the release of large amounts of glutamine into the blood. The kidneys take up and catabolize the glutamine generating NH_3 in the process. The NH_3 is converted to NH_4^+ by secreted H^+ and is excreted (see Figure). [Note: When ketone bodies are plentiful, enterocytes shift to using them as a fuel instead of glutamine. This increases the amount of glutamine going to the kidney.]

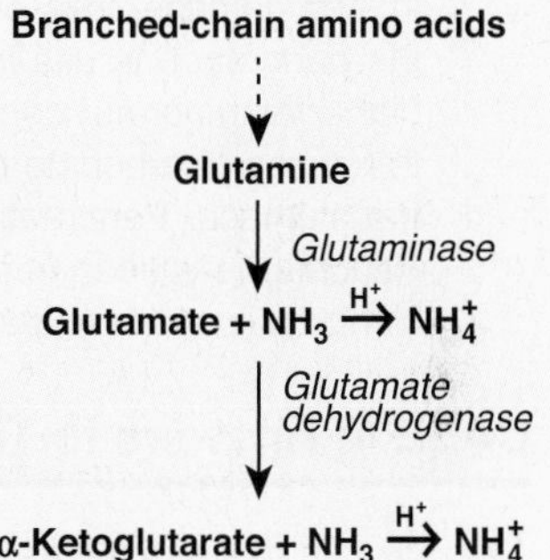

TQ6. Because fatty acid β-oxidation supplies the acetyl CoA substrate for ketogenesis, impaired β-oxidation decreases the ability to make ketone bodies. Ketone bodies are an alternate to the use of glucose, and, thus, dependence on glucose increases. Because fatty acid β-oxidation supplies the NADH and the nucleoside triphosphates needed for gluconeogenesis, glucose production decreases. The result is a hypoketotic hypoglycemia. Recall that this was seen with medium-chain acyl CoA dehydrogenase (MCAD) deficiency.

CASE 4: Answers to Review Questions

RQ1. Answer = D. The rise in reduced nicotinamide adenine dinucleotide (NADH) in the mitochondria decreases the tricarboxylic acid (TCA) cycle, fatty acid oxidation, and gluconeogenesis. NADH inhibits the isocitrate dehydrogenase reaction, the key regulated step of the TCA cycle, and the α-ketoglutarate dehydrogenase reaction (see Figure). It also favors the reduction of oxaloacetate to malate (not malate to oxaloacetate), decreasing the availability of oxaloacetate for condensation with acetyl coenzyme A (CoA) in the TCA cycle and for gluconeogenesis. Fatty acid oxidation requires NAD^+ for the 3-hydroxyacyl CoA dehydrogenase step and, thus, is inhibited by the rise in NADH. The decrease in fatty acid oxidation decreases the production of adenosine triphosphate (ATP) and acetyl CoA (the allosteric activator of pyruvate carboxylase) needed for gluconeogenesis. Lipolysis is activated in fasting as a consequence of the fall in insulin and the rise in catecholamines that result in activation of hormone-sensitive lipase.

Acetyl CoA
Citrate synthase
Oxaloacetate
Citrate
TCA cycle
Malate
Isocitrate
NADH
ATP
Isocitrate dehydrogenase
Fumarate
α-Ketoglutarate
NADH
Succinyl CoA
Succinate
Succinyl CoA

RQ2. Answer = E. The irreversible, oxidative portion of the pentose phosphate pathway provides the nicotinamide adenine dinucleotide phosphate (NADPH) that supplies the reducing equivalents needed for activity of cytochrome P450 (CYP) proteins and for the regeneration of functional (reduced) glutathione. It is also an important source of NADPH for reductive biosynthetic processes in the cytosol, such as fatty acid and cholesterol synthesis. CYP proteins are monooxygenases (mixed-function oxidases). They incorporate one O atom from O_2 into the substrate as the other is reduced to water. It is the CYP proteins of the smooth endoplasmic reticulum membrane that are involved in detoxification reactions. Those of the inner mitochondrial membrane are involved in the synthesis of steroid hormones, bile acids, and calcitriol. Reactive oxygen species are reduced by glutathione peroxidase as glutathione is oxidized.

RQ3. Answer = C. Serotonin is released by activated platelets and causes vasoconstriction and platelet aggregation. [Note: Platelets do not synthesize serotonin, but they take up serotonin that was made in the intestine and secreted into the blood.] Serotonin is associated with a feeling of well-being. It is degraded by monoamine oxidase (MAO) that catalyzes oxidative deamination. It is catechol-O-methyl transferase (COMT) that catalyzes the methylation step in the degradation of the catecholamines. Serotonin is synthesized from tryptophan in a two-step process that utilizes tetrahydrobiopterin-requiring tryptophan hydroxylase and a pyridoxal phosphate (PLP)-requiring decarboxylase (see Figure).

CH_2CHCOO^- NH_3^+

Tryptophan

Tetrahydro-biopterin → O_2 *Hydroxylase* → Dihydro-biopterin + H_2O

HO CH_2CHCOO^- NH_3^+

5-Hydroxy-tryptophan

Aromatic amino acid decarboxylase PLP → CO_2

HO $CH_2CH_2NH_2$

Serotonin

RQ4. Answer = B. The exocrine pancreas secretes enzymes required for the digestion of dietary carbohydrate, protein, and fat. The endocrine pancreas secretes the peptide hormones insulin and glucagon. Damage that affects the functions of the pancreas would lead to diabetes (decreased insulin) and steatorrhea (fatty stool), with the latter the consequence of maldigestion of dietary fat. As was seen with the rise of troponins in a myocardial infarction and transaminases in liver damage, loss of cellular integrity (as would be seen in autodigestion of the pancreas) results in proteins that normally are intracellular being found in higher-than-normal concentrations in the blood. Secretin causes the pancreas to release bicarbonate to raise the pH of the chyme coming to the intestine from the stomach. Pancreatic enzymes work best at neutral or slightly alkaline pH. Pancreatitis is seen in individuals with hypertriglyceridemia as a result of a deficiency in lipoprotein lipase or its coenzyme, apolipoprotein C-II.

CASE 4: Answers to Thought Questions

TQ1. A. The rise in cytosolic NADH seen with ethanol metabolism inhibits glycolysis. The glyceraldehyde 3-phosphate dehydrogenase step requires NAD^+, which gets reduced as glyceraldehyde 3-phosphate gets oxidized. With the rise in NADH, glyceraldehyde 3-phosphate accumulates.

B. The glyceraldehyde 3-phosphate from glycolysis is converted to glycerol 3-phosphate, the initial acceptor of fatty acids in triacylglycerol (TAG) synthesis (see Figure). Fatty acids are available because of increased synthesis (from acetyl CoA, which is increased as a result of both increased production from the acetate product of acetaldehyde and decreased use in the TCA cycle), increased availability from lipolysis in adipose tissue, and decreased degradation. The TAGs produced in the liver accumulate (due, in part, to decreased production of very-low-density lipoproteins) and cause fatty liver (steatosis). Hepatic steatosis is an early (and reversible) stage in alcohol-induced liver disease. Subsequent stages are alcohol-related hepatitis (sometimes reversible) and cirrhosis (irreversible).

Glycerol 3-phosphate

Fatty acyl CoA → CoA *Acyltransferase*

Lysophosphatidic acid

Fatty acyl CoA → CoA *Acyltransferase*

Phosphatidic acid (DAG phosphate)

H_2O → P_i *Phosphatase*

Diacylglycerol (DAG)

Fatty acyl CoA → CoA *Acyltransferase*

Triacylglycerol (TAG)

TQ2. The rise in NADH favors the reduction of pyruvate to lactate by lactate dehydrogenase. Lactate decreases the renal excretion of uric acid, thereby causing hyperuricemia, a necessary step in an acute gouty attack. [Note: The shift from pyruvate to lactate decreases the availability of pyruvate, a substrate for gluconeogenesis. This contributes to the hypoglycemia seen in the patient.]

TQ3. Prothrombin time (PT) measures the time it takes for plasma to clot after the addition of tissue factor (FIII), thereby allowing evaluation of the extrinsic (and common) pathways of coagulation (see Figure). In the extrinsic pathway, FIII activates FVII. FVII, like most of the proteins of clotting, is made by the liver. Alcohol-induced liver damage can decrease its synthesis. Additionally, FVII has a short half-life and, as a γ-carboxyglutamate (Gla)-containing protein, its synthesis requires vitamin K. Poor nutrition can result in decreased availability of vitamin K and, therefore, decreased ability to clot. [Note: Severe liver disease results in prolonged PT and activated partial thromboplasin time, or aPPt.]

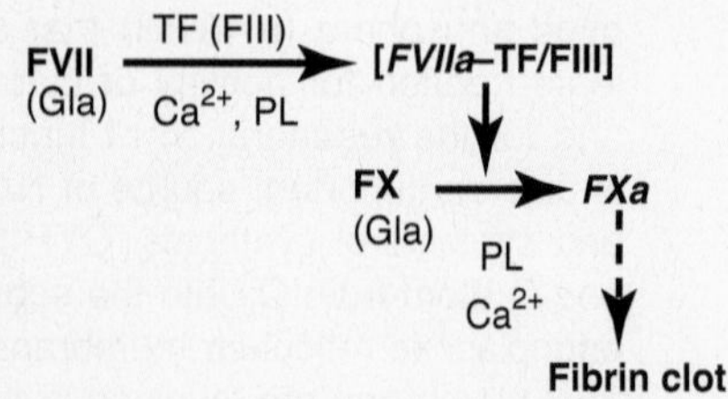

TQ4. Administration of folate can mask a deficiency in vitamin B_{12} by reversing the hemotologic manifestations of the deficiency. However, folate has no effect on the neurologic damage caused by B_{12} deficiency. Over time, then, the neurologic effects can become severe and irreversible. Thus, folate can mask a deficiency of B_{12} and prevent treatment until the neuropathy is apparent.

III. FOCUSED CASES

CASE 1: MICROCYTIC ANEMIA

Patient Presentation: JS is a 24-year-old man who is being evaluated as a follow-up to a pre-placement medical evaluation he had prior to starting his new job.

Focused History: JS has no significant medical issues. His family history is unremarkable, but he knows little of the health status of those family members who remain in Greece.

Pertinent Findings: The physical examination was normal. Routine analysis of his blood included the following results:

	Patient	Reference Range
Red blood cells	$4.8 \times 10^6/mm^3$	4.3–5.9
Hemoglobin	9.6 g/dl (**L**)	13.5–7.5 (men)
Mean corpuscular volume	70 μm^3 (**L**)	80–100
Serum iron	150 µg/dl	50–170

Based on the data, hemoglobin (Hb) electrophoresis was performed. The results:

	Patient	Reference Range
HbA*	90% (**L**)	96–98
HbA_2	6% (**H**)	<3
HbF	4% (**H**)	<2
*Includes HbA_{1c}	**H** = High; **L** = Low.	

Diagnosis: JS has β-thalassemia trait (β-thalassemia minor) that is causing a microcytic anemia (see Image). Ethnicity (such as being of Mediterranean origin) influences the risk for thalassemia.

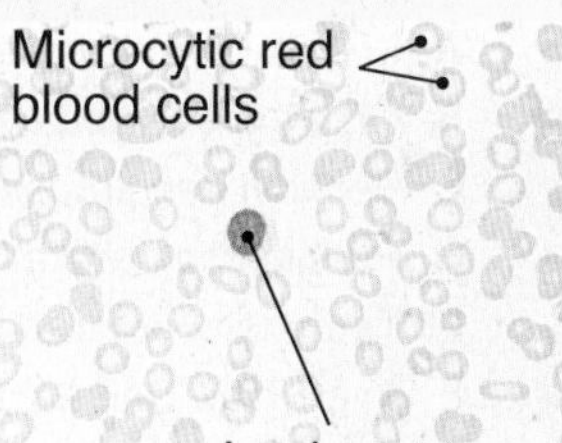

Treatment: None is required at this time. Patients are advised that iron supplements will not prevent their anemia.

Prognosis: β-thalassemia trait does not cause mortality or significant morbidity. Patients should be informed of the genetic nature of their autosomal recessive condition for family planning considerations because homozygous β-thalassemia (Cooley anemia) is a serious disorder.

CASE-RELATED QUESTIONS: Choose the ONE best answer.

Q1. Mutations to the gene for β globin that result in decreased production of the protein are the cause of β-thalassemia. The mutations primarily affect gene transcription or posttranscriptional processing of the messenger RNA (mRNA) product. Which of the following statements concerning mRNA is correct?

A. Eukaryotic mRNA is polycistronic.

B. mRNA synthesis involves trans-acting factors binding to cis-acting elements.

C. mRNA synthesis is terminated at the DNA base sequence thymine adenine guanine (TAG).

D. Polyadenylation of the 5' end of eukaryotic mRNA requires a methyl donor.

E. Splicing of eukaryotic mRNA involves removal of exons and joining of introns by the proteasome.

Q2. Hemoglobin A (HbA), a tetramer of 2 α and 2 β globin chains, delivers O_2 from the lungs to the tissues and protons and CO_2 from the tissues to the lungs. Increased concentration of which of the following will result in decreased O_2 delivery by HbA?

A. 2,3-Bisphosphoglycerate

B. Carbon dioxide

C. Carbon monoxide

D. Protons

Q3. What is the basis for the increase in HbA_2 and HbF in the β-thalassemias?

Q4. Why is the allele-specific oligonucleotide (ASO) hybridization technique useful in the diagnosis of all cases of sickle cell anemia but not all cases of β-thalassemia?

CASE 2: SKIN RASH

Patient Presentation: KL is a 34-year-old woman who presents with a red, nonitchy rash on her left thigh and flulike symptoms.

Focused History: KL reports that the rash first appeared a little over 2 weeks ago. It started out small but has gotten larger. She also thinks she is getting the flu because her muscles and joints ache (myalgia and arthralgia, respectively), and she has had a headache for the last few days. Upon questioning, KL tells you she and her husband took a camping trip through New England last month.

Pertinent Findings: The physical examination is remarkable for the presence of a red, circular, flat lesion about 11 cm in size that resembled a bullseye (erythema migrans) (see image). KL also has a low-grade fever.

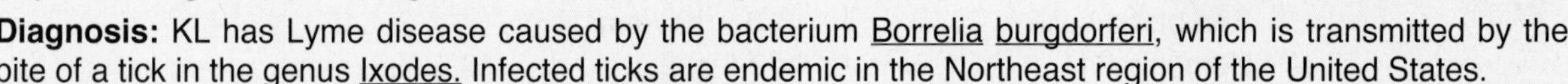

Diagnosis: KL has Lyme disease caused by the bacterium Borrelia burgdorferi, which is transmitted by the bite of a tick in the genus Ixodes. Infected ticks are endemic in the Northeast region of the United States.

Treatment: The patient is prescribed doxycycline, an antibiotic in the tetracycline family. Monitoring of KL will continue until all symptoms have completely resolved. Blood is drawn for clinical laboratory tests.

Prognosis: Patients treated with the appropriate antibiotic in the early stages of Lyme disease typically recover quickly and completely.

CASE-RELATED QUESTIONS: Choose the ONE best answer.

Q1. Antibiotics in the tetracycline class inhibit protein synthesis (translation) at the initiation step. Which of the following statements about translation is correct?

A. In eukaryotic translation, the initiating amino acid is formylated methionine.
B. Only the charged initiating transfer RNA goes directly to the ribosomal A site.
C. Peptidyl transferase is a ribozyme that forms the peptide bond between two amino acids.
D. Prokaryotic translation can be inhibited by the phosphorylation of initiation factor 2.
E. Termination of translation is independent of guanosine triphosphate hydrolysis.
F. The Shine-Dalgarno sequence facilitates the binding of the large ribosomal subunit to eukaryotic messenger RNA (mRNA).

Q2. The Centers for Disease Control and Prevention recommends a two-tier testing procedure for Lyme disease that involves a screening enzyme-linked immunosorbent assay (ELISA) follow by a confirmatory Western blot analysis on any sample with a positive or equivocal ELISA result. Which of the following statements about these testing procedures is correct?

A. Both techniques are used to detect specific mRNAs.
B. Both techniques involve the use of antibodies.
C. ELISAs require the use of electrophoresis.
D. Western blots require use of the polymerase chain reaction.

Q3. Why are eukaryotic cells unaffected by antibiotics in the tetracycline class?

CASE 3: BLOOD ON THE TOOTHBRUSH

Patient Presentation: LT is an 84-year-old man whose gums have been bleeding for several months.

Focused History: LT is a widower and lives alone in a suburban community on the East Coast. He no longer drives. His two children live on the West Coast and come east infrequently. Since the death of his wife 11 months ago, he has been isolated and finds it hard to get out of the house. His appetite has changed, and he is content with cereal, coffee, and packaged snacks. Chewing is difficult.

Pertinent Findings: The physical examination was remarkable for the presence of swollen dark-colored gums (see Image). Several of the patient's teeth were loose, including one that anchors his dental bridge. Several black and blue marks (ecchymoses) were noted on the legs, and an unhealed sore was present on the right wrist. Inspection of his scalp revealed tiny red spots (petechia) around some of the hair follicles. Blood was drawn for testing.

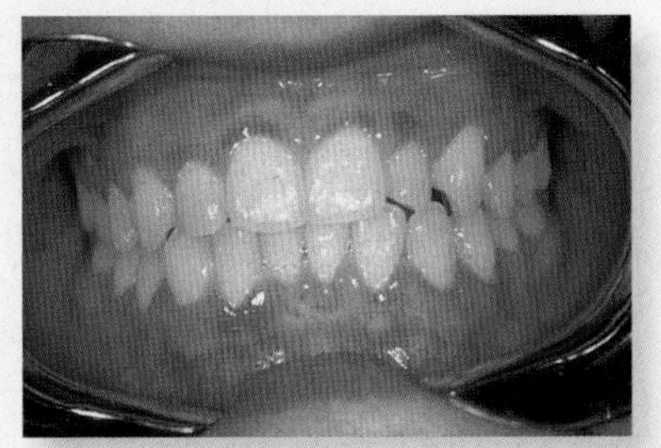

Results of tests on the patient's blood:

	Patient	Reference Range
Red blood cells	$4.0 \times 10^6/mm^3$ (**L**)	4.3–5.9
Hemoglobin	10 g/dl (**L**)	13.5–17.5 (men)
Mean corpuscular volume	78 μm^3 (**L**)	80–100
Serum iron	40 µg/dl (**L**)	50–170
Platelets	250×10^9/l	$150–350 \times 10^9$

The test for blood in his stool (occult blood test) was negative.

Results of follow-up tests (obtained several days after the appointment) included:

	Patient	Reference Range
Vitamin C (plasma)	0.16 mg/dl (**L**)	0.2–2

H = High; **L** = Low

Diagnosis: Vitamin C deficiency with a microcytic, hypochromic anemia secondary to the deficiency

Treatment: LT was prescribed Vitamin C (as oral ascorbic acid) and iron (as oral ferrous sulfate) supplements. He will also be referred to social services.

Prognosis: The prognosis for recovery is excellent.

CASE-RELATED QUESTIONS: Choose the ONE best answer.

Q1. Which of the following statements about vitamin C is correct? Vitamin C is:

A. a competitor of iron absorption in the intestine.
B. a fat-soluble vitamin with a 3-month supply typically stored in adipose tissue.
C. a coenzyme in several enzymic reactions such as the hydroxylation of proline.
D. required for the cross-linking of collagen.

Q2. In contrast to the microcytic anemia characteristic of iron deficiency (common in older adults), a macrocytic anemia is seen with deficiencies of vitamin B_{12} and/or folic acid. These vitamin deficiencies are also common in older adults. Which of the following statements concerning these vitamins is correct?

A. An inability to absorb B_{12} results in pernicious anemia.
B. Both vitamins cause changes in gene expression.
C. Folic acid plays a key role in energy metabolism in most cells.
D. Treatment with methotrexate can result in toxic levels of the coenzyme form of folic acid.
E. Vitamin B_{12} is the coenzyme for enzymes catalyzing amino acid deaminations, decarboxylations, and transaminations.

Q3. How do hemolytic anemias differ from nutritional anemias?

CASE 4: RAPID HEART RATE, HEADACHE, AND SWEATING

Patient Presentation: BE is a 45-year-old woman who presents with concerns about sudden (paroxysmal), intense, brief episodes of headache, sweating (diaphoresis), and a racing heart (palpitations).

Focused History: BE reports that the attacks started about 3 weeks ago. They last from 2 to 10 minutes, during which time she feels quite anxious. During the attacks it feels as though her heart is skipping beats (arrhythmia). At first she thought the attacks were related to recent stress at work and maybe even menopause. The last time it happened, she was in the drug store and had her blood pressure taken. She was told it was 165/110 mm Hg. BE notes that she has lost weight (about 8 lbs) in this period even though her appetite has been good.

Pertinent Findings: The physical examination was remarkable for the patient's thin, pale appearance. Blood pressure was elevated (150/100 mm Hg), as was the heart rate (110–120 beats/minute). Based on the patient's history, blood levels of normetanephrine and metanephrine were ordered. They were found to be elevated.

Diagnosis: Pheochromocytoma, a rare catecholamine-secreting tumor of the adrenal medulla

Treatment: Imaging studies of the abdomen were performed to locate the tumor. Surgical resection of the tumor was performed. The tumor was found to be nonmalignant. Follow-up measurement of plasma metanephrines was performed 2 weeks later and was in the normal range.

Prognosis: The 5-year survival rate for nonmalignant pheochromocytomas is over 95%.

CASE-RELATED QUESTIONS: Choose the ONE best answer.

Q1. Pheochromocytomas secrete norepinephrine and epinephrine. Which of the following statements concerning the synthesis and degradation of these two biogenic amines is correct?

A. The substrate for their synthesis is tryptophan, which is hydroxylated to 3,4-dihydroxyphenylalanine (DOPA) by tetrahydrobiopterin-requiring tryptophan hydroxylase.

B. The conversion of DOPA to dopamine utilizes a pyridoxal phosphate–requiring carboxylase.

C. The conversion of norepinephrine to epinephrine requires vitamin C.

D. Degradation involves methylation by catechol-O-methytransferase and produces normetanephrine from norepinephrine and metanephrine from epinephrine.

E. Normetanephrine and metanephrine are oxidatively deaminated to homovanillic acid by monoamine oxidase.

Q2. Which of the following statements concerning the actions of epinephrine and/or norepinephrine are correct?

A. Norepinephrine functions as a neurotransmitter and a hormone.

B. They are initiated by autophosphorylation of select tyrosine residues in their receptors.

C. They are mediated by binding to adrenergic receptors, which are a class of nuclear receptors.

D. They result in the activation of glycogen and triacylglycerol synthesis.

Q3. Norepinephrine bound to certain receptors causes vasoconstriction and an increase in blood pressure. Why might norepinephrine be used clinically in the treatment of septic shock?

CASE 5: SUN SENSITIVITY

Patient Presentation: AZ is a 6-year-old boy who is being evaluated for freckle-like areas of hyperpigmentation on his face, neck, forearms, and lower legs.

Focused History: AZ's father reports that the boy has always been quite sensitive to the sun. His skin turns red (erythema) and his eyes hurt (photophobia) if he is exposed to the sun for any period of time.

Pertinent Findings: The physical examination was remarkable for the presence of thickened, scaly areas (actinic keratosis) and hyperpigmented areas on skin exposed to ultraviolet (UV) radiation from the sun. Small dilated blood vessels (telangiectasia) were also seen. Tissue from several sites on his face was biopsied, and two were later determined to be squamous cell carcinomas.

Diagnosis: Xeroderma pigmentosum, a rare defect in nucleotide excision repair of DNA

Treatment: Protection from sunlight through use of sunscreens such as protective clothing that reflect UV radiation and chemicals that absorb it is essential. Frequent skin and eye examinations are recommended.

Prognosis: Most patients with xeroderma pigmentosum die at an early age from skin cancers. However, survival beyond middle age is possible.

CASE-RELATED QUESTIONS: Choose the ONE best answer.

Q1. Which of the following statements about DNA repair mechanisms is correct? DNA repair:

A. is performed only by eukaryotes.

B. of double-strand breaks is error free.

C. of mismatched bases involves repair of the parental strand.

D. of ultraviolet radiation–induced pyrimidine dimers involves removal of a short oligonucleotide containing the dimer.

E. of uracil produced by the deamination of cytosine requires the actions of endo- and exonucleases to remove the uracil base.

Q2. Which one of the following statements about DNA synthesis (replication) is correct? Replication:

A. in both eukaryotes and prokaryotes requires an RNA primer.

B. in eukaryotes requires condensation of chromatin.

C. in prokaryotes is accomplished by a single DNA polymerase.

D. is initiated at random sites in the genome.

E. produces a polymer of deoxyribonucleoside monophosphates linked by 5'→3' phosphodiester bonds.

Q3. What is the difference between DNA proofreading and repair?

CASE 6: DARK URINE AND YELLOW SCLERAE

Patient Presentation: JF is a 13-year-old girl who presents with fatigue and yellow sclerae.

Focused History: JF began treatment about 4 days ago with a sulfonamide antibiotic and a urinary analgesic for a urinary tract infection. She had been told that her urine would change color (become reddish) with the analgesic, but she reports that it has gotten darker (more brownish) over the last 2 days. Last night her mother noticed that her eyes had a yellow tint. JF says she feels as though she has no energy.

Pertinent Findings: The physical examination was remarkable for the pale appearance of the patient, mild scleral icterus (jaundice), mild splenomegaly, and an increased heart rate (tachycardia). JF's urine tested positive for hemoglobin (hemoglobinuria). A peripheral blood smear reveals a lower-than-normal number of red blood cells (RBCs), with some containing precipitated hemoglobin (Heinz bodies; see Image), and a higher-than-normal number of reticulocytes (immature RBCs). Results of the complete blood count (CBC) and blood chemistry tests are pending.

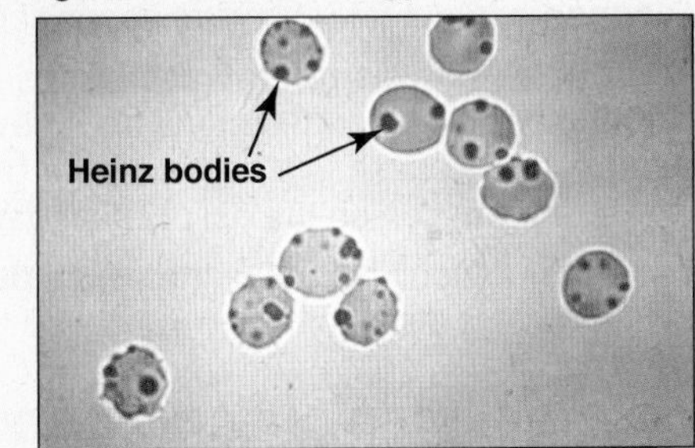

Diagnosis: *Glucose 6-phosphate dehydrogenase* (*G6PD*) deficiency, an X-linked disorder that causes hemolysis (RBC lysis)

Treatment: *G6PD* deficiency can result in a hemolytic anemia in affected individuals exposed to oxidative agents. JF will be switched to a different antibiotic. She will be advised that she is susceptible to certain drugs (for example, sulfa drugs), foods (fava or broad beans), and certain chemicals (for example, naphthalene), and must avoid exposure to them.

Prognosis: In the absence of exposure to oxidative agents, *G6PD* deficiency does not cause mortality or significant morbidity.

CASE-RELATED QUESTIONS: Choose the ONE best answer.

Q1. Glucose 6-phosphate dehydrogenase (G6PD) catalyzes the regulated step in the pentose phosphate pathway. Which of the following statements concerning G6PD and the pentose phosphate pathway is correct?

A. Deficiency of G6PD occurs only in red blood cells.

B. Deficiency of G6PD results in an inability to keep glutathione in its functional, reduced form.

C. The pentose phosphate pathway includes one reversible reductive reaction followed by a series of phosphorylated sugar interconversions.

D. The reduced nicotinamide adenine dinucleotide phosphate (NADPH) product of the pentose phosphate pathway is utilized in processes such as fatty acid oxidation.

Q2. When received, the results of the blood count were consistent with a hemolytic anemia. Blood chemistry tests revealed an elevation in the bilirubin level. Which of the following statements concerning bilirubin is correct?

A. Hyperbilirubinemia can cause deposition of bilirubin in the skin and sclerae resulting in jaundice.

B. The solubility of bilirubin is increased by conjugating it with two molecules of ascorbic acid in the liver.

C. The conjugated form of bilirubin increases in the blood with a hemolytic anemia.

D. Phototherapy can increase the solubility of the excess bilirubin generated in the porphyrias.

Q3. Why is urinary urobilinogen increased relative to normal in hemolytic jaundice and absent in obstructive jaundice?

CASE 7: JOINT PAIN

Patient Presentation: BJ is a 22-year-old male who presents for follow-up 10 days after having been treated in the Emergency Department (ED) for severe inflammation at the base of his thumb.

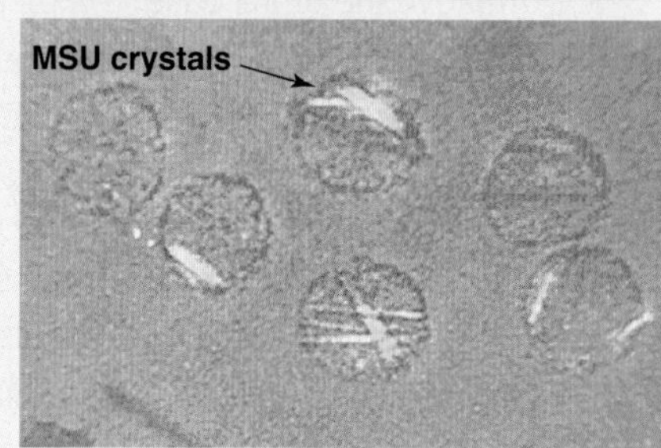

Focused History: This was BJ's first occurrence of severe joint pain. In the ED, he was given an anti-inflammatory medication. Fluid aspirated from the carpometacarpal joint of the thumb was negative for organisms but positive for needle-shaped monosodium urate (MSU) crystals (see Image). The inflammatory symptoms have since resolved. BJ reports he is in good health otherwise, with no significant past medical history. His body mass index (BMI) is 31. No tophi (deposits of MSU crystals under the skin) were detected in the physical examination.

Pertinent Findings: Results on a 24-hour urine specimen and blood tests requested in advance of this visit reveal that BJ is not an undersecretor of uric acid. His blood urate was 8.5 mg/dl (reference = 2.5–8.0). The unusually young age of presentation is suggestive of an enzymopathy of purine metabolism, and additional blood tests are ordered.

Diagnosis: Gout (MSU crystal deposition disease), a type of inflammatory arthritis

Treatment: BJ was given prescriptions for allopurinol and colchicine. The treatment goals are to reduce his blood urate levels to <6.0 mg/dl and prevent additional attacks. He was advised to lose weight because being overweight or obese is a risk factor for gout. His BMI of 31 puts him in the obese category. He was also given written information on the association between diet and gout.

Prognosis: Gout increases the risk of developing renal stones. It is also associated with hypertension, diabetes, and heart disease.

CASE-RELATED QUESTIONS: Choose the ONE best answer.

Q1. Allopurinol is converted in the body to oxypurinol, which functions as a noncompetitive inhibitor of an enzyme in purine metabolism. Which of the following statements concerning purine metabolism and its regulation is correct?

A. As a noncompetitive inhibitor, oxypurinol increases the apparent Michaelis constant (K_m) of the target enzyme.

B. Colchicine inhibits xanthine oxidase, an enzyme of purine degradation.

C. Glutamate provides two of the nitrogen atoms of the purine ring.

D. In purine nucleotide synthesis, the ring system is first constructed and then attached to ribose 5-phosphate.

E. Oxypurinol inhibits the amidotransferase that initiates degradation of the purine ring system.

F. Partial or complete enzymic deficiencies in the salvage of purine bases are characterized by hyperuricemia.

Q2. Purines are one type of nitrogenous base found in nucleotides. Pyrimidines are the other. Which of the following statements is true of the pyrimidines?

A. Carbamoyl phosphate synthetase I is the regulated enzymic activity in pyrimidine ring synthesis.

B. Methotrexate decreases synthesis of the pyrimidine nucleotide thymidine monophosphate.

C. Orotic aciduria is a pathology of pyrimidine degradation.

D. Pyrimidine nucleotide synthesis is independent of 5-phosphoribosyl-1-pyrophosphate (PRPP).

Q3. BJ is subsequently shown to have a form of PRPP synthetase that shows increased enzymic activity. Why does this result in hyperuricemia?

CASE 8: NO BOWEL MOVEMENT

Patient Presentation: MW is a 48-hour-old female who has not yet had a bowel movement.

Focused History: MW is the full-term product of a normal pregnancy and delivery. She appeared normal at birth. MW is the first child of parents of Northern European ethnicity. The parents are both in good health, and their family histories are unremarkable.

Pertinent Findings: MW has a distended abdomen. She recently vomited small amounts of bilious (green-colored) material.

Diagnosis: Meconium ileus (obstruction of the ileum by meconium, the first stool produced by newborns) was confirmed by abdominal x-rays. About 98% of full-term newborns with meconium ileus have cystic fibrosis (CF). Diagnosis of CF was subsequently confirmed with a chloride sweat test.

Treatment: The ileus was successfully treated nonsurgically. For management of the CF, the family was referred to the CF center at the regional children's hospital.

Prognosis: CF is the most common life-limiting autosomal-recessive disease in Caucasians.

CASE-RELATED QUESTIONS: Choose the ONE best answer.

Q1. CF is the result of mutations to the gene that codes for the cystic fibrosis transmembrane conductance regulator (CFTR) protein that functions as a chloride channel in the apical membrane of epithelial cells on a mucosal surface. Which of the following statements concerning CF is correct?

A. Clinical manifestations of CF are the consequence of chloride retention with increased water reabsorption that causes mucous on the epithelial surface to be excessively thick and sticky.

B. Excessive pancreatic secretion of insulin commonly results in hypoglycemia.

C. Genetic testing for CF may involve the use of a set of probes for the most common mutations, a technique known as restriction fragment length polymorphism analysis.

D. Some mutations result in premature degradation of the CFTR protein through tagging with ubiquinone followed by proteasome-mediated proteolysis.

E. The most common mutation, ΔF508, results in the loss of a codon for phenylalanine and is classified as a frameshift mutation.

Q2. The CFTR protein is an intrinsic plasma membrane glycoprotein. Targeting of proteins destined to function as components of membranes:

A. includes transport to and through the Golgi.

B. involves an amino-terminal signal sequence that is retained in the functional protein.

C. occurs after the protein has been completely synthesized (that is, posttranslationally).

D. requires the presence of mannose 6-phosphate residues on the protein.

Q3. Why might steatorrhea be seen with CF?

CASE 9: ELEVATED AMMONIA

Patient Presentation: RL is a 40-hour-old male with signs of cerebral edema.

Focused History: RL is the full-term product of a normal pregnancy and delivery. He appeared normal at birth. At age 36 hours he became irritable, lethargic, and hypothermic. He fed only poorly and vomited. He also displayed tachypneic (rapid) breathing and neurologic posturing. At age 38 hours he had a seizure.

Pertinent Findings: Respiratory alkalosis (increased pH, decreased CO_2 [hypocapnia]), increased ammonia level, and decreased blood urea nitrogen level were found. An amino acid screen revealed that argininosuccinate was increased more than 60-fold over baseline, and citrulline was increased 4-fold. Glutamine was elevated, and arginine was decreased relative to normal.

Diagnosis: Urea cycle enzyme defect with neonatal onset

Treatment: Hemodialysis was performed to remove ammonia. Sodium phenylacetate and sodium benzoate were administered to aid in excretion of waste nitrogen, as was arginine. Long-term treatment will include lifelong limitation of dietary protein; supplementation with essential amino acids; and administration of arginine, sodium phenylacetate, and sodium phenylbutyrate.

Prognosis: Survival into adulthood is possible. The degree of neurologic impairment is related to the degree and extent of the hyperammonemia.

CASE-RELATED QUESTIONS: Choose the ONE best answer.

Q1. Based on the findings, which enzyme of the urea cycle is most likely to be deficient in this patient?

A. Arginase
B. Argininosuccinate lyase
C. Argininosuccinate synthetase
D. Carbamoyl phosphate synthetase I
E. Ornithine transcarbamoylase

Q2. Why is arginine supplementation helpful in this case?

Q3. In individuals with partial (milder) deficiency of urea cycle enzymes, the level of which one of the following would be expected to be decreased during periods of physiologic stress?

A. Alanine
B. Ammonia
C. Glutamine
D. Insulin
E. pH

CASE 10: CALF PAIN

Patient Presentation: CR is a 19-year-old female who is being evaluated for pain and swelling in her right calf.

Focused History: Ten days ago, CR had her spleen removed following a bicycle accident in which she fractured her tibial eminence, necessitating immobilization of the right knee. She has had a good recovery from the surgery. CR is no longer taking pain medication but has continued her oral contraceptives.

Pertinent Findings: CR's right calf is reddish in color (erythematous) and warm to the touch. It is visibly swollen. The left calf is normal in appearance and is without pain. An ultrasound is ordered.

Diagnosis: CR has a deep venous thrombosis (DVT). Oral contraceptives are a risk factor for DVT, as are surgery and immobilization.

Treatment (Immediate): Heparin and warfarin are administered.

Prognosis: In the 10 years following a DVT, about one third of individuals have a recurrence.

CASE-RELATED QUESTIONS: Choose the ONE best answer.

Q1. A deep venous thrombosis is a blood clot that occludes the lumen of a deep vein, most commonly in the leg. Which of the following statements about the clotting cascade is correct?

A. A deficiency in factor (F)IX of the intrinsic pathway results in hemophilia A.
B. FIII of the extrinsic pathway is a serine protease.
C. Formation of the fibrin meshwork is referred to as primary hemostasis.
D. Thrombin proteolytically activates components of the extrinsic, intrinsic, and common pathways.
E. Vitamin K is required for the activation of fibrinogen.

Q2. Which one of the following would increase the risk of thrombosis?

A. Excess production of antithrombin
B. Excess production of protein S
C. Expression of FV Leiden
D. Hypoprothrobinemia
E. von Willebrand disease

Q3. Compare and contrast the actions of heparin and warfarin.

IV. FOCUSED CASES: ANSWERS TO CASE-BASED QUESTIONS

CASE 1: Anemia with β-Thalassemia Minor

Q1. Answer = B. Transcription (synthesis of single-stranded RNA from the template strand of double-stranded DNA) requires the binding of proteins (trans-acting factors) to sequences on the DNA (cis-acting elements). Eukaryotic messenger RNA (mRNA) is monocistronic because it contains information from just one gene (cistron). The base sequence TAG (thymine adenine guanine) in the coding strand of DNA is U(uracil)AG in the mRNA. UAG is a signal that terminates translation (protein synthesis), not transcription. It is formation of the 5' cap of eukaryotic mRNA that requires methylation (using S-adenosylmethionine), not 3' polyadenylation. Splicing is the spliceosome-mediated process by which introns are removed from eukaryotic mRNA and exons joined.

Q2. Answer = C. Carbon monoxide (CO) increases the affinity of hemoglobin (Hb)A for O_2, thereby decreasing the ability of HbA to offload O_2 in the tissues. CO stabilizes the R (relaxed) or oxygenated form and shifts the O_2 dissociation curve to the left (see Figure). The other choices decrease the affinity for O_2, stabilize the T (tense) or deoxygenated form, and cause a right shift in the curve.

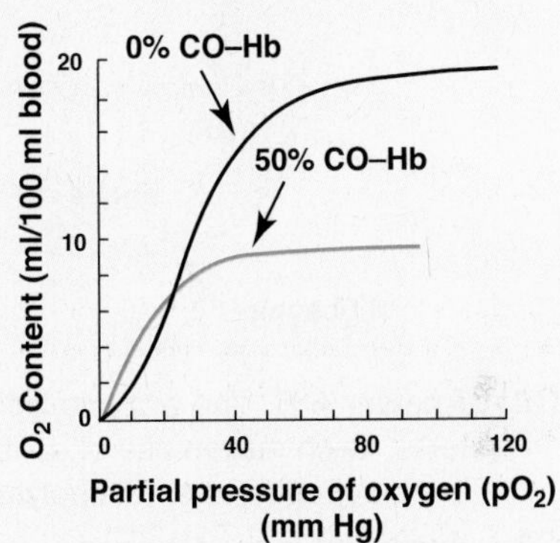

Q3. HbA_2 and HbF do not contain β globin. As β globin production decreases, synthesis of HbA_2 ($\alpha_2\delta_2$) and HbF ($\alpha_2\gamma_2$) increases.

Q4. Sickle cell anemia is caused by a single point mutation (A→T) in the gene for β globin that results in the replacement of glutamate by valine at the sixth amino acid position in the protein. Mutational analysis using allele-specific oligonucleotide (ASO) probes for that mutation (β^S) and for the normal sequence (β^A) is used in diagnosis (see Figure). β-Thalassemia, in contrast, is caused by hundreds of different mutations. Mutational analysis using ASO probes can assess common mutations, including point mutations, in at-risk populations (for example, those of Greek ancestry). However, less common mutations are often not included in the panel and can be detected only by DNA sequencing.

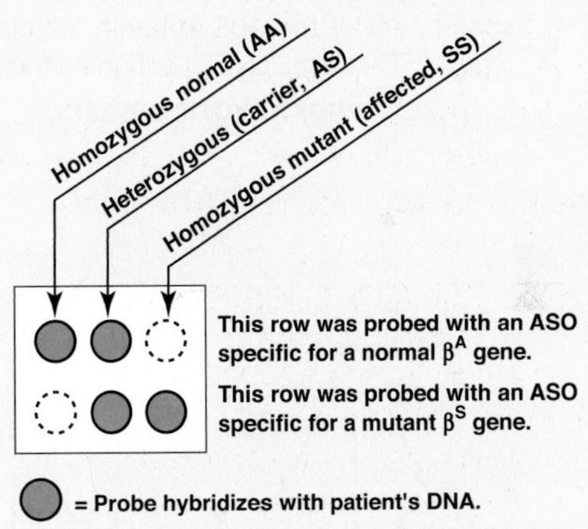

CASE 2: Skin Rash with Lyme Disease

Q1. Answer = C. Peptide bond formation between the amino acid in the A site of the ribosome and the amino acid last added to the growing peptide in the P site is catalyzed by an RNA of the large ribosomal subunit. Any RNA with catalytic activity is referred to as a ribozyme (see Figure below). Formylated methionine is used to initiate prokaryotic translation. The charged initiating transfer RNA (tRNA) is the only tRNA that goes directly to the P site, leaving the A site available for the tRNA carrying the next amino acid of the protein being made. Eukaryotic translation is inhibited by the phosphorylation of initiation factor 2 (eIF-2). The Shine-Dalgarno (SD) sequence is found in prokaryotic messenger RNA (mRNA) and facilitates the interaction of the mRNA with the small ribosomal subunit. In eukaryotes, the cap-binding proteins perform that task.

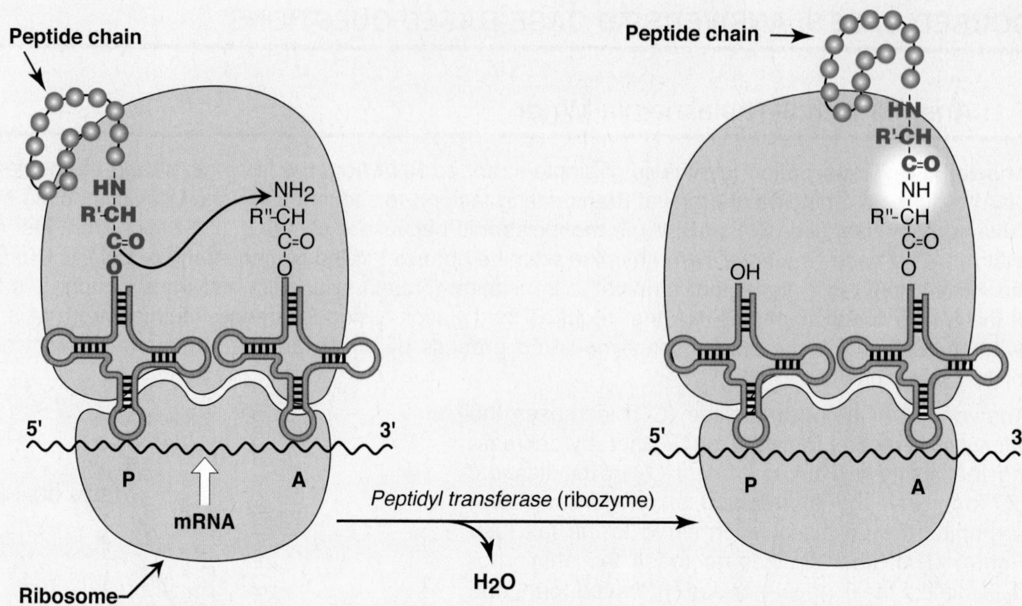

Q2. **Answer = B.** The enzyme-linked immunosorbent assay (ELISA) and Western blot are used to analyze proteins. Each makes use of antibodies to detect and quantify the protein of interest. It is Western blots that utilize electrophoresis. The polymerase chain reaction (PCR) is used to amplify DNA.

Q3. Antibiotics in the tetracycline family inhibit protein synthesis by binding to and blocking the A site of the small ribosomal subunit (30S) in prokaryotes. Tetracycline specifically interacts with the 16S ribosomal RNA (rRNA) component of the 30S subunit, inhibiting translation initiation. Eukaryotes do not contain 16S rRNA (see Figure). Their small (40S) subunit contains 18S rRNA, which does not bind tetracycline.

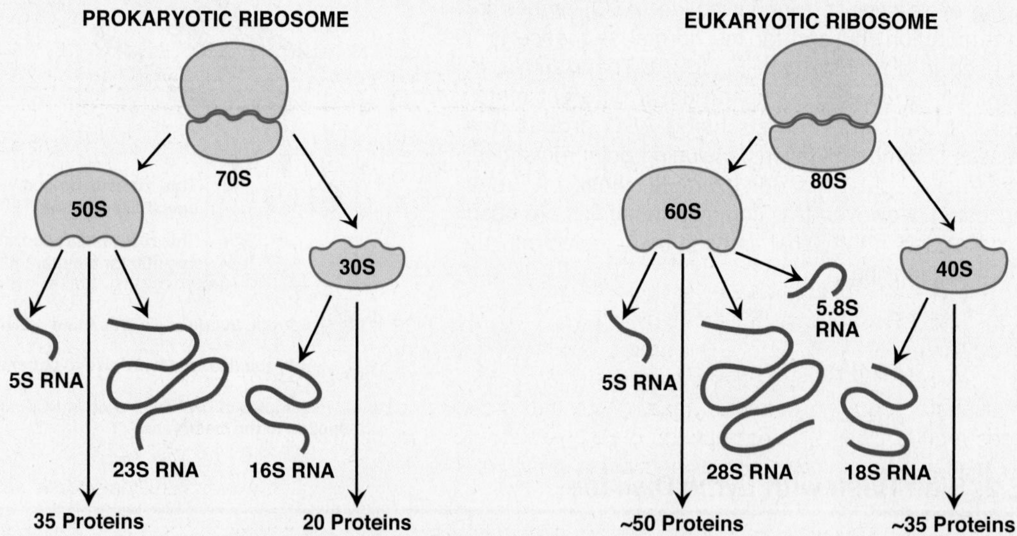

CASE 3: Blood on the Toothbrush with Vitamin C Deficiency

Q1. **Answer = C.** Vitamin C (ascorbic acid) functions as a coenzyme in the hydrolylation of proline and lysine in the synthesis of collagen, a fibrous protein of the extracellular matrix. Vitamin C reduces dietary iron from the ferric (Fe^{3+}) to the ferrous (Fe^{2+}) form that is required for absorption. With a deficiency of vitamin C, uptake of dietary iron is impaired and results in a microcytic, hypochromic anemia. As a water-soluble vitamin, vitamin C is not stored. Cross-linking of collagen by lysyl oxidase requires copper, not vitamin C.

Q2. **Answer = A.** An inability to absorb vitamin B_{12} leads to pernicious anemia and is most commonly caused by decreased production of intrinsic factor (IF) by the parietal cells of the stomach (see Figure). Vitamins D and A, in complex with their receptors, bind to DNA and alter gene expression. Thiamine (vitamin B_1) is a coenzyme in the oxidative decarboxylation of pyruvate and α-ketoglutarate and, therefore, is important in energy metabolism in most cells. Methotrexate inhibits dihydrofolate reductase, the enzyme required to reduce dihydrofolate to tetrahydrofolate (THF), the functional coenzyme form of folate. This results in decreased availability of THF. It is pyridoxine (vitamin B_6) as pyridoxal phosphate (PLP) that is the coenzyme for most reactions involving amino acids. (Note that tetrahydrobioptrin is required by aromatic amino acid hydroxylases.)

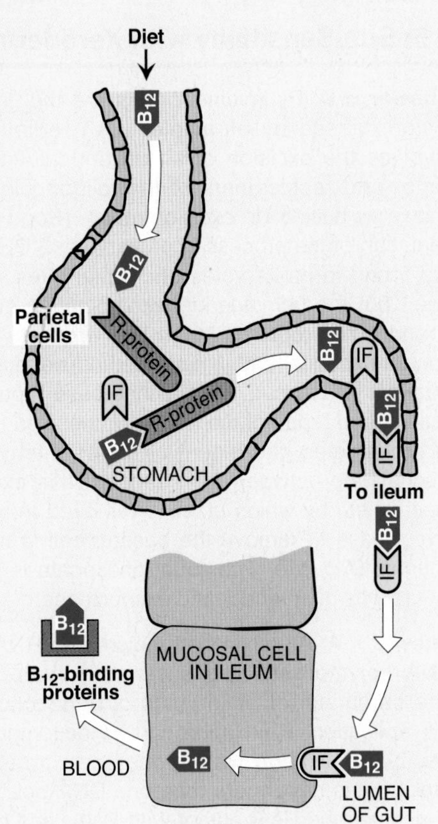

Q3. Nutritional anemias are characterized by either increased red blood cell (RBC) size (folate and B_{12} deficiencies) or decreased RBC size (iron and vitamin C deficiencies). In hemolytic anemias, such as is seen in glucose 6-phosphate dehydrogenase and pyruvate kinase deficiencies and in sickle cell anemia, RBC size typically is normal and RBC number is decreased.

CASE 4: Rapid Heart Rate, Headache, and Sweating with a Pheochromocytoma

Q1. **Answer = D.** Degradation of both epinephrine and norepinephrine involves methylation by catechol-O-methytransferase (COMT) that produces normetanephrine from norepinephrine and metanephrine from epinephrine (see Figure). Both of these products are deaminated to vanillylmandelic acid by monoamine oxidase (MAO). The substrate for the synthesis of the catecholamines is tyrosine, which gets hydroxylated to 3,4-dihydroxyphenylalanine (DOPA) by tetrahydrobiopterin-requiring tyrosine hydroxylase. DOPA is converted to dopamine by a pyridoxal phosphate–requiring decarboxylase. (Note that most carboxylases require biotin.) Norepinephrine is converted to epinephrine by methylation, and S-adenosylmethionine provides the methyl group.

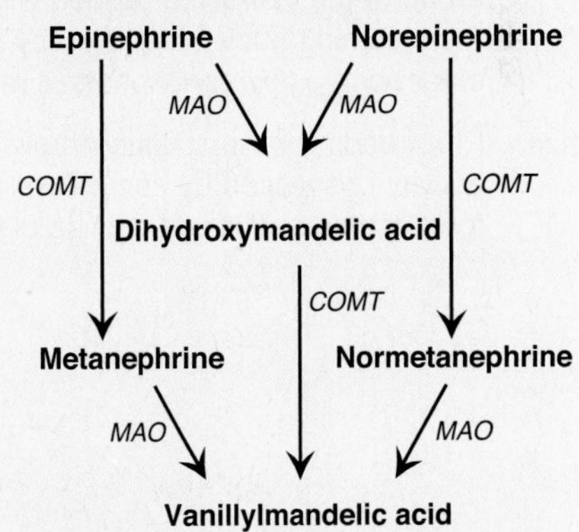

Q2. **Answer = A.** Norepinephrine released from the sympathetic nervous system functions as a neurotransmitter that acts on postsynaptic neurons and causes, for example, increased heart rate. It is also released from the adrenal medulla and, along with epinephrine, functions as a counterregulatory hormone that results in mobilization of stored fuels (for example, glucose and triacylglycerols). These actions are mediated by the binding of norepinephrine to adrenergic receptors, which are G protein–coupled receptors of the plasma membrane, and not to nuclear receptors like those of steroid hormones or membrane tyrosine kinase receptors like that of insulin.

Q3. Septic shock is vasodilatory hypotension (low blood pressure caused by blood vessel dilation) resulting from the production of large amounts of nitric oxide by inducible nitric oxide synthase (iNOS) in response to infection. Norepinephrine bound to receptors on smooth muscle cells causes vasoconstriction and, thus, raises blood pressure.

CASE 5: Sun Sensitivity with Xeroderma Pigmentosum

Q1. Answer = D. Pyrimidine dimers are the characteristic DNA lesion caused by ultraviolet (UV) radiation. Their repair involves the excision of an oligonucleotide containing the dimer and replacement of that oligonucleotide, a process known as nucleotide excision repair. (See Figure for a representation of the process in prokaryotes.) DNA repair systems are found in prokaryotes and eukaryotes. Nothing is "error free," but the homologous-recombination method of double-strand break repair is much less prone to error than is the nonhomologous–end-joining method because any DNA that was lost is replaced. Mismatched-base repair involves identification and repair of the newly synthesized (daughter) strand. In prokaryotes, the extent of strand methylation is used to discriminate between the strands. Base excision repair, the mechanism by which uracil is removed from DNA, utilizes a glycosylase to remove the base, creating an apyrimidinic or apurinic (AP) site. The sugar-phosphate is then removed by the actions of an endo- and exonuclease.

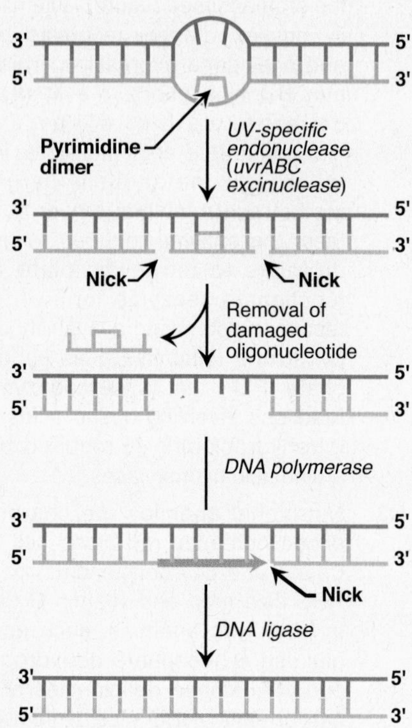

Q2. Answer = A. All replication requires an RNA primer because DNA polymerases (pols) cannot initiate DNA synthesis. The chromatin of eukaryotes gets decondensed (relaxed) for replication. Relaxation can be accomplished, for example, by acetylation via histone acetyltransferases (HATs). Prokaryotes have more than one DNA pol. For example, pol III extends the RNA primer with DNA, and pol I removes the primer and replaces it with DNA. Replication is initiated at specific locations (one in prokaryotes, many in eukaryotes) that are recognized by proteins (for example, DnaA in prokaryotes). Deoxynucleoside monophosphates (dNMPs) are joined by a phosphodiester bond that links the 3'-hydroxyl group of the last dNMP added with the 5'-phosphate group of the incoming nucleotide, thereby forming a 3'→5' phosphodiester bond as pyrophosphate is released.

Q3. Proofreading occurs during replication in the S phase of the cell cycle and involves the 3'→5' exonuclease activity possessed by some DNA pols (see Figure). Repair can occur independently of replication and, therefore, can be performed outside of the S phase.

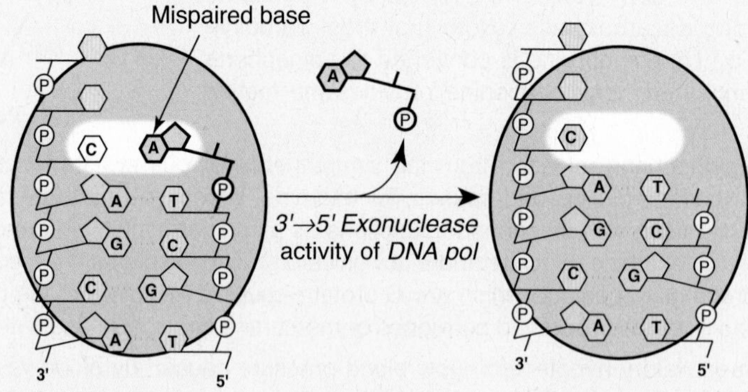

CASE 6: Dark Urine and Yellow Sclerae with Glucose 6-Phosphate Dehydrogenase Deficiency

Q1. Answer = B. Glutathione in its reduced form (G-SH) is an important antioxidant. The enzyme glutathione peroxidase reduces hydrogen peroxide (a reactive oxygen species) to water as glutathionine is oxidized (G-S-S-G). Reduced nicotinamide adenine dinucleotide phosphate (NADPH)-requiring glutathionine reductase regenerates the reduced, functional form of glutathione (see Figure A). The NADPH is supplied by the oxidative reactions of the pentose phosphate pathway (see Figure B), which is regulated by the availability of NADPH at the glucose 6-phosphate dehydrogenase (G6PD)-catalyzed step (the first step). Deficiency of G6PD occurs in all cells, but the effects are seen in red blood cells where the pentose phosphate pathway is the only source of NADPH. The pathway involves two irreversible oxidative reactions, each of which generates NADPH. The NADPH is used in reductive processes such as fatty acid synthesis (not oxidation) as well as steroid hormone and cholesterol synthesis.

A.

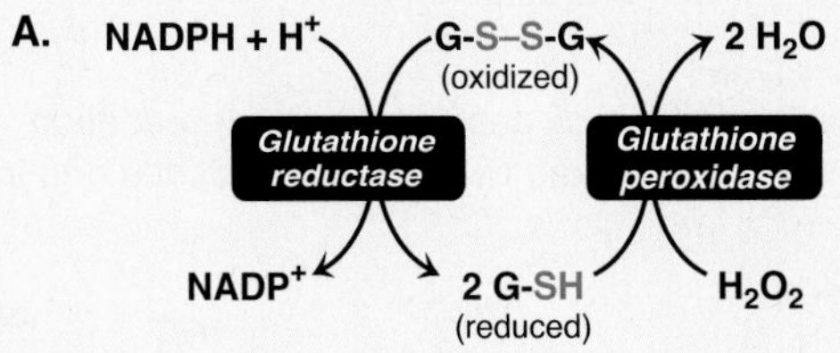

B.

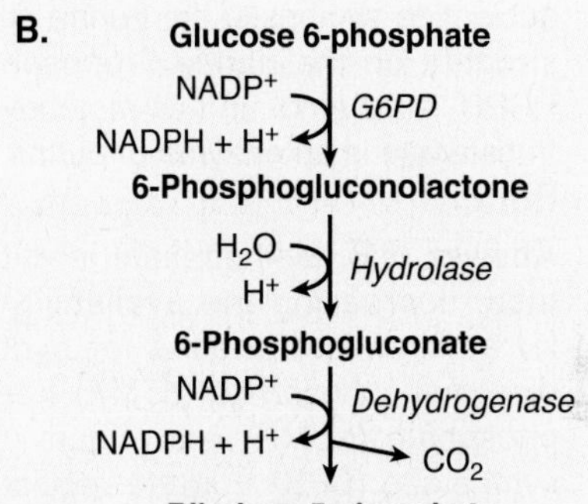

Q2. Answer = A. Jaundice (icterus) refers to the yellow color of the skin, nail beds, and sclerae that results from the deposition of bilirubin when the bilirubin level in the blood is elevated (hyperbilirubinemia; see Image C). Bilirubin has low solubility in aqueous solutions, and its solubility is increased by conjugation with uridine diphosphate (UDP)-glucuronic acid in the liver, forming bilirubin diglucuronide or conjugated bilirubin (CB). In hemolytic conditions, such as G6PD deficiency, both conjugated and unconjugated bilirubin (UCB) are increased, but it is UCB that is found in the blood. CB is sent into the intestine. Phototherapy is used to treat unconjugated hyperbilirubinemia because it converts bilirubiin to isomeric forms that are more water soluble. Bilirubin is the product of heme degradation in cells of the reticuloendothelial system, particularly in the liver and the spleen. The porphyrias are pathologies of heme synthesis and, therefore, are not characterized by hyperbilirubinemia.

C.

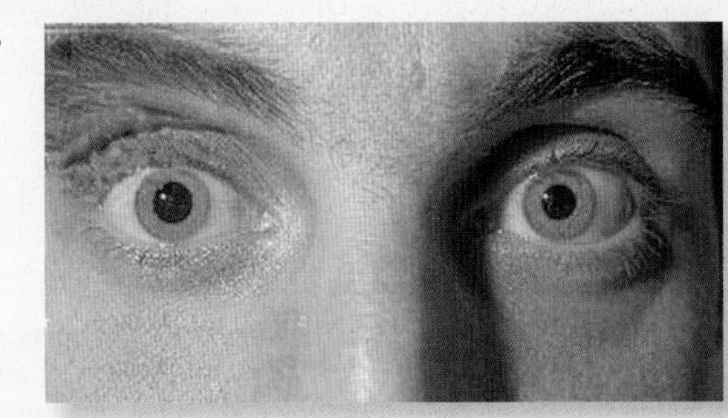

D.

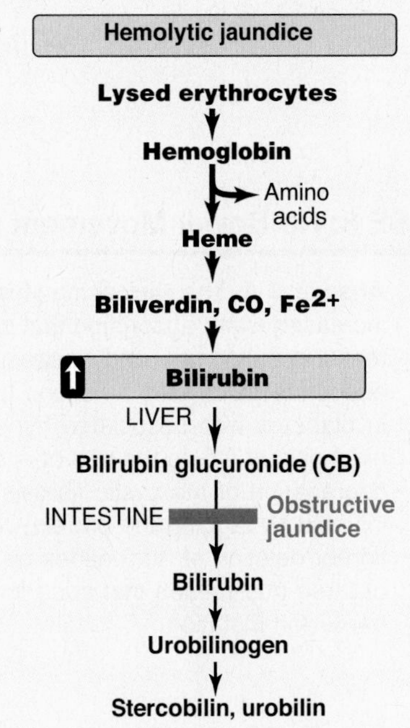

Q3. With hemolysis, more bilirubin is produced and conjugated. CB is sent to the intestine where it is converted to urobilinogen, some of which is reabsorbed, enters the portal blood, and travels to the kidney. Because the source of urinary urobilinogen is intestinal urobilinogen, urinary urobilinogen will be low in obstructive jaundice because intestinal urobilinogen will be low as a result of the obstruction of the common bile duct (see Figure D).

CASE 7: Joint Pain with Gout

Q1. Answer = F. Salvage of the purine bases hypoxanthine and guanine to the purine nucleotides inosine monophosphate (IMP) and guanosine monophosphate (GMP) by hypoxanthine-guanine phosphoribosyltransferase (HGPRT) requires 5-phosphoribosyl-1-pyrophosphate (PRPP) as the source of the ribose 1-phosphate. Salvage decreases the amount of substrate available for degradation to uric acid. Therefore, a deficiency in salvage results in hyperuricemia (see figure). Noncompetitive inhibitors such as oxypurinol have no effect on the Michaelis constant (K_m) but decrease the apparent maximal velocity (V_{max}). Colchicine is an anti-inflammatory drug. It has no effect on the enzymes of purine synthesis or degradation. Glutamine (not glutamate) is a nitrogen source for purine ring synthesis. In purine nucleotide synthesis, the purine ring system is constructed on the ribose 5-phosphate provided by PRPP. Allopurinol and its metabolite, oxypurinol, inhibit xanthine oxidase of purine degradation. The amidotransferase is an enzyme of purine synthesis. Its activity is decreased by purine nucleotides and increased by PRPP.

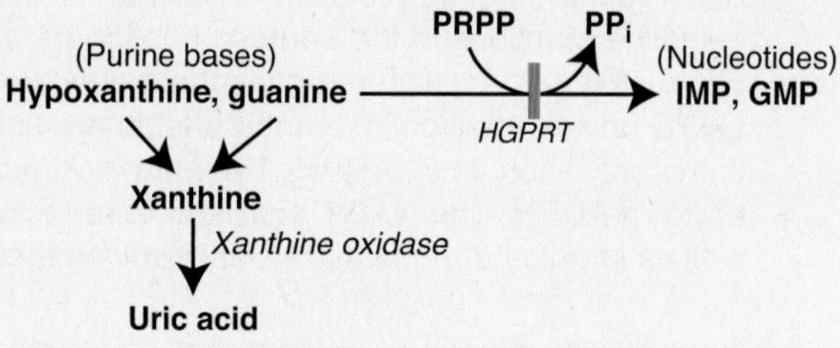

Q2. Answer = B. Methotrexate inhibits dihydrofolate reductase, decreasing the availability of N^5,N^{10}-methylene tetrahydrofolate needed for synthesis of deoxythymidine monophosphate (dTMP) from deoxyuridine monophosphate (dUMP); see Figure. Carbamoyl phosphate synthetase (CPS) II is the regulated enzymic activity of pyrimidine biosynthesis in humans. CPS I is an enzyme of the urea cycle. Orotic aciduria is a rare pathology of pyrimidine synthesis caused by a deficiency in one or both enzymic activities of bifunctional uridine monophosphate synthase. Pyrimidine nucleotide synthesis, like purine synthesis and salvage, requires PRPP.

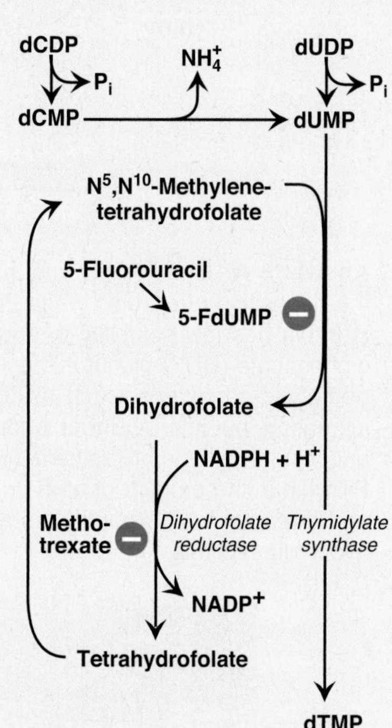

Q3. Increased activity of PRPP synthetase results in increased synthesis of PRPP. This results in an increase in purine nucleotide synthesis beyond need. The excess purine nucleotides get degraded to uric acid, thereby causing hyperuricemia.

CASE 8: No Bowel Movement with Cystic Fibrosis

Q1. Answer = A. The clinical manifestations of cystic fibrosis (CF) are the consequence of chloride retention with increased water absorption that causes mucus on an epithelial surface to be excessively thick and sticky. The result is pulmonary and gastrointestinal problems such as respiratory infection and impaired exocrine and endocrine pancreatic functions (pancreatic insufficiency). Impaired endocrine pancreatic function can result in diabetes with associated hyperglycemia. The genetic testing technique described, and one used in the diagnosis of CF, is the use of allele-specific oligonucleotides (ASOs). Some mutations do result in increased degradation of the cystic fibrosis transmembrane conductance regulator (CFTR) protein, but degradation is initiated by tagging the protein with ubiquitin. Frameshift mutations alter the reading frame through the addition or deletion of nucleotides by a number not divisible by three. The ΔF509 mutation is caused by the loss of three nucleotides that code for phenylalanine at position 509 in the CFTR protein and, therefore, is not a frameshift mutation.

Q2. Answer = A. Targeting of proteins destined to function as components of the plasma membrane is an example of cotranslational targeting. It involves the initiation of translation on cytosolic ribosomes; the recognition of the amino (N)-terminal signal sequence in the protein; the movement of the protein-synthesizing complex to the outer face of the membrane of the endoplasmic reticulum (ER); and the continuation of protein synthesis such that the protein is threaded into the lumen of the ER, packaged into vesicles that travel to and through the Golgi, and eventually fuse with the plasma membrane. The N-terminal signal sequence is removed by a peptidase in the lumen of the ER. Mannose 6-phosphate is the signal that posttranslationally targets proteins to the matrix of the lysosome where they function as acid hydrolases.

Q3. The pancreatic insufficiency seen in some patients with CF results in a decreased ability to digest food, and digestion is required for absorption. Dietary fats move through the intestine and are excreted in the stool, which is foul-smelling and bulky and may float (see Figure). Patients are at risk for malnutrition and deficiencies in fat-soluble vitamins. Oral supplementation of pancreatic enzymes is the treatment.

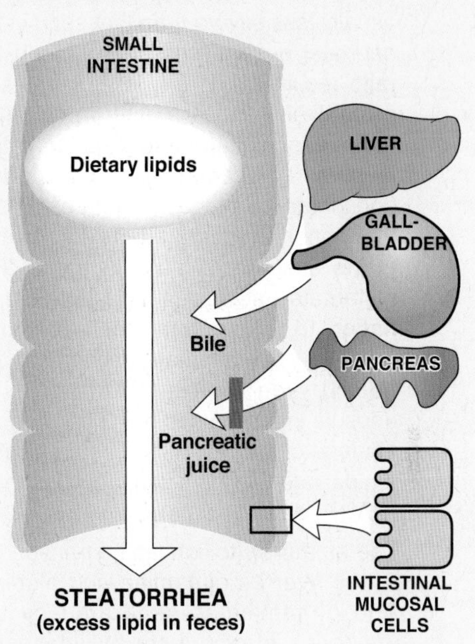

CASE 9: Hyperammonemia with a Urea Cycle Defect

Q1. **Answer = B.** Argininosuccinate lyase (ASL) cleaves argininosuccinate to arginine and fumarate. The increase in argininosuccinate and citrulline and the decrease in arginine seen in the patient indicate a deficiency in ASL (see Figure below). With arginase deficiency, arginine would be increased, not decreased. Additionally, with arginase deficiency, the hyperammonemia would be less severe. Deficiency of argininosuccinate synthetase (ASS) would also cause an increase in citrulline, but argininosuccinate would be low to absent. Deficiency of carbamoyl phosphate synthetase (CPS) I is characterized by low levels of arginine and citrulline. Deficiency of ornithine transcarbamoylase (OTC), the only X-linked enzyme of the urea cycle, would result in low levels of arginine and citrulline and elevated levels of urinary orotic acid. [Note: The orotic acid is elevated because the carbamoyl phosphate (CP) substrate of OTC is being used in the cytosol as a substrate for pyrimidine synthesis.]

MITOCHONDRION
$NH_3 + CO_2$
2ATP
2 ADP + P_i
CPSI
Ornithine + Carbamoyl phosphate
in *OTC* deficiency
Carbamoyl phosphate
OTC
Citrulline
Orotic acid (pyrimidine)
CYTOSOL
Citrulline
Aspartate
ATP
ASS
AMP + PP_i
Ornithine
Argininosuccinate
Arginase
ASL
Urea
H_2O
Arginine
Fumarate

Q2. Arginine supplementation is helpful because the arginine will be hydrolyzed to urea plus ornithine by arginase. The ornithine will be combined with carbamoyl phosphate to form citrulline (see Figure above). With ASL (and ASS) deficiency, citruline accumulates and is excreted, thereby carrying waste nitrogen out of the body.

Q3. Answer = D. In individuals with milder (partial) deficiencies in the enzymes of the urea cycle, hyperammonemia may be triggered by physiologic stress (for example, an illness or prolonged fasting) that decreases the insulin-to-counterregulatory hormone ratio. [Note: The degree of the hyperammonemia is usually less severe than that seen in the neonatal onset forms.] The shift in the ratio results, in part, in skeletal muscle proteolysis, and the amino acids that are released get degraded. Degradation involves transamination by pyridoxal phosphate–requiring aminotransferases that generate the α-keto acid derivative of the amino acid plus glutamate. The glutamate undergoes oxidative deamination to α-ketoglutarate and ammonia (NH_3) by glutamate dehydrogenase (GDH): see Figure. [Note: GDH is unusual in that it uses both nicotinamide adenine dinucleotide (NAD) and nicotinamide adenine dinucleotide phosphate (NADP) as coenzymes.]

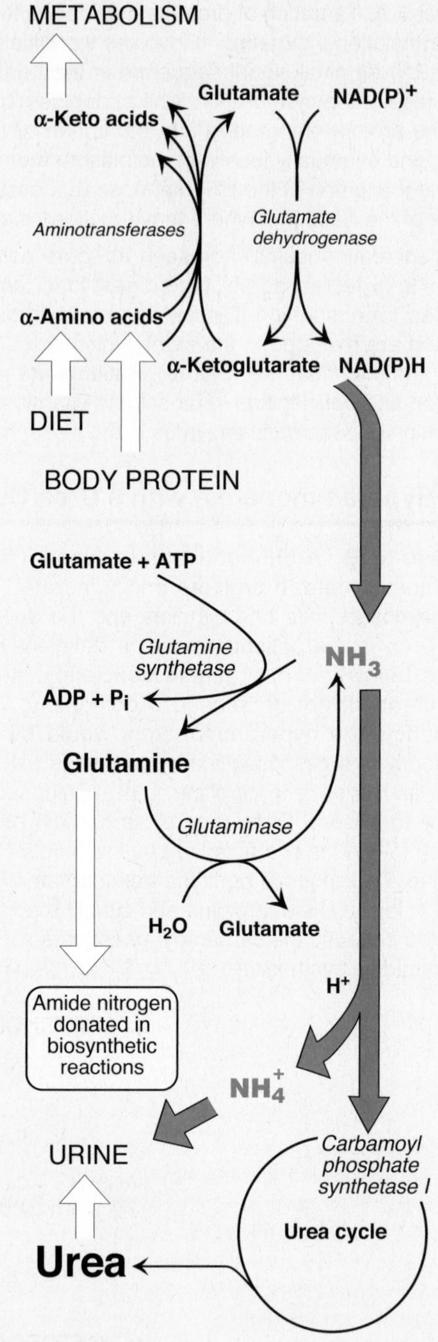

The ammonia (toxic) can be transported to the liver as glutamine and alanine. The glutamine is generated by the amination of glutamate by adenosine triphosphate–requiring glutamine synthetase. In the liver, the enzyme glutaminase removes the ammonia, which can be converted to urea by the urea cycle (see Figure). Glutamine, then, is a nontoxic vehicle of ammonia transport in the blood. Alanine is generated in skeletal muscle from the catabolism of the branched-chain amino acids. In the liver, alanine is transaminated to pyruvate (used in gluconeogenesis) and glutamate. Thus, alanine carries nitrogen to the liver for conversion to urea. Therefore, defects in the urea cycle would result in an elevation in ammonia, glutamine, and alanine. The elevated ammonia drives respiration, and the hyperventilation causes a rise in pH (respiratory alkalosis). [Note: Hyperammonemia is toxic to the nervous system. Although the exact mechanisms are not completely understood, it is known that the metabolism of large amounts of ammonia to glutamine (in the astrocytes of the brain) results in osmotic effects that cause the brain to swell. Additionally, the rise in glutamine decreases the availability of glutamate, an excitatory neurotransmitter.]

CASE 10: Swollen, Painful Calf with Deep Venous Thrombosis

Q1. Answer = D. Thrombin, a serine protease, is activated by the prothrombinase complex of factor (F)Xa + FVa. Once formed, activated thrombin proteolytically activates components of the extrinsic (FVII) and intrinsic (FXI, FVIII) pathways, generating FXa. Thrombin can also activate FV, FI, and FXIII of the common pathway (see Figure below). Hemophilia A is caused by a deficiency in FVIII. FIX deficiency results in hemophilia B. FIII, also known as tissue factor (TF), is a transmembrane glycoprotein of the vascular endothelium. It functions as an accessory protein and not a protease. Formation of the platelet plug is primary hemostasis, and formation of the fibrin meshwork is secondary hemostasis. Vitamin K is required for the activation (γ-carboxylation) of FII, FVII, FIX, and FX but not for FI (fibrinogen).

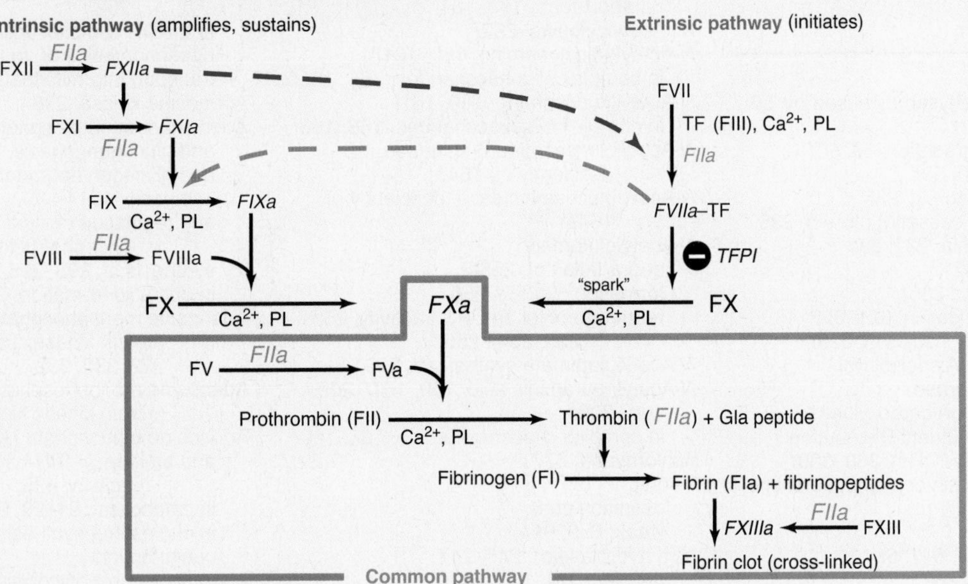

Q2. Answer = C. FV Leiden is a mutant form of FV that is resistant to proteolysis by the activated protein C complex. Decreased ability to degrade FV allows continued production of activated thrombin and leads to an increased risk of clot formation or thrombophilia. Antithrombin III (ATIII) and protein S are proteins of anticoagulation. Increased, not decreased, production of prothrombin would result in thrombophilia. Deficiency of von Willebrand factor causes a coagulopathy or a deficiency in clotting through effects on FVIII and platelets.

Q3. Heparin and warfarin are anticoagulants. Heparin, a glycosaminoglycan, increases the affinity of ATIII for thrombin. Binding of ATIII removes thrombin from the blood and prevents it from converting fibrinogen to fibrin. Warfarin, a synthetic analog of vitamin K, inhibits vitamin K epoxide reductase and prevents the regeneration of the functional hydroquinone form of the vitamin that is required for the γ-carboxylation of glutamate residues to γ-carboxyglutamate (Gla) residues in FII, FVII, FIX, and FX (see Figures).

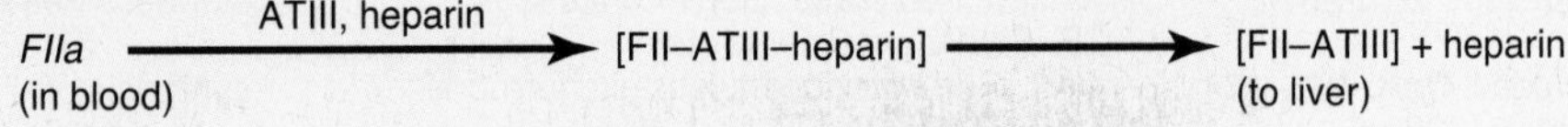

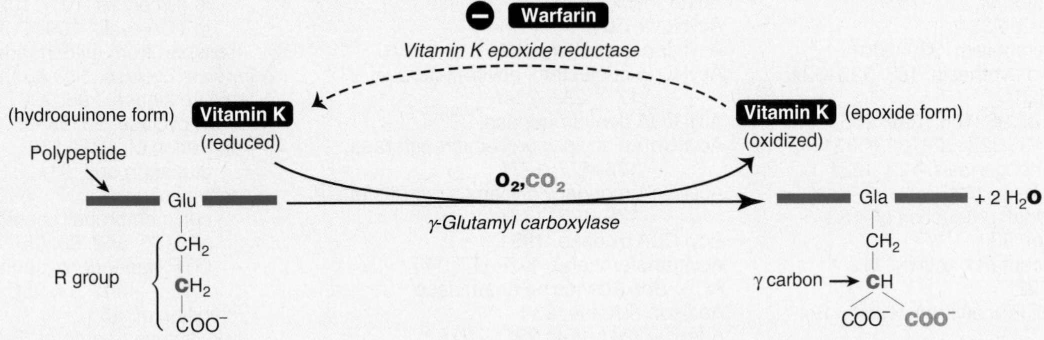

Index

Note: Page numbers followed by *f* and *t* indicate figures and tables, respectively.

A

D

E

F

G

I

J

K

L

M

N

O

P

S

T

Figure Sources

Figure 2.12: Modified from Garrett, R. H. and Grisham, C. M. *Biochemistry*. Saunders College Publishing, 1995. Figure 6.36, p. 193.

Figure 2.13 (panel C, top): Abdulla, S. Basic mechanisms of protein folding disease. Nature Publishing Group.

Figure 3.1A: Illustration: Irving Geis. Rights owned by Howard Hughes Medical Institute. Not to be used without permission

Figure 3.20: Photo curtesy of Photodyne Incorporated, Hartland, WI.

Figure 3.21: Corbis

Figure 4.3: Electron micrograph of collagen: Natural Toxin Research Center. Texas A&M University-Kingsville. Collagen molecule modified from Mathews, C. K., van Holde, K. E. and Ahern, K. G. *Biochemistry, 3rd Ed.*, Addison Wesley Longman, Inc. 2000. Figure 6.13, p.175.

Figure 4.4: modified from Yurchenco, P. D., Birk, D. E., and Mecham, R. P., eds. (1994) *Extracellular Matrix Assembly and Structure*, Academic Press, San Diego, California

Figure 4.8: Kronauer and Buhler, Images in Clinical Medicine, *N Engl J Med*, June 15, 1995 , Vol. 332, No. 24, p.1611.

Figure 4.10: Photo from Web site Derma.de

Figure 4.11: Jorde, L. B., Carey, J. C., Bamshad, M. J. and White, R. L. *Medical Genetics, 2nd Ed.* http://medgen.genetics.utah.edu/index.htm

Question 4.3: from Berge LN, Marton V, Tranebjaerg L, Kearney MS, Kiserud T, Oian P. Prenatal diagnosis of osteogenesis imperfecta. *Acta Obstetricia et Gynecologica Scandinavica.* 74(4):321-3, 1995 Apr.

Figure 13.11: The Crookston Collection, University of Toronto.

Figure 17.13: *Urbana Atlas of Pathology*, University of Illinois College of Medicine at Urbana-Champaign. Image number 26.

Figure 17.19: Interactive Case Study Companion to Robbins Pathologic Basis of Disease.

Figure 18.12: Custom Medical Stock Photo.

Figure 20.20: Success in MRCO phth. http://www.mrcophth.com/iriscases/albinism.html

Figure 20.22 (top): Rubin, E. and Farber, J. L. *Pathology, 2nd Ed.* J. B. Lippinoctt. 194. Figure 6-30, p. 244.

Figure 20.22 (bottom): Gilbert-Barness, E. and Barness L. *Metabolic Disease.* Eaton Publishing, 2000. Figure 15, p.42.

Figure 21.6: Rich, M. W. Porphyria cutanea tarda, *Postgraduate Medicine*, 105: 208-214 (1999).

Figure 21.7: Department of Dermatlogy, University of Pittsburgh. http://www.upmc.edu/dermatology/MedStudentInfo/introLecture/enlarged/vespct.htm.

Figure 21.11: Custom Medical Stock Photo, Inc.

Figure 21.14: Phototake.

Figure 22.16: Wuthrich, D. A., and Lebowitz. Tophaceous gout. Images in clinical Medicine. *N Engl J Med*, 332:646, 1995.

Figure 22.18: WebMD Inc. http://www.samed.com/sam/forms/index.htm

Figure 23.2: Childs, G. http://www.cytochemistry.net/.

Figure 23.13: Modified from Cryer, P. E., Fisher, J. N. and Shamoon, H. Hypoglycemia. *Diabetes Care* 17:734-753, 1994.

Figure 24.5: Phototake.

Figure 26.5: Corbis.

Figure 26.6: Gibson W, et al. *The Journal of Clinical Endocrinology & Metabolism* 89 (10):4821, 2004.

Figure 27.22 A + B: Centers for Disease Control and Prevention Public Health Image Library, Atlanta, Georgia, USA.

Figure 28.4: Matthews, J. H. Queen's University Department of Medicine, Division of Hematology/Oncology, Kingston, Canada.

Figure 29.7: Nolan, J., Department of Biochemistry, Tulane University, New Orleans, LA.

Figure 34.10: Foerster J, Lee G, Lukens J, et al. *Wintrobe's Clinical Hematology, 10th Ed.* Philadelphia. Lippincott Williams & Wilkins, 1998.

Figure 34.20: Cohen BJ, Taylor JJ. *Memmler's The Human Body in Health and Disease, 10th Ed.* Baltimore. Lippincott Williams & Wilkins, 2005.

Appendix p. 489: Gold DH, MD, and Weingeist TA, MD, PhD. *Color Atlas of the Eye in Systemic Disease.* Baltimore. Lippincott Williams & Wilkins, 2001.

Appendix p. 506: Goodheart HP, MD. *Goodheart's Photographs of Common Skin Disorders, 2nd Ed.* Philadelphia. Lippincott Williams & Wilkins, 2003.

Appendix p. 510: Thomas H. McConnell. *The Nature of Disease Pathology for the Health Professions.* Philadelphia. Lippincott Williams & Wilkins, 2007.